Handbook of Critical Care Nephrology

Visual Abstracts created by:

Edgar V. Lerma, MD
University of Illinois at Chicago/Advocate Christ Medical Center
Associates in Nephrology
Chicago, Illinois

Michelle G. A. Lim, MBChB
Royal Infirmary of Edinburgh
Edinburgh, United Kingdom

Sinead Stoneman, MB, BCh, BAO
Beaumont Hospital
Dublin, Ireland

Handbook of Critical Care Nephrology

Jay L. Koyner, MD
Professor of Medicine
Medical Director, Acute Dialysis
Director, ICU Nephrology
Section of Nephrology
University of Chicago
Chicago, Illinois

Joel M. Topf, MD
Assitant Clinical Professor
William Beaumont School of Medicine
Oakland University
Rochester, Michigan

Edgar V. Lerma, MD, FACP, FASN, FPSN (Hon)
Clinical Professor of Medicine
Section of Nephrology
University of Illinois at Chicago College of Medicine/ Advocate Christ Medical Center
Oak Lawn, Illinois

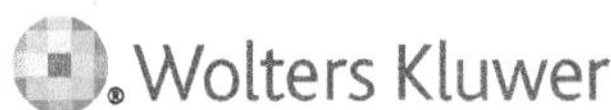

Philadelphia • Baltimore • New York • London
Buenos Aires • Hong Kong • Sydney • Tokyo

Acquisitions Editor: Colleen Dietzler
Development Editor: Ariel Winter
Editorial Coordinator: Ann Francis
Marketing Manager: Kirsten Watrud
Production Project Manager: David Saltzberg
Design Coordinator: Steve Druding
Manufacturing Coordinator: Beth Welsh
Prepress Vendor: S4Carlisle Publishing Services

9 8 7 6 5 4

Printed in the United States of America

Library of Congress Cataloging-in-Publication Data

ISBN-13: 978-1-9751-4409-8

ISBN-10: 1-9751-4409-0

Library of Congress Control Number: 2021905606

---

shop.lww.com

JLK: Dedicated to Robyn, Henry, and Ruby; thank you for your love, support, patience, laughter and all of the family couch time.

JMT: Dedicated to my wife, Cathy, who is always patient with me.

EVL: I dedicate this book to my wife Michelle and my two daughters Anastasia and Isabella, all of whom have been exceedingly patient and immensely supportive of all of my endeavors ... truly, they continue to serve as my daily inspiration.

CONTRIBUTING AUTHORS

Hussain Aboud, MD
Assistant Professor
Critical Care and Pulmonology Department
Central Michigan University
Staff Intensivist
Critical Care and Pulmonology Department
Ascension St. Mary's Hospital
Saginaw, Michigan

Paul Mark Adams, MD
Fellow Physician
Nephrology, Bone and Mineral Metabolism
University of Kentucky Medical Center
Lexington, Kentucky

Waleed E. Ali, MD
Hypertension Fellow
Department of Medicine
University of Chicago
Chicago, Illinois

Mohammad Y. Alsawah, MD
Attending Nephrologist
Department of Nephrology
Detroit Medical Center
Detroit, Michigan

Tanima Arora, MBBS
Postdoctoral Researcher
Department of Internal Medicine
Yale University School of Medicine
New Haven, Connecticut

Bourne Lewis Auguste, MD, MSc
Assistant Professor
Department of Medicine
University of Toronto
Toronto, Ontario, Canada

Sean M. Bagshaw, MD, MSc, FRCP(C)
Chair and Professor
Department of Critical Care Medicine
University of Alberta
Edmonton, Alberta, Canada

George L. Bakris, MD
Professor of Medicine
Department of Medicine
University of Chicago
Chicago, Illinois

Andrew B. Barker, MD
Assistant Professor
Department of Anesthesiology
University of Alabama at Birmingham
Birmingham, Alabama

Anthony P. Basel, DO, MAJ
Assistant Professor
Department of Medicine
Uniformed Services University
Bethesda, Maryland
Director of Burn Intensive Care Unit
Department of Surgery
United States Army Institute for Surgical Research
Fort Sam Houston, Texas

Rajit K. Basu, MD, MS, FCCM
Associate Professor of Pediatrics
Emory School of Medicine
Children's Healthcare of Atlanta—Egleston Hospital
Atlanta, Georgia

Ayham Bataineh, MD
Renal Fellow
University of Pittsburgh School of Medicine
Pittsburgh, Pennsylvania

Garrett W. Britton, DO
Medical Intensivist
US Army Institute of Surgical Research Burn Center
JBSA-Fort Sam Houston
Houston, Texas

Winn Cashion, MD, PhD
Physician
Renal Electrolytes Division
University of Pittsburgh
Pittsburgh, Pennsylvania

Armando Cennamo, MD
Department of Critical Care
Guy's & St. Thomas' Hospital
London, United Kingdom

Kalyani Chandra, MD
Transplant Nephrology Fellow
University of California Davis School of Medicine
Sacramento, California

Huiwen Chen, MD
Renal Fellow
Renal-Electrolyte Division
Department of Medicine
University of Pittsburgh
Pittsburgh, Pennsylvania

Ling-Xin Chen, MD, MS
Assistant Professor
Division of Transplant Nephrology
University of California Davis School of Medicine
Sacramento, California

Kevin K. Chung, MD
Professor and Chair
Department of Medicine
Uniformed Services
University of the Health Sciences
Bethesda, Maryland

Nathan J. Clendenen, MD, MS
Assistant Professor
Department of Anesthesiology
University of Colorado Hospital
Aurora, Colorado

Steven Coca, DO, MS
Associate Professor of Medicine
Department of Medicine
Icahn School of Medicine at Mount Sinai
New York, New York

Camilo Cortesi, MD
Clinical Fellow
Division of Nephrology
University of California San Francisco
San Francisco, California

Wilfred Druml, MD
Professor
Division of Nephrology
Medical University of Vienna
Chief (Retired)
Department of Medicine III, Division of Nephrology
Vienna General Hospital
Vienna, Austria

Stephen Duff, MD, MCAI
Newman Fellow
School of Medicine
University College Dublin
Dublin, Ireland

Francois Durand, MD
Professor of Hepatology
Department of HepatoGastroenterology
University of Paris
Paris, France
Head of the Liver and Intensive Care Unit
Department of Hepatology and Liver Intensive Care
Hospital Beaujon
Clichy, France

Sarah Faubel, MD
Professor of Medicine
Division of General Internal Medicine
University of Colorado Denver—Anschutz Medical Campus
Aurora, Colorado

Lui G. Forni, BSc, MB, PhD
Intensive Care Physician, Critical Care
Royal Surrey County Hospital NHS Foundation Trust
Guildford, United Kingdom

Claire Francoz, MD, PhD
Physician
Department of Hepatology
Hospital Beaujon
Clichy, France

Anna Gaddy, MD
Assistant Professor
Department of Medicine
Medical College of Wisconsin
Faculty
Department of Medicine
Froedtert Hospital
Milwaukee, Wisconsin

Michael George, MD
Resident
Department of Medicine
University of Pittsburgh Medical Center
Pittsburgh, Pennsylvania

Jaime Glorioso, MD
Assistant Professor of Surgery
Department of Surgery
Thomas Jefferson University Hospital
Philadelphia, Pennsylvania

Fernando D. Goldenberg, MD
Associate Professor of Neurology and Surgery (Neurosurgery)
Department of Neurology
University of Chicago
Chicago, Illinois

Benjamin R. Griffin, MD
Assistant Professor
Department of Medicine
University of Iowa Hospitals and Clinics
Iowa City, Iowa

Gaurav Gulati, MD
Fellow
Division of Cardiology
Tufts Medical Center
Boston, Massachusetts

Ryan W. Haines, MBBS
Clinical Research Fellow
William Harvey Research Institute
Queen Mary University of London
London, United Kingdom

Michael Heung, MD, MS
Professor
Division of Nephrology
Department of Medicine
University of Michigan
Ann Arbor, Michigan

Michelle A. Hladunewich, MD
Professor
Department of Medicine
University of Toronto
Toronto, Ontario, Canada

Luke E. Hodgson, MBBS, MRCP, FFICM, MD(Res)
Intensive Care Physician
Department of Anaesthetics
Western Sussex Hospitals NHS Foundation Trust
West Sussex, United Kingdom

Soo Min Jang, PharmD
Assistant Professor, Pharmacy Practice
School of Pharmacy, Loma Linda University
Loma Linda, California

Aron Jansen, MD
PhD Candidate
Radboudumc Intensive Care
Nijmegen, The Netherlands

David N. Juurlink, MD, PhD
Professor
Department of Medicine
Faculty of Medicine, University of Toronto
Toronto, Ontario, Canada

Aalok K. Kacha, MD, PhD
Assistant Professor
Department of Anesthesiology and Critical Care
University of Chicago
Chicago, Illinois

Kamyar Kalantar-Zadeh, MD, MPH, PhD
Professor and Chief
Nephrologist Faculty
Nephrology, Hypertension and Kidney Transplantation
University of California Irvine Medical Center
Orange, California

Mina El Kateb, MD
Core Teaching Faculty
Department of Nephrology
Ascension St. John Hospital
Detroit, Michigan

John A. Kellum, MD
Professor
Department of Critical Care Medicine
University of Pittsburgh
Pittsburgh, Pennsylvania

John S. Kim, MD, MS
Assistant Professor of Pediatrics–Cardiology
Department of Pediatrics
University of Colorado School of Medicine
Cardiologist and Intensivisit
Cardiac Intensive Care Unit, Heart Institute
Children's Hospital Colorado
Aurora, Colorado

Elizabeth A. King, MD, PhD
Assistant Professor
Department of Surgery
Johns Hopkins University
Baltimore, Maryland

Neal R. Klauer, MD
Medical Instructor
Department of Internal Medicine
Duke University
Durham, North Carolina

Benjamin Ko, MD
Associate Professor
Section of Nephrology
Department of Medicine
University of Chicago
Chicago, Illinois

Ravi Kodali, MD
Instructor
Department of Internal Medicine
Yale University School of Medicine
New Haven, Connecticut

Andrew Kowalski, MD
Clinical Attending, Nephrology
MacNeal Hospital
Berwyn, Illinois

Christopher Kramer, MD
Assistant Professor
Department of Neurology
University of Chicago
Chicago, Illinois

Danielle Laufer, MD
Clinical Fellow
Department of Anesthesia and Perioperative Care
University of California San Francisco
San Francisco, California

Christos Lazaridis, MD, EDIC
Associate Professor
Department of Neurology and Neurosurgery
University of Chicago
Chicago, Illinois

Kathleen Liu, MD, PhD
Professor of Medicine
Division of Nephrology, Departments of Medicine and Anesthesia
University of California, San Francisco
San Francisco, CA

Sai Sudha Mannemuddhu, MD, FAAP
Assistant Professor
Department of Medicine
University of Tennessee
Nephrologist
Department of Pediatrics
East Tennessee Children's Hospital
Knoxville, Tennessee

David Mariuma, DO
Assistant Professor
Department of Medicine
Icahn School of Medicine at Mount Sinai
New York, New York

Blaithin A. McMahon, MD, PhD
Assistant Professor
Department of Medicine
College of Medicine
Medical University of South Carolina
Charleston, South Carolina

Gearoid M. McMahon, MB, BCh
Associate Physician
Department of Medicine
Brigham and Women's Hospital
Boston, Massachusetts

Priti Meena, MBBS, MD, DNB
Assistant Professor
Department of Nephrology
AIIMS, Bhubaneswar
Bhubaneswar, India

Alejandro Y. Meraz-Munoz, MD
Clinical Fellow
Division of Nephrology
University Health Network
Toronto, Ontario, Canada

Dennis G. Moledina, MD, PhD
Assistant Professor
Department of Internal Medicine
Yale University School of Medicine
New Haven, Connecticut

Alvin H. Moss, MD
Professor
Department of Medicine
Health Sciences Center
West Virginia University
Morgantown, West Virginia

Bruce A. Mueller, PharmD
Associate Dean of Academic Affairs
University of Michigan School of Pharmacy
Ann Arbor, Michigan

Kathleen M. Mullane, DO, PharmD, FIDSA, FAST
Professor
Section of Infectious Diseases
Department of Medicine
Section of Infectious Diseases
University of Chicago
Chicago, Illinois

Patrick T. Murray, MD, FASN, FRCPI, FJFICMI
Consultant nephrologist/clinical pharmacologist
Professor of Clinical Pharmacology
School of Medicine
University College Dublin
Dublin, Ireland

Mitra K. Nadim, MD, FASN
Professor of Clinical Medicine
Department of Medicine
Keck School of Medicine
University of Southern California
Los Angeles, California

Javier A. Neyra, MD
Assistant Professor
Nephrology, Bone and Mineral Metabolism
University of Kentucky Medical Center
Lexington, Kentucky

Michael F. O'Connor, MD, FCCM
Professor
Department of Anesthesia and Critical Care Medicine
University of Chicago
Chicago, Illinois

Marlies Ostermann, MD, PhD
Professor and Consultant
King's College
Department of Critical Care
Guy's & St. Thomas Hospital
London, United Kingdom

Paul M. Palevsky, MD
Chief, Renal Section
VA Pittsburgh Healthcare System
Pittsburgh, Pennsylvania

Neesh Pannu, MD, SM
Professor
Department of Medicine
University of Alberta School of Public Health
Edmonton, Alberta, Canada

Bhakti K. Patel, MD
Assistant Professor
Section of Pulmonary and Critical Care Medicine
Department of Medicine
University of Chicago
Chicago, Illinois

Sharad Patel, MD
Assistant Professor
Intensivist
Department of Critical Care
Cooper-Rowan Medical School
Cooper Hospital
Camden, New Jersey

Steven D. Pearson, MD
Fellow
Section of Pulmonary and Critical Care Medicine
Department of Medicine
University of Chicago
Chicago, Illinois

Mark A. Perazella, MD
Professor of Medicine
Department of Internal Medicine
Yale University School of Medicine
New Haven, Connecticut

Zane Perkins, MBBCh, PhD
Consultant Trauma Surgeon
Major Trauma Centre
Barts Health NHS Trust
London, United Kingdom

Alfredo Petrosino, MD
Critical Care
Guy's and Saint Thomas' NHS Foundation Trust
London, United Kingdom

Peter Pickkers, MD, PhD
Full Professor
Radboudumc Intensive Care
Nijmegen, The Netherlands

Jason T. Poston, MD
Associate Professor
Section of Pulmonary and Critical Care Medicine
Department of Medicine
University of Chicago
Chicago, Illinois

John R. Prowle, MD
Senior Lecturer in Intensive Care Medicine
Barts and The London School of Medicine and Dentistry
William Harvey Research Institute
London, United Kingdom

Madhuri Ramakrishnan, MD
Fellow
Division of Nephrology
Washington University in Saint Louis
St. Louis, Missouri

Nirali Ramani, MD
Resident, Internal Medicine
MacNeal Hospital
Berwyn, Illinois

Anis Abdul Rauf, DO, FASN
Associate Professor
Chicago College of Osteopathic Medicine, Midwestern University
Hinsdale, Illinois

Nathaniel C. Reisinger, MD, FASN
Assistant Professor of Medicine
Internal Medicine—Nephrology
Rowan University Cooper Medical School
Camden, New Jersey

Claudia Rodriguez Rivera, MD
Fellow Physician
Department of Nephrology
University of Illinois in Chicago
Chicago, Illinois

Roger A. Rodby, MD
Professor of Medicine
Division of Nephrology
Rush University Medical Center
Chicago, Illinois

Bethany Roehm, MD
Fellow
Division of Nephrology
Tufts Medical Center
Boston, Massachusetts

Claudio Ronco, MD
Full Professor of Nephrology
Department of Medicine
Università degli Studi di Padova
Director
Department of Nephrology Dialysis and Transplantation
San Bortolo Hospital
Vicenza, Italy

Alan J. Schurle, MD
Assistant Professor
Department of Anesthesia and Critical Care Medicine
University of Chicago
Chicago, Illinois

Nicholas Michael Selby, BMedSci, BMBS, MRCP, DM
Associate Professor of Nephrology
Centre for Kidney Research and Innovation
University of Nottingham School of Medicine
Derby, United Kingdom

Pratik B. Shah, MD, FASN, FACP
Nephrologist
US Department of Veterans Affairs
Mather, California

Gurkeerat Singh, MBBS, MD
Critical Care Specialist
Piedmont Columbus Regional Critical Care
Columbus, Georgia

Krishna Sury, MD
Assistant Professor
Department of Internal Medicine
Yale University School of Medicine
New Haven, Connecticut

Jessica Sheehan Tangren, MD
Assistant Professor
Department of Medicine
Harvard University
Boston, Massachusetts

Anam Tariq, DO, MHS
Nephrology Fellow
Johns Hopkins School of Medicine
Baltimore, Maryland

Emily Temple-Woods, DO
Resident Physician
Family Medicine
Advocate Lutheran General Hospital
Park Ridge, Illinois

Kevin C. Thornton, MD
Clinical Professor
Department of Anesthesia and Perioperative Care
University of California San Francisco
San Francisco, California

Maria Clarissa Tio, MD
Fellow
Department of Medicine
Brigham and Women's Hospital
Boston, Massachusetts

Ashita J. Tolwani, MD, MSc
Professor
Department of Medicine
University of Alabama at Birmingham
Birmingham, Alabama

Joel M. Topf, MD
Assistant Clinical Professor
William Beaumont School of Medicine, Oakland University
Rochester, Michigan

Anitha Vijayan, MD
Professor of Medicine
Division of Nephrology
Washington University in Saint Louis
St. Louis, Missouri

Ron Wald, MDCM, MPH, BSc
Staff Physician and Professor of Medicine
Division of Nephrology
St. Michael's Hospital
Toronto, Ontario, Canada

Jacqueline Garonzik Wang, MD, PhD
Associate Professor
Department of Surgery
Johns Hopkins University School of Medicine
Baltimore, Maryland

Daniel E. Weiner, MD, MS
Nephrologist
Division of Nephrology
Tufts Medical Center
Boston, Massachusetts

Steven D. Weisbord, MD, MSc
Staff Physician, Renal Section
VA Pittsburgh Healthcare System
Pittsburgh, Pennsylvania

Raphael Weiss, MD
Department of Anesthesiology, Intensive Care and Pain Medicine
University Hospital Münster
Münster, Germany

Francis Perry Wilson, MD, MSCE
Associate Professor of Medicine
Department of Internal Medicine
Yale University School of Medicine
New Haven, Connecticut

Hunter Witt, MD
Chief
Surgical Resident
Wellspan York Hospital
York, Pennsylvania

Krysta S. Wolfe, MD
Assistant Professor
Section of Pulmonary and Critical Care Medicine
Department of Medicine
University of Chicago
Chicago, Illinois

Awais Zaka, MD, FACP
Hospitalist
Department of Internal Medicine
Henry Ford Macomb Hospital
Clinton Township, Michigan

Alexander Zarbock, MD
Chair and Professor,
Department of Anesthesiology, Intensive Care and Pain Medicine
University Hospital Münster
Münster, Germany

Yan Zhong, MD, PhD
Assistant Professor
Division of Nephrology and Hypertension
Keck School of Medicine
University of Southern California
Los Angeles, California

Jonathan S. Zipursky, MD
Physician
Department of Medicine
University of Toronto
Toronto, Ontario, Canada

Anna L. Zisman, MD
Associate Professor
Section of Nephrology
Department of Medicine
University of Chicago
Chicago, Illinois

FOREWORD

Over two decades ago, Rinaldo Bellomo, MBBS, MD, and I decided to write a commentary entitled "Critical Care Nephrology: The Time Has Come." This published manuscript was a summary of experiences matured in our long-standing collaborations to try to improve the outcome of critically ill patients with kidney problems. In the 1980s, continuous kidney replacement therapies were only sporadically performed in critically ill patients at select centers. Back then, the super-majority of patients were treated with standard intermittent hemodialysis with poor outcomes and an unacceptably high rate of complications. The reason for this was a mentality of "us and them" developed over years of narrow vision and lack of collaboration between nephrologists and critical care physicians. In spite of historical reasons for the limited interaction between nephrology and intensive care, new evidence emerged from our initial publications that a strict collaboration with improved cross-pollination was bringing better patient outcomes. The time for a new bridge between critical care and nephrology had come and many observations were supporting this new vision: exchange of competencies and knowledge, technologic transfer and exchange, better understanding of the pathophysiology of acute kidney injury (AKI), and, thus, better management and patient care. In the 1990s, new machines and new techniques for kidney replacement therapy were proposed, developed, and applied. Finally, the new millennium brought important studies on dose and efficacy of kidney replacement, advantages of continuous kidney replacement therapies, combined pharmacologic and artificial organ support, and so forth. These advances were further strengthened through adoption and systematic investigation by groups such as the Acute Disease Quality Initiative (ADQI). These groups have furthered the collaboration between nephrology and critical care and generated significant lines of evidence for prevention, diagnosis, classification, and treatment of AKI. In parallel with the ADQI consensus conferences, an impressive number of studies were published and many of them had in the key words the term "critical care nephrology." Books were made available as a source of information and training for the newer generations who became experienced specialists in both disciplines, being transfected by the common knowledge in critical care and nephrology. The present book by Jay L. Koyner, Edgar Lerma, and Joel M. Topf is a clear example of this sharing of ideas, information, and knowledge. The authors should be commended for the effort to create a useful new *Handbook of Critical Care Nephrology* edited by Wolters Kluwer. The handbook includes more than 50 chapters covering a wide array of critical care nephrology topics. Each chapter is written by a top expert in the field with long-lasting experience, and this guarantees a practical and immediate acquisition of the fundamental information by the reader. Over the years, experts like John Kellum, Pat Murray, Lui Forni, Paul Palevsky, Marlies Ostermann, Kathleen Lui, Alex Zarbock, and the other authors of the book chapters have become the reference authors for the most important publications in the field. The critical care nephrology community has established a relationship that goes beyond the pure professional collaboration. We have become close friends and we learned to share more than clinical cases and treatment protocols. We learned to work together for the benefit of our patients through mutual help and understanding, through close relationships with our fellows and residents, through a strong willingness to transform critical care nephrology into a real new discipline. This *Handbook of Critical Care Nephrology* edited by Koyner, Lerma, and Topf is the proof that the seeds were planted in the right environment and they have germinated and grown to flourish in the name of interdisciplinary collaboration, friendship, and science.

Claudio Ronco
Università degli Studi di Padova
and San Bortolo Hospital
Vicenza, Italy

PREFACE

Since the beginning of modern scientifically-based medicine, there has been a progression from generalists to specialists. Surgeons and internists divided up with surgical steel on one side and pharmaceuticals on the other. Then the internists Balkanized their field by organ system, with doctors identifying as cardiologists, pulmonologist, endocrinologists, and nephrologists among others. From there the specialization continued with subspecialists in hepatology, electrophysiology, and diabetology, expanding our vocabulary. For a long time, nephrology resisted the siren call of further specialization, but the last few decades have seen resistance crumble as nephrologists differentiated into transplant nephrologists, interventional nephrologists, and most importantly (given the book you are holding) critical care nephrologists.

The intersection of the intensive care unit (ICU) and nephrology is decades old. Although the role of the nephrologist in the ICU has morphed over the past 50 years, it is clear ICU patients are getting more complex and the modern nephrologist needs to understand the impact of critical care on the kidney as well as be aware of any advances that benefit the critically ill. It is with this backdrop that we created the first edition of *The Handbook of Critical Care Nephrology*.

The Handbook of Critical Care Nephrology covers a breadth of topics. Whereas some chapters cover bread-and-butter nephrology topics such as the prevention and care of acute kidney injury or the timing, dose, and modality of kidney replacement therapy in the ICU, this handbook offers much more. It covers a wealth of critical care topics including chapters on shock, acute respiratory distress syndrome (ARDS), and the care of transplant patients in the ICU. Beyond these, there are chapters dedicated to electrolytes and acid–base abnormalities in critically ill patients. We have attempted to create a handbook that reinforces the basic tenets of nephrology care in the ICU while expanding on aspects of critical care that nephrologists (and others) are less familiar with, including but not limited to extracorporeal membrane oxygenation (ECMO), intoxications, and left ventricular assist devices.

We have compiled 56 chapters with the goal that each chapter can be read in a single sitting. The chapters have been written by international experts, many of whom have published research on their chapter topic. These chapters average less than 3,000 words and are chock-full of clinical pearls. In addition to easy-to-digest chapters, when possible we have constructed visual abstracts for two or three of the major studies/trials for that topic. We specifically targeted older papers that do not have preexisting visual abstracts. As an added bonus, the PDFs of these visual abstracts can be used in talks or to bludgeon the other side in your latest evidence-based Twitter feud.

The Handbook of Critical Care Nephrology is a streamlined introduction to the complex care of patients in the ICU with kidney issues. This book is not meant to be exhaustive. It is geared toward medical students, interns, and residents who are interested in developing a broad knowledge base. In addition, we expect that internists, surgeons, anesthetists, advanced practice nurses, physician assistants, and pharmacists will find this book useful. Given the visual abstracts for many of the older classic studies and trials, nephrologists and intensivists may find them useful as teaching tools. Regardless, we hope you enjoy it.

Jay L. Koyner
Edgar V. Lerma
Joel M. Topf

CONTENTS

Contributing Authors vii
Foreword xv
Preface xvii

I. Critical Care and Intensive Care Unit Monitoring 1

1 Hemodynamic Monitoring in the Intensive Care Unit 3
2 Overview of the Management of Shock 12
3 Principles of Mechanical Ventilation 24
4 Acute Respiratory Distress Syndrome 36

II. Acute Kidney Injury in the Intensive Care Unit 45

5 Definitions and Etiologies of Acute Kidney Injury 47
6 Epidemiology of Acute Kidney Injury 58
7 Acute Kidney Injury and Non–Acute Kidney Injury Risk Scores in the Intensive Care Unit 67
8 Prevention of Acute Kidney Injury 81
9 Treatment of Acute Kidney Injury 90

III. Drugs and Blood Products in the Intensive Care Unit Setting .. 101

10 Resuscitation Fluids: Which One, How Much, and How to Assess 103
11 Transfusion Medicine in the Intensive Care Unit 118
12 Diuretics and Acute Kidney Injury 131
13 Vasoactive Medications 145
14 Anticoagulants in the Intensive Care Unit 159
15 The Metabolic Management and Nutrition of Acute Kidney Injury 169

IV Special Labs 181

16 Biomarkers of Acute Kidney Injury 183

17 Biomarkers of Critical Illness 192

V Imaging in the Intensive Care Unit 199

18 Ultrasound Imaging in the Intensive Care Unit 201

VI Electrolytes and Acid-Base Disorders 215

19 Sodium Homeostasis and Hyponatremia in the Intensive Care Unit 217

20 Hypernatremia in the Intensive Care Unit 230

21 Dyskalemias in the Intensive Care Unit 236

22 Calcium Management in the Intensive Care Unit 245

23 Phosphorus Management in the Intensive Care Unit 254

24 Magnesium Management in the Intensive Care Unit 264

25 Acid-Base Management in the Intensive Care Unit 273

VII Poisonings and Intoxications 281

26 Drug Dosing in Acute Kidney Injury 283

27 Drugs and Antidotes 292

28 Extracorporeal Therapy for Poisonings and Intoxications 309

VIII Extracorporeal Therapies 329

29 Vascular Access for Kidney Replacement Therapy 331

30 Dosing of Kidney Replacement Therapy 340

31 Timing of Kidney Replacement Therapy 348

32 Modality Selection of Kidney Replacement Therapy 360

33 Anticoagulation and Kidney Replacement Therapy 375

34 Blood Purification in the Intensive Care Unit 387

35 Extracorporeal Membrane Oxygenation in the Intensive Care Unit 398

IX Specific Conditions 413

36 Sepsis-Associated Acute Kidney Injury 415

37 Diabetic Ketoacidosis 427

38 Obstetric Acute Kidney Injury 436

39 Postcardiac Surgery Acute Kidney Injury 444

40 Cardiorenal Syndrome 453

41 Left Ventricular Assist Devices in the Intensive Care Unit 463

42 Acute Kidney Injury in Liver Disease 473

43 Abdominal Compartment Syndrome 483

44 Contrast-Associated Acute Kidney Injury 491

45 Hypertensive Emergency 504

46 Acute Kidney Injury in Burns Patients 520

47 Trauma-Associated Acute Kidney Injury 528

48 Neurologic Emergencies in the Intensive Care Unit 537

49 Rhabdomyolysis 550

50 Onconephrology Emergencies 561

51 Caring for Patients After Acute Kidney Injury 575

X Organ Transplantation 587

52 Perioperative Management of Kidney Transplant Recipients 589

53 Acute Kidney Injury in Patients with Kidney Transplants 597

54 Infectious Complications in Patients with Kidney Transplant 606

55 Care for the Brain-Dead Organ Donor 613

XI Ethics/Palliative Care 625

56 Shared Decision-Making/Time-Limited Trials of Kidney Replacement Therapy 627

Index 639

SECTION I

Critical Care and Intensive Care Unit Monitoring

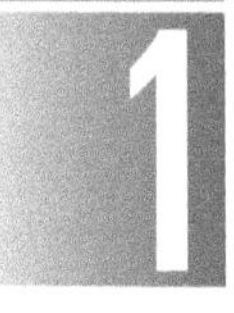

1 Hemodynamic Monitoring in the Intensive Care Unit

Alan J. Schurle and Michael F. O'Connor

INADEQUATE CIRCULATION

The evaluation of hemodynamics in critical care focuses on the assessment of shock, or globally inadequate tissue oxygenation and organ dysfunction. Clinical signs of shock include altered mentation, oliguria, and sluggish capillary refill. Hypotension is often a relatively late indicator of a suboptimal circulation. As hypotension develops, dynamic indicators such as pulse pressure variation (PPV) and systolic pressure variation (SPV) are the most useful predictors of response to volume infusion. More conventional parameters including heart rate, blood pressure, pulse pressure, and central venous pressure (CVP) can be used in concert to help identify the etiology of shock. Adequacy of resuscitation can be evaluated by appropriate improvement in lactic acid and mixed or central venous saturation.

Static Markers

Basic hemodynamic parameters including heart rate, blood pressure, and pulse pressure (the difference between systolic and diastolic pressure) can be used to formulate an initial differential diagnosis of a shock state and a plan for its management. Tachycardia, hypotension, and narrow pulse pressure are consistent with a low cardiac output caused by hypovolemia, cardiogenic shock, and obstructive shock. An increased pulse pressure is especially useful for distinguishing vasodilated shock from the other causes of shock (**Figure 1.1**). CVP is by far the most popular parameter used to make inference about the adequacy of the circulating volume and predict volume responsiveness. Without exception, all studies have demonstrated that CVP is a poor predictor of volume responsiveness; a 2008 meta-analysis of 24 studies relating CVP to either circulating volume or cardiac output augmentation by fluid challenge concluded that CVP's relationship to volume responsiveness generated an area under the curve (AUC) of 0.56, equivalent to flipping a coin.[1] An elevated CVP and PPV in a hypotensive patient can suggest a diagnosis of obstructive shock or right ventricular failure.[1] Peripheral venous pressure (PVP), transduced from peripheral intravenous (IV) rather than central line, correlates very well with CVP and may be used as a proxy by practitioners who may want to use a CVP measurement for the diagnosis or management of obstructive shock[2] (**Figure 1.2, Visual Abstract 1.1**). Finally, peripheral intravenous volume analysis (PIVA) is a technique where heart rate and respiratory variations in continuously monitored PVP are analyzed by a proprietary algorithm to generate a "PIVA signal." This signal, when compared either between different patients or in a single patient before and after volume removal with diuresis or dialysis, may be an emerging method to analyze an individual's volume status.[3]

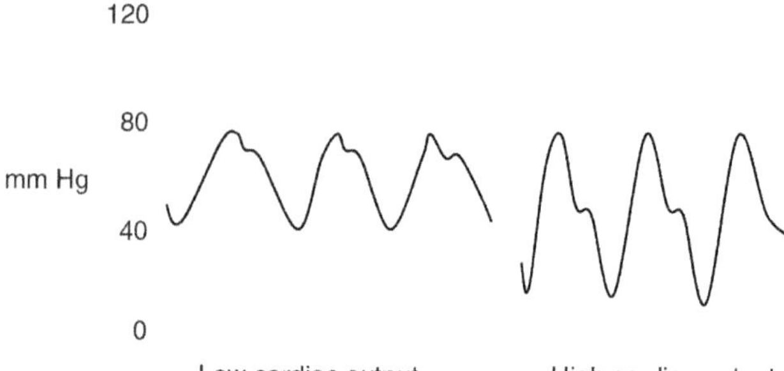

FIGURE 1.1: Utilization of pulse pressure to distinguish vasodilated shock from low cardiac output shock.

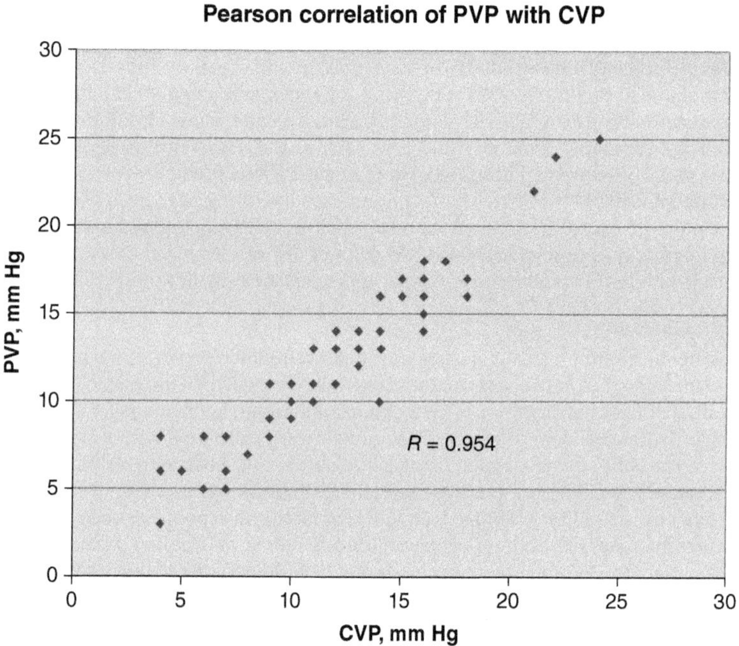

FIGURE 1.2: Correlation of PVP with CVP in ICU patients (unpublished data from University of Chicago Medicine ICUs). CVP, central venous pressure; ICU, intensive care unit; PVP, peripheral venous pressure.

Dynamic Markers

Hemodynamic parameters that change with an intervention such as mechanical ventilation or autotransfusion (as in the case of straight leg raise) are described as dynamic markers. These parameters can predict an improvement in cardiac output after fluid administration.

The straight leg raise test is designed to facilitate gravitational venous drainage from the lower extremities back into the systemic circulation, leading to an increase in venous return. After raising either a supine or semi-recumbent patient's leg to 45 degrees above the bed, an increase of approximately 15% in indices of cardiac output as measured by aortic blood flow via esophageal Doppler, stroke volume via echocardiography, or cardiac index by pulse contour monitoring is taken as a positive sign that predicts a similar increase in these variables with an IV fluid administration of around 500 mL, though the specificity and sensitivity are lower than that of SPV or PPV (discussed below). The benefits of this test include its ease of use and applicability across both mechanically ventilated and spontaneously breathing patients. Contraindications to this test include immobilized lower extremities as in the case of traumatic injury or an inability to lie supine as in the case of orthopnea or elevated intracranial pressure (ICP).[4]

Both SPV and PPV are commonly used to guide fluid administration. Changes in pleural pressures throughout the respiratory cycle are transmitted to the mediastinal structures, which cause fluctuations in venous return (**Figure 1.3**). These changes in preload lead to changes in stroke volume, which is reflected in a change in the pulse pressure of an arterial pressure tracing over the course of the respiratory cycle.[5] These measurements require sinus rhythm, patients synchronous with mechanical ventilation with tidal volumes of 8 mL/kg (ideal body weight), and an arterial catheter. A PPV of greater than 12% to 15% is predictive of fluid responsiveness; the higher the PPV, the more the cardiac output will be increased with a fluid bolus. Though there is no widely recognized ideal volume or type of fluid administration, common boluses are around 500 mL of either crystalloid or colloid. Dynamic indicators of volume responsiveness like PPV, SPV, and stroke volume variation (SVV) outperform all static methods to predict volume responsiveness, and of these three, PPV performs the best with an AUC of 0.94 compared with 0.86 to 0.84 for SPV and SVV. All three outperform CVP, with an AUC of 0.55[6] (**Table 1.1, Visual Abstract 1.2**). Pathologic states that elevate PPV, such as pulmonary hypertension or obstructive shock (tension

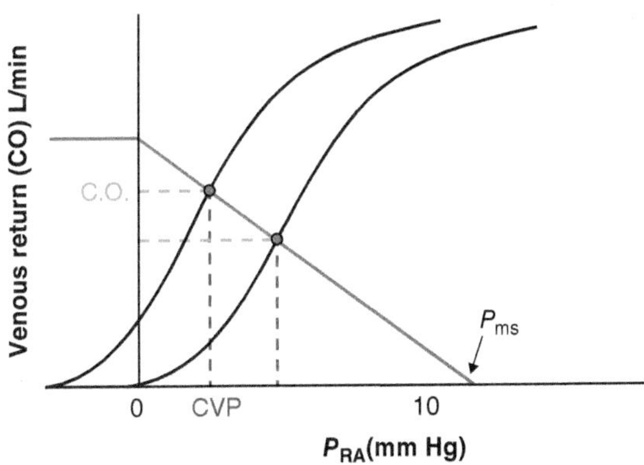

FIGURE 1.3: Fluctuations in pleural pressure produce fluctuations in venous return and variations in pulse pressure. CO, cardiac output; CVP, central venous pressure; P_{ms}, mean systemic pressure; P_{RA}, right atrial pressure.

TABLE 1.1 Approximate Area Under the Curve (AUC) of Variables Used to Predict Volume Responsiveness

Parameter	AUC
PPV	0.94
SPV	0.86
SVV	0.84
CVP	0.55

CVP, central venous pressure; PPV, pulse pressure variation; SPV, systolic pressure variation; SVV, stroke volume variation.

Adapted from Marik PE, Baram M, Vahid B. Does central venous pressure predict fluid responsiveness? A systematic review of the literature and the tale of seven mares. *Chest.* 2008;134:172-178.

pneumothorax, cardiac tamponade, abdominal compartment syndrome, auto-positive end-expiratory pressure [PEEP]), will lead to a false prediction of fluid responsiveness.[7] These dynamic indicators have been well studied in mechanically ventilated patients either paralyzed or compliant with the ventilator because the thoracic pressure changes required to produce a tidal volume are reproducible over multiple respiratory cycles. In spontaneously breathing patients, however, venous return from one respiratory cycle to the next can change because of variability in the thoracic pressures generated by the patient's breathing rather than changes in intravascular fluid status. Thus, PPV in spontaneously breathing patients is not currently as well-validated as in mechanically ventilated patients.[8,9] Additionally, pulse oximetry waveform variations over the course of the respiratory cycle, as analyzed by an algorithm similar to PPV, may offer similar data to PPV as a noninvasive alternative.[10] The possibility of using a pulse oximetry waveform in this way to make inference about volume responsiveness in a non-intubated spontaneously breathing patient could dramatically increase the use of dynamic indicators to assess volume responsiveness.

Assessment of Resuscitation

Over the past 20 years, central venous saturation and serum lactates have been strongly advocated and widely used to assess the adequacy of the resuscitation of shock.[11] Serum lactate, or lactic acid, is produced by normal cellular processes but can be pathologically elevated from either inadequate oxygen delivery or disrupted oxygen extraction (as in sepsis). Because of its association with anaerobic metabolism, lactate is useful as a surrogate for inadequate tissue perfusion. A serum sample can be obtained from an arterial blood gas. Restoration of a normal serum lactate is widely accepted as an indicator of an adequate and successful resuscitation.[12]

Central venous oxygen saturations ($ScvO_2$) obtained from a catheter positioned in the superior vena cava (SVC) have been used as surrogate for the mixed venous oxygen saturation (MvO_2) for the past 20 years. MvO_2, sampled from the pulmonary artery, requires the use of a pulmonary artery catheter. $ScvO_2$, drawn from the SVC or right atrium (RA) with a standard central venous catheter, have been shown to correlate with MvO_2.[13,14] There is evidence that mixed venous and central venous saturations may not be as interchangeable as widely believed.[15-17] The restoration of a central venous saturation of 65% to 70% is a commonly used target of resuscitation.[12]

Protocols that employ serial measurement of lactate or central venous saturation have been developed, studied, and disseminated as effective tools for the resuscitation of patients with shock.[18,19] Though other widely publicized protocol-driven resuscitation trials for septic shock such as PROCESS, PROMISE, and ARISE were not associated with improved mortality in the protocol-driven care group, it is possible that standard care has evolved to include targeted resuscitation endpoints as a matter of course.[20-23]

Clinical Endpoints

Historically, bedside practitioners have always asserted that a bedside assessment of a patient provided essential and otherwise impossible to obtain information about a patient's condition. Bedside assessments have included serial evaluation of the mental status and urine volume. Altered mentation is subjective and difficult to assess in the intensive care unit (ICU) where many patients are sedated, encephalopathic, or delirious despite having an otherwise adequate circulation. Oliguria, similarly, has a broad differential in the ICU that includes inadequate perfusion, nephrotoxic medications, disease states such as sepsis, and obstruction. In spite of these limitations, both have been studied and are well-accepted indicators of patient well-being. Other elements of bedside evaluation have not been systematically studied, and thus have heretofore been discounted.

Capillary refill time (CRT), measured by applying pressure to a glass slide overlying a patient's fingernail until the underlying skin became white then holding pressure for ten seconds before releasing it to time the return of blood flow, is quick, easily performed, and a long-standing component of the physical exam. Renewed interest in the utility of capillary refill time in guiding resuscitation in sepsis has led to a randomized controlled trial (RCT) suggesting that serial assessment of nail bed return every 30 minutes until CRT is less than 3 seconds is as efficacious a guide to resuscitation as serial measurement of serum lactate every 2 hours until either normalization or decrease by more than 20%. These targets were achieved in septic patients with mean arterial pressure (MAP) less than 65 by a protocolized approach first by fluid administration, second by norepinephrine infusion, and finally by starting either dobutamine or milrinone.[24] This result reaffirms the importance of serial bedside patient evaluations and may offer a quicker, more cost-effective method to guide resuscitation in septic patients with inadequate circulation, especially in resource-limited settings (**Visual Abstract 1.3**).

CONCLUSION

Hemodynamic monitoring is used to evaluate and manage shock. Dynamic parameters have supplanted traditional static parameters over the past 20 years. Simple hemodynamic endpoints for resuscitation (e.g., blood pressure and heart rate) have been supplanted by serial monitoring of central venous saturation, serum lactate, and nail bed return.

Acknowledgment

The authors thank Zdravka Zafirova, MD, for creating the PVP and CVP correlation graph.

References

1. Marik PE, Baram M, Vahid B. Does central venous pressure predict fluid responsiveness? A systematic review of the literature and the tale of seven mares. *Chest.* 2008;134:172-178.
2. Munis JR, Bhatia S, Lozada L. Peripheral venous pressure as a hemodynamic variable in neurosurgical patients. *Anesth Analg.* 2001;92:172-179.
3. Miles M, Alvis B, Hocking K, et al. Peripheral intravenous volume analysis (PIVA) for quantitating volume overload in patients hospitalized with acute decompensated heart failure—a pilot study. *J Cardiac Fail.* 2018;24:525-532.
4. Chernapath TGV, Hirsch A, Geerts BF, et al. Predicting fluid responsiveness by passive leg raising: a systematic review and meta-analysis of 23 clinical trials. *Crit Care Med.* 2016;44:981-991.
5. Michard F. Changes in arterial pressure during mechanical ventilation. *Anesthesiology.* 2005;103:419-428.
6. Marik PE, Cavallazzi R, Vasu T, et al. Dynamic changes in arterial waveform derived variables and fluid responsiveness in mechanically ventilated patients: a systematic review of the literature. *Crit Care Med.* 2009;37:2642-2647.
7. Wyler von Ballmoos M, Takala J, Roeck M, et al. Pulse-pressure variation and hemodynamic response in patients with elevated pulmonary artery pressure: a clinical study. *Crit Care.* 2010;14:R111.
8. Zollei E, Bertalan V, Nemeth A, et al. Non-invasive detection of hypovolemia or fluid responsiveness in spontaneously breathing subjects. *BMC Anesthesiol.* 2013;13:40.
9. Hong DM, Lee JM, Seo JH, et al. Pulse pressure variation to predict fluid responsiveness in spontaneously breathing patients: tidal vs forced inspiratory breathing. *Anaesthesia.* 2014;69:717-722.
10. Nanadoumgar H, Loupec TL, Frasca DF, et al. Pleth variability index predicts fluid responsiveness in critically ill patients. *Crit Care Med.* 2011;39:294-299.
11. Simpson SQ, Gaines M, Hussein Y, et al. Early goal-directed therapy for severe sepsis and septic shock: a living systematic review. *J Crit Care.* 2016; 36:43-48.
12. Rhodes A, Evans LE, Alhazzani W, et al. Surviving sepsis campaign: international guidelines for management of sepsis and septic shock: 2016. *Intensive Care Med.* 2017; 43:304-377.
13. Rivers EP, Ander DS, Powell D. Central venous oxygen saturation monitoring in the critically ill patient. *Curr Opin Crit Care.* 2001;7:204-211.
14. Ladakis C, Myrianthefs P, Karabinis A, et al. Central venous and mixed venous oxygen saturation in critically ill patients. *Respiration.* 2001;68:279-285.
15. Chawla LS, Hasan Z, Gutierrez G, et al. Lack of equivalence between central and mixed venous oxygen saturation. *Chest.* 2004;126:1891-1896.
16. Varpula M, Karlsson S, Ruokonen E, et al. Mixed venous oxygen saturation cannot be estimated with central venous oxygen saturation in septic shock. *Intensive Care Med.* 2006;32:1336-1343.
17. Sander M, Spies CD, Foer A, et al. Agreement of central venous saturation and mixed venous saturation in cardiac surgery patients. *Intensive Care Med.* 2007;33:1719-1725.
18. Jansen TC, Van Bommel J, Schoonderbeek FJ, et al. Early lactate-guided therapy in intensive care unit patients: a multicenter, open-label, randomized controlled trial. *Am J Respir Crit Care Med.* 2010;182:752-761.
19. Jones AE, Shapiro NI, Trzeciak S, et al. Lactate clearance vs central venous oxygen saturation as goals of early sepsis therapy: a randomized clinical trial. *JAMA.* 2010;303:739-746.
20. Yealy DM, Kellum JA, Huang DT, et al. A randomized trial of protocol-based care for early septic shock. *N Engl J Med.* 2014;370(18):1683-1693.
21. Mouncey PR, Osborn TM, Power GS, et al. Trial of early, goal-directed resuscitation for septic shock. *N Engl J Med.* 2015;372(14):1301-1311.
22. Peake SL, Delaney A, Bailey M, et al. Goal-directed resuscitation for patients with early septic shock. *N Engl J Med.* 2014;371(16):1496-1506.
23. Levy MM. Early goal-directed therapy: what do we do now? *Crit Care.* 2014;18(6):705.
24. Hernandez G, Ospina-Tascón GA, Damiani LP, et al. Effect of a resuscitation strategy targeting peripheral perfusion status vs serum lactate levels on 28-day mortality among patients with septic shock. *JAMA.* 2019;321:654-664.

Correlation between central venous pressure (CVP) and peripheral venous pressure (PVP) in neurosurgical patients

PVP was compared with CVP across 1026 paired measurements

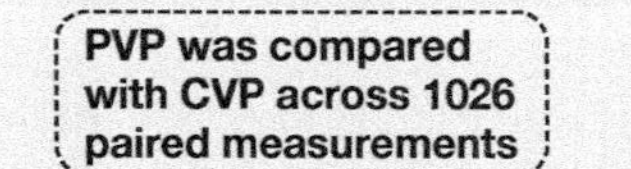
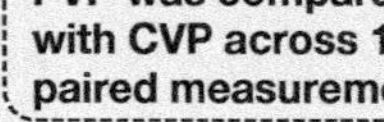

Craniotomy *(supine)* **n = 8**

Complex Spine Surgery *(prone)* **n = 7**

Hypotheses

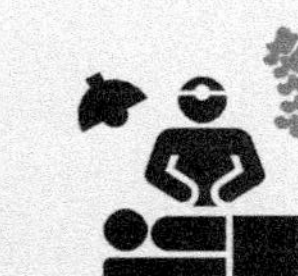

PVP trends parallel CVP trends and this relationship is independent of patient position

During planned circulatory arrest, PVP approximates mean systemic pressure (circulatory arrest pressure)

Peripheral Venous Pressure (PVP) 13.19± 3.68

Central Venous Pressure (PVP) 10.19± 3.72

0.819

Correlation between PVP and CVP was best demonstrated

Estimated Blood Loss > 1000 mL 0.885

Hemodynamic Instability (SD of CVP > 2) 0.923

Correlation coefficient

Conclusion: The results are consistent with the hypothesis that PVP reflects mean systemic pressure; and therefore PVP measurement may provide a method of estimating mean systemic pressure during normal circulatory function.

Munis JR, Bhatia S, Lozada LJ. ***Peripheral venous pressure as a hemodynamic variable in neurosurgical patients.*** Anesth Analg. 2001 Jan;92(1):172-9.

VISUAL ABSTRACT 1.1

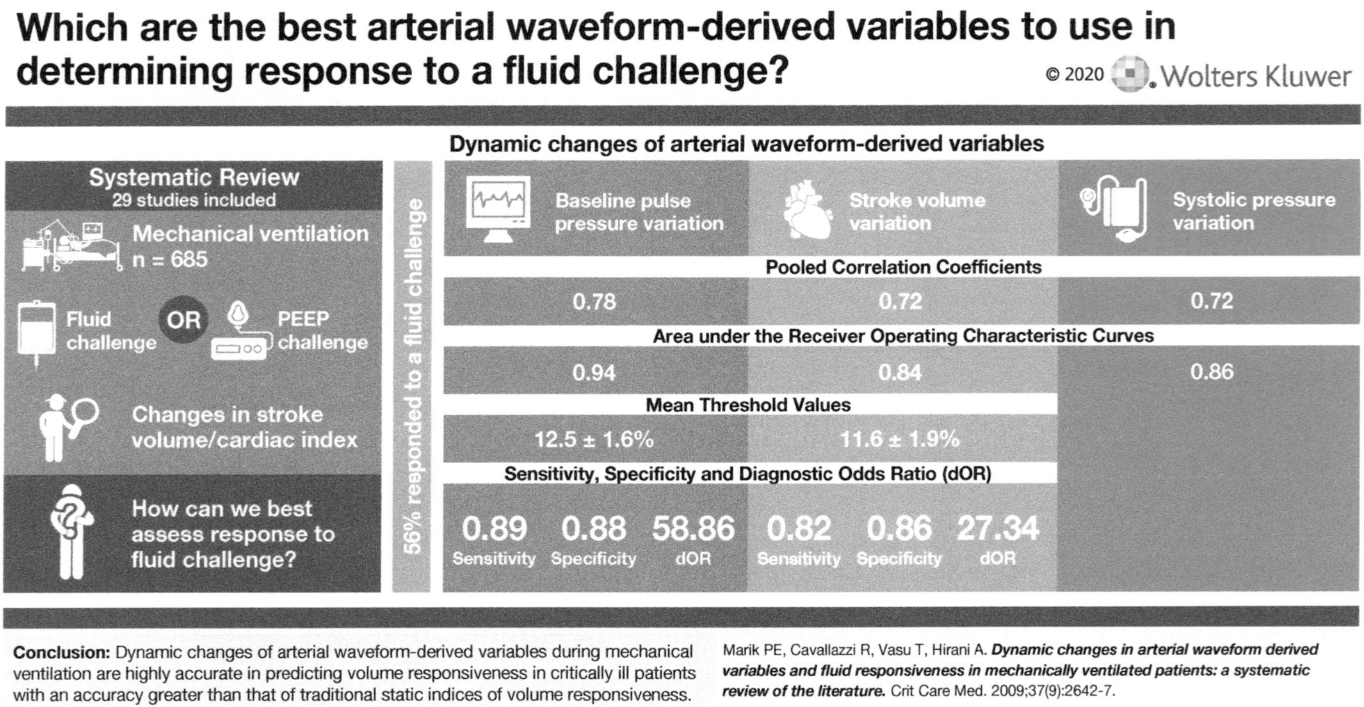

Which are the best arterial waveform-derived variables to use in determining response to a fluid challenge?

 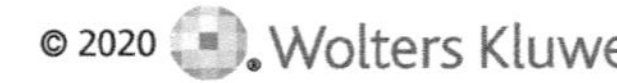

Systematic Review
29 studies included

Mechanical ventilation
n = 685

Fluid challenge OR PEEP challenge

Changes in stroke volume/cardiac index

How can we best assess response to fluid challenge?

56% responded to a fluid challenge

Dynamic changes of arterial waveform-derived variables

	Baseline pulse pressure variation	Stroke volume variation	Systolic pressure variation
Pooled Correlation Coefficients	0.78	0.72	0.72
Area under the Receiver Operating Characteristic Curves	0.94	0.84	0.86
Mean Threshold Values	12.5 ± 1.6%	11.6 ± 1.9%	
Sensitivity, Specificity and Diagnostic Odds Ratio (dOR)	0.89 Sensitivity, 0.88 Specificity, 58.86 dOR	0.82 Sensitivity, 0.86 Specificity, 27.34 dOR	

Conclusion: Dynamic changes of arterial waveform-derived variables during mechanical ventilation are highly accurate in predicting volume responsiveness in critically ill patients with an accuracy greater than that of traditional static indices of volume responsiveness.

Marik PE, Cavallazzi R, Vasu T, Hirani A. ***Dynamic changes in arterial waveform derived variables and fluid responsiveness in mechanically ventilated patients: a systematic review of the literature.*** Crit Care Med. 2009;37(9):2642-7.

VISUAL ABSTRACT 1.2

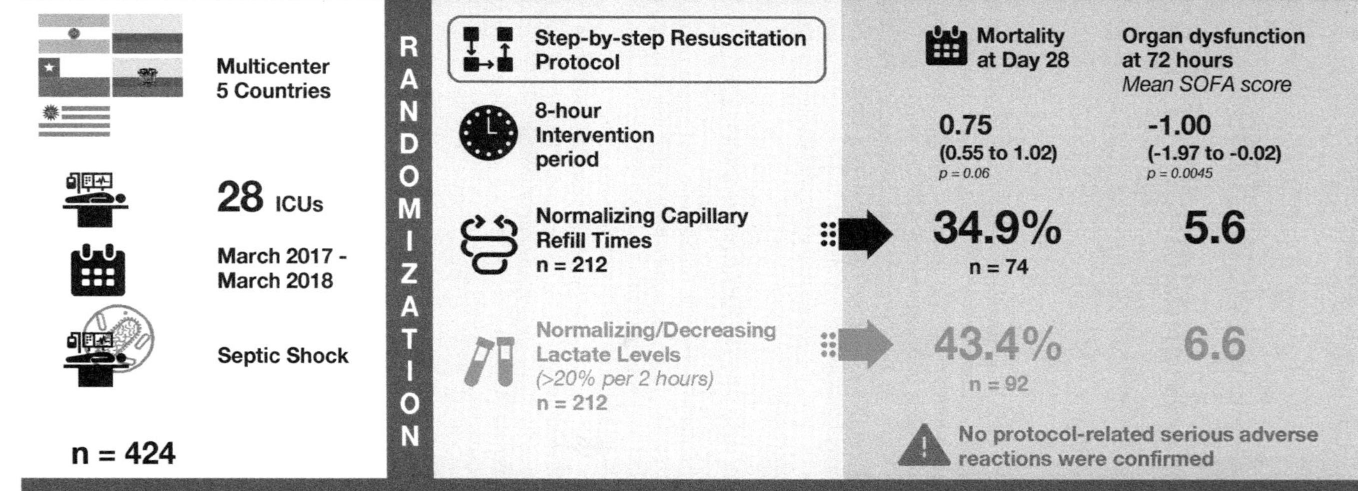

Conclusion: Among patients with septic shock, a resuscitation strategy targeting normalization of capillary refill time, compared with a strategy targeting serum lactate levels, did not reduce all-cause 28-day mortality.

Hernandez G, Ospina-Tascon GA, Damiani LP, Estenssoro E, et al. ***Effect of a Resuscitation Strategy Targeting Peripheral Perfusion Status vs Serum Lactate Levels on 28-Day Mortality Among Patients With Septic Shock: The ANDROMEDA-SHOCK Randomized Clinical Trial.*** JAMA 2019 Feb 19;321(7):654-664.

VISUAL ABSTRACT 1.3

Overview of the Management of Shock

Michael George and John A. Kellum

INTRODUCTION

Circulatory shock is a common intensive care problem, affecting up to one-third of admissions to an intensive care unit (ICU).[1] It represents the end point of a multitude of different pathophysiologic processes, leading to hypotension (relative or absolute) and imbalance between oxygen delivery and oxygen consumption in end-organ tissue. Key to management of this condition is rapid differentiation of the type of shock and elucidation of its underlying cause. Although we will discuss general management of this problem, it must be emphasized that these treatments serve as temporizing measures while the underlying cause is sought out and, if possible, reversed.

PATHOPHYSIOLOGY AND DIFFERENTIATION OF SHOCK STATES

The fundamental problem in shock is inadequate end-organ perfusion. In this section, we will outline the basic pathophysiology of shock utilizing the cardiac output (CO) equation and then use this to highlight the major hemodynamic differences leading to inadequate perfusion in each subset of shock, broadly divided into primarily low CO and low systemic vascular resistance (SVR) states. It is worth noting that although we will focus on circulatory shock that results in decreased oxygen delivery to end organs, any mismatch between oxygen consumption and delivery can cause a state of shock (e.g., carbon monoxide poisoning leading to decreased oxygen delivery).

Cardiac Output Equation

The fundamentals of circulatory shock physiology can be understood by examining the CO equation where mean arterial pressure (MAP) is equal to CO multiplied by SVR. CO can be further broken down into heart rate (HR) times stroke volume (SV) (**Table 2.1**). Under normal conditions, decreases in either CO or SVR will lead to automatic and compensatory increases in the other variable, therefore the patient in shock will either have had an extremely profound decrease in one variable (e.g., severe hemorrhagic shock with SV and CO rapidly approaching nil) or loss of the ability to compensate on the other side of the equation (e.g., the patient with advanced heart failure and high baseline SVR progressing to low-output heart failure).

Low Cardiac Output States

Hypovolemic Shock

Hypovolemic shock is due to a relative or absolute decrease in intravascular volume. Absolute hypovolemia is most commonly seen in patients with hemorrhagic shock, although it may also be due to excessive fluid losses from other means,

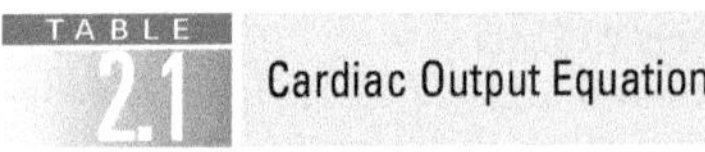

Cardiac Output Equation

Cardiac Output Equation: MAP = CO × SVR; CO = HR × SV

Low SVR Shock (Distributive)	**High SVR Shock**	
	Low SV	**Low HR**
Adrenal crisis	Arrhythmia (ventricular, SVT)	Bradyarrhythmia
Anaphylaxis	Cardiomyopathy (ischemic, nonischemic)	
Decreased sympathetic tone (neurogenic)	Hypovolemia (relative, absolute)	
Sepsis	Obstructive (pulmonary embolism, tamponade, tension pneumothorax)	
Systemic inflammatory response		
Vasoplegic crisis		

CO, cardiac output; HR, heart rate; MAP, mean arterial pressure; SV, stroke volume; SVR, systemic vascular resistance; SVT, supraventricular tachycardia.

such as increased insensible fluid loss from the skin in burn victims, the gastrointestinal (GI) tract with severe diarrhea or vomiting, or excessive third spacing (e.g., severe pancreatitis). Relative hypovolemia can occur with increased venous capacitance, resulting in a larger proportion of the circulating blood volume being on the venous side and thus decreasing venous return for the same total volume. Certain drugs (e.g., nitrates, anesthetics) are potent venodilators and can produce this effect. Whether absolute or relative, a profound loss of intravascular volume leads to progressively decreased SV, and when this cannot be compensated by increasing HR, shock occurs.

Cardiogenic Shock

Cardiogenic shock occurs because of aberrations in cardiac pump function. This is often due to heart failure, leading to low SV and thus CO. Another subset of this type of shock includes mechanical disruptions within the heart, such as acute mitral regurgitation, leading to decreased SV. Also included in this category are tachy- and bradyarrhythmias. Severe bradyarrhythmias decrease HR with a fixed SV, whereas tachyarrhythmias lead to ineffective diastolic filling and decreased SV.

Obstructive Shock

Obstructive shock occurs when an abnormal mechanical force within the thorax interferes with normal CO. This includes obstruction of normal left ventricular filling (and thus decreased SV) such as cardiac tamponade, pericarditis, or restrictive cardiomyopathy. Within the lungs, a pulmonary embolism can decrease flow through pulmonary vasculature or a tension pneumothorax can impede filling of the RV, both again leading to decreased SV and CO. A milder form of obstructive shock can occur simply from positive pressure ventilation, particularly when some degree of hypovolemia is also present.

Low Systemic Vascular Resistance States/Distributive Shock

Distributive shock is the most common form of shock seen in the ICU, often because of sepsis.[2] The hallmark of distributive shock is decreased SVR. In septic shock, this is mediated by both bacterial endotoxins and excessive release of the body's own inflammatory mediators. These signaling pathways lead to vasodilation, increased vascular bed permeability, and decreased cardiac function.[3] A closely related condition mechanistically is vasoplegic syndrome. Most commonly seen after cardiac surgery, this syndrome consists of an inappropriate balance between molecular mediators of vasoconstriction and vasodilation, leading to refractory shock.[4] Other causes of distributive shock include loss of sympathetic tone (neurogenic shock), decreased glucocorticoid/mineralocorticoid production (adrenal crisis), and severe hypersensitivity reactions (anaphylactic shock).

EVALUATION

Early identification of shock is key to successful management. For example, the strongest predictor of mortality in sepsis is time to antibiotic administration—one study demonstrated a 7.6% increase in mortality *per hour* before antibiotic administration in septic shock.[5] We will thus start with clinical evaluation for shock.

Bedside Evaluation

Assessment of shock starts at the bedside. Subjective findings may be common to multiple types of shock (e.g., altered mental status because of decreased central nervous system [CNS] perfusion) or relatively specific (crushing, substernal chest pain in the patient with a myocardial infarction and cardiogenic shock). Physical examination findings may provide the first clue to differentiating between low-output and distributive states. Classically, early distributive shock leads to warm extremities and even a flushed appearance because of decreased SVR, whereas low CO states that increase vasoconstriction tend to cause pallor, decreased capillary refill, and cool/dusky extremities. Certain shock states have even more specific findings: Anaphylactic shock often features diffuse cutaneous wheals, edema of the face/lips, and inspiratory stridor because of laryngeal edema. Cardiogenic shock findings can include lower extremity edema, lung crackles, extra heart sounds or new murmurs, and elevated jugular venous pulsations (JVP). Clues to obstructive shock include elevated JVP, distant heart sounds, or absent/asymmetric breath sounds.

The Role of Screening Algorithms in Septic Shock

Many clinicians are familiar with the systemic inflammatory response syndrome (SIRS) and quick Sequential Organ Failure Assessment (qSOFA) screening criteria (**Table 2.2**). Although either can be useful in the appropriate context, they each suffer from flaws: SIRS may be highly sensitive but lacks specificity, whereas qSOFA may lack sensitivity for early sepsis or septic shock.[6-9] This again highlights the importance of high clinical suspicion for shock.

Laboratory Findings

Laboratory evaluation should focus on screening for and identifying end-organ dysfunction. A basic metabolic panel should be performed, which may help assess changes in kidney function (keeping in mind changes in urine output will usually occur first) and to identify a new or enlarging anion gap. All patients with suspected circulatory shock should also have serum lactate drawn as shock may

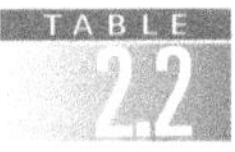

SIRS/qSOFA Criteria

Screening Test	Values	Positive Result
SIRS	Temperature: >38°C or <36°C Heart rate: >90 beats/min Tachypnea: respiratory rate >20 or $PaCO_2$ <32 mm Hg White blood cell count: >12,000/mm³ or <4,000/mm³ or >10% immature neutrophils	2/4
qSOFA	Respiratory rate ≥22 Altered mental status (GCS ≤15) Systolic blood pressure ≤100 mm Hg	2/3

GCS, Glasgow Coma Scale; $PaCO_2$, partial pressure of carbon dioxide; qSOFA, quick Sequential Organ Failure Assessment; SIRS, systemic inflammatory response syndrome.

initially present with conserved blood pressure (BP), particularly in patients with chronic hypertension. When elevated, lactate should also be trended to assess resolution of shock and help gauge resuscitation. An arterial blood gas can confirm suspected acid-base abnormalities. Other markers of end-organ injury such as liver function tests or troponin should be ordered on a case-by-case basis based on clinical judgment.

MANAGEMENT

Management of circulatory shock follows per the type of shock identified. Fluid resuscitation is the fundamental treatment of hypovolemic shock, whereas the therapy for cardiogenic shock will focus on the cardiac pathology that is present (acute ischemia, dysrhythmia, etc.). Treatment for distributive shock emphasizes reversal of absolute and relative hypovolemia as well as addressing vasomotor paralysis. Given that septic shock is the most common cause of distributive shock management, principles will be largely reflective of the Surviving Sepsis Campaign guidelines for resuscitation, while acknowledging areas of uncertainty in the current literature.

Goals of Resuscitation

Blood Pressure

BP should be monitored frequently, with a goal of MAP greater than or equal to 65 mm Hg. Placement of an arterial line is often useful to provide a real-time measure of BP. Studies of higher BP targets have not found a benefit of routinely resuscitating to higher targets.[10] However, clinicians should individualize therapy based on medical history and response to therapy. Patients with chronic hypertension may require higher pressures, whereas younger patients with lower baseline BP may tolerate lower pressure targets.

Lactate

Serum lactate is used as a surrogate measure of tissue hypoperfusion. Although the true physiologic basis for lactate elevation in shock has been debated, it is clear that elevated lactate is a marker of increased in-hospital mortality.[11]

Elevated lactate is a predictor of mortality even in the absence of hypotension, making this value useful in patients on the cusp of developing shock or already on vasopressors.[12] If elevated (typically >2 mmol/L), this should be repeated every 2 to 4 hours until normalized.

Oxygenation

The end goal of normalizing BP is ultimately to ensure adequate oxygen delivery. Additionally, patients with shock may have coexisting pulmonary abnormalities and are at increased risk of acute respiratory distress syndrome. Thus, intermittent or continuous pulse oximetry should be used to ensure adequate arterial oxygen saturation. If basic laboratory assessment suggests acid-base disturbances, an arterial blood gas should be sent for further evaluation. Central venous oxygen saturation ($ScvO_2$), although of questionable utility for guiding resuscitation, may be useful in delineating the type of shock. Typically, in distributive shock, $ScvO_2$ will remain high because of shunting and impaired oxygen extraction in peripheral tissues, whereas cardiogenic shock is associated with near-maximal oxygen extraction and reduced $ScvO_2$. Routine use of pulmonary artery catheterization has not been found to be superior to other means of assessing hemodynamics and is thus reserved for specialized circumstances (e.g., advanced cardiogenic shock).[13]

Early Goal-Directed Therapy

In 2001, a relatively small, single-center study popularized protocolized resuscitation—early goal-directed therapy (EGDT)—of patients with septic shock.[14] These interventions included early placement of a central venous catheter (CVC) with fluid resuscitation targeted to a central venous pressure (CVP) of 8 to 12 mm Hg and blood product and inotrope infusion to a $ScvO_2$ of 70% or greater. In 2014, three high-quality, multicenter studies demonstrated equivalent outcomes with more conservative care, most notably removing CVP and $ScvO_2$ targets.[15-17] Among the differences between the study groups in these trials were increased fluid and inotrope administration in the EGDT group without any mortality benefit. Although use of EGDT per se has been refuted, the basic principles including early fluid administration directed to improving tissue perfusion remains unchanged (**Visual Abstract 2.1**).

Fluid Resuscitation

Only about half of critically ill patients will have a significant response in CO to a fluid challenge.[18] Although the question of the best way to predict responsiveness or amount of fluid to be given remains unanswered, the clear dangers of inappropriate fluid administration demand that fluids be given thoughtfully.

Determining Fluid Responsiveness

Passive Leg Raise

One simple and easily reversible test of fluid responsiveness is the passive leg raise (PLR), in which a patient's torso is laid flat while elevating the legs to 45 degrees for approximately 60 seconds. This has been validated using several hemodynamic parameters—most readily accessible to the clinician at the bedside is an increase of systolic BP of 8% after PLR, correlating with subsequent response to fluid bolus.[19] Caution should be exercised to avoid causing pain or agitation as these may also raise BP.

Central Venous Pressure

As previously mentioned, CVP is not a reliable predictor of volume status. Readings may be impacted by thoracic pressure alterations during positive pressure ventilation, and although high readings (>20 mm Hg) may reflect volume overload, normal to near-normal values are not clinically useful.[20,21]

Ultrasonography and Fluid Responsiveness

With the increasing popularity of point-of-care ultrasound (POCUS), there is increasing interest in its use to predict fluid responsiveness. Inferior vena cava (IVC) diameter variability is easily obtainable, but is a relatively poor predictor of response. Stroke volume variation (SVV) and pulse pressure variation (PPV) are more accurate predictors but are limited by the requirement that a patient be intubated and ventilated, and it varies with both tidal volume and abdominal pressure.[22,23] Other elements of POCUS such as cardiac ultrasound may be invaluable in delineating causes of shock, but implementation varies based on machine availability and provider experience.

Choice of Fluid

Crystalloids remain the ideal fluid to give for volume expansion, except in select circumstances. Some colloids (e.g., starch) have been shown to be ineffective or dangerous compared to crystalloids. The most readily available colloid, albumin, has not been shown to provide a benefit over crystalloid for shock resuscitation.[24] Between crystalloids, there is increasing evidence that more physiologic solutions such as Lactated Ringers are more kidney protective than 0.9% saline (**Visual Abstract 2.2**).[25] Additional information on resuscitation fluids is found in Chapter 10.

Amount of Volume Expansion

The amount of fluid to administer in any given patient in circulatory shock is not easily determined. In sepsis and septic shock, guidelines continue to support an initial bolus of 30 mL/kg body weight. However, this recommendation is not based on rigorous evidence. Excessive fluid administration increases the risk of respiratory distress and acute lung injury, and increases intra-abdominal pressure and cerebral edema. An increasingly robust body of literature has demonstrated that a positive fluid balance in septic shock is an independent predictor of mortality.[26,27] Additional consideration to fluid administration should be given to patients with known derangements of cardiac or kidney function. These considerations support assessing for fluid responsiveness after early boluses, attention to overall fluid balance throughout a patient's stay, and early use of vasopressors when hypotension persists despite volume expansion.

Vasopressors/Inotropes

When shock is refractory to initial fluid resuscitation, it is appropriate to consider vasopressor support. Distributive shock requires alpha-adrenergic stimulation to promote vasoconstriction and raise SVR. In most cases of septic shock, norepinephrine (NE) is the first-line agent because it also provides some beta-adrenergic stimulation. Additional vasopressors, both adrenergic and nonadrenergic, should be considered if BPs are refractory to this first-line agent—a brief overview of these agents can be seen in **Table 2.3**. See Chapter 13 for a detailed review.

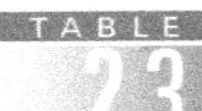

TABLE 2.3 Vasopressors/Inotropes

Class	Agent	Vasoactive Properties	Indications/Unique Features	Limitations
Adrenergic vasopressors	Norepinephrine	Alpha- > beta-adrenergic agonist, increases systemic vascular resistance and cardiac output	First-line vasopressor for distributive shock, may be used as adjunct for low CO shock	Disproportionate increases in SVR may lead to kidney and peripheral hypoperfusion[35]
	Epinephrine	Alpha/beta-adrenergic agonist	Most potent adrenergic stimulation of all vasopressors	Large increases in serum lactate, concerns for excessive splanchnic and peripheral vasoconstriction
	Dopamine	Acts on dopamine, beta, alpha receptors	Theoretical benefit on kidney and splanchnic circulation although not clinically significant	Increased mortality, more arrhythmogenic compared to norepinephrine[36]
	Phenylephrine	Selective alpha-1 agonist, increases SVR	Short half-life with rapid effect, possibly less arrhythmogenic than mixed alpha/beta agonists	Little data on continuous infusions, more modest BP increases than other agents
Nonadrenergic vasopressors	Vasopressin	Activates peripheral V1 leading to vasoconstriction	Validated as an adjunct to norepinephrine in distributive shock, may decrease catecholaminergic requirements[28,29]	Only validated as second-line vasopressor, limited range of titration
	Angiotensin II	Binds AT-1 in vascular smooth muscle causing vasoconstriction	Only available agent targeting the RAS system, may decrease need for high-dose adrenergic agents[30]	May be cost-prohibitive, few large-scale trials to date
Inotropes	Dobutamine	Beta-1/2 agonist, increases CO	Cardiogenic shock, may lead to less hypotension than milrinone[37]	Tachycardia, hypotension, arrhythmia, and increased mortality (long term)
	Milrinone	PDE-3 inhibitor increases myocardial contractility, CO	Cardiogenic shock, may cause less tachycardia than dobutamine, not affected by beta blockade[37]	Hypotension, tachycardia, arrhythmia, and increased mortality (long term)

AT-1, angiotensin-1; BP, blood pressure; CO, cardiac output; PDE, phosphodiesterase; RAS, renin-angiotensin system; SVR, systemic vascular resistance; V1, vasopressin receptor 1

Refractory Shock

Low Cardiac Output States

In the case of refractory cardiogenic shock, some specialized centers may place mechanical assist devices, such as intra-aortic balloon pumps or left ventricular assist devices depending on the nature of the cardiac disease. These devices may also be used as a bridge to more definitive therapy including heart transplant.

Low Systemic Vascular Resistance States

Corticosteroids

Corticosteroids in septic shock have been theorized to mitigate hypotension by addressing relative adrenal insufficiency in severe illness and attenuate the aberrant inflammatory cascade, leading to hemodynamic instability. Large-scale studies of steroids in septic shock have reached conflicting results, variably showing small benefit or no effect.[31-33] Based on existing data, most clinicians consider use of steroids when shock is refractory to high-dose or multiple vasopressors (**Visual Abstract 2.3**).

Novel Agents

Numerous therapeutics have been trialed in refractory vasodilatory shock, including increasing calcium signaling (calcium chloride), decreasing nitric oxide signaling (methylene blue, hydroxocobalamin), improving vasopressor/renin-angiotensin-aldosterone system (RAAS) signaling molecule synthesis (ascorbic acid), but at this time they cannot be recommended as standard of care.[34]

References

1. Sakr Y, Reinhart K, Vincent JL, et al. Does dopamine administration in shock influence outcome? Results of the Sepsis Occurrence in Acutely Ill Patients (SOAP) Study. *Crit Care Med.* 2006;34(3):589-597.
2. Vincent JL, De Backer D. Circulatory shock. *N Engl J Med.* 2013;369:1726-1734.
3. Russel JA, Rush B, Boyd J. Pathophysiology of septic shock. *Crit Care Clin.* 2018;34(1):43-61.
4. Liu H, Yu, L, Yang L, et al. Vasoplegic syndrome: an update on perioperative considerations. *Clin Anesth.* 2017;40:63-71.
5. Kumar A, Roberts D, Wood KE, et al. Duration of hypotension before initiation of effective antimicrobial therapy is the critical determinant of survival in human septic shock. *Crit Care Med.* 2006;34(6):1589-1596.
6. Luo J, Jiang W, Weng L, et al. Usefulness of qSOFA and SIRS scores for detection of incipient sepsis in general ward patients: a prospective cohort study. *J Crit Care.* 2019;51:13-18.
7. Dykes LA, Heintz SJ, Heintz BH, et al. Contrasting qSOFA and SIRS criteria for early sepsis identification in a veteran population. *Fed Pract.* 2019;36(Suppl 2):S21-S24.
8. Singer M, Deutschman CS, Seymour CW, et al. The Third International Consensus Definitions for Sepsis and Septic Shock (Sepsis-3). *JAMA.* 2016;315(8):801-810.
9. Dorsett M, Kroll M, Smith CS, et al. qSOFA has poor sensitivity for prehospital identification of severe sepsis and septic shock. *Prehosp Emerg Care.* 2017;21(4):489-497.
10. Asfar P, Meziani F, Hamel JF, et al. High versus low blood-pressure target in patients with septic shock. *N Engl J Med.* 2014;370(17):1583-1593.
11. Casserly B, Phillips GS, Schorr C, et al. Lactate measurements in sepsis-induced tissue hypoperfusion: results from the Surviving Sepsis Campaign database. *Crit Care Med.* 2015;43(3):567-573.
12. Bou Chebl R, El Khuri C, Shami A, et al. Serum lactate is an independent predictor of hospital mortality in critically ill patients in the emergency department: a retrospective study. *Scand J Trauma Resusc Emerg Med.* 2017;25:69.
13. Simmons J, Ventetuolo CE. Cardiopulmonary monitoring of shock. *Curr Opin Crit Care.* 2017;23(3):223-231.
14. Rivers E, Nguyen, B, Havstad S, et al. Early goal-directed therapy in the treatment of severe sepsis and septic shock. *N Engl J Med.* 2001;345:1368-1377.
15. Yealy DM, Kellum JA, Huang DT, et al. A randomized trial of protocol-based care for early septic shock. *N Engl J Med.* 2014;370(18):1683-1693.

16. Peake SL, Delaney A, Bailey M, et al. Goal-directed resuscitation for patients with early septic shock. *N Engl J Med.* 2014;371(16):1496-1506.
17. Mouncey PR, Osborn TM, Power GS, et al. Trial of early, goal-directed resuscitation for septic shock. *N Engl J Med.* 2015;372(14):1301-1311.
18. Michard F, Teboul JL. Predicting fluid responsiveness in ICU patients: a critical analysis of the evidence. *Chest.* 2002;121(6):2000-2008.
19. Pickett JD, Bridges E, Kritek PA, et al. Passive leg-raising and prediction of fluid responsiveness: systematic review. *Crit Care Nurse.* 2017;37(2):32-47.
20. Marik PE, Baram M, Vahid B. Does central venous pressure predict fluid responsiveness?: A systematic review of the literature and the tale of seven mares. *Chest.* 2008;134(1):172-178.
21. Long E, Oakley E, Duke T, et al. Does respiratory variation in inferior vena cava diameter predict fluid responsiveness: a systematic review and meta-analysis. *Shock.* 2017;47(5):550-559.
22. Michard F, Lopes M, Auler JC. Pulse pressure variation: beyond the fluid management of patients with shock. *Crit Care.* 2007;11(3):131.
23. Jan Vos J, Poterman M, Papineau Salm P, et al. Noninvasive pulse pressure variation and stroke volume variation to predict fluid responsiveness at multiple thresholds: a prospective observational study. *Can J Anaesth.* 2015;62(11):1153-1160.
24. Finfer S, Bellomo R, Boyce N, et al. A comparison of albumin and saline for fluid resuscitation in the intensive care unit. *N Engl J Med.* 2004;350(22):2247-2256.
25. Semler MW, Self WH, Wanderer JP, et al. Balanced crystalloids versus saline in critically ill adults. *N Engl J Med.* 2018;378(9):829-839.
26. Sirvent JM, Ferri C, Baro A, et al. Fluid balance in sepsis and septic shock as a determining factor of mortality. *Am J Emerg Med.* 2015;33(2):186-189.
27. Tigabu BM, Davari M, Kebriaeezadeh A, et al. Fluid volume, fluid balance and patient outcome in severe sepsis and septic shock: a systematic review. *J Crit Care.* 2018;48:153-159.
28. Sharshar T, Blanchard A, Paillard M, et al. Circulating vasopressin levels in septic shock. *Crit Care Med.* 2003;31(6):1752-1758.
29. Russell JA, Walley KR, Singer J, et al. Vasopressin versus norepinephrine infusion in patients with septic shock. *N Engl J Med.* 2008;358(9):877-887.
30. Khanna A, English SW, Wang XS, et al. Angiotensin II for the treatment of vasodilatory shock. *N Engl J Med.* 2017;377(5):419-430.
31. Venkatesh B, Finfer S, Cohen J, et al. Adjunctive glucocorticoid therapy in patients with septic shock. *N Engl J Med.* 2018;378(9):797-808.
32. Annane D, Renault A, Brun-Buisson C. Hydrocortisone plus fludrocortisone for adults with septic shock. *N Engl J Med.* 2018;378(9):809-818.
33. Sprung CL, Annane D, Keh D. Hydrocortisone therapy for patients with septic shock. *N Engl J Med.* 2008;358(2):111-124.
34. Jentzer JC, Vallabhajosyula S, Khanna AK, et al. Management of refractory vasodilatory shock. *Chest.* 2018;154(2):416-426.
35. Hollenberg SM. Vasopressor support in septic shock. *Chest.* 2007;132(5):1678-1687.
36. Rui Q, Jiang Y, Chen M, et al. Dopamine versus norepinephrine in the treatment of cardiogenic shock. *Medicine (Baltimore).* 2017;96(43):e8402.
37. Francis GS, Bartos JA, Adatya S. Inotropes. *J Am Coll Cardiol.* 2014;63(20):2069-2078.

Does a protocol-based resuscitation of patients diagnosed with septic shock improve outcomes?

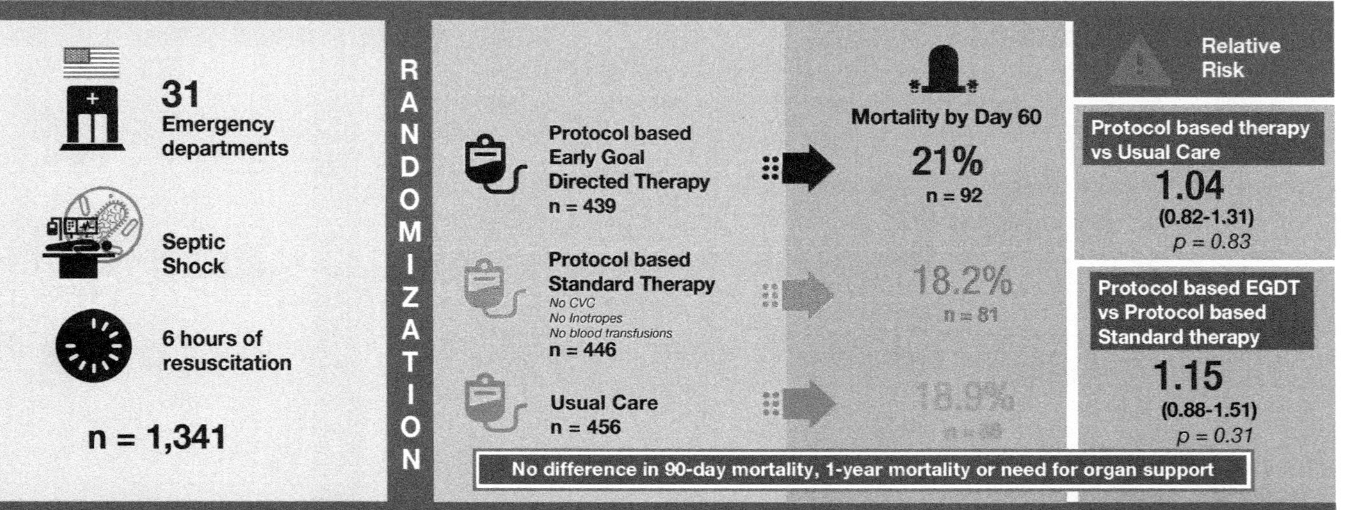

Conclusion: In a multicenter trial conducted in the tertiary care setting, protocol-based resuscitation of patients in whom septic shock was diagnosed in the emergency department did not improve outcomes.

ProCESS invesigators, Yealy DM, Kellum JA, Huang DT, et al. ***A randomized trial of protocol-based care for early septic shock.*** N Engl J Med 2014 May 1;370(18):1683-93.

VISUAL ABSTRACT 2.1

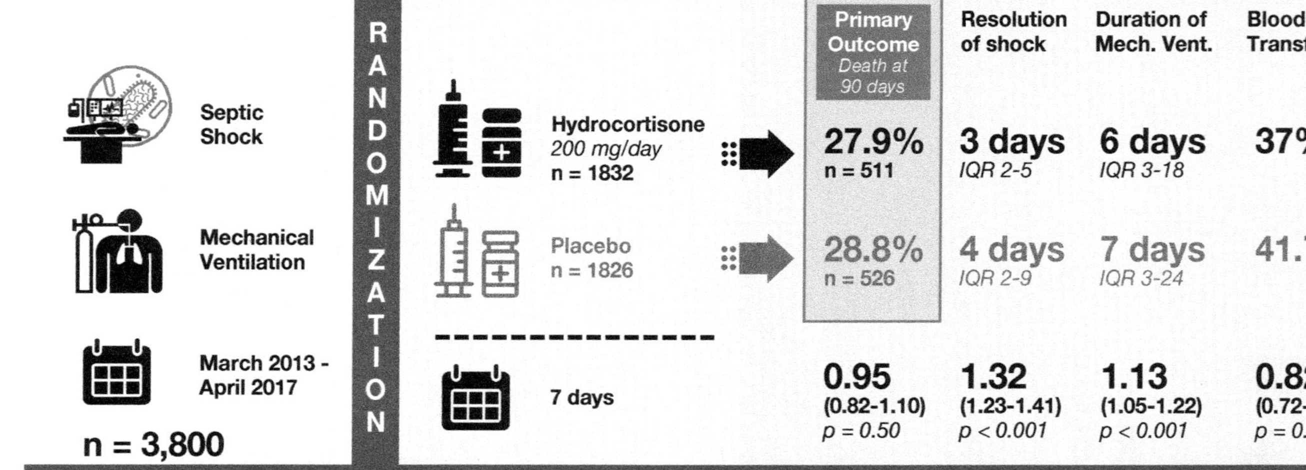

VISUAL ABSTRACT 2.2

Comparative clinical effects of balanced crystalloids and saline in critically ill patients cared for inside an intensive care unit (ICU)

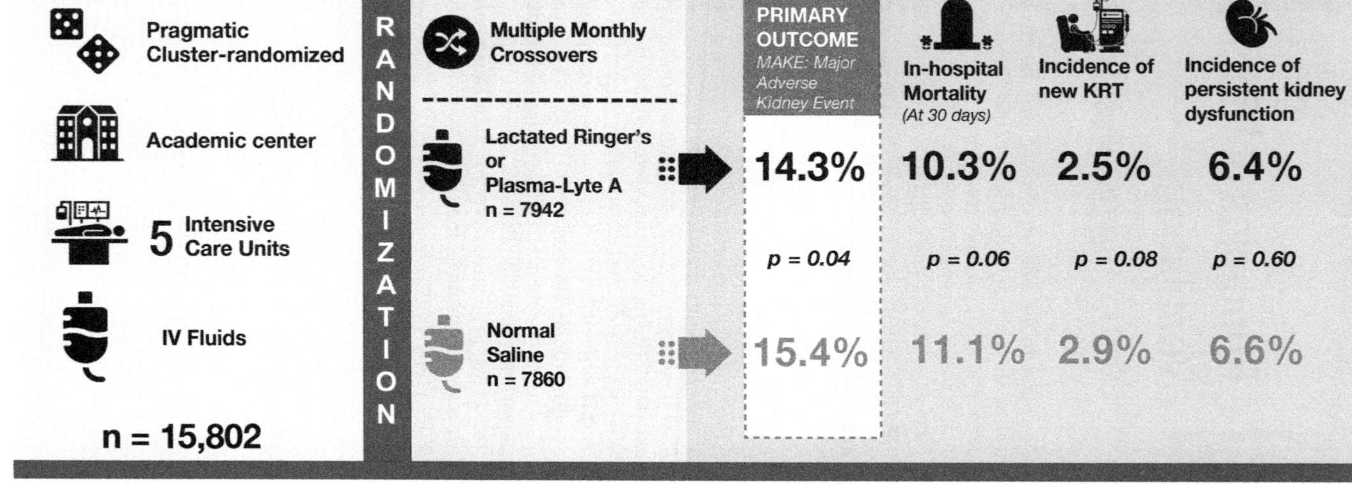

Conclusion: Among critically ill adults, the use of balanced crystalloids for intravenous fluid administration resulted in a lower rate of the composite outcome of death from any cause, new kidney-replacement therapy, or persistent renal dysfunction than the use of saline.

Semler MW, Self WH, Wanderer JP, Wanderer JP, et al. SMARRT Investigators. ***Balanced Crystalloids versus Saline in Critically Ill Adults.*** N Engl J Med 2018; 378:829-839

VISUAL ABSTRACT 2.3

3 Principles of Mechanical Ventilation

Krysta S. Wolfe and Bhakti K. Patel

Mechanical ventilation refers to the delivery of supported breaths either through a mask (noninvasive) or through an endotracheal tube (invasive). Mechanical ventilation is indicated in acute or chronic respiratory failure resulting from insufficient oxygenation, inadequate ventilation, or inability to maintain an airway (**Table 3.1**). It can be used to fully or partially replace spontaneous breathing to improve gas exchange and decrease the work of breathing.

MODES OF MECHANICAL VENTILATION

Modes of mechanical ventilation differ in the types of breaths delivered to the patient (**Table 3.2**). In all modes, a breath is triggered by either a timer (ventilator-initiated breaths at a set respiratory rate) or patient effort. After a breath is triggered, air flows into the lungs at a predetermined flow rate or pressure limit. The breath is terminated at end inspiration as signaled by the delivery of a set tidal volume, completion of set inspiratory time, or decrease in flow to a predetermined percentage of its peak value. The mode of mechanical ventilation used is dependent on physician preference and the level of ventilatory support the patient needs. Modes of ventilation that support breaths at a minimum set respiratory rate are referred to as assist-control mode. The majority of patients are initially ventilated using a volume-control mode, in which ventilator-initiated breaths are delivered at a set tidal volume with termination of the breath once that volume is delivered. In this mode, the airway pressure is determined by the patient's respiratory mechanics, including airway resistance, lung compliance, and chest wall compliance. Full ventilatory support can also be provided by the ventilator in a pressure-control mode in which breaths are delivered with a set pressure limit for a given inspiratory time, resulting in variable tidal volumes related to compliance

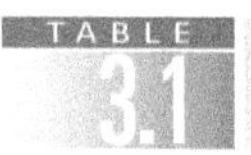

TABLE 3.1 Indications for Invasive Mechanical Ventilation

Indications for Invasive Mechanical Ventilation
Refractory hypoxemia
Ventilation impairment
Altered mental status/airway protection
Secretion management
Other: airway protection during procedure, metabolic acidosis, and shock

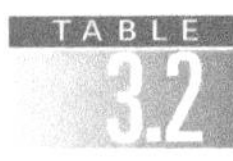

Common Modes of Mechanical Ventilation

Mode	Breath Target	Set Parameters	Measured Parameters	Cycle (Breath Termination Signal)	Comments
Assist control	Volume control	TV, RR, flow, PEEP	Peak and plateau pressures	Volume	Provides mandatory and assisted breaths
	Pressure control	Inspiratory pressure, PEEP inspiratory time, RR	TV	Time	Provides mandatory and assisted breaths
Pressure support ventilation	Pressure limited	Inspiratory pressure, PEEP	TV, RR, flow	Flow, time, or pressure	Assisted breaths triggered by patient
Continuous positive airway pressure		Continuous airway pressure		Flow	Spontaneous breaths
Synchronized intermittent mandatory ventilation	Volume limited	TV, RR, flow, PEEP	Peak and plateau pressures		Additional breaths above set rate can be spontaneous or assisted (pressure support added)

PEEP, positive end-expiratory pressure; RR, respiratory rate; TV, tidal volume.

and airway resistance. In pressure support ventilation (PSV), the ventilator provides a driving pressure (inspiratory pressure and positive end-expiratory pressure [PEEP]) to support patient-initiated breaths.

INITIAL VENTILATOR SETTINGS

Tidal Volume

The goal tidal volume, or amount of air delivered with each breath, is one that allows for adequate minute ventilation while minimizing the risks associated with volumes that are too high (overdistension) or too low (atelectasis). In patients with acute respiratory distress syndrome (ARDS), the use of a lung-protective strategy with tidal volumes less than or equal to 6 mL/kg of predicted (or ideal) body weight (PBW) is recommended (see Chapter 4). The optimal tidal volume in mechanically ventilated patients without ARDS is less clear.[1] In most patients, a tidal volume of 6 to 8 mL/kg PBW is an appropriate initial setting. In patients undergoing abdominal surgery, the use of intraoperative tidal volumes of 6 to 8 mL/kg PBW as compared with higher volumes (10 to 12 mL/kg PBW) was associated with a reduction in adverse pulmonary events, need for postoperative mechanical ventilation, and length of stay.[2]

Respiratory Rate

An initial rate of 12 to 16 breaths/min is often chosen and then adjusted to achieve the desired minute ventilation for a patient (guided by pH and $Paco_2$). In patients with ARDS, a higher respiratory rate is often needed to maintain adequate ventilation in the setting of low tidal volumes. Alternatively, in patients with severe obstructive lung disease, the respiratory rate may need to be decreased to minimize air trapping.

Positive End-Expiratory Pressure

Extrinsic PEEP is typically set at 5 cm H_2O. This level of PEEP is applied to prevent end-expiratory alveolar collapse or atelectasis. Higher levels of PEEP may be required to improve oxygenation in acute hypoxemic respiratory failure, with careful attention to limit the plateau pressure to less than 30 cm H_2O to prevent barotrauma.

Fraction of Inspired Oxygen

The fraction of inspired oxygen (Fio_2) is set by the physician in all modes of mechanical ventilation. It is often initially set to 100%, but should be weaned quickly to the minimum level needed to maintain adequate oxygenation. An Fio_2 of 60% or less is preferred to minimize injury that may result from prolonged exposure to higher levels of oxygen.[3,4]

MONITORING PATIENTS ON THE VENTILATOR

Routine management of patients receiving mechanical ventilation includes evaluation of the respiratory system mechanics and waveform analysis. This approach provides information regarding the underlying pathology leading to respiratory failure, can be used to assess the response to therapeutic interventions, and can guide the physician in adjusting the ventilator settings to optimize the level of support provided.

Ventilator Waveforms

The use of a volume-control mode of ventilation with a square wave and constant flow (typically 60 L/min) allows for a rapid assessment of ventilator waveforms and respiratory mechanics in patients without ventilator dyssynchrony. The peak inspiratory pressure (PIP) is measured at the airway opening and is composed of the inspiratory resistance (P_{res}), the pressure required to expand the alveoli against the elastic recoil of the lung and chest wall (elastic pressure), and the PEEP. To determine the relative contributions of the resistive and elastic pressures, an end-inspiratory hold is performed to measure the plateau pressure (P_{plat}) (see **Figure 3.1**). When the PIP is elevated (>25 cm H_2O), the difference between the peak and plateau pressures can be used to determine whether the elevation is because of an increase in resistance or a decrease in compliance (see **Figure 3.2**).

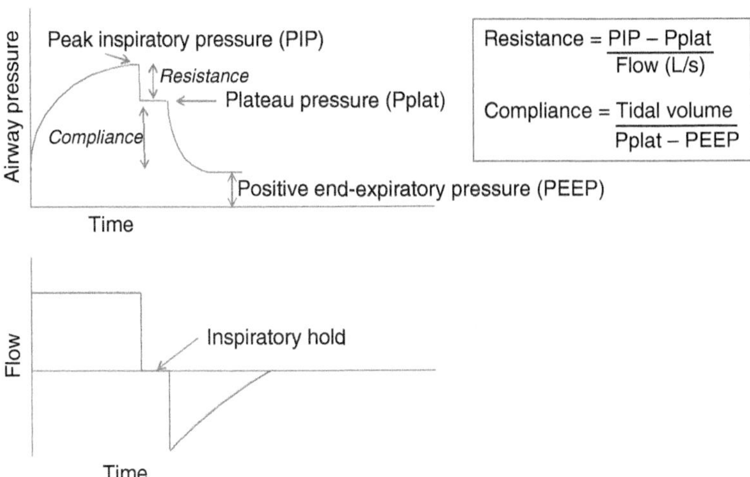

FIGURE 3.1: Ventilator waveform during constant flow, volume-control mode of ventilation in a passive patient. An inspiratory pause is shown, allowing for the determination of peak inspiratory and plateau pressures. The difference between the peak and plateau pressures is reflective of resistance. The plateau pressure is used to determine compliance.

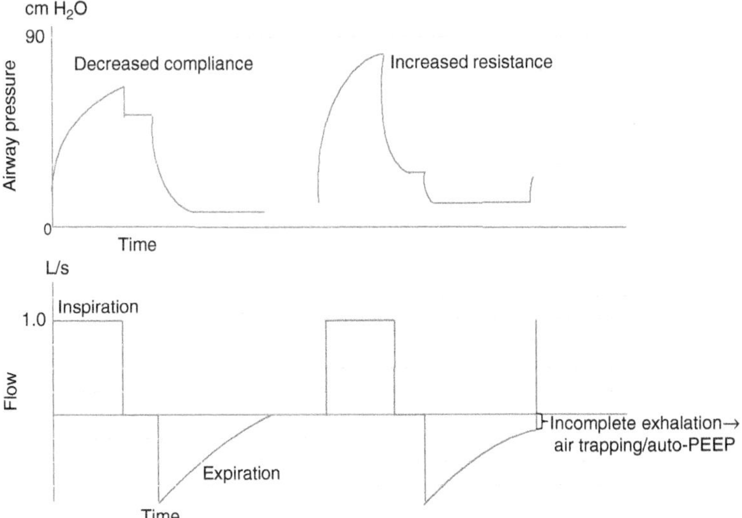

FIGURE 3.2: On the left is a patient with decreased lung compliance ("stiff" lungs) due to acute respiratory distress syndrome, as illustrated by an elevated plateau pressure measured during an inspiratory hold. On the right is an obstructed patient with increased airway resistance (large difference between peak inspiratory and plateau pressure) due to status asthmaticus. The patient continues to have flow at end expiration (bottom panel), indicating the presence of auto-PEEP. PEEP, positive end-expiratory pressure.

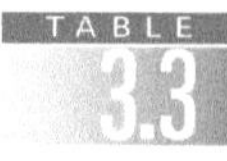

Differential Diagnosis for Elevated Peak Inspiratory Pressure

Increased Resistance	Increased Elastic Pressure (or Decreased Compliance)
High flow	Pulmonary hemorrhage
Bronchospasm	Chest wall restriction (musculoskeletal, pleural, obesity, abdominal distension)
Chronic obstructive pulmonary disease	Interstitial lung disease
Mucus plugging/secretions	Pulmonary edema
Airway edema	Atelectasis
Airway obstruction (tumor, foreign body)	Pneumonia
Obstructed endotracheal tube	Tension pneumothorax

Normal resistance is less than 10 cm H_2O/L/s. A difference between the peak and plateau pressures greater than 10 cm H_2O/L/s indicates increased resistance to airflow. Common etiologies of increased resistance include bronchospasm, mucus plugging, or endotracheal tube obstruction. Alternatively, increased PIP in the setting of normal airway resistance is due to an elevation in the elastic pressure of the lung resulting from lung stiffness or restriction from the chest wall or diaphragm (e.g., tense ascites). Compliance is the inverse of elastance; therefore, high elastic pressure is the same as low compliance. The differential for elevated resistance or elastic pressure is given in **Table 3.3.**

Auto–Positive End-Expiratory Pressure

Auto-PEEP is the intrinsic PEEP. End-expiratory pressure is created when inspiration begins before expiration is complete, leading to air trapping (see Figure 3.2). This can be measured by performing an end-expiratory hold on the ventilator. Under normal conditions, the pressure measured at the end of an expiratory hold maneuver should equal the PEEP applied. If the pressure is higher than the PEEP, then auto-PEEP is present. This commonly occurs in patients with obstructive lung disease, particularly status asthmaticus. If present, decreasing the respiratory rate and tidal volume or increasing the inspiratory flow rate to allow more time in exhalation prevents hemodynamic compromise because of auto-PEEP. If hypotension occurs, patients should be temporarily disconnected from the ventilator until hypotension resolves and volume resuscitated in addition to adjustment of ventilator settings.

CARE OF THE MECHANICALLY VENTILATED PATIENT

Mechanically ventilated patients are at risk for complications, such as ventilator-associated pneumonia (VAP), immobilization, and adverse effects of sedatives (**Table 3.4**). Simple measures should be employed to potentially reduce the risk of VAPs, such as elevation of head of bed to 30 to 45 degrees.[5,6] To minimize the risk of venous thromboembolism associated with immobility, prophylaxis should be used in all patients without a contraindication. "Bundles" are commonly used to promote adherence to evidence-based interventions to reduce risk associated

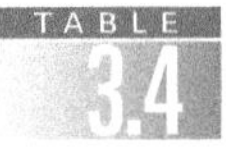

TABLE 3.4 Complications of Mechanical Ventilation
Nosocomial pneumonia
Barotrauma
Intensive care unit–acquired weakness
Delirium
Ventilator-associated lung injury
Ventilator-induced diaphragm dysfunction
Sinusitis
Airway injury

with invasive mechanical ventilation. The ABCDEF bundle promotes an assessment and management strategy for pain (A), daily sedative interruption (**Visual Abstract 3.1**) and spontaneous breathing trials (SBTs) (B), choosing an optimal sedation strategy (C), prevention and assessment of delirium (D), early mobilization (E), and family engagement (F). Adherence to the ABCDEF bundle is associated with decreased hospital death, delirium, and mechanical ventilation use.[7]

LIBERATION FROM MECHANICAL VENTILATION

Prolonged duration of mechanical ventilation is associated with increased mortality and risk for complications.[8] The most successful strategies for mechanical ventilation liberation include a daily assessment of readiness to wean and minimization of sedative use.[9] Clinicians tend to underestimate a patient's readiness for liberation; therefore, objective clinical criteria for readiness are recommended,[10,11] which include improvement in the cause of respiratory failure, adequate oxygenation, arterial pH greater than 7.25, hemodynamic stability, and the ability to initiate an inspiratory effort.[12] If a patient meets these criteria, then a weaning test should be performed. Performance of daily SBTs reduces the duration of weaning from mechanical ventilation compared to all other methods.[10]

During an SBT, the ventilator is switched to a spontaneous breathing mode for 30 minutes (up to 2 hours) either using a T-piece that provides no ventilatory support or at a low level of pressure support (typically inspiratory pressure of 5 to 8 cm H_2O or continuous positive airway pressure [CPAP]).[13] A recent study showed that an SBT consisting of 30 minutes of PSV, compared to a 2-hour T-piece trial, resulted in a higher rate of successful extubation (**Visual Abstract 3.2**).[13] If a patient passes an SBT, the patient should be assessed for an adequate cough, secretions, and mental status prior to extubation. A peak cough flow less than 60 L/min, secretions greater than 2.5 mL/hr, and the inability to complete four simple commands are associated with increased risk of extubation failure.[14] The application of noninvasive ventilation (NIV) after extubation may be beneficial in patients with severe chronic obstructive pulmonary disease (COPD) or heart failure who are at high risk for extubation failure.[15]

NONINVASIVE VENTILATION

NIV has been shown to reduce the need for endotracheal intubation in select patients with acute respiratory failure. The benefit of this approach is the ability to provide ventilatory assistance via a tight-fitting mask while reducing the risks associated with invasive mechanical ventilation. The benefits of NIV are greatest among patients with COPD exacerbations with hypercapnic acidosis and cardiogenic pulmonary edema. NIV is commonly delivered as either CPAP or bilevel positive airway pressure (BPAP). Failure of NIV has been associated with increased mortality; therefore, identification of patients most likely to benefit from NIV is critical. Indications for converting from NIV to intubation include inability to tolerate NIV, progressive hypercapnia associated with a pH less than 7.25, requirement for high airway pressures (>20 cm H_2O), refractory hypoxemia, altered mental status, and concern for inability to protect airway. Contraindications to NIV include the following:

- Cardiopulmonary arrest
- Severely impaired consciousness
- Facial surgery, trauma, or deformity
- High aspiration risk
- Prolonged duration of mechanical ventilation anticipated
- Recent esophageal anastomosis

Acute on Chronic Hypercapnic Respiratory Failure

The use of NIV in the treatment of acute exacerbations of COPD has been shown to decrease mortality, reduce the need for intubation, decrease treatment failure, reduce treatment complications, and have a shorter hospital length of stay (**Visual Abstract 3.3**).[16,17] The success rate of NIV in acute exacerbations of COPD is approximately 80% to 85% and is, therefore, recommended as a first-line therapy.[18]

Acute Cardiogenic Pulmonary Edema

NIV can improve the work of breathing and cardiovascular function in patients with cardiogenic pulmonary edema. Improvement in cardiac function results from afterload reduction and reduction of right and left ventricular preload.[19,20] The use of NIV is associated with reduced rates of endotracheal intubation in this patient population.[21]

Hypoxemic Respiratory Failure

Although NIV is often used in the treatment of hypoxemic respiratory failure, there is conflicting evidence about its benefit. The benefit of NIV in hypoxemic respiratory failure is in part because of the ability to provide PEEP to improve respiratory mechanics and gas exchange. In a meta-analysis, NIV use in acute hypoxemic nonhypercapnic respiratory failure was associated with decreased intubation rate and hospital mortality.[22] However, caution must be exercised when applying this strategy in patients with ARDS due to high failure rates and an association with increased mortality in patients with moderate-to-severe ARDS.[23]

Immunocompromised Patients

There are conflicting results regarding NIV use in immunocompromised patients with acute respiratory failure. Early studies indicated a potential benefit with less need for intubation, less infectious complications, and decreased mortality in patients receiving NIV,[24,25] although more recent trials have not replicated these results and show that NIV may in fact be associated with harm in this patient population.[26,27]

References

1. Simonis FD, Serpa Neto A, Binnekade JM, et al. Effect of a low vs intermediate tidal volume strategy on ventilator-free days in intensive care unit patients without ARDS: a randomized clinical trial. *JAMA.* 2018;320(18):1872-1880.
2. Futier E, Constantin JM, Paugam-Burtz C, et al. A trial of intraoperative low-tidal-volume ventilation in abdominal surgery. *N Engl J Med.* 2013;369(5):428-437.
3. Elliott CG, Rasmusson BY, Crapo RO, Morris AH, Jensen RL. Prediction of pulmonary function abnormalities after adult respiratory distress syndrome (ARDS). *Am Rev Respir Dis.* 1987;135(3):634-638.
4. Deneke SM, Fanburg BL. Normobaric oxygen toxicity of the lung. *N Engl J Med.* 1980;303(2):76-86.
5. Drakulovic MB, Torres A, Bauer TT, Nicolas JM, Nogué S, Ferrer M. Supine body position as a risk factor for nosocomial pneumonia in mechanically ventilated patients: a randomised trial. *Lancet.* 1999;354(9193):1851-1858.
6. van Nieuwenhoven CA, Vandenbroucke-Grauls C, van Tiel FH, et al. Feasibility and effects of the semirecumbent position to prevent ventilator-associated pneumonia: a randomized study. *Crit Care Med.* 2006;34(2):396-402.
7. Pun BT, Balas MC, Barnes-Daly MA, et al. Caring for critically ill patients with the ABCDEF bundle: results of the ICU liberation collaborative in over 15,000 adults. *Crit Care Med.* 2019;47(1):3-14.
8. Funk GC, Anders S, Breyer MK, et al. Incidence and outcome of weaning from mechanical ventilation according to new categories. *Eur Respir J.* 2010;35(1):88-94.
9. Girard TD, Kress JP, Fuchs BD, et al. Efficacy and safety of a paired sedation and ventilator weaning protocol for mechanically ventilated patients in intensive care (Awakening and Breathing Controlled trial): a randomised controlled trial. *Lancet.* 2008;371(9607):126-134.
10. Esteban A, Frutos F, Tobin MJ, et al. A comparison of four methods of weaning patients from mechanical ventilation. Spanish Lung Failure Collaborative Group. *N Engl J Med.* 1995;332(6):345-350.
11. Brochard L, Rauss A, Benito S, et al. Comparison of three methods of gradual withdrawal from ventilatory support during weaning from mechanical ventilation. *Am J Respir Crit Care Med.* 1994;150(4):896-903.
12. MacIntyre NR, Cook DJ, Ely EW, et al. Evidence-based guidelines for weaning and discontinuing ventilatory support: a collective task force facilitated by the American College of Chest Physicians; the American Association for Respiratory Care; and the American College of Critical Care Medicine. *Chest.* 2001;120(6 Suppl):375s-395s.
13. Subira C, Hernández G, Vázquez A, et al. Effect of pressure support vs T-piece ventilation strategies during spontaneous breathing trials on successful extubation among patients receiving mechanical ventilation: a randomized clinical trial. *JAMA.* 2019;321(22):2175-2182.
14. Salam A, Tilluckdharry L, Amoateng-Adjepong Y, Manthous CA. Neurologic status, cough, secretions and extubation outcomes. *Intensive Care Med.* 2004;30(7):1334-1339.
15. Rochwerg B, Brochard L, Elliott MW, et al. Official ERS/ATS clinical practice guidelines: noninvasive ventilation for acute respiratory failure. *Eur Respir J.* 2017;50(2):1602426.
16. Ram FS, Picot J, Lightowler J, Wedzicha JA. Non-invasive positive pressure ventilation for treatment of respiratory failure due to exacerbations of chronic obstructive pulmonary disease. *Cochrane Database Syst Rev.* 2004;(1):CD004104.
17. Brochard L, Mancebo J, Wysocki M, et al. Noninvasive ventilation for acute exacerbations of chronic obstructive pulmonary disease. *N Engl J Med.* 1995;333(13):817-822.
18. Vogelmeier CF, Criner GJ, Martinez FJ, et al. Global strategy for the diagnosis, management, and prevention of chronic obstructive lung disease 2017 report. GOLD executive summary. *Am J Respir Crit Care Med.* 2017;195(5):557-582.
19. Lenique F, Habis M, Lofaso F, Dubois-Randé JL, Harf A, Brochard L. Ventilatory and hemodynamic effects of continuous positive airway pressure in left heart failure. *Am J Respir Crit Care Med.* 1997;155(2):500-505.
20. Chadda K, Annane D, Hart N, Gajdos P, Raphaël JC, Lofaso F. Cardiac and respiratory effects of continuous positive airway pressure and noninvasive ventilation in acute cardiac pulmonary edema. *Crit Care Med.* 2002;30(11):2457-2461.
21. Vital FM, Ladeira MT, Atallah AN. Non-invasive positive pressure ventilation (CPAP or bilevel NPPV) for cardiogenic pulmonary oedema. *Cochrane Database Syst Rev.* 2013;(5):CD005351.

22. Xu XP, Zhang XC, Hu SL, et al. Noninvasive ventilation in acute hypoxemic nonhypercapnic respiratory failure: a systematic review and meta-analysis. *Crit Care Med.* 2017;45(7):e727-e733.
23. Bellani G, Laffey JG, Pham T, et al. Noninvasive ventilation of patients with acute respiratory distress syndrome. Insights from the LUNG SAFE study. *Am J Respir Crit Care Med.* 2017;195(1):67-77.
24. Hilbert G, Gruson D, Vargas F, et al. Noninvasive ventilation in immunosuppressed patients with pulmonary infiltrates, fever, and acute respiratory failure. *N Engl J Med.* 2001;344(7):481-487.
25. Antonelli M, Conti G, Bufi M, et al. Noninvasive ventilation for treatment of acute respiratory failure in patients undergoing solid organ transplantation: a randomized trial. *JAMA.* 2000;283(2):235-241.
26. Frat JP, Ragot S, Girault C, et al. Effect of non-invasive oxygenation strategies in immunocompromised patients with severe acute respiratory failure: a post-hoc analysis of a randomised trial. *Lancet Respir Med.* 2016;4(8):646-652.
27. Lemiale V, Mokart D, Resche-Rigon M, et al. Effect of noninvasive ventilation vs oxygen therapy on mortality among immunocompromised patients with acute respiratory failure: a randomized clinical trial. *JAMA.* 2015;314:1711-1719.

Is it safe and beneficial to wean both sedation and ventilation in mechanically ventilated patients in ICU?

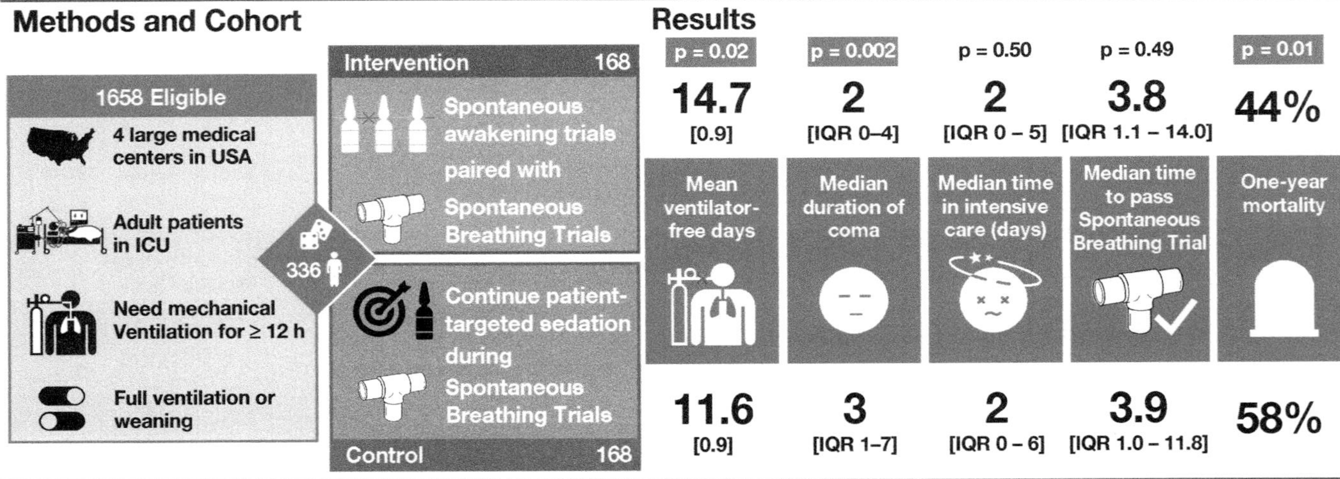

Conclusion: This randomized control trial in mechanically ventilated ICU patients showed that a paired sedation and ventilator weaning protocol resulted in more ventilator-free days.

Girard TD, Kress JP, Fuchs BD, et al. ***Efficacy and safety of a paired sedation and ventilator weaning protocol for mechanically ventilated patients in intensive care (Awakening and Breathing Controlled trial): a randomised controlled trial.*** Lancet. 2008;371(9607):126-34.

VISUAL ABSTRACT 3.1

Is pressure support or T-piece ventilation better as a strategy for spontaneous breathing trials?

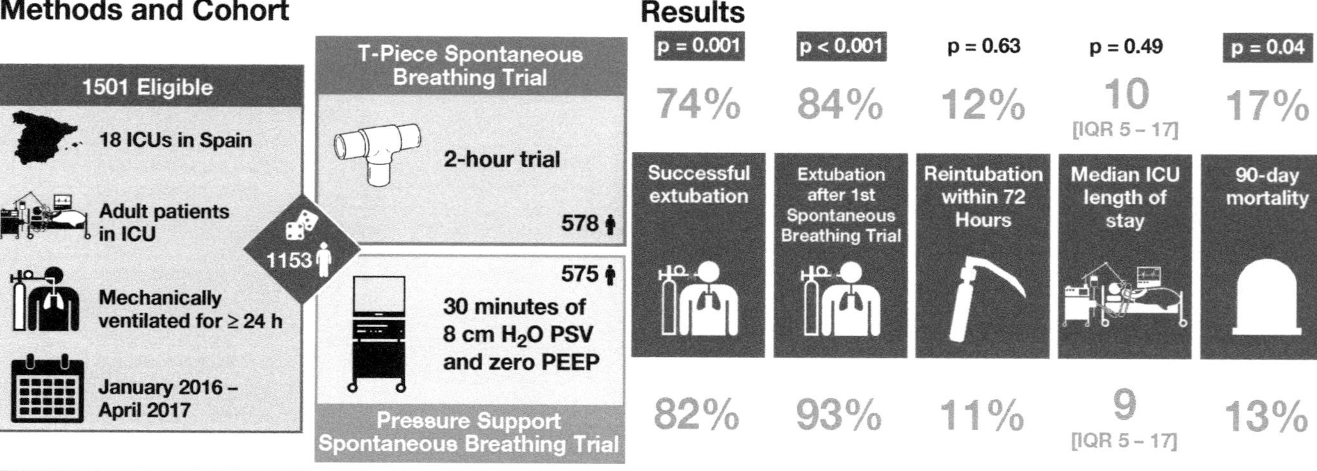

Conclusion: In this randomized trial, a 30-minute PSV spontaneous breathing trial resulted in a significantly higher rate of successful extubation than a 2-hour T-piece spontaneous breathing trial without significantly increasing reintubation.

Subirà C, Hernández G, Vázquez A, et al. ***Effect of Pressure Support vs T-Piece Ventilation Strategies During Spontaneous Breathing Trials on Successful Extubation Among Patients Receiving Mechanical Ventilation: A Randomized Clinical Trial***. JAMA. 2019;321(22):2175-2182.

VISUAL ABSTRACT 3.2

Can noninvasive ventilation reduce need for mechanical ventilation and improve outcomes in COPD?

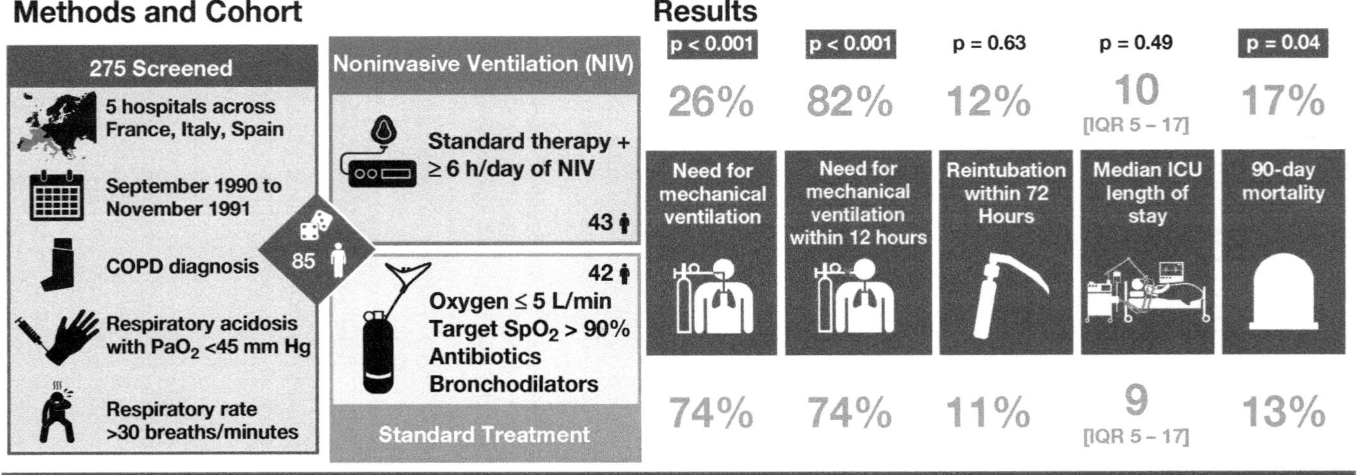

Conclusion: In selected patients with acute exacerbations of chronic obstructive pulmonary disease, non-invasive ventilation can reduce the need for endotracheal intubation, the length of the hospital stay, and the in-hospital mortality rate.

Brochard L, Mancebo J, Wysocki M, et al. ***Noninvasive ventilation for acute exacerbations of chronic obstructive pulmonary disease.*** N Engl J Med. 1995;333(13):817-22.

VISUAL ABSTRACT 3.3

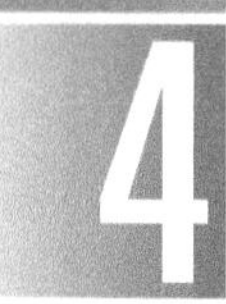

Acute Respiratory Distress Syndrome

Camilo Cortesi and Kathleen Liu

INTRODUCTION

The acute respiratory distress syndrome (ARDS) has an incidence of 10.4% in the intensive care unit (ICU) setting, and it is associated with mortality rates in the range of 40% to 50% in its severe forms.[1] There is significant overlap between patients with acute respiratory failure and acute kidney injury (AKI), with the latter present in one-third of patients with ARDS. This highlights the importance of an integrative approach when managing these patients. This chapter aims to provide an overview and guidance from a kidney perspective to nephrologists and critical care health practitioners, in particular with regard to lung and kidney cross talk. Insights about how kidney hemodynamics and function might be affected by ARDS pathophysiology and management are critical when providing recommendations from a kidney perspective.

DEFINITION, ETIOLOGIES, AND DIFFERENTIAL DIAGNOSIS

ARDS is characterized by an acute pulmonary inflammatory response, leading to an increase in pulmonary vascular permeability and subsequent alveolar and interstitial noncardiogenic pulmonary edema. ARDS should be suspected in the presence of a known trigger plus the development of acute onset (hours to less than 7 days) of respiratory symptoms, increased oxygen requirements, and radiologic evidence of bilateral lung infiltrates not completely attributed to acute heart failure or volume overload. There are several known ARDS triggers, including sepsis, pneumonia, pancreatitis, trauma, extensive burns, pulmonary inhalation injury, aspiration of gastric contents, thoracic surgery, blood product transfusion, and administration of certain types of chemotherapy. Conditions that can present with ARDS-like picture should be taken into consideration early on during evaluation, especially in the absence of a known trigger condition. ARDS mimics can include acute cardiogenic pulmonary edema, bilateral pneumonia, pulmonary vasculitis, exacerbation of idiopathic fibrosis, and metastatic malignancy, among others.

CLASSIFICATION

The original definition for ARDS, along with acute lung injury, was proposed by the American-European Consensus Conference in 1994. More recently, this definition was revised and is now referred to as the "Berlin" definition.[2] The Berlin definition classified ARDS into three different categories, based on the ratio of the partial pressure of arterial oxygen/fraction of inspired oxygen (Pao_2/Fio_2) levels in patients on ventilatory support ($\geq$5 cm H_2O of positive end-expiratory pressure [PEEP] or continuous positive airway pressure [CPAP]) as follows:

- Mild ARDS: $Pao_2/Fio_2 > 200$ mm Hg and ≤ 300 mm Hg
- Moderate ARDS: $Pao_2/Fio_2 > 100$ mm Hg and ≤ 200 mm Hg
- Severe ARDS: $Pao_2/Fio_2 \leq 100$ mm Hg

LUNG-KIDNEY CROSS TALK IN ACUTE RESPIRATORY DISTRESS SYNDROME

Nephrology and critical care practitioners should be aware of the lung-kidney cross talk when evaluating an ARDS patient. These interactions can have an impact on kidney function and hemodynamics that might then worsen ARDS and its outcomes (**Figure 4.1**). AKI can be triggered or worsened by the following factors/situations:

1. Effects of oxygenation, hypercarbia, and acidosis on kidney hemodynamics:
   a) Hypoxemia: importantly, these changes likely occur predominantly in the setting of severe hypoxemia (e.g., $Pao_2 < 40$ mm Hg) and not during the mild hypoxemia that often occurs during ARDS.
      i. In the lung, severe hypoxemia may result in pulmonary artery vasoconstriction and pulmonary hypertension. Over time, this may result in right heart failure with associated renal venous congestion and decreased glomerular filtration rate (GFR).
      ii. In the kidney, severe hypoxemia may result in impairment of the endothelin, nitric oxide, angiotensin II, and bradykinin pathways, leading to sympathetic systemic activation and a reduction in renal blood flow.
   b) Hypercarbia
      i. CO_2 is a direct pulmonary vasoconstrictor independent of oxygen concentration.
      ii. In the kidney, severe hypercarbia can result in renal artery vasoconstriction, sympathetic nervous system activation (via norepinephrine), systemic vasodilation, and renin-angiotensin-aldosterone system activation, leading to a reduction in renal blood flow.

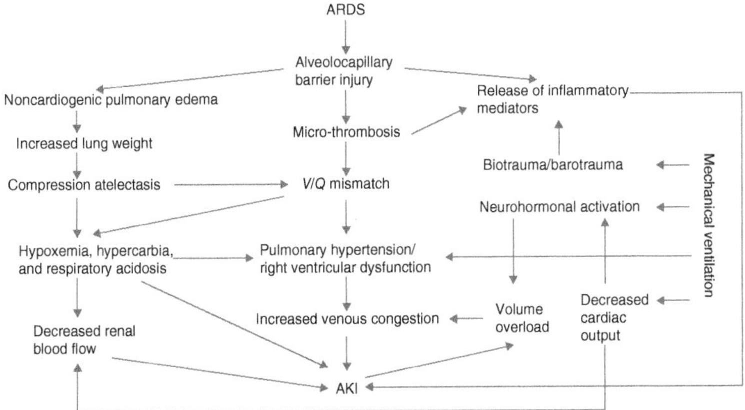

FIGURE 4.1: Lung and kidney interactions. AKI, acute kidney injury; ARDS, acute respiratory distress syndrome.

   c) A moderate degree of acidosis may result in renal vasodilation, with more severe acidosis resulting in renal vasoconstriction. However, it has also been proposed that permissive hypercarbia and acidosis may have a cytoprotective and anti-inflammatory effect.
2. Effects of volume overload, increased right-sided pressures of the heart, and venous congestion on kidney function:
   a) Volume overload is quite common in the setting of ARDS and AKI; this can exacerbate right ventricular dysfunction and venous congestion, leading to interstitial edema in the kidney, decreased perfusion pressure and oxygen delivery within in the kidney, and AKI.
   b) Volume overload may also dilute serum creatinine (by increasing the volume of distribution) and therefore mask AKI.
3. Effects of mechanical ventilation on the kidneys. In particular with high levels of PEEP, mechanical ventilation can reduce preload and decrease cardiac output. Mechanical ventilation can also increase intrathoracic pressure and pulmonary vascular resistance. In addition, during mechanical ventilation, a number of forms of injury to the lung can occur, including barotrauma, volutrauma, and atelectrauma, which can lead to release of proinflammatory cytokines, systemic inflammation, and AKI.

In sum, understanding lung-kidney cross talk highlights the importance of avoiding or promptly addressing extreme hypoxia, hypercarbia, and acidosis; implementing a lung-protective strategy to reduce the risk of further lung injury; and understanding hemodynamic and neurohormonal changes given their implications in the development of AKI in ARDS patients.

PREDICTIVE BIOMARKERS IN ACUTE RESPIRATORY DISTRESS SYNDROME

Multiple biomarkers have been linked to ARDS severity and the development of adverse outcomes. More recently, these biomarkers have been used to identify hypo- and hyperinflammatory subphenotypes of ARDS.[3] These subphenotypes appear to have a differential risk of death and other adverse outcomes (those with the hyperinflammatory phenotype have poorer outcomes). More intriguingly, in reanalysis of a number of negative randomized clinical trials, there appears to be a differential treatment effect, with some novel therapies appearing to have benefit in patients with the hyperinflammatory subphenotype.

With regard to the development of AKI in the context of ARDS, associations between elevated levels of plasma biomarkers—plasminogen activator inhibitor-1 (PAI-I), interleukin 6 (IL-6), and tumor necrosis factor receptor I and II—and the development of AKI in ARDS patients have been described. The mechanism of injury remains unclear.[4] Finally, a novel biomarker that identifies patients at increased risk for AKI has recently been developed, the Nephrocheck (bioMérieux). This biomarker is discussed in detail in Chapter 16; of note, the initial validation studies were performed in critically ill patients with respiratory or cardiovascular failure, many of whom likely had ARDS.

EVIDENCE-BASED ACUTE RESPIRATORY DISTRESS SYNDROME THERAPY

ARDS therapies can be separated into treatment of the underlying cause and supportive care. Prompt treatment of the underlying cause of ARDS is a critical first step in management, especially when ARDS is related to sepsis. Second, supportive therapy for ARDS, which has been shown to be beneficial and may reduce further lung injury, is key. The cornerstone of supportive care is lung-protective ventilation. Multiple trials have shown that low tidal volumes (4 to 6 mL/kg of predicted body weight [PBW], targeting plateau pressures ≤30 cm H_2O) are associated with reducing mortality and better outcomes (**Visual Abstract 4.1**).[5] PBW is related to height, with different formulas used in men and women:

1. Male PBW (kg) = 50 + 2.3 (height [in] – 60)
2. Female PBW (kg) = 45.5 + 2.3 (height [in])

In contrast, the impact of lower or higher PEEP levels is more controversial; a number of randomized clinical trials have not shown a benefit to a higher PEEP strategy.[6] However, meta-analyses have had varying findings,[7] and a subgroup analysis suggested that the hyperinflammatory ARDS subphenotype benefited from a higher PEEP strategy. Further studies are likely needed to define whether a subgroup of ARDS patients would benefit from a higher PEEP strategy.

With regard to other ventilatory strategies, prone ventilation has been associated with improvement in oxygenation and survival in patients with moderate to severe ARDS with PaO_2/FiO_2 less than 120 mm Hg.[8] In contrast, although a French randomized clinical trial showed mortality benefit in patients with moderate-severe ARDS (PaO_2/FiO_2 < 150 mm Hg[9]) randomized to receive neuromuscular blockade, a larger, more recent US clinical trial did not demonstrate any benefit with early neuromuscular blockade in a similar population.[10] There are some notable differences between the two trials, with the latter trial comparing neuromuscular blockade to usual care including a higher PEEP strategy and sedation to tolerate mechanical ventilation, rather than to deep sedation (which was required in the French trial because it was a blinded study; the US study was unblinded).

A fluid conservative management algorithm implemented after the resolution of shock has been associated with improvement in lung function (as measured by oxygenation index), an increase in ventilator-free days (a composite of mortality and time on the ventilator in survivors), and a decrease in length of ICU stay. This was associated with a trend toward improved mortality at 60 days that was not statistically significant (**Visual Abstract 4.2**).[11] In the original clinical trial, the fluid conservative algorithm was driven by bedside measures of end-organ perfusion including urine output along with cardiac filling pressures (central venous pressures or pulmonary capillary wedge pressures). Simplified versions of the protocol that do not rely on the presence of a central venous catheter to make invasive hemodynamic measurements have been subsequently developed. Although there was a slight increase in the risk of stage 1 AKI in those in the fluid conservative arm in the original trial, after accounting for differences in fluid balance in participants in the two arms, this risk was largely attenuated.[12]

Finally, in settings where it is available, extracorporeal membrane oxygenation (ECMO) can be applied to patients with refractory ARDS. Its role in the management of ARDS remains controversial, as it has been associated with an improvement in ventilator-free days,[13] but it has not been shown to improve survival in severe ARDS.[14] ECMO in ARDS should be considered with refractory hypoxemia (PaO_2/FiO_2 < 80 mm Hg), uncorrectable respiratory acidosis (pH < 7.15), persistent high end-inspiratory plateau pressures more than 35 cm H_2O, and Murray score greater than 3 despite management for more than 6 hours if no absolute contraindications. For more details about this topic, refer to Chapter 35.

In sum, therapy goals for ARDS include an oxygen saturation of 88% to 95% or PaO_2 55 to 80 mm Hg (to avoid oxygenation toxicity), pH 7.30 to 7.45, plateau pressure 30 cm H_2O or less, and euvolemia (after initial resuscitation, aiming for at least even to negative fluid balance with the goal of approximately even fluid balance over the first week or so of ARDS). A protocolized guide for mechanical ventilation setup and adjustments based on the National Heart Lung and Blood Institute (NHLBI) ARDS Network clinical trials, including FiO_2/PEEP combinations, is available at www.ardsnet.org/tools.shtml. PEEP titration and optimal PEEP remain subjects of greater controversy.

With regard to pharmacologic interventions, multiple therapeutic alternatives have been studied and have shown no evidence of benefit (and in some cases potential for harm). Some of the most relevant of these include: inhaled and intravenous beta-2 agonists, with the rationale of increasing alveolar fluid clearance and resolution of edema,[15] statins, and surfactant replacement. Corticosteroids have been studied extensively, with the rationale that these may decrease inflammation and fibrosis; however, their use is not associated with a reduction in mortality rates and steroids may be harmful, especially if started late in the ARDS course.[16] However, there is now considerable interest in steroids in the setting of COVID-19-associated hypoxemic respiratory failure, where dexamethasone has been shown to reduce mortality.[17] High-frequency oscillatory ventilation has been of much interest as a rescue therapy, but has not been associated with improved survival in several large randomized clinical trials.[18] Inhaled nitric oxide has been used as rescue therapy for refractory hypoxemia, but has not been shown to improve mortality rates. Inhaled nitric oxide has also been associated with several adverse outcomes, including an increased rate of AKI.[19]

INDICATIONS FOR KIDNEY REPLACEMENT THERAPY IN ACUTE RESPIRATORY DISTRESS SYNDROME

Indications for kidney replacement therapy (KRT) in ARDS are similar to other critical illnesses, perhaps with a greater emphasis on volume management. One of the main goals of supportive therapy is to avoid or manage interstitial lung edema that may lead to increased ventilator-associated lung injury. See Chapters 30 to 32 for discussions around timing, dosing, and modality of KRT.

References

1. Bellani G, Laffey JG, Pham T, et al. Epidemiology, patterns of care, and mortality for patients with acute respiratory distress syndrome in intensive care units in 50 countries. *JAMA*. 2016;315(8):788-800.
2. Ranieri VM, Rubenfeld GD, Thompson BT, et al. Acute respiratory distress syndrome: the Berlin definition. *JAMA*. 2012;307(23):2526-2533.
3. Calfee CS, Delucchi K, Parsons PE, et al. Subphenotypes in acute respiratory distress syndrome: latent class analysis of data from two randomised controlled trials. *Lancet Respir Med*. 2014; 2(8):611-620.
4. Liu KD, Glidden DV, Eisner MD, et al. Predictive and pathogenetic value of plasma biomarkers for acute kidney injury in patients with acute lung injury. *Crit Care Med*. 2007;35(12):2755-2761.
5. Acute Respiratory Distress Syndrome Network. Ventilation with lower tidal volumes as compared with traditional tidal volumes for acute lung injury and the acute respiratory distress syndrome. *N Engl J Med*. 2000;342(18):1301-1308.
6. The National Heart, Lung, and Blood Institute ARDS Clinical Trials Network. Higher versus lower positive end-expiratory pressures in patients with the acute respiratory distress syndrome. *N Engl J Med*. 2004;351(4):327-336.
7. Briel M, Meade M, Mercat A, et al. Higher vs lower positive end-expiratory pressure in patients with acute lung injury and acute respiratory distress syndrome. *JAMA*. 2010;303(9):865-873.
8. Guérin C, Reignier J, Richard J-C, et al. Prone positioning in severe acute respiratory distress syndrome. *N Engl J Med*. 2013;368(23):2159-2168.

9. Papazian L, Forel J-M, Gacouin A, et al. Neuromuscular blockers in early acute respiratory distress syndrome. *N Engl J Med.* 2010;363(12):1107-1116.
10. The National Heart, Lung, and Blood Institute PETAL Clinical Trials Network. Early neuromuscular blockade in the acute respiratory distress syndrome. *N Engl J Med.* 2019;380(21):1997-2008.
11. The National Heart, Lung, and Blood Institute ARDS Clinical Trials Network. Comparison of two fluid-management strategies in acute lung injury. *N Engl J Med.* 2006;354(24):2564-2575.
12. Liu KD, Thompson BT, Ancukiewicz M, et al. Acute kidney injury in patients with acute lung injury: impact of fluid accumulation on classification of acute kidney injury and associated outcome. *Crit Care Med.* 2011;39(12):2665-2671.
13. Bein T, Weber-Carstens S, Goldmann A, et al. Lower tidal volume strategy (≈3 ml/kg) combined with extracorporeal CO_2 removal versus "conventional" protective ventilation (6 ml/kg) in severe ARDS. *Intensive Care Med.* 2013;39(5):847-856.
14. Combes A, Hajage D, Capellier G, et al. Extracorporeal membrane oxygenation for severe acute respiratory distress syndrome. *N Engl J Med.* 2018;378(21):1965-1975.
15. The National Heart, Lung, and Blood Institute ARDS Clinical Trials Network. Randomized, placebo-controlled clinical trial of an aerosolized β_2-agonist for treatment of acute lung injury. *Am J Respir Crit Care Med.* 2011;184(5):561-568.
16. The National Heart, Lung, and Blood Institute ARDS Clinical Trials Network. Efficacy and safety of corticosteroids for persistent acute respiratory distress syndrome. *N Engl J Med.* 2006;354(16):1671-1684.
17. The RECOVERY Collaborative Group. Dexamethasone in hospitalized patients with Covid-19—preliminary report. *N Engl J Med.* 2020. doi:10.1056/NEJMoa2021436
18. Ferguson ND, Cook DJ, Guyatt GH, et al. High-frequency oscillation in early acute respiratory distress syndrome. *N Engl J Med.* 2013;368(9):795-805.
19. Adhikari NKJ, Burns KEA, Friedrich JO, Granton JT, Cook DJ, Meade MO. Effect of nitric oxide on oxygenation and mortality in acute lung injury: systematic review and meta-analysis. *BMJ.* 2007;334(7597):779. doi:10.1136/bmj.39139.716794.55

Suggested Reading

Matthay MA, Zemans RL. The acute respiratory distress syndrome: pathogenesis and treatment. *Annu Rev Pathol.* 2011;6:147-163.

Thompson BT, Chambers RC, Liu KD. Acute respiratory distress syndrome. *N Engl J Med.* 2017;377:562-572.

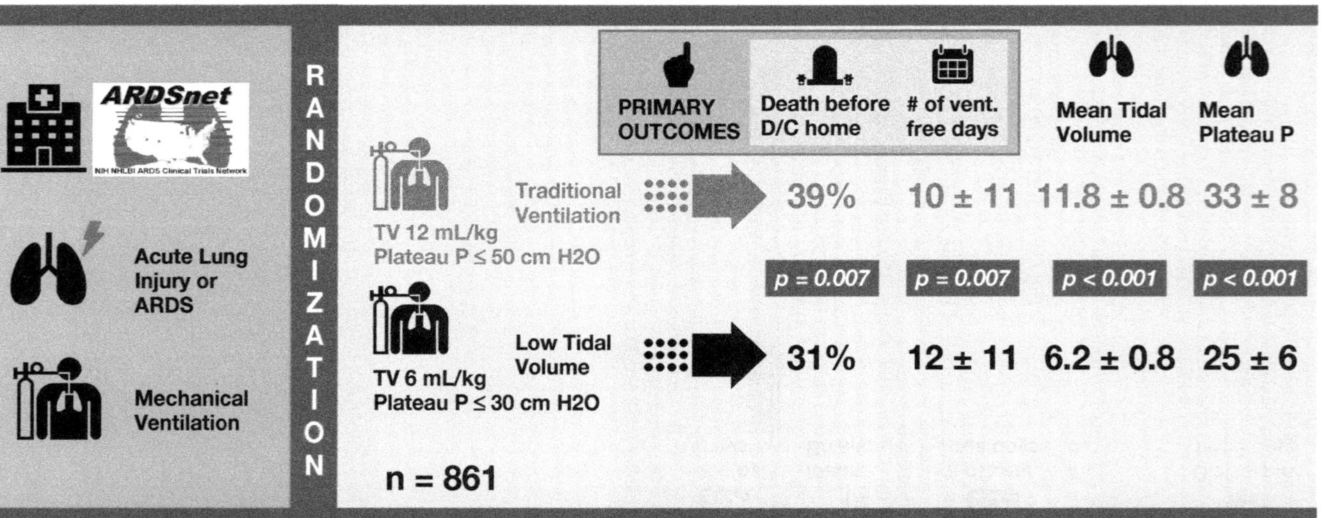

Conclusion: In patients with acute lung injury and the acute respiratory distress syndrome, mechanical ventilation with a lower tidal volume than is traditionally used results in decreased mortality and increases the number of days without ventilator use

Acute Respiratory Distress Syndrome Network, Brower RG, Matthay MA, Morris A, et al. ***Ventilation with lower tidal volumes as compared with traditional tidal volumes for acute lung injury and the acute respiratory distress syndrome.*** N Engl J Med 2000 May 4;342(18): 1301-8.

VISUAL ABSTRACT 4.1

Effects of two fluid-management strategies on lung function and extrapulmonary-organ perfusion

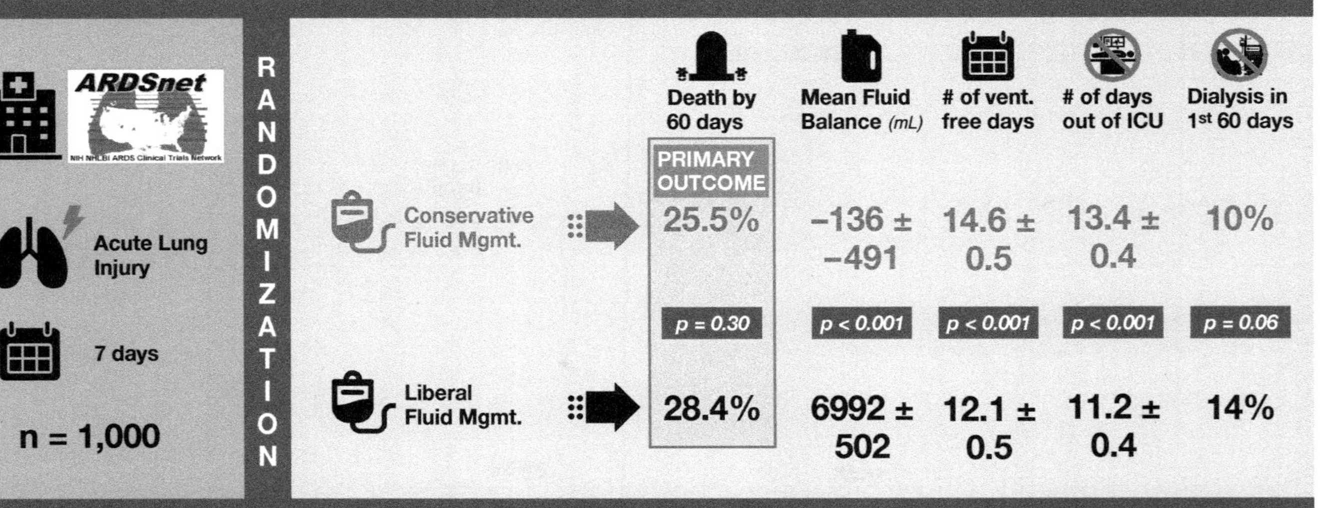

Conclusion: Although there was no significant difference in the primary outcome of 60-day mortality, the conservative strategy of fluid management improved lung function and shortened the duration of mechanical ventilation and intensive care without increasing nonpulmonary-organ failures.

NHLBI Acute Respiratory Distress Syndrome (ARDS) Clinical Trials Network, Widemann HP, Wheeler AP, Bernard GR, at al. ***Comparison of two fluid-management strategies in acute lung injury.*** N Engl J Med 2006 Jun 15;354(24):2564-75.

SECTION II

Acute Kidney Injury in the Intensive Care Unit

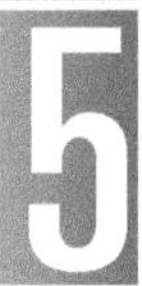

Definitions and Etiologies of Acute Kidney Injury

Armando Cennamo, Alfredo Petrosino, and Marlies Ostermann

BACKGROUND

Acute kidney injury (AKI) is a syndrome characterized by an abrupt decrease in kidney function over the course of hours to days. The clinical manifestations are related to the decline in kidney function (i.e., retention of waste products; disruption of fluid, electrolyte, and acid-base homeostasis; and reduced clearance of toxins, including drugs). Extrarenal complications, such as nonrenal organ dysfunction, fluid overload, and immunosuppression, may also occur.[1-3] AKI is often multifactorial, especially in the context of critical illness. Most patients with AKI recover kidney function, but survivors of AKI remain at risk for serious long-term complications, including the development of chronic kidney disease (CKD), cardiovascular morbidity, and premature mortality.[4] The epidemiology depends on the criteria used to define AKI, patient population, and clinical setting.

DIAGNOSTIC CRITERIA OF ACUTE KIDNEY INJURY

Traditionally, the diagnosis of AKI is based on a rise in serum creatinine or a fall in urine output. Serum creatinine and urine output are surrogate markers of glomerular filtration rate (GFR) and have the advantage of being widely available and easy to measure.

In the past two decades, the definition of AKI has evolved from the RIFLE (Risk, Injury, Failure, Loss, End-stage kidney disease) criteria to the Acute Kidney Injury Network (AKIN) classification in 2007 to the Kidney Disease Improving Global Outcomes (KDIGO) criteria in 2012[1,2,5] (**Table 5.1**). Accordingly, AKI is diagnosed if serum creatinine increases by 0.3 mg/dL (26.5 µmol/L) or more in 48 hours or rises to at least 1.5-fold from baseline within 7 days or urine output falls to less than 0.5 mL/kg/hr for 6 hours or more. AKI stages are defined by the maximum change of either serum creatinine or urine output. Outcome prediction is best when both criteria are used to define AKI.[6]

Several studies in various patient populations have confirmed an association between the different AKI classifications and short- and long-term outcomes.[7-9]

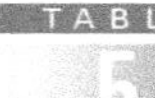

TABLE 5.1 Classifications of Acute Kidney Injury

	RIFLE (2004)[4]		AKIN (2007)[1]			KDIGO (2012)[11]		
AKI Class	**SCr or GFR**	**Urine Output**	**AKI Stage**	**SCr**	**Urine Output**	**AKI Stage**	**SCr**	**Urine Output**
Risk	SCr $\times$ 1.5 times or GFR decrease $<$ 25% from baseline (in a 7-d period)	$<$0.5 mL/kg/hr for $\geq$6 hr	1	Increase $\geq$0.3 mg/dL (26.5 μmol/L) in 48 hr or $\times$ 1.5-2 times baseline in a 7-d period	$<$0.5 mL/kg/hr for $\geq$6 hr	1	Increase $\geq$0.3 mg/dL (26.5 μmol/L) in 48 hr or $\times$1.5-2 times baseline in a 7-d period	$<$0.5 mL/kg/hr for $\geq$6 hr
Injury	SCr $\times$ 2 or GFR decrease $<$50%	$<$0.5 mL/kg/hr for $\geq$12 hr	2	2-3 times baseline	$<$0.5 mL/kg/hr for $\geq$12 hr	2	2.0-2.9$\times$ baseline	$<$0.5 mL/kg/hr for $\geq$12 hr
Failure	SCr $\times$ 3 or $\geq$4.0 mg/dL (with an acute increase of at least 0.5 mg/dL) or GFR decrease $>$75%	$<$0.3 mL/kg/hr for $\geq$24 hr or anuria for $\geq$12 hr	3	$>$3 times baseline or $\geq$4.0 mg/dL (with an acute increase of at least 0.5 mg/dL) or initiation of KRT	$<$0.3 mL/kg/hr for $\geq$24 hr or anuria for $\geq$12 hr	3	3.0$\times$ baseline or $\geq$4.0 mg/dL or initiation of KRT	$<$0.3 mL/kg/hr for $\geq$24 hr or anuria for $\geq$12 hr

AKI, acute kidney injury; AKIN, Acute Kidney Injury Network; GFR, glomerular filtration rate; KDIGO, Kidney Disease Improving Global Outcomes; RIFLE, Risk, Injury, Failure, Loss, End-stage; KRT, kidney replacement therapy; SCr, serum creatinine.

LIMITATIONS AND CHALLENGES OF CURRENT ACUTE KIDNEY INJURY CRITERIA

Serum creatinine and urine output are markers of excretory function only. They do not indicate early structural changes within the kidneys. In addition, they do not provide any information about any other roles of the kidney, that is, metabolic, endocrine, or immunologic functions, and are not renal specific.

CREATININE

Serum creatinine is a metabolite of creatine, a molecule that is synthesized from the amino acids glycine and arginine in the liver, pancreas, and kidneys and serves as an energy reservoir in skeletal muscle. Apart from kidney function, the key factors that affect serum creatinine concentration are as follows:

i. Change in liver function and muscle bulk
ii. Age
iii. Race
iv. Presence of sepsis (large and sustained falls in creatinine production may occur in sepsis)[10]
v. Acute changes in volume of distribution, including aggressive fluid administration and fluid overload (leading to dilution of creatinine concentration)
vi. Administration of drugs that compete with creatinine tubular secretion
vii. An acute rise in serum creatinine without associated changes in GFR (i.e., cimetidine and trimethoprim)
viii. Laboratory interference of creatinine measurement (e.g., by bilirubin)

The diagnosis and staging of AKI are based on a change from baseline, but premorbid creatinine results may not always be available. Three different strategies of defining baseline kidney function have been suggested:

i. Use of mean or median outpatient creatinine value within a year before AKI[11-13]
ii. Back-estimation of baseline creatinine with Modification of Diet in Renal Disease (MDRD) formula (assuming that baseline kidney function was normal)
iii. Use of first creatinine measurement during hospitalization. This approach carries the risk of underestimating or not recognizing AKI in patients with a creatinine rise prior to hospital admission.[10,14]

These different methods can inflate as well as reduce the true incidence of AKI. At present, there is no shared approach of determining baseline kidney function.

Finally, creatinine-based criteria for AKI do not take into account underlying kidney reserve. In patients with normal kidney function, a rise in serum creatinine by 0.3 mg/dL may be due to an important reduction in GFR. However, in patients with underlying CKD, absolute rises in serum creatinine represent variable changes in GFR, and a rise by 0.3 mg/dL may be within the acceptable daily variation and simply reflect an inconsequential change in GFR.

Therefore, any change in serum creatinine needs to be interpreted within the clinical context. It is possible that a patient's kidney function declines without an obvious change in serum creatinine concentration (for instance, patients with severe liver failure). Similarly, a patient's serum creatinine concentration may rise despite stable kidney function (for instance, in patients taking cimetidine).

LIMITATIONS OF URINE OUTPUT CRITERIA

A fall in urine output is complementary to a rise in creatinine criteria and independently associated with an increased risk of mortality. Furthermore, the number of episodes of oliguria and the duration of oliguria are also associated with increased mortality.[15] However, similar to creatinine, urine output is not specific to the kidneys. It may be appropriately reduced in the setting of fluid depletion or in conditions associated with antidiuretic hormone (ADH) release. Furthermore, it can be influenced by diuretics.[5,6,16-18] It also remains unclear whether ideal rather than actual body weight should be used for the diagnosis of oliguria.[14] Using actual body weight can result in an overdiagnosis of AKI in obese patients.

ACUTE KIDNEY DISEASE AND DISORDERS

The term "acute kidney disease and disorders" (AKD) describes conditions that are characterized by acute functional and structural changes of the kidneys that last up to 90 days and include AKI and other conditions that do not meet the CKD criteria[5,19] (**Table 5.2** and **Figure 5.1**). For instance, epidemiologic studies and

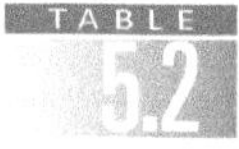

TABLE 5.2 AKD Criteria and Comparison With AKI and CKD Criteria

	Functional Criteria	Structural Criteria
AKI	• SCr ≥ 0.3 mg/dL (26.5 µmol/L) in 48 hr, or • ×1.5-2 times baseline in a 7-d period, or • UO < 0.5 mL/kg/hr ≥ 6 hr	No structural criteria
AKD	• AKI criteria • Decrease in GFR > 35% or increase in SCr > 25% for <3 mo • GFR < 60 mL/kg/1.73 m^2 for <3 mo	Kidney damage for <3 mo
CKD	• GFR < 60 mL/kg/1.73 m^2 for >3 mo	Kidney damage for >3 mo

AKD, acute kidney disease and disorders; AKI, acute kidney injury; CKD, chronic kidney disease; GFR, glomerular filtration rate; KRT, kidney replacement therapy; mo, months; SCr, serum creatinine; UO, urine output.

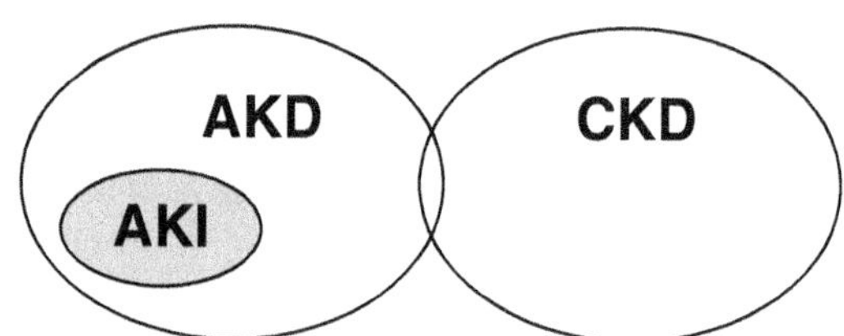

FIGURE 5.1: Acute kidney injury as a subset of acute kidney diseases and disorders. AKD, acute kidney diseases and disorders; AKI, acute kidney injury; CKD, chronic kidney disease.

From Kidney Disease: Improving Global Outcomes (KDIGO) Acute Kidney Injury Work Group. KDIGO clinical practice guideline for acute kidney injury. *Kidney Int Suppl.* 2012;2:1-138.

histologic case series have shown that some patients have a slow but persistent (creeping) rise in serum creatinine over days or weeks without fulfilling the consensus criteria for AKI.

In fact, AKD is more common than AKI and is associated with significant long-term complications.[20] Similar to AKI, AKD syndromes comprise multiple different etiologies and rarely occur in isolation but usually in the context of other acute illnesses and often on the background of profound chronic comorbidities.

RECOVERY FROM ACUTE KIDNEY INJURY

There is no consensus on the definition of recovery from AKI. It is commonly defined as return to previous baseline creatinine. However, serum creatinine at time of discharge may not be representative of kidney function because of potential muscle loss and may, therefore, lead to an overestimation of kidney function. It has been proposed that serum creatinine at 3 months after discharge from hospital may be more representative.[21]

ETIOLOGIES OF ACUTE KIDNEY INJURY

The exact etiologies of AKI vary depending on geography, setting, and patient population. There are multiple factors that contribute to the increased risk of AKI, including CKD, chronic heart failure, vascular disease, chronic respiratory failure, chronic liver disease, human immunodeficiency virus (HIV), and cancer. Frequently, AKI is multifactorial, involving several different pathophysiologic mechanisms occurring simultaneously or sequentially (**Table 5.3**).

TABLE 5.3 Pathophysiologic Mechanisms of AKI

Mechanism	Description	Common Clinical Conditions
Hemodynamic instability	Reduction of kidney perfusion	Hypovolemia Cardiogenic shock
Microcirculatory dysfunction	Heterogeneity of flow to the kidneys, causing areas of micro-ischemia Redistribution of intra-kidney blood flow Hypoxic damage and ROS generation	Sepsis Inflammatory diseases
Endothelial dysfunction	Loss of integrity in the structure of endothelial barrier, resulting in increased permeability Increased capillary permeability, leading to interstitial edema and impairment of oxygen Release of proinflammatory cytokines by endothelial cells Leukocyte transmigration into the interstitium	Sepsis Vasculitis

(*continued*)

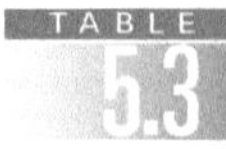

Pathophysiologic Mechanisms of AKI (*continued*)

Mechanism	Description	Common Clinical Conditions
Formation of microvascular thrombi	Inflammation-induced activation of procoagulant factors along with decrease in production of natural anticoagulants Amplification of coagulation cascade by damaged endothelial cells Complement activation	Sepsis HUS/TTP Preeclampsia
Inflammation	Activation of resident inflammatory cells Recruitment of neutrophils from the bloodstream	Sepsis
Tubular cell injury	Tubular injury as a result of microcirculatory dysfunction Direct exposure of tubules to inflammatory substances/toxins	Acute tubular injury
Renal venous congestion	Increased backward renal pressure owing to elevated central venous pressure, resulting in reduction of GFR	Congestive heart failure Cardiorenal syndrome
Obstruction	Blockade of urine flow at any stage along the urinary tract from tubule to the urethra Ureteric obstruction because of intrinsic or extrinsic causes Intratubular cast/crystal formation	Nephrolithiasis Retroperitoneal fibrosis Crystal nephropathy Myoglobinuria/ hemoglobinuria
Autoimmune processes	Circulating or in situ immune complexes that deposit in glomeruli	SLE Glomerulonephritis
Hypersensitivity immune reactions	Development of inflammatory infiltrates	Drugs Inflammatory diseases Malignancies
Intra-abdominal hypertension	Reduction of venous drainage, resulting in venous congestion	Abdominal compartment syndrome

AKI, acute kidney injury; GFR, glomerular filtration rate; HUS, hemolytic uremic syndrome; ROS, reactive oxygen species; SLE, systemic lupus erythematosus; TTP, thrombotic thrombocytopenic purpura.

COMMON ETIOLOGIES OF ACUTE KIDNEY INJURY

Hypoperfusion

Adequate kidney perfusion is essential for maintaining a normal GFR and a normal urinary output. The kidneys receive up to 25% of cardiac output. Conditions that compromise systemic perfusion, such as hypovolemia, cardiac failure, and systemic vasodilatation, can potentially lead to functional AKI. It is often reversible, but prolonged hypoperfusion can result in acute tubular ischemia.

Sepsis-Associated Acute Kidney Injury

Sepsis-associated AKI is common in critically ill patients, accounting for up to 50% of cases of AKI. It often occurs despite normal or increased global renal blood flow.[22,23] Various pathophysiologic processes play a role, including macrovascular and microvascular alterations, endothelial dysfunction and capillary leak, inflammation, tubular injury, and intrarenal shunting.[24] Non-sepsis-related factors such as nephrotoxic drugs or venous congestion may also contribute.

Cardiac Surgery–Associated Acute Kidney Injury

AKI is a common complication following cardiac surgery, affecting up to 45% of patients.[25] The pathogenesis is multifactorial. Hemodynamic perturbations such as exposure to cardiopulmonary bypass, cross-clamping of the aorta, and high doses of exogenous vasopressors contribute. Other mechanisms, including cholesterol embolization and neurohormonal activation, are also relevant, as is hemolysis and the release of free hemoglobin and free iron.[26-28]

Drug-Induced Acute Kidney Injury

Approximately 20% of the drugs prescribed in the intensive care unit (ICU) are nephrotoxic via multiple different mechanisms[29-31] (**Table 5.4**). The adverse impact of drug-induced AKI on patient outcomes can be severe, with hospital mortality rates reported between 18% and 50%.[32,33]

TABLE 5.4 Mechanisms Involved in Drug-Induced Nephrotoxicity

	Mechanism of Nephrotoxicity	Examples
Hemodynamic alteration	Vasoconstriction of afferent arteriole	NSAIDs Vasopressors Calcineurin inhibitors
	Vasodilatation of efferent arteriole	ACE-I ARBs
Vascular damage	Thrombotic microangiopathy	Chemotherapeutic agents ARBs IFN-α Ticlopidine mTOR inhibitors Calcineurin inhibitors
	Vasculitis of renal vessels	Penicillamine Allopurinol Anti–TNF-α Cocaine-containing levamisole Hydralazine
	Atheroembolism	Anticoagulants

(*continued*)

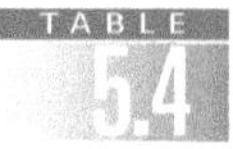

Mechanisms Involved in Drug-Induced Nephrotoxicity (*continued*)

	Mechanism of Nephrotoxicity	**Examples**
Glomerular damage	Minimal change disease	NSAIDs Lithium Quinolones Penicillins Interferon Pamidronate Gold
	Focal segmental glomerulosclerosis	Lithium Bisphosphonates Heroin IFNs
Tubular damage	ATI	Aminoglycosides Vancomycin Foscarnet Polymyxins Amphotericin Acyclovir, tenofovir, indinavir, atazanavir Cisplatin and other chemotherapeutic agents Hyperosmolar radiocontrast Warfarin Statin Fibrates
	Acute osmotic nephropathy	Starch Dextran Mannitol
Interstitial damage	Interstitial nephritis	Proton pump inhibitor NSAIDs β-Lactams Fluoroquinolones Vancomycin Allopurinol
Tubular obstruction	Formation of intratubular crystals	Methotrexate Acyclovir Indinavir Ciprofloxacin Sulfonamides

ACE-I, angiotensin-converting enzyme inhibitor; ARB, angiotensin receptor blocker; ATI, Acute Tubular Injury; IFN, interferon; mTOR, mammalian target of rapamycin; NSAID, nonsteroidal anti-inflammatory drug; TNF, tumor necrosis factor.

Rhabdomyolysis

Rhabdomyolysis is a condition characterized by muscle necrosis secondary to many causes, including crush injury, immobilization, hyperthermia, exercise, drugs, and toxins, resulting in the leakage of intracellular constituents (i.e., myoglobin, creatine kinase, aspartate aminotransferase [AST]) into the circulation (see Chapter 49).[34] AKI is one of the most common complications.[35] Different mechanisms are involved in the pathogenesis: (a) myoglobin concentrates in the urine, and its interaction with Tamm-Horsfall protein forms casts, which can precipitate, leading to tubular obstruction. (b) The heme group of myoglobin may induce the production of reactive oxygen species (ROS).

Contrast-Associated Acute Kidney Injury

Contrast agents can have a toxic effect on kidney via direct and indirect mechanisms, including early tubular epithelial injury and intrarenal vasoconstriction (see Chapter 44).[36,37] Contrast-associated AKI is often listed as a common cause of hospital-acquired AKI, but the incidence is relatively low and dependent on underlying kidney function and the degree of acute comorbidities.

Obstructive Acute Kidney Injury

Acute obstruction of the urinary flow can occur at any level from the intratubular lumen to the urethra. Typical intrinsic and extrinsic causes include kidney stones, drugs, retroperitoneal fibrosis, pelvic malignancies, and bladder outflow obstruction.

Primary Kidney Diseases

Primary kidney disease characterized by glomerular inflammation is a rare cause of AKI in the ICU setting, but it can manifest. Potential presentations are small-vessel vasculitis, hemolytic uremic syndrome or thrombotic thrombocytopenic purpura, lupus nephritis, anti–glomerular basement membrane (anti-GBM) disease, or a flare-up of an underlying glomerulonephritis. Overall, the prevalence is relatively low.

Hepatorenal Syndrome

Hepatorenal syndrome (HRS) is characterized by kidney injury in the context of liver disease (see Chapter 42). In this setting, AKI has been traditionally considered a purely functional form of AKI because of splanchnic vasodilatation and relative hypovolemia induced by cirrhosis.[38,39]

New evidence, however, suggests a role for systemic inflammation and structural kidney damage in the pathogenesis of HRS. Bacterial translocation would lead to the release of bacterial products and inflammatory cytokines, resulting in tubular and microvascular dysfunction, similar to sepsis. In addition, bilirubin may cause direct tubular damage, as documented by both kidney biopsy and damage biomarkers.[40]

CONCLUSIONS

AKI represents a multifactorial syndrome involving a variety of etiologies, pathophysiologic mechanisms, and clinical manifestations. The definition of AKI is currently based on functional criteria only but may evolve in the future, given the expanding information about the dynamic course, pathophysiology, and the discovery of new kidney biomakers.

References

1. Mehta RL, Kellum JA, Shah SV, et al. Acute kidney injury network: report of an initiative to improve outcomes in acute kidney injury. *Crit Care.* 2007;11(2):R31. doi:10.1186/cc5713
2. Singbartl JK, Joannidis M. Short-term effects of acute kidney injury. *Crit Care Clin.* 2015;31(4):751-762. doi:10.1016/j.ccc.2015.06.010
3. Ostermann M, Joannidis M. Acute kidney injury 2016: diagnosis and diagnostic workup. *Crit Care.* 2016;20(1):299. doi:10.1186/s13054-016-1478-z
4. Ronco C, Bellomo R, Kellum JA. Acute kidney injury. *Lancet.* 2019;394(10212):1949-1964.
5. Kidney Disease: Improving Global Outcomes (KDIGO) Acute Kidney Injury Work Group. KDIGO clinical practice guideline for acute kidney injury. *Kidney Int Suppl.* 2012;2:1-138.
6. Kellum JA, Sileanu FE, Murugan R, Lucko N, Shaw AD, Clermont G. Classifying AKI by urine output versus serum creatinine level. *J Am Soc Nephrol.* 2015;26(9):2231-2238. doi:10.1681/ASN.2014070724
7. Joannidis M, Metnitz B, Bauer P, et al. Acute kidney injury in critically ill patients classified by AKIN versus RIFLE using the SAPS 3 database. *Intensive Care Med.* 2009;35(10):1692-1702. doi:10.1007/s00134-009-1530-4
8. Fujii T, Uchino S, Takinami M, Bellomo R. Validation of the kidney disease improving global outcomes criteria for AKI and comparison of three criteria in hospitalized patients. *Clin J Am Soc Nephrol.* 2014;9(5):848-854. doi:10.2215/CJN.09530913
9. Chu R, Li C, Wang S, Zou W, Liu G, Yang L. Assessment of KDIGO definitions in patients with histopathologic evidence of acute renal disease. *Clin J Am Soc Nephrol.* 2014;9(7):1175-1182. doi:10.2215/CJN.06150613
10. Thomas ME, Blaine C, Dawnay A, et al. The definition of acute kidney injury and its use in practice. *Kidney Int.* 2015;87(1):62-73. doi:10.1038/ki.2014.328
11. Bellomo R, Ronco C, Kellum JA, Mehta RL, Palevsky P; Acute Dialysis Quality Initiative Workgroup. Acute renal failure—definition, outcome measures, animal models, fluid therapy and information technology needs: the Second International Consensus Conference of the Acute Dialysis Quality Initiative (ADQI) Group. *Crit Care.* 2004;8(4):R204-R212. doi:10.1186/cc2872
12. Kashani K, Al-Khafaji A, Ardiles T, et al. Discovery and validation of cell cycle arrest biomarkers in human acute kidney injury. *Crit Care.* 2013;17(1):R25. doi:10.1186/cc12503
13. Siew ED, Ikizler TA, Matheny ME, et al. Estimating baseline kidney function in hospitalized patients with impaired kidney function. *Clin J Am Soc Nephrol.* 2012;7(5):712-719. doi:10.2215/CJN.10821011
14. Fliser D, Laville M, Covic A, et al; The Ad-hoc Working Group of ERBP. A European Renal Best Practice (ERBP) position statement on the Kidney Disease Improving Global Outcomes (KDIGO) clinical practice guidelines on acute kidney injury: part 1: definitions, conservative management and contrast-induced nephropathy. *Nephrol Dial Transplant.* 2012;27(12):4263-4272. doi:10.1093/ndt/gfs375
15. Macedo E, Malhotra R, Bouchard J, Wynn SK, Mehta RL. Oliguria is an early predictor of higher mortality in critically ill patients. *Kidney Int.* 2011;80(7):760-767. doi:10.1038/ki.2011.150
16. Thurau K, Boylan JW. Acute renal success. The unexpected logic of oliguria in acute renal failure. *Am J Med.* 1976;61(3):308-315.
17. Solomon AW, Kirwan CJ, Alexander NDE, Nimako K, Jurukov A, Forth RJ; on behalf of the Prospective Analysis of Renal Compensation for Hypohydration in Exhausted Doctors (PARCHED) Investigators. Urine output on an intensive care unit: case-control study. *BMJ.* 2010;341:c6761. doi:10.1136/bmj.c6761
18. Lehner GF, Forni LG, Joannidis M. Oliguria and biomarkers of acute kidney injury: star struck lovers or strangers in the night? *Nephron.* 2016;134(3):183-190. doi:10.1159/000447979
19. Chawla LS, Bellomo R, Bihorac A, et al. Acute kidney disease and renal recovery: consensus report of the Acute Disease Quality Initiative (ADQI) 16 Workgroup. *Nat Rev Nephrol.* 2017;13(4):241-257. doi:10.1038/nrneph.2017.2
20. James MT, Levey AS, Tonelli M, et al. Incidence and prognosis of acute kidney diseases and disorders using an integrated approach to laboratory measurements in a universal health care system. *JAMA Network Open.* 2019;2(4):e191795. doi:10.1001/jamanetworkopen.2019.1795
21. Forni LG, Darmon M, Ostermann M, et al. Renal recovery after acute kidney injury. *Intensive Care Med.* 2017;43(6):855-866. doi:10.1007/s00134-017-4809-x
22. Bellomo R, Kellum JA, Ronco C, et al. Acute kidney injury in sepsis. *Intensive Care Med.* 2017;43(6):816-828. doi:10.1007/s00134-017-4755-7
23. Keir I, Kellum JA. Acute kidney injury in severe sepsis: pathophysiology, diagnosis, and treatment recommendations: acute kidney injury and sepsis. *J Vet Emerg Crit Care (San Antonio).* 2015;25(2):200-209. doi:10.1111/vec.12297
24. Poston JT, Koyner JL. Sepsis associated acute kidney injury. *BMJ.* 2019;364:k4891. doi:10.1136/bmj.k4891

25. Hobson CE, Yavas S, Segal MS, et al. Acute kidney injury is associated with increased long-term mortality after cardiothoracic surgery. *Circulation.* 2009;119(18):2444-2453. doi:10.1161/CIRCULATIONAHA.108.800011
26. Lau G, Wald R, Sladen R, Mazer D. Acute kidney injury in cardiac surgery and cardiac intensive care. *Semin Cardiothorac Vasc Anesth.* 2015;19(4):270-287. doi:10.1177/1089253215593177
27. Vives M, Wijeysundera D, Marczin N, Monedero P, Rao V. Cardiac surgery-associated acute kidney injury. *Interact Cardiovasc Thorac Surg.* 2014;18(5):637-645. doi:10.1093/icvts/ivu014
28. Nadim MK, Forni LG, Bihorac A, et al. Cardiac and vascular surgery-associated acute kidney injury: the 20th International Consensus Conference of the ADQI (Acute Disease Quality Initiative) Group. *J Am Heart Assoc.* 2018;7(11):e008834. doi:10.1161/JAHA.118.008834
29. Cavanaugh C, Perazella MA. Urine sediment examination in the diagnosis and management of kidney disease: core curriculum 2019. *Am J Kidney Dis.* 2019;73(2):258-272. doi:10.1053/j.ajkd.2018.07.012
30. Perazella MA, Luciano RL. Review of select causes of drug-induced AKI. *Expert Rev Clin Pharmacol.* 2015;8(4):367-371. doi:10.1586/17512433.2015.1045489
31. Kodner CM, Kudrimoti A. Diagnosis and management of acute interstitial nephritis. *Am Fam Phys.* 2003;67(12):2527-2534.
32. Kane-Gill SL, Goldstein SL. Drug-induced acute kidney injury: a focus on risk assessment for prevention. *Crit Care Clin.* 2015;31(4):675-684. doi:10.1016/j.ccc.2015.06.005
33. Wu TY, Jen MH, Bottle A, et al. Ten-year trends in hospital admissions for adverse drug reactions in England 1999-2009. *J R Soc Med.* 2010;103(6):239-250. doi:10.1258/jrsm.2010.100113
34. Huerta-Alardín AL, Varon J, Marik PE. Bench-to-bedside review: rhabdomyolysis—an overview for clinicians. *Crit Care.* 2005;9(2):158-169. doi:10.1186/cc2978
35. Bosch X, Poch E, Grau JM. Rhabdomyolysis and acute kidney injury. *N Engl J Med.* 2009;361(1):62-72. doi:10.1056/NEJMra0801327
36. Scharnweber T, Alhilali L, Fakhran S. Contrast-induced acute kidney injury. *Magn Res Imaging Clin N Am.* 2017;25(4):743-753. doi:10.1016/j.mric.2017.06.012
37. Mehran R, Dangas GD, Weisbord SD. Contrast-associated acute kidney injury. *N Engl J Med.* 2019;380(22):2146-2155. doi:10.1056/NEJMra1805256
38. Durand F, Graupera I, Ginès P, Olson JC, Nadim MK. Pathogenesis of hepatorenal syndrome: implications for therapy. *Am J Kidney Dis.* 2016;67(2):318-328. doi:10.1053/j.ajkd.2015.09.013
39. Mattos ÂZ, Schacher FC, Mattos AA. Vasoconstrictors in hepatorenal syndrome—a critical review. *Ann Hepatol.* 2019;18(2):287-290. doi:10.1016/j.aohep.2018.12.002
40. Angeli P, Garcia-Tsao G, Nadim MK, Parikh CR. News in pathophysiology, definition and classification of hepatorenal syndrome: a step beyond the International Club of Ascites (ICA) Consensus document. *J Hepatol.* 2019;71(4):811-822. doi:10.1016/j.jhep.2019.07.002

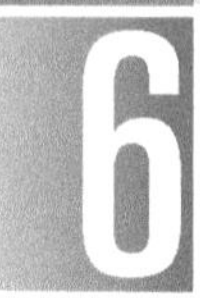

Epidemiology of Acute Kidney Injury

Neesh Pannu

Acute kidney injury (AKI) is a clinical syndrome characterized by retention of waste products; impaired acid-base, fluid, and electrolyte homeostasis; and altered drug metabolism resulting from a reduction in kidney function. The spectrum of AKI is broad, ranging from small changes in biomarkers to overt kidney failure requiring kidney replacement therapy (KRT). Over the past decade, AKI has been identified as a potent predictor of outcomes in critical illness. It is common in critically ill patients and, regardless of etiology, is associated with an increased risk of adverse short- and long-term outcomes, including prolonged mechanical ventilation, hospitalization, development or progression of chronic kidney disease (CKD), and death.[1] The epidemiology of AKI has changed with advances in the science of critical care medicine. This chapter reviews the incidence, risk factors, and outcomes associated with AKI in the intensive care unit (ICU).

DEFINITION OF ACUTE KIDNEY INJURY

Although current definitions of AKI, as discussed in detail in Chapter 5 (see **Table 6.1**)[2], are largely reliant on changes in serum creatinine (SCr) levels, in the ICU, oliguria and anuria are often the sole markers of kidney injury. Furthermore, these biomarkers are relatively insensitive to changes in kidney function and fail to discriminate true kidney injury from hemodynamic changes in kidney function, which are common in critical illness. These definitions inform, but do not replace clinical judgment in establishing an AKI diagnosis. Clinical context, evaluation of urine sediment, ultrasound of the kidneys, and ancillary supportive testing (biomarkers—see Chapter 16) can help distinguish kidney injury from other conditions as well as identify the etiology of AKI.

INCIDENCE OF ACUTE KIDNEY INJURY

The epidemiology of AKI has been described using administrative data and through prospective, retrospective, and cross-sectional cohort studies using a variety of definitions. A systematic review of 312 cohort studies, which included 49 million patients across the world, found that one in five adults and one in three children hospitalized with acute illness will develop some form of AKI.[3] The incidence of AKI in unselected hospitalized patients in the developed world is between 0.4% and 18% depending on the definition used and accounts for 1% to 4% of all hospital admissions.[4] Several large studies suggest that the incidence of AKI in hospitalized patients has increased by approximately 13% per year over the past three decades.[5,6] Notably, the incidence was identified by diagnostic codes,

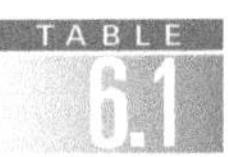

TABLE 6.1 Recent Consensus Definitions of Stage 1 AKI

Definitions	Serum Creatinine Criteria	Urine Output Criteria
RIFLE (2003)	Increase in SCr × 1.5 or decrease in GFR by 25% within 48 hr	Urine volume <0.5 mL/kg/hr for 6 hr
AKIN (2007)	Increase in SCr × 1.5 or by ≥0.3 mg/dL (≥26.5 μmol/L) within 48 hr	Urine volume <0.5 mL/kg/hr for 6 hr
KDIGO (2012)	Increase in SCr by ≥0.3 mg/dL (≥26.5 μmol/L) within 48 hr Increase in SCr to ≥1.5 times baseline, which is known or presumed to have occurred within the prior 7 d Severity staging after initial criteria met	Urine volume <0.5 mL/kg/hr for 6 hr

AKI, acute kidney injury; AKIN, Acute Kidney Injury Network; GFR, glomerular filtration rate; KDIGO, Kidney Disease Improving Global Outcomes; RIFLE, Risk, Injury, Failure, Loss, End-stage; SCr, serum creatinine.

which are highly specific for AKI (97%) but are relatively insensitive (35.4%),[7] and thus these studies likely underestimate the true incidence. Similar increases have been observed in the incidence of severe AKI (requiring KRT) between 2000 and 2009 and a doubling in the number of deaths attributable to AKI.[6] The increased incidence is likely related to increasing patient age and a higher burden of comorbidity, including a higher prevalence of CKD.

AKI is particularly common in the setting of critical illness; approximately 50% of ICU patients will develop at least stage 1 AKI. The incidence of AKI in a number of large cohort studies of critically ill patients is presented in **Table 6.2**.[8] Multicenter studies have reported the incidence of AKI to be between 10% and 67%, likely reflecting differences in case mix between patients, health care systems, and countries.[9] A large cross-sectional multinational study (Acute Kidney Injury-Epidemiologic Prospective Investigation or AKI-EPI) reported the incidence of AKI to be 57% using Kidney Disease Improving Global Outcomes (KDIGO) criteria.[9] Between 5% and 11% of critically ill patients will require KRT; this is dependent on AKI etiology, with less than 5% of patients undergoing cardiac surgery requiring KRT versus approximately 15% of patients with sepsis.[10]

CAUSES OF ACUTE KIDNEY INJURY

AKI in the ICU context is most commonly due to acute tubular necrosis (nephrotoxic and ischemic) and prerenal causes.[11] Other potentially modifiable causes discussed in detail elsewhere include radiocontrast nephropathy and nephrotoxicity from nonsteroidal anti-inflammatories, angiotensin-converting enzyme (ACE) inhibitors, angiotensin receptor blockers, diuretics, and chemotherapeutic agents.[4] Patients may present to the ICU with AKI (community-acquired) or develop AKI while in hospital. Hospital-acquired AKI is generally associated with a worse prognosis.[12]

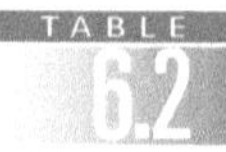

Incidence of AKI in Critically Ill Patients

Author	Year	# ICU	Patients (*n*)	Criteria	Creatinine Criteria/ Urine Output Criteria	Incidence (%)
Hoste et al[62]	2006	7	5,383	RIFLE	Both	67
Ostermann and Chang[63]	2007	22	41,972	RIFLE	Creatinine	35.8
Ostermann et al[64]	2008	22	22,303	AKIN	Creatinine	35.4
Bagshaw et al[65]	2008	57	120,123	RIFLE/AKIN	Both	37.1
Joannidis et al[66]	2009	303	16,784	RIFLE/AKIN	Both	35.5
Mandelbaum et al[67]	2011	7	14,524	AKIN	Both	57
Nisula et al[68]	2013	17	2,091	AKIN	Both	39.3
Liborio et al[69]	2014	1	18,410	KDIGO	Both	55.6
Kellum[70]	2014	8	32,045	KDIGO	Both	74.5
Hoste et al[9]	2015	97	1,802	KDIGO	Both	57.3
Bouchard et al[71]	2015	9	6,637	AKIN	Creatinine	19.2

AKI, acute kidney injury; AKIN, Acute Kidney Injury Network; ICU, intensive care unit; KDIGO, Kidney Disease Improving Global Outcomes; RIFLE, Risk, Injury, Failure, Loss, End-stage.

Taken from Bellomo R, Ronco C, Mehta RL, et al. Acute kidney injury in the ICU: from injury to recovery: reports from the 5th Paris International Conference. *Ann Intensive Care*. 2017;7(1):49.

RISK FACTORS FOR ACUTE KIDNEY INJURY

Risk factors for AKI have been determined in a variety of clinical settings, including cardiac surgery, contrast-induced AKI, and critically ill populations. Nonmodifiable and illness-specific risk factors common to all populations are summarized in **Table 6.3** and discussed elsewhere.

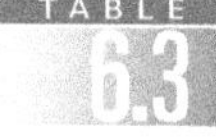

AKI Risk Factors

Patient-Specific Risk Factors for AKI	Illness-Specific Risk Factors for AKI
• Age • Gender (male) • Chronic kidney disease • Proteinuria • Diabetes • Congestive heart failure • Chronic liver disease	• Drug exposures (nephrotoxins) • Septic/cardiogenic/hypovolemic shock • Multiorgan dysfunction • Surgery

AKI, acute kidney injury.

Age

Multiple studies have shown that AKI is more common in elderly individuals, and many have shown an independent association between AKI and older age.[13] In a community-based prospective study, the very elderly (aged 80-89) were 55 times more likely to develop AKI than adults younger than 50 years.[14] Possible explanations for this association include (1) structural and functional changes associated with age that lead to diminished nephron reserve and reduced capacity of the kidneys for autoregulation; (2) accumulation of comorbidity, which increases susceptibility to AKI (vascular disease, diabetes, hypertension, CKD); and (3) increased exposure among the elderly to medications and procedures that predispose to AKI.[13]

Reduced Estimated Glomerular Filtration Rate

Preexisting reduction in estimated glomerular filtration rate (eGFR) is a potent risk factor for AKI following exposure to radiocontrast,[15] major surgery, and medical illness,[16] although the pathophysiology underlying this association is poorly understood. Hsu and colleagues found that the odds of developing dialysis requiring AKI were increased at lower baseline eGFR: the excess risk as compared to normal eGFR was approximately 2-fold in patients with baseline eGFR 45 to 60 mL/min/1.73 m^2 but more than 40-fold for patients with baseline eGFR <15 mL/min/1.73 m^2.[17] These associations were confirmed in several recent systematic reviews, demonstrating strong independent associations between the risk of AKI and lower baseline eGFR.[18-20] Although these analyses support a causal association between CKD and hospitalization-associated AKI, little is known about how this association may be modified by the presence of one or more comorbidities such as heart failure or whether all causes of CKD confer similar risk of AKI.

Proteinuria

Proteinuria is also strongly associated with AKI risk. A case-control study of over 600,000 patients identified proteinuria as an independent predictor for AKI,[17] which was replicated in multiple settings, including postcardiac surgery in Taiwan and a general population studies from the United States and Canada.[21-23]

ASSOCIATIONS BETWEEN ACUTE KIDNEY INJURY AND ADVERSE OUTCOMES

AKI is associated with high costs and adverse clinical outcomes, including excess mortality, increased length of hospital stay, development and/or progression of CKD, requirement for chronic dialysis in survivors, and a greater requirement for posthospitalization care.[24,25]

Mortality

Multiple observational studies demonstrate increased mortality among patients who experience AKI during hospitalization; nearly 50% of critically ill patients with severe AKI will die during hospital admission.[26] A meta-analysis of eight studies of hospitalized patients (most of whom were critically ill or had heart failure) confirms a graded relationship between increasing severity of AKI and short-term mortality.[27] Most importantly, it confirms that even mild forms of AKI are clinically relevant; an increase in SCr of 26 µmol/L (0.3 mg/dL) was associated with a short-term relative risk for death of 2.3 (95% confidence interval [CI], 1.8-3.0). The association between AKI and mortality is likely influenced by several factors, including the presence of underlying CKD, duration and severity of AKI, and degree of recovery of kidney function.[28] A recent analysis of postoperative AKI comparing kidney and survival outcomes in those subjects (3.7%) with and without preexisting CKD (defined as eGFR < 45 mL/min/1.73 m^2) found a lower attributable mortality due to AKI (hazard ratio [HR] 1.26 [95% CI, 1.09-1.78]) when subjects with prior CKD but no AKI were used as reference.[29] However, not all changes in serum creatinine have been linked to increased mortality.[30] Setting and timing of AKI diagnosis also have important prognostic significance; weekend admission for AKI has been consistently associated with increased mortality[31] as well as hospital size.

Although the incidence of AKI continues to climb, there has been a corresponding improvement in survival. A recent analysis reported a 19% decrease in mortality between 2000 and 2009 in subjects requiring acute dialysis.[6] Whether this represents a move toward earlier and more aggressive use of dialysis (rather than a true improvement in survival) requires further investigation.

Chronic Kidney Disease

An increasing number of recent studies have linked AKI survivorship to the development of CKD or end-stage kidney disease (ESKD). A meta-analysis of 13 cohort studies reported that the HRs for patients with CKD and ESKD were 8.8 (95% CI, 3.1-25.5) and 3.1 (95% CI, 1.9-5.0), respectively, compared to subjects without AKI.[32] Depending on AKI severity and the presence of CKD, between 2% and 30% of AKI survivors will progress to ESKD within 2 to 5 years of hospital discharge.[33-36] Baseline kidney function, AKI severity, and nonrecovery of kidney function are potent predictors of de novo CKD and CKD progression.[37,38] A recently published population-based risk prediction score of CKD progression after AKI in hospitalized patients additionally identified proteinuria, age, and sex as risk factors.[39] The prospective cohort study has also identified pre-AKI proteinuria as a potent predictor of CKD progression.[40] However, the risk of CKD is evident even in transient stage 1 AKI and in those with normal baseline kidney function.[41] Recurrent episodes of AKI further increase the risk of progressive CKD: each additional AKI event after the first episode appears to double the risk of progression to stage 4 CKD.[42]

Cardiovascular Risk

AKI has long been associated with an increased risk of cardiovascular events in patients with underlying or suspect cardiovascular disease.[43,44] Several large retrospective cohort studies of patients undergoing both vascular and nonvascular major surgeries have recently confirmed an association between postoperative AKI and cardiovascular mortality.[45,46] Further, a recent systematic review by Odutayo and colleagues analyzed data from 25 cohort studies of patients (n = 254,408) with and without AKI and reported that AKI is associated with an 86% increased risk of cardiovascular mortality, a 38% increased risk of major adverse cardiovascular event (MACE), and a 40% increased risk of heart failure.[47] The association between AKI and both incident heart failure and increased risk of hospitalization for heart failure is particularly striking and is perhaps the most plausible in the context of decreased water and solute clearance associated with AKI and the post-AKI period.[48,49] Consistent with these observations, the use of statins and renin-angiotensin blockade in AKI survivors has been associated with reduced mortality.[50-52]

The development of AKI in critical illness identifies a cohort of patients at high risk for adverse outcomes. However, US data suggest that only 5% of AKI survivors saw a nephrologist after hospital discharge,[36] and AKI survivors with CKD and proteinuria often do not receive treatment with ACE inhibitors/angiotensin receptor blockers after hospital discharge.[53] Given this, longitudinal follow-up of AKI survivors is recommended.

Quality of Life

There are conflicting data regarding the impact of AKI on the quality of life in ICU survivors. Whereas early studies suggested that these patients had poor long-term quality of life relative to non-AKI survivors,[54,55] recent studies suggest that critically ill patients have low quality of life prior to ICU admission and that AKI does not significantly change this.[56,57]

Costs

Several studies have evaluated the costs associated with the development of AKI in hospitalized patients. A single-center study of AKI in hospitalized patients demonstrated a direct relationship between the severity of AKI and associated hospital length of stay and hospital costs.[58] AKI defined as a 0.3 mg/dL (24 μmol/L) increase in SCr was associated with an incremental total hospitalization cost of $4,886; a doubling of SCr was associated with an incremental cost of $9,000. Studies of specific populations of hospitalized patients support these findings; a recent study of the cost of AKI postcardiac surgery suggests that the average difference in postoperative costs ranges between $9,000 and 14,000 depending on AKI severity. Postoperative AKI in noncardiac surgery is similarly associated with an $11,308 increase in the median cost.[59] However, none of these studies accounted for the impact of CKD on AKI and attendant costs, which is likely to be significant.[60] A recent Canadian study of hospitalized patients with AKI identified incremental costs associated with increasing KDIGO AKI stage, with a 3-fold increase in hospital costs and doubling of hospital length of stay in those requiring dialysis. Additional costs, increasing by AKI stage, were also seen over a 1-year period after hospital admission.[61]

AKI is a common and serious complication of critical illness that is associated with high hospital mortality and poor short- and long-term outcomes in AKI survivors. Increasing age and the presence of CKD are important risk factors for AKI. As critical care improves and patient complexity increases, the incidence of AKI and AKI survivorship continues to increase. Longitudinal care for AKI survivors is warranted.

References

1. Srisawat N, Kellum JA. Acute kidney injury: definition, epidemiology, and outcome. *Curr Opin Crit Care.* 2011;17(6):548-555.
2. Thomas ME, Blaine C, Dawnay A, et al. The definition of acute kidney injury and its use in practice. *Kidney Int.* 2015;87(1):62-73.
3. Susantitaphong P, Cruz DN, Cerda J, et al. World Incidence of AKI: a meta-analysis. *Clin J Am Soc Nephrol.* 2013;8(9):1482-1493.
4. Lameire N, Van Biesen W, Vanholder R. The changing epidemiology of acute renal failure. *Nat Clin Pract Nephrol.* 2006;2(7):364-377.
5. Waikar SS, Curhan GC, Wald R, McCarthy EP, Chertow GM. Declining mortality in patients with acute renal failure, 1988 to 2002. *J Am Soc Nephrol.* 2006;17(4):1143-1150.
6. Hsu RK, McCulloch CE, Dudley RA, Lo LJ, Hsu C-Y. Temporal changes in incidence of dialysis-requiring AKI. *J Am Soc Nephrol.* 2013;24(1):37-42.
7. Waikar SS, Wald R, Chertow GM, et al. Validity of International Classification of Diseases, Ninth Revision, clinical modification codes for acute renal failure. *J Am Soc Nephrol.* 2006;17(6):1688-1694.

8. Bellomo R, Ronco C, Mehta RL, et al. Acute kidney injury in the ICU: from injury to recovery: reports from the 5th Paris International Conference. *Ann Intensive Care.* 2017;7(1):49.
9. Hoste EA, Bagshaw SM, Bellomo R, et al. Epidemiology of acute kidney injury in critically ill patients: the multinational AKI-EPI study. *Intensive Care Med.* 2015;41(8):1411-1423.
10. Hoste EAJ, Kellum JA, Selby NM, et al. Global epidemiology and outcomes of acute kidney injury. *Nat Rev Nephrol.* 2018;14(10):607-625.
11. Nash K, Hafeez A, Hou S. Hospital-acquired renal insufficiency. *Am J Kidney Dis.* 2002;39(5):930-936.
12. Wonnacott A, Meran S, Amphlett B, Talabani B, Phillips S. Epidemiology and outcomes in community-acquired versus hospital-acquired AKI. *Clin J Am Soc Nephrol.* 2014;9(6):1007-1014.
13. Coca SG. Acute kidney injury in elderly persons. *Am J Kidney Dis.* 2010;56(1):122-131.
14. Feest TG, Round A, Hamad S. Incidence of severe acute renal failure in adults: results of a community based study. *BMJ.* 1993;306(6876):481-483.
15. Pannu N, Wiebe N, Tonelli M. Prophylaxis strategies for contrast-induced nephropathy 1. *JAMA.* 2006;295(23):2765-2779.
16. Mehta RL, Pascual MT, Gruta CG, et al. Refining predictive models in critically ill patients with acute renal failure. *J Am Soc Nephrol.* 2002;13(5):1350-1357.
17. Hsu CY, Ordonez JD, Chertow GM, Fan D, McCulloch CE, Go AS. The risk of acute renal failure in patients with chronic kidney disease. *Kidney Int.* 2008;74(1):101-107.
18. James MT, Grams ME, Woodward M, et al. A meta-analysis of the association of estimated GFR, albuminuria, diabetes mellitus, and hypertension with acute kidney injury. *Am J Kidney Dis.* 2015;66(4):602-612.
19. Grams ME, Sang Y, Ballew SH, et al. A meta-analysis of the association of estimated GFR, albuminuria, age, race, and sex with acute kidney injury. *Am J Kidney Dis.* 2015;66(4):591-601.
20. Gansevoort RT, Matsushita K, van der Velde M, et al. Lower estimated GFR and higher albuminuria are associated with adverse kidney outcomes. A collaborative meta-analysis of general and high-risk population cohorts. *Kidney Int.* 2011;80(1):93-104.
21. Huang TM, Wu VC, Young GH, et al. Preoperative proteinuria predicts adverse renal outcomes after coronary artery bypass grafting. *J Am Soc Nephrol.* 2011;22(1):156-163.
22. Grams ME, Astor BC, Bash LD, Matsushita K, Wang Y, Coresh J. Albuminuria and estimated glomerular filtration rate independently associate with acute kidney injury. *J Am Soc Nephrol.* 2010;21(10):1757-1764.
23. James MT, Hemmelgarn BR, Wiebe N, et al. Glomerular filtration rate, proteinuria, and the incidence and consequences of acute kidney injury: a cohort study. *Lancet.* 2010; 376(9758):2096-2103.
24. Liangos O, Wald R, O'Bell JW, Price L, Pereira BJ, Jaber BL. Epidemiology and outcomes of acute renal failure in hospitalized patients: a national survey. *Clin J Am Soc Nephrol.* 2006;1(1):43-51.
25. Xue JL, Daniels F, Star RA, et al. Incidence and mortality of acute renal failure in Medicare beneficiaries, 1992 to 2001. *J Am Soc Nephrol.* 2006;17(4):1135-1142.
26. Liano F, Pascual J; Madrid Acute Renal Failure Study Group. Epidemiology of acute renal failure: a prospective, multicenter, community-based study. *Kidney Int.* 1996;50(3):811-818.
27. Coca SG, Peixoto AJ, Garg AX, Krumholz HM, Parikh CR. The prognostic importance of a small acute decrement in kidney function in hospitalized patients: a systematic review and meta-analysis. *Am J Kidney Dis.* 2007;50(5):712-720.
28. Pannu N, James M, Hemmelgarn BR, et al. Modification of outcomes after acute kidney injury by the presence of CKD. *Am J Kidney Dis.* 2011;58(2):206-213.
29. Wu VC, Huang TM, Lai CF, et al. Acute-on-chronic kidney injury at hospital discharge is associated with long-term dialysis and mortality. *Kidney Int.* 2011;80(11):1222-1230.
30. Coca SG, Zabetian A, Ferket BS, et al. Evaluation of short-term changes in serum creatinine level as a meaningful end point in randomized clinical trials. *J Am Soc Nephrol.* 2016;27(8):2529-2542.
31. James MT, Wald R, Bell CM, et al. Weekend hospital admission, acute kidney injury, and mortality. *J Am Soc Nephrol.* 2010;21(5):845-851.
32. Coca SG, Singanamala S, Parikh CR. Chronic kidney disease after acute kidney injury: a systematic review and meta-analysis. *Kidney Int.* 2012;81(5):442-448.
33. Pannu N, James M, Hemmelgarn B, Klarenbach S; Alberta Kidney Disease Network. Association between AKI, recovery of renal function, and long-term outcomes after hospital discharge. *Clin J Am Soc Nephrol.* 2013;8(2):194-202.
34. Ishani A, Xue JL, Himmelfarb J, et al. Acute kidney injury increases risk of ESRD among elderly. *J Am Soc Nephrol.* 2009;20(1):223-228.
35. Mehta RL, Kellum JA, Shah SV, et al. Acute kidney injury network: report of an initiative to improve outcomes in acute kidney injury. *Crit Care.* 2007;11(2):R31.
36. United States Renal Data System. USRDS Annual Data Report. 2015. https://www.usrds.org/media/1541/vol1_05_aki_15.pdf

37. James MT, Ghali WA, Tonelli M, et al. Acute kidney injury following coronary angiography is associated with a long-term decline in kidney function. *Kidney Int.* 2010;78(8):803-809.
38. Lo LJ, Go AS, Chertow GM, et al. Dialysis-requiring acute renal failure increases the risk of progressive chronic kidney disease. *Kidney Int.* 2009;76(8):893-899.
39. James MT, Pannu N, Hemmelgarn BR, et al. Derivation and external validation of prediction models for advanced chronic kidney disease following acute kidney injury. *JAMA.* 2017;318(18):1787-1797.
40. Lee BJ, Go AS, Parikh R, et al. Pre-admission proteinuria impacts risk of non-recovery after dialysis-requiring acute kidney injury. *Kidney Int.* 2018;93(4):968-976.
41. Bucaloiu ID, Kirchner HL, Norfolk ER, Hartle JE II, Perkins RM. Increased risk of death and de novo chronic kidney disease following reversible acute kidney injury. *Kidney Int.* 2012;81(5):477-485.
42. Holmes J, Geen J, Williams JD, Phillips AO. Recurrent acute kidney injury: predictors and impact in a large population-based cohort. *Nephrol Dial Transplant.* 2019;35(8):1361-1369.
43. Chawla LS, Amdur RL, Shaw AD, Faselis C, Palant CE, Kimmel PL. Association between AKI and long-term renal and cardiovascular outcomes in United States veterans. *Clin J Am Soc Nephrol.* 2014;9(3):448.
44. Chawla LS, Eggers PW, Star RA, Kimmel PL. Acute kidney injury and chronic kidney disease as interconnected syndromes. *N Engl J Med.* 2014;371(1):58-66.
45. Ozrazgat-Baslanti T, Thottakkara P, Huber M, et al. Acute and chronic kidney disease and cardiovascular mortality after major surgery. *Ann Surg.* 2016;264(6):987-996.
46. Huber M, Ozrazgat-Baslanti T, Thottakkara P, Scali S, Bihorac A, Hobson C. Cardiovascular-specific mortality and kidney disease in patients undergoing vascular surgery. *JAMA Surg.* 2016;151(5):441-450.
47. Odutayo A, Wong CX, Farkouh M, et al. AKI and long-term risk for cardiovascular events and mortality. *J Am Soc Nephrol.* 2016;28(1):377-387.
48. Bansal N, Matheny ME, Greevy RA Jr, et al. Acute kidney injury and risk of incident heart failure among US veterans. *Am J Kidney Dis.* 2018;71(2):236-245.
49. Go AS, Hsu CY, Yang J, et al. Acute kidney injury and risk of heart failure and atherosclerotic events. *Clin J Am Soc Nephrol.* 2018;13(6):833-841.
50. Brar S, Ye F, James MT, et al. Association of angiotensin-converting enzyme inhibitor or angiotensin receptor blocker use with outcomes after acute kidney injury. *JAMA Intern Med.* 2018;178(12):1681-1690.
51. Brar S, Ye F, James M, Hemmelgarn B, Klarenbach S, Pannu N. Statin use and survival after acute kidney injury. *Kidney Int Rep.* 2016;1(4):279-287.
52. Gayat E, Hollinger A, Cariou A, et al. Impact of angiotensin-converting enzyme inhibitors or receptor blockers on post-ICU discharge outcome in patients with acute kidney injury. *Intensive Care Med.* 2018;44(5):598-605.
53. Leung KC, Pannu N, Tan Z, et al. Contrast-associated AKI and use of cardiovascular medications after acute coronary syndrome. *Clin J Am Soc Nephrol.* 2014;9(11):1840-1848.
54. Ahlstrom A, Tallgren M, Peltonen S, Räsänen P, Pettilä V. Survival and quality of life of patients requiring acute renal replacement therapy. *Intensive Care Med.* 2005;31(9):1222-1228.
55. Noble JS, Simpson K, Allison ME. Long-term quality of life and hospital mortality in patients treated with intermittent or continuous hemodialysis for acute renal and respiratory failure. *Ren Fail.* 2006;28(4):323-330.
56. Hofhuis JG, van Stel HF, Schrijvers AJ, Rommes JH, Spronk PE. The effect of acute kidney injury on long-term health-related quality of life: a prospective follow-up study. *Crit Care.* 2013;17(1):R17.
57. Nisula S, Vaara ST, Kaukonen KM, et al. Six-month survival and quality of life of intensive care patients with acute kidney injury. *Crit Care.* 2013;17(5):R250.
58. Chertow GM, Burdick E, Honour M, Bonventre JV, Bates DW. Acute kidney injury, mortality, length of stay, and costs in hospitalized patients. *J Am Soc Nephrol.* 2005;16(11):3365-3370.
59. Dimick JB, Pronovost PJ, Cowan JA, Lipsett PA. Complications and costs after high-risk surgery: where should we focus quality improvement initiatives? *J Am Coll Surg.* 2003;196(5):671-678.
60. Smith DH, Gullion CM, Nichols G, Keith DS, Brown JB. Cost of medical care for chronic kidney disease and comorbidity among enrollees in a large HMO population. *J Am Soc Nephrol.* 2004;15(5):1300-1306.
61. Collister D, Pannu N, Ye F, et al. Health care costs associated with AKI. *Clin J Am Soc Nephrol.* 2017;12(11):1733-1743.
62. Hoste EA, Clermont G, Kersten A, et al. RIFLE criteria for acute kidney injury are associated with hospital mortality in critically ill patients: a cohort analysis 8. *Crit Care.* 2006;10(3):R73.
63. Ostermann M, Chang RW. Acute kidney injury in the intensive care unit according to RIFLE. *Crit Care Med.* 2007;35(8):1837-1843; quiz 52.

64. Ostermann M, Chang R; Riyadh ICU Program Users Group. Correlation between the AKI classification and outcome. *Crit Care.* 2008;12(6):R144.
65. Bagshaw SM, George C, Bellomo R; ANZICS Database Management Committee. Early acute kidney injury and sepsis: a multicentre evaluation. *Crit Care.* 2008;12(2):R47.
66. Joannidis M, Metnitz B, Bauer P, et al. Acute kidney injury in critically ill patients classified by AKIN versus RIFLE using the SAPS 3 database. *Intensive Care Med.* 2009;35(10):1692-1702.
67. Mandelbaum T, Scott DJ, Lee J, et al. Outcome of critically ill patients with acute kidney injury using the Acute Kidney Injury Network criteria. *Crit Care Med.* 2011;39(12):2659-2664.
68. Nisula S, Kaukonen KM, Vaara ST, et al. Incidence, risk factors and 90-day mortality of patients with acute kidney injury in Finnish intensive care units: the FINNAKI study. *Intensive Care Med.* 2013;39(3):420-428.
69. Liborio AB, Branco KM, Torres de Melo Bezerra C. Acute kidney injury in neonates: from urine output to new biomarkers. *Biomed Res Int.* 2014;2014:601568.
70. Kellum JA, Sileanu FA, Murugan R, et al. Classifying AKI by urine output versus serum creatinine level. *J Am Soc Nephrol.* 2015;26(9):2231-2238.
71. Bouchard J, Acharya A, Cerda J, et al. A prospective international multicenter study of AKI in the intensive care unit. *Clin J Am Soc Nephrol.* 2015;10(8):1324-1331.

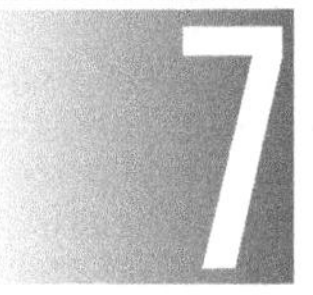

Acute Kidney Injury and Non–Acute Kidney Injury Risk Scores in the Intensive Care Unit

Luke E. Hodgson and Lui G. Forni

INTRODUCTION TO PREDICTION MODELS

Prognostic prediction research investigates the ability of combinations of variables to predict a future outcome in the form of a prediction model.[1] Such models are intended to enhance decision making by providing objective estimates of probability.[2]

MODEL PERFORMANCE

Following data collection, model performance is assessed initially in the original derivation data set. Quantifying the effect of using a model on patient and physician behaviors and outcomes is termed *impact analysis*. The TRIPOD guidelines through the equator network (www.equator-network.org) provide a useful reference to judge the quality of reporting of such model studies. The overall performance of a model may be quantified using various pseudo-R^2 measures; the Brier score is commonly employed.[3] *Discrimination* refers to the ability of a model to distinguish individuals with and without the outcome of interest.[3] It can be quantified by the concordance (c) statistic, which is identical to the area under the receiver operating characteristic curve (AUROC) for logistic models.[4] The c statistic can be interpreted as the chance a patient with the outcome of interest is assigned a higher probability of the outcome by the model than a randomly chosen patient without the outcome: a value of 0.5 indicates the model does not perform better than chance, whereas a value of 1 indicates perfect discrimination.[4] *Calibration* refers to agreement between outcome probability predicted and the observed outcome frequency.[5] It can be investigated graphically by plotting observed outcome frequencies against the predicted outcome probabilities for subjects grouped by quantiles of predicted probabilities.[6] A calibration plot on the 45 degree line denotes perfect agreement. Calibration can be formally assessed by modeling a regression line with intercept (α) and slope (β),[3] which can be estimated in a logistic regression model with the observed outcome as the dependent variable and the linear prediction as the only independent variable. The intercept is 0 and the calibration slope is 1 for well-calibrated models. Although commonly used, the Hosmer-Lemeshow goodness-of-fit test may lack statistical power to reject poor calibration.[5]

INTENSIVE CARE UNIT PREDICTION MODELS

Acute Physiology and Chronic Health Evaluation

Since the 1980s, many complex scoring systems have been described to predict intensive care unit (ICU) mortality. The most well-known is the Acute Physiology and Chronic Health Evaluation (APACHE) score.[7] The model was revised and simplified (from 34 to 12 physiologic variables, age, and chronic health status) to create APACHE II, the most widely used severity of illness score.[8] The worst value recorded during the first 24 hours of admission to the ICU is used for each variable, and the principal diagnosis leading to ICU admission is added as a category weight so that predicted mortality is computed based on the APACHE II score and principal diagnosis. APACHE III was developed in 1991,[9] and most recently, APACHE IV was developed with the same physiologic variables and weights but with different predictor variables.[10] Unfortunately, such scores are time consuming—for example, APACHE IV, with a maximum score of 286, is said to take 37 minutes to calculate. A score of 56 corresponds to a mortality risk estimate of 10%, and a score of 132 predicts a mortality of 90%. Commonly employed ICU prediction models are presented in **Table 7.1**.

Simplified Acute Physiology Score

Simplified Acute Physiology Score (SAPS), developed and validated in France in 1984, used 13 weighted physiologic variables measured in the first 24 hours of ICU admission.[11] This was updated to develop SAPS II, including 12 physiologic variables, age, type of admission, and 3 variables related to underlying disease.[12] SAPS III was created in 2005 and includes 20 variables divided into three subscores related to patient characteristics: prior to admission, admission reason, and the degree of physiologic derangement less than 1 hour pre- or post-ICU admission.[13] The score ranges from 0 to 217, with a score of 40 corresponding to a mortality risk estimate of less than 10% and a score of 120 predicting a mortality of more than 90%. SAPS III includes customized equations for prediction of hospital mortality in different geographical regions and has also been used to examine variability in resource use between ICUs.[14]

Mortality Probability Model

The first Mortality Probability Model (MPM) consisted of an admission model using seven admission variables and a 24-hour model using seven variables.[15] MPM II appeared in 1993 using logistic regression from a database of 12,610 ICU patients from 12 countries.[16] Unlike APACHE or SAPS, in MPM II, each variable is designated present or absent (except age). A further iteration MPM0-III has been derived and includes 16 variables, including 3 physiologic parameters, obtained within one hour of ICU admission.[17]

Intensive Care National Audit and Research Centre Score

In the United Kingdom, the Intensive Care National Audit and Research Centre (ICNARC) score was derived using a UK-wide database and calibrated for adult critically ill patients admitted to ICUs in the United Kingdom.[18] This score, ranging from 0 to 100, uses elements of the APACHE, SAPS, and MPM systems and performed better (c statistic 0.87 on development and validation samples) than SAPS II, APACHE II and APACHE III, and MPM II.[18] A score of 10 corresponded to a mortality risk estimate of less than 10%, and a score of 50 carried a mortality

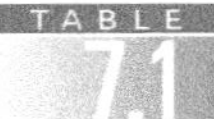

General ICU Mortality Prediction Models

	APACHE (1981)	APACHE II (1985)	APACHE III (1991)	APACHE IV (2006)	SAPS (1984)	SAPS II (1993)	SAPS III (2005)	MPM (1985)	MPM II (1993)	MPM III (2007)	ICNARC (2007)	ICNARC Update (2015)
Countries	1	1	1	1	1	12	35	1	12	1	1	1
ICUs	2	13	40	104	8	137	303	1	140	135	163	232
Patients	705	5,815	17,440	110,558	679	12,997	16,784	2,783	19,124	124,855	216,626	245,246
Age	No	Yes	Yes	Yes	Yes	Yes	Yes	Yes	Yes	Yes	Yes	Yes
Origin	No	No	Yes	Yes	No	No	Yes	No	No	No	No	No
Surgical status	No	Yes	Yes	Yes	No	Yes	Yes	Yes	Yes	Yes	Yes	Yes
Chronic health	Yes	Yes	Yes	Yes	No	Yes	Yes	Yes	Yes	Yes	No	Yes
Physiology	Yes	Yes	Yes	Yes	Yes	Yes	Yes	Yes	Yes	Yes	Yes	Yes
Acute diagnosis	No	Yes	Yes	Yes	No	No	Yes	No	Yes	Yes	Yes	Yes
Variables	34	17	26	142	14	17	20	11	15	16	19	18
Score	Yes	Yes	Yes	Yes	Yes	Yes	Yes	No	No	No	Yes	Yes
Mortality prediction	No	Yes	Yes	Yes	No	Yes	Yes	Yes	Yes	Yes	Yes	Yes

APACHE, Acute Physiology and Chronic Health Evaluation; ICNARC, Intensive Care National Audit and Research Centre; ICU, intensive care unit; MPM, Mortality Probability Model; SAPS, Simplified Acute Physiology Score.

risk of more than 90%. The ICNARC score has subsequently been updated and has demonstrated improved discrimination and overall performance compared to the original model (c-index 0.89 vs 0.87).[19]

External Validation

Data derived from ICUs (n = 10,393) in Scotland compared APACHE II and APACHE III, SAPS II, and MPM0 and MPM24.[20] All models demonstrated good discrimination, although observed mortality was significantly different from that predicted (poor calibration). SAPS II had the best overall performance, but APACHE II demonstrated better calibration. From an American cohort, the coefficients for APACHE IV, MPM0-III, and SAPS II scores were reestimated and applied to assess risk-adjusted mortality rates.[21] Discrimination and calibration were adequate (AUROC 0.892 for APACHE IV, 0.873 for SAPS II, and 0.809 for MPM0-III). Harrison et al, in a large UK external validation (n = 141,106), found moderate discrimination (c statistic for APACHE II 0.80, APACHE III 0.83, SAPS II 0.82, and MPM II 0.82); however, all demonstrated imperfect calibration requiring recalibration.[22]

Limitations of Intensive Care Unit Mortality Models

General models are likely to perform best in groups of patients close to the derivation population. Accuracy of all the models is dependent on the quality of input, such as definitions, time of data collection, and rules for missing data. Most models are created from ICUs, specifically interested in measuring and improving performance, and, as a consequence, may not be generalizable, and the predicted outcome is usually vital status at discharge rather than longer term outcomes, such as health-related quality of life and resource use. The statistical methodology used to assess calibration, most commonly the Hosmer-Lemeshow statistic, is influenced by the number of covariates assessed, the manner in which observations with equal probabilities are sorted, and sample size.[23] It is thus recommended when assessing calibration in validation studies to produce calibration plots.[24] Although discrimination is often adequate, calibration deteriorates in most external validations, requiring additional recalibration. The use of automatic data management systems can, by changing the sampling rate for the physiologic variables, change model accuracy. Finally, there is little clinical evidence of benefit for using such scoring systems, which is important as there are potential drawbacks such as self-fulfilling "poor outcome" conclusions that could be drawn when these models are employed.

ORGAN DYSFUNCTION SCORES

Organ failure scores are designed to describe the degree of organ dysfunction rather than to predict survival and account for time and severity. Three of the most commonly used are the Multiple Organ Dysfunction Score (MODS),[25] the Sequential Organ Failure Assessment (SOFA),[26] and Logistic Organ Dysfunction System (LODS) (**Table 7.2**).[27] Each uses six organ systems: pulmonary, cardiovascular, renal, neurologic, hematologic/coagulation, and hepatic.

Logistic Organ Dysfunction System

LODS was developed using a database from 137 ICUs in 12 countries, with 12 variables selected using logistic regression with the worst value in the first 24 hours

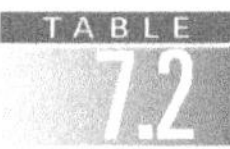

TABLE 7.2 Organ Dysfunction Scores

System	MODS (1995)	LODS (1996)	SOFA (1996)
Respiratory	$Pa{O_2}/Fi{O_2}$ ratio	$Pa{O_2}/Fi{O_2}$ ratio, MV	$Pa{O_2}/Fi{O_2}$ ratio, MV
Cardiovascular	Pressure-adjusted HR	HR, SBP	MAP, vasopressor use
Renal	Creatinine	Urea, creatinine, urine output	Creatinine, urine output
Neurologic	GCS	GCS	GCS
Hepatic	Bilirubin	Bilirubin, PT	Bilirubin
Hematologic	Platelet count	WBC, platelet count	Platelet count

$Fi{O_2}$, fractional inspired concentration of O_2; GCS, Glasgow coma scale; HR, heart rate; LODS, Logistic Organ Dysfunction System; MAP, mean arterial blood pressure; MODS, Multiple Organ Dysfunction Score; MV, mechanical ventilation; $Pa{O_2}$, arterial oxygen partial pressure; PT, prothrombin time; SBP, systolic blood pressure; SOFA, Sequential Organ Failure Assessment; WBC, white blood cell.

of admission selected. In the derivation population, a maximum score[22] carried a mortality of 99.7%. [27] On validation, increased LODS was associated with higher mortality,[28] and in a French study, LODS demonstrated an AUC (area under the curve) of 0.72 to predict mortality.[29]

Sequential Organ Failure Assessment

SOFA is the predominant score in current use being developed during a 1994 consensus conference.[26,30] The worst value on each day is recorded. Unlike LODS and MODS, cardiovascular system includes a treatment-related variable: vasopressor dose. Initially validated in a mixed ICU population,[26,31] SOFA has subsequently been validated in multiple patient groups, including cardiac surgery, burns, and sepsis.[32-35] In one study, a score greater than 15 is correlated with a mortality rate of 90%.[36] In another study, an increase in the score during the first 48 hours predicted a mortality rate greater than 50%, whereas a decrease was associated with a mortality rate of 27%.[37] In a multicenter study of those older than 60 years, a maximum score greater than 13 on any of the first 5 days, a minimum SOFA greater than 10 at all times, and a positive or unchanged SOFA over the first 5 days had 100% mortality.[38] The updated Sepsis-3 definitions incorporate SOFA (see Chapter 35), with organ dysfunction identified as an acute change in total SOFA score greater than or equal to 2 points consequent to infection.[30]

Multiple Organ Dysfunction Score

MODS was based on a literature review of publications that had characterized organ dysfunction with seven organ systems initially selected for consideration (pulmonary, cardiovascular, renal, neurologic, hematologic, hepatic, and gastrointestinal). No accurate descriptors of gastrointestinal function were identified; thus, this system was not included. The score was developed in one surgical ICU

(n = 336) and validated on the same ICU (n = 356). For each system, the first parameters of the day are used with a maximum score of 24. Change in MODS (difference between admission MODS and maximum score) may be more predictive of outcome than individual scores.

External Validations of Organ Dysfunction Scores

Similar discriminative power of SOFA, APACHE III, LODS, and MODS to predict hospital mortality has been described.[39,40] SOFA in patients with brain injury has been reported to have superior discriminative ability for hospital mortality and unfavorable neurologic outcome compared to MODS.[41]

ACUTE KIDNEY INJURY INTENSIVE CARE UNIT PREDICTION MODELS

Acute kidney injury (AKI), defined as an abrupt decline in kidney function, is common in the ICU with an estimated prevalence of 57% and is associated with increased risk of mortality, prolonged length of stay, and development of chronic kidney disease (CKD).[42-44] Early risk stratification for AKI in the ICU is challenging, but is essential in developing novel, sophisticated strategies for the prevention and treatment of AKI.[45] Several investigators have developed and validated clinical risk prediction models for AKI or predict mortality in those who have developed AKI, among heterogeneous groups of critically ill patients.

Mortality Prediction in Patients With Acute Kidney Injury

A 2017 systematic review of mortality prediction scores in patients with AKI included 12 derivation studies (7 in ICU populations, the most recent published in 2011) and 9 external validations.[46] Two studies,[47,48] although classed as validations in the systematic review, also derived a model and are included in **Table 7.3.** Although good performance was reported for internal validation, most prediction models had poor discrimination (AUROC $<$ 0.7 on external validation) and variable performance compared to general ICU models.

Recent Acute Kidney Injury Prediction Studies and Future Directions

AKI prediction in the ICU can be challenging with such a high incidence, potential for prior insults to not yet be reflected in serum creatinine changes, and frequent lack of accurate baseline kidney function. A number of small studies were described predating Kidney Disease Improving Global Outcomes (KDIGO) definitions.[49-51] A number of recent studies since the publication of KDIGO definitions[52] have proposed models predicting the onset of AKI or more severe AKI (**Table 7.4**). Three models employed random forest (RF) plots, an ensemble classifier that aggregates the results of multiple decision trees via majority voting with machine learning (ML).[53-55] Such techniques have been reported to perform well in other areas of the ICU[56] and for AKI prediction in the wider hospital up to a 72-hour time frame.[57] One model reported an AUROC of 0.88 using the same variables as in the SAPS II general ICU mortality model.[54]

The concept of renal angina was described a decade ago[58] and subsequently operationalized to describe a renal angina index (RAI) in children with promising performance to predict AKI (AUROC 0.74-0.81).[59] The RAI uses a combination of risk (such as ventilated) and signs of injury (fluid overload) and has recently been validated in adults.[60] Functional markers may in the future be incorporated into risk prediction. For example, the furosemide stress test (FST)

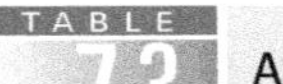
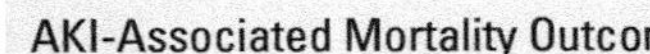

TABLE 7.3 AKI-Associated Mortality Outcome Model Studies

Study	Centers	Sample Size	KRT	Mortality[a]	AKI Definition	Variables	AUROC
Schaefer et al (1991)[66] Germany	1	126	100%	57%	KRT	MV, hypotension	–
Paganini et al (1996)[67] CCF, the United States	1	506	100%	67%	KRT	MV, male, hematologic dysfunction[b], bilirubin, medical, SCr[c], increasing organ failure, urea	–
Lins et al (2000)[68] SHARF, Belgium	1	197	26%	53%	SCr $>$ 2 mg/dL or $>$50% baseline	Age, MV, albumin, PT time, HF	0.87-0.90
Mehta et al (2002)[69] the United States	4	605	50%	52%	SCr $>$ 2 mg/dL, urea $>$40 mg/dL, or rise in SCr $>$1 if preexisting kidney disease	Age, male, respiratory, liver and hematologic failure, SCr, urea, UO, HR	0.83
D'Avila et al (2004)[48]	1	280	100%	85%	KRT	Male, unconscious, liver, respiratory failure, vasoactives, sepsis	0.815
Lins et al (2004)[70] SHARF II, Belgium	8	293	37%	51%	SCr $>$ 3 or $>$50% increase in mild-to-moderate kidney disease	Age, albumin, PT, bilirubin, HF, hypotension, sepsis	0.82-0.83

(continued)

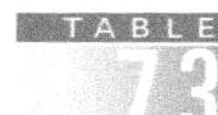

TABLE 7.3 AKI-Associated Mortality Outcome Model Studies (*continued*)

Study	Centers	Sample Size	KRT	Mortality[a]	AKI Definition	Variables	AUROC
Chertow et al (2006)[71] the United States	5	618	64%	37%	SCr > 0.5 mg/dL, baseline SCr < 1.5 mg/dL, or rise >1 if baseline >1.5 and <5 mg/dL	Initial: age, oliguria, liver, respiratory failure, sepsis, and thrombocytopenia; at KRT: age, liver, respiratory failure, sepsis, higher urea, lower SCr	0.62-0.72
Lin et al (2008)[47] Taiwan	4	398	100%	63%-66%	KRT	MV, age, lactate, SOFA, TPN, CPR, sepsis	0.80-0.84
Demirjian et al (2011)[72] the United States	27	1,122	99%	50%	Ischemic or nephrotoxic ATN, oliguria, SCr >2 mg/dL in males or >1.5 mg/dL in females	MV, age, chronic hypoxemia, CVD, malignancy, immunosuppressive therapy, ischemic AKI, postsurgery, HR, MAP, urine volume, FiO_2, pH, pO_2, SCr, HCO_3, PO_4, albumin, bilirubin, INR, platelet count	0.85 (0.83-0.88)

[a]Hospital mortality.

[b]Platelet count <50,000, leukocyte count <2,500, or bleeding diathesis.

[c]On first dialysis treatment day.

AKI, acute kidney injury; ATN, acute tubular necrosis; AUROC, area under the receiver operating characteristic curve; BUN, blood urea nitrogen; CCF, Cleveland Clinic Foundation; CPR, cardiopulmonary resuscitation; CVD, cardiovascular disease; FiO_2, fractional inspired concentration of O_2; HCO_3, serum bicarbonate; HF, heart failure; HR, heart rate; MAP, mean arterial pressure; MV, mechanical ventilation; PO_4, serum phosphate; PT, prothrombin time; KRT, kidney replacement therapy; SCr, serum creatinine; SHARF, Stuivenberg Hospital Acute Renal Failure; SOFA, Sequential Organ Failure Assessment; TPN, total parenteral nutrition; UO, urine output.

TABLE 7.4 Recent AKI Prediction Studies on ICU

Study	Outcome, Design, Sample Size	Variable	AUROCs
Malhotra et al (2017)[45] US dual center	Outcome: KDIGO AKI mortality Forward stepwise logistic regression Derivation: $n = 573$, validation: $n = 144$	MV, CKD, liver disease, HF, HTN, CVD, pH ≤ 7.30, nephrotoxins, sepsis, anemia	Derivation: 0.79 (0.70-0.89); external validation: 0.81 (0.78-0.83)
Flechet et al (2017)[53] Multicenter	Outcome: KDIGO AKI and stages 2-3 ICU admission and 24 hr RF ML-final variable selection determined incrementally for each time-based model via bootstrapped backward elimination Derivation: $n = 2,123$, validation: $n = 2,367$ AKI occurred in 29% and stages 2-3 15%	AKI: age, baseline SCr, diabetes, admission type Stages 2-3: additionally height and weight	AKI: 0.75 (0.75-0.75) 24 hr: 0.82 (0.82-0.82); AKI 2-3: 0.77 (0.77-0.77) 24 hr: 0.84 (95% CI, 0.83-0.84)
Haines et al (2018)[73] Trauma ICU patients, UK single center	KDIGO AKI Logistic regression Derivation: $n = 830$, validation: $n = 564$ AKI occurred in 163 (19.6%) of 830, with 42 (5.1%) receiving KRT	Age, SCr day 1, PO_4, units blood transfused, Charlson score	AKI 0.77 (0.72-0.81), validation: 0.70 (0.64-0.77) Stages 2-3: development: 0.81 (0.75-0.88), validation: 0.83 (0.74-0.92) KRT: development: 0.92 (0.88-0.96), validation: 0.91 (0.86-0.97)

(*continued*)

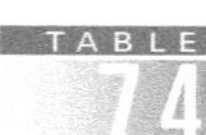

Recent AKI Prediction Studies on ICU (*continued*)

Study	Outcome, Design, Sample Size	Variable	AUROCs
McKown et al (2017)[74] **US single center**	Outcome: MAKE30 Logistic regression $n = 10{,}983$. Outcome: $n = 1{,}489$ (13.6%)	MV, age, UHSC expected mortality, baseline SCr, fluid, race, male, admitting service, unit, source, vasopressors, KRT prior, AKI at ICU admission, CKD, Elixhauser coding algorithms kidney failure	0.90 after bootstrapping
Chiofolo et al (2019)[54]	RF ML for a continuous AKI risk score Derivation: $n = 4{,}572$, validation: $n = 1{,}958$ AKI in 30%	Age, urea, pH, DBP, MAP, temperature, HCT, Na^+, K^+, eGFR, UO 12, 24 hr, SI, PP, TV, P/F ratio, fluid balance, total N. Saline fluid dose	AUC 0.88 For AKI stages 2-3: 91% sensitivity, 71% specificity, and 53% detection of AKI cases at least 6 hr before AKI onset
Lin et al (2019)[55]	RF ML using MIMIC III database 19,044 with AKI—mortality 13.6%	Used same variables as SAPS II	0.866 (95% CI, 0.862-0.870)

AKI, acute kidney injury; AUC, area under the curve; AUROC, area under the receiver operating characteristic curve; CI, confidence interval; CKD, chronic kidney disease; CVD, cardiovascular disease; DBP, diastolic blood pressure; eGFR, estimated glomerular filtration rate; HCT, hematocrit; HF, heart failure; HR, heart rate; HTN, hypertension; ICU, intensive care unit; K^+, serum potassium; KDIGO, Kidney Disease Improving Global Outcomes; MAKE30, Major Adverse Kidney Events within 30 days—composite of persistent kidney dysfunction, KRT, and in-hospital mortality; MAP, mean arterial pressure; ML, machine learning; MV, mechanical ventilation; Na^+, serum sodium; P/F, Pao_2/Fio_2; PO_4, serum phosphate; PP, pulse pressure; RF, random forest; KRT, kidney replacement therapy; SAPS, Simplified Acute Physiology Score; SCr, serum creatinine; SI, shock index; UHSC, University Health System Consortium; UO, urine output.

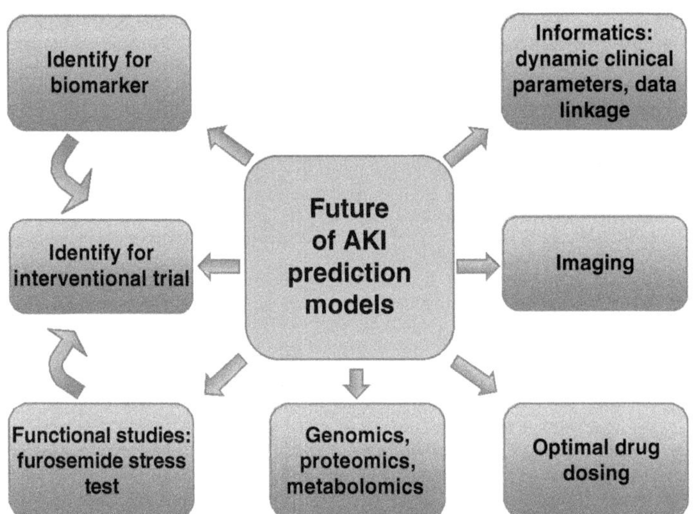

FIGURE 7.1: A schematic outlining the potential development of AKI prediction models.

predicts progression to more severe stages of AKI (**Figure 7.1**).[61] The number of AKI biomarkers continues to grow and has been described in concert with prediction models to recognize those at highest risk[62] and enable tailored interventions[63] (see Chapter 16).

A major challenge limiting AKI prediction and prognostication is its multifactorial origin, further complicated by the fact that the changes of molecular expression induced by AKI are difficult to distinguish from those of the diseases associated or causing AKI, such as sepsis.[64] A large genome-wide association study (GWAS) by Zhao et al identified two genetic loci associated with increased risk of AKI that could reveal novel pathways for early diagnosis and subsequent therapeutic development.[65] Addition of genomic profiling to prediction model assessments promises further enhancement of risk modeling.

References

1. Moons KG, Royston P, Vergouwe Y, Grobbee DE, Altman DG. Prognosis and prognostic research: what, why, and how? *BMJ.* 2009;338:b375.
2. Concato J, Feinstein AR, Holford TR. The risk of determining risk with multivariable models. *Ann Intern Med.* 1993;118(3):201-210.
3. Steyerberg EW, Vickers AJ, Cook NR, et al. Assessing the performance of prediction models: a framework for traditional and novel measures. *Epidemiology.* 2010;21(1):128-138.
4. Harrell FJ. *Regression Modeling Strategies.* Springer; 2001.
5. Moons KG, Kengne AP, Grobbee DE, et al. Risk prediction models: II. External validation, model updating, and impact assessment. *Heart.* 2012;98(9):691-698.
6. Royston P, Moons KG, Altman DG, Vergouwe Y. Prognosis and prognostic research: developing a prognostic model. *BMJ.* 2009;338:b604.
7. Knaus WA, Zimmerman JE, Wagner DP, Draper EA, Lawrence DE. APACHE-acute physiology and chronic health evaluation: a physiologically based classification system. *Crit Care Med.* 1981;9(8):591-597.
8. Knaus WA, Draper EA, Wagner DP, Zimmerman JE. APACHE II: a severity of disease classification system. *Crit Care Med.* 1985;13(10):818-829.
9. Knaus WA, Wagner DP, Draper EA, et al. The APACHE III prognostic system. Risk prediction of hospital mortality for critically ill hospitalized adults. *Chest.* 1991;100(6):1619-1636.

10. Zimmerman JE, Kramer AA, McNair DS, Malila FM. Acute Physiology and Chronic Health Evaluation (APACHE) IV: hospital mortality assessment for today's critically ill patients. *Crit Care Med.* 2006;34(5):1297-1310.
11. Le Gall JR, Loirat P, Alperovitch A, et al. A simplified acute physiology score for ICU patients. *Crit Care Med.* 1984;12(11):975-977.
12. Le Gall JR, Lemeshow S, Saulnier F. A new Simplified Acute Physiology Score (SAPS II) based on a European/North American multicenter study. *JAMA.* 1993;270(24):2957-2963.
13. Moreno RP, Metnitz PG, Almeida E, et al. SAPS 3—From evaluation of the patient to evaluation of the intensive care unit. Part 2: Development of a prognostic model for hospital mortality at ICU admission. *Intensive Care Med.* 2005;31(10):1345-1355.
14. Rothen HU, Stricker K, Einfalt J, et al. Variability in outcome and resource use in intensive care units. *Intensive Care Med.* 2007;33(8):1329-1336.
15. Lemeshow S, Teres D, Pastides H, Avrunin JS, Steingrub JS. A method for predicting survival and mortality of ICU patients using objectively derived weights. *Crit Care Med.* 1985;13(7):519-525.
16. Lemeshow S, Teres D, Klar J, Avrunin JS, Gehlbach SH, Rapoport J. Mortality Probability Models (MPM II) based on an international cohort of intensive care unit patients. *JAMA.* 1993;270(20):2478-2486.
17. Higgins TL, Teres D, Copes WS, Nathanson BH, Stark M, Kramer AA. Assessing contemporary intensive care unit outcome: an updated Mortality Probability Admission Model (MPM0-III). *Crit Care Med.* 2007;35(3):827-835.
18. Harrison DA, Parry GJ, Carpenter JR, Short A, Rowan K. A new risk prediction model for critical care: the Intensive Care National Audit & Research Centre (ICNARC) model. *Crit Care Med.* 2007;35(4):1091-1098.
19. Harrison DA, Ferrando-Vivas P, Shahin J, Rowan KM. *Ensuring Comparisons of Health-Care Providers Are Fair: Development and Validation of Risk Prediction Models for Critically Ill Patients.* NIHR Journals Library. Queen's Printer and Controller of HMSO; 2015.
20. Livingston BM, MacKirdy FN, Howie JC, Jones R, Norrie JD. Assessment of the performance of five intensive care scoring models within a large Scottish database. *Crit Care Med.* 2000;28(6):1820-1827.
21. Kuzniewicz MW, Vasilevskis EE, Lane R, et al. Variation in ICU risk-adjusted mortality: impact of methods of assessment and potential confounders. *Chest.* 2008;133(6):1319-1327.
22. Harrison DA, Brady AR, Parry GJ, Carpenter JR, Rowan K. Recalibration of risk prediction models in a large multicenter cohort of admissions to adult, general critical care units in the United Kingdom. *Crit Care Med.* 2006;34(5):1378-1388.
23. Kramer AA, Zimmerman JE. Assessing the calibration of mortality benchmarks in critical care: the Hosmer-Lemeshow test revisited. *Crit Care Med.* 2007;35(9):2052-2056.
24. Moons KG, Altman DG, Reitsma JB, et al. Transparent reporting of a multivariable prediction model for Individual Prognosis or Diagnosis (TRIPOD): explanation and elaboration. *Ann Intern Med.* 2015;162(1):W1-W73.
25. Marshall JC, Cook DJ, Christou NV, Bernard GR, Sprung CL, Sibbald WJ. Multiple organ dysfunction score: a reliable descriptor of a complex clinical outcome. *Crit Care Med.* 1995;23(10):1638-1652.
26. Vincent JL, Moreno R, Takala J, et al. The SOFA (Sepsis-related Organ Failure Assessment) score to describe organ dysfunction/failure. On behalf of the Working Group on Sepsis-Related Problems of the European Society of Intensive Care Medicine. *Intensive Care Med.* 1996;22(7):707-710.
27. Le Gall JR, Klar J, Lemeshow S, et al; The Logistic Organ Dysfunction system. A new way to assess organ dysfunction in the intensive care unit. ICU Scoring Group. *JAMA.* 1996;276(10):802-810.
28. Metnitz PG, Lang T, Valentin A, Steltzer H, Krenn CG, Le Gall JR. Evaluation of the logistic organ dysfunction system for the assessment of organ dysfunction and mortality in critically ill patients. *Intensive Care Med.* 2001;27(6):992-998.
29. Timsit JF, Fosse JP, Troche G, et al. Calibration and discrimination by daily Logistic Organ Dysfunction scoring comparatively with daily Sequential Organ Failure Assessment scoring for predicting hospital mortality in critically ill patients. *Crit Care Med.* 2002;30(9):2003-2013.
30. Singer M, Deutschman CS, Seymour CW, et al. The Third International Consensus Definitions for Sepsis and Septic Shock (Sepsis-3). *JAMA.* 2016;315(8):801-810.
31. Moreno R, Vincent JL, Matos R, et al. The use of maximum SOFA score to quantify organ dysfunction/failure in intensive care. Results of a prospective, multicentre study. Working Group on Sepsis related Problems of the ESICM. *Intensive Care Med.* 1999;25(7):686-696.
32. Ceriani R, Mazzoni M, Bortone F, et al. Application of the sequential organ failure assessment score to cardiac surgical patients. *Chest.* 2003;123(4):1229-1239.
33. Lorente JA, Vallejo A, Galeiras R, et al. Organ dysfunction as estimated by the sequential organ failure assessment score is related to outcome in critically ill burn patients. *Shock.* 2009;31(2):125-131.

34. Vosylius S, Sipylaite J, Ivaskevicius J. Sequential organ failure assessment score as the determinant of outcome for patients with severe sepsis. *Croat Med J.* 2004;45(6):715-720.
35. Jentzer JC, Bennett C, Wiley BM, et al. Predictive value of the sequential organ failure assessment score for mortality in a contemporary cardiac intensive care unit population. *J Am Heart Assoc.* 2018;7(6):e008169.
36. Vincent JL, de Mendonca A, Cantraine F, et al. Use of the SOFA score to assess the incidence of organ dysfunction/failure in intensive care units: results of a multicenter, prospective study. Working group on "sepsis-related problems" of the European Society of Intensive Care Medicine. *Crit Care Med.* 1998;26(11):1793-1800.
37. Ferreira FL, Bota DP, Bross A, Mélot C, Vincent J-L. Serial evaluation of the SOFA score to predict outcome in critically ill patients. *JAMA.* 2001;286(14):1754-1758.
38. Cabre L, Mancebo J, Solsona JF, et al. Multicenter study of the multiple organ dysfunction syndrome in intensive care units: the usefulness of Sequential Organ Failure Assessment scores in decision making. *Intensive Care Med.* 2005;31(7):927-933.
39. Pettila V, Pettila M, Sarna S, Voutilainen P, Takkunen O. Comparison of multiple organ dysfunction scores in the prediction of hospital mortality in the critically ill. *Crit Care Med.* 2002;30(8):1705-1711.
40. Peres Bota D, Melot C, Lopes Ferreira F, Nguyen Ba V, Vincent JL. The Multiple Organ Dysfunction Score (MODS) versus the Sequential Organ Failure Assessment (SOFA) score in outcome prediction. *Intensive Care Med.* 2002;28(11):1619-1624.
41. Zygun D, Berthiaume L, Laupland K, Kortbeek J, Doig C. SOFA is superior to MOD score for the determination of non-neurologic organ dysfunction in patients with severe traumatic brain injury: a cohort study. *Crit Care.* 2006;10(4):R115.
42. Uchino S, Bellomo R, Bagshaw SM, Goldsmith D. Transient azotaemia is associated with a high risk of death in hospitalized patients. *Nephrol Dial Transplant.* 2010;25(6):1833-1839.
43. Coca SG, Peixoto AJ, Garg AX, Krumholz HM, Parikh CR. The prognostic importance of a small acute decrement in kidney function in hospitalized patients: a systematic review and meta-analysis. *Am J Kidney Dis.* 2007;50(5):712-720.
44. Hoste EA, Bagshaw SM, Bellomo R, et al. Epidemiology of acute kidney injury in critically ill patients: the multinational AKI-EPI study. *Intensive Care Med.* 2015;41(8):1411-1423.
45. Malhotra R, Kashani KB, Macedo E, et al. A risk prediction score for acute kidney injury in the intensive care unit. *Nephrol Dial Transplant.* 2017;32(5):814-822.
46. Ohnuma T, Uchino S. Prediction models and their external validation studies for mortality of patients with acute kidney injury: a systematic review. *PLoS One.* 2017;12(1):e0169341.
47. Lin YF, Ko WJ, Wu VC, et al. A modified sequential organ failure assessment score to predict hospital mortality of postoperative acute renal failure patients requiring renal replacement therapy. *Blood Purif.* 2008;26(6):547-554.
48. D'Avila DO, Cendoroglo NM, dos Santos OF, Schor N, Poli de Figueiredo CE. Acute renal failure needing dialysis in the intensive care unit and prognostic scores. *Ren Fail.* 2004;26(1):59-68.
49. Coritsidis GN, Guru K, Ward L, Bashir R, Feinfeld DA, Carvounis CP. Prediction of acute renal failure by "bedside formula" in medical and surgical intensive care patients. *Ren Fail.* 2000;22(2):235-244.
50. Hoste EA, Lameire NH, Vanholder RC, Benoit DD, Decruyenaere JM, Colardyn FA. Acute renal failure in patients with sepsis in a surgical ICU: predictive factors, incidence, comorbidity, and outcome. *J Am Soc Nephrol.* 2003;14(4):1022-1030.
51. Chawla LS, Abell L, Mazhari R, et al. Identifying critically ill patients at high risk for developing acute renal failure: a pilot study. *Kidney Int.* 2005;68(5):2274-2280.
52. Kidney International. KDIGO Clinical Practice Guideline for Acute Kidney Injury. *Kidney Int Suppl.* 2012;2(1):1-136.
53. Flechet M, Guiza F, Schetz M, et al. AKI predictor, an online prognostic calculator for acute kidney injury in adult critically ill patients: development, validation and comparison to serum neutrophil gelatinase-associated lipocalin. *Intensive Care Med.* 2017;43(6):764-773.
54. Chiofolo C, Chbat N, Ghosh E, Eshelman L, Kashani K. Automated continuous acute kidney injury prediction and surveillance: a random forest model. *Mayo Clin Proc.* 2019;94(5):783-792.
55. Lin K, Hu Y, Kong G. Predicting in-hospital mortality of patients with acute kidney injury in the ICU using random forest model. *Int J Med Inform.* 2019;125:55-61.
56. Van Poucke S, Zhang Z, Schmitz M, et al. Scalable predictive analysis in critically ill patients using a visual open data analysis platform. *PLoS One.* 2016;11(1):e0145791.
57. Koyner JL, Carey KA, Edelson DP, Churpek MM. The development of a machine learning inpatient acute kidney injury prediction model. *Crit Care Med.* 2018;46(7):1070-1077.
58. Goldstein SL, Chawla LS. Renal angina. *Clin J Am Soc Nephrol.* 2010;5(5):943-949.
59. Basu RK, Zappitelli M, Brunner L, et al. Derivation and validation of the renal angina index to improve the prediction of acute kidney injury in critically ill children. *Kidney Int.* 2014;85(3):659-667.

60. Cruz DN, Ferrer-Nadal A, Piccinni P, et al. Utilization of small changes in serum creatinine with clinical risk factors to assess the risk of AKI in critically ill adults. *Clin J Am Soc Nephrol.* 2014;9(4):663-672.
61. Rewa OG, Bagshaw SM, Wang X, et al. The furosemide stress test for prediction of worsening acute kidney injury in critically ill patients: a multicenter, prospective, observational study. *J Crit Care.* 2019;52:109-114.
62. Hodgson LE, Venn RM, Short S, et al. Improving clinical prediction rules in acute kidney injury with the use of biomarkers of cell cycle arrest: a pilot study. *Biomarkers.* 2018;24:1-21.
63. Meersch M, Schmidt C, Hoffmeier A, et al. Prevention of cardiac surgery-associated AKI by implementing the KDIGO guidelines in high risk patients identified by biomarkers: the PrevAKI randomized controlled trial. *Intensive Care Med.* 2017;43(11):1551-1561.
64. Marx D, Metzger J, Pejchinovski M, et al. Proteomics and metabolomics for AKI diagnosis. *Semin Nephrol.* 2018;38(1):63-87.
65. Zhao B, Lu Q, Cheng Y, et al. A genome-wide association study to identify single-nucleotide polymorphisms for acute kidney injury. *Am J Respir Crit Care Med.* 2017;195(4):482-490.
66. Schaefer JH, Jochimsen F, Keller F, Wegscheider K, Distler A. Outcome prediction of acute renal failure in medical intensive care. *Intensive Care Med.* 1991;17(1):19-24.
67. Paganini EP, Halstenberg WK, Goormastic M. Risk modeling in acute renal failure requiring dialysis: the introduction of a new model. *Clin Nephrol.* 1996;46(3):206-211.
68. Lins RL, Elseviers M, Daelemans R, et al. Prognostic value of a new scoring system for hospital mortality in acute renal failure. *Clin Nephrol.* 2000;53(1):10-17.
69. Mehta RL, Pascual MT, Gruta CG, Zhuang S, Chertow GM. Refining predictive models in critically ill patients with acute renal failure. *J Am Soc Nephrol.* 2002;13(5):1350-1357.
70. Lins RL, Elseviers MM, Daelemans R, et al. Re-evaluation and modification of the Stuivenberg Hospital Acute Renal Failure (SHARF) scoring system for the prognosis of acute renal failure: an independent multicentre, prospective study. *Nephrol Dial Transplant.* 2004;19(9):2282-2288.
71. Chertow GM, Soroko SH, Paganini EP, et al. Mortality after acute renal failure: models for prognostic stratification and risk adjustment. *Kidney Int.* 2006;70(6):1120-1126.
72. Demirjian S, Chertow GM, Zhang JH, et al. Model to predict mortality in critically ill adults with acute kidney injury. *Clin J Am Soc Nephrol.* 2011;6(9):2114-2120.
73. Haines RW, Lin S-P, Hewson R, et al. Acute kidney injury in trauma patients admitted to critical care: development and validation of a diagnostic prediction model. *Sci Rep.* 2018;8(1):3665.
74. McKown AC, Wang L, Wanderer JP, et al. Predicting major adverse kidney events among critically ill adults using the electronic health record. *J Med Syst.* 2017;41(10):156.

8 Prevention of Acute Kidney Injury

Nicholas Michael Selby

INTRODUCTION

Prevention is the action of stopping something from happening, which in medical terms is to prevent disease before its onset. This implies several things: that patients at risk can be identified, that there is a window of opportunity to act prior to disease onset, and that effective preventative interventions exist. When it comes to acute kidney injury (AKI) in the intensive care unit (ICU), these elements are not always apparent. It is also important to recognize that AKI is not a single condition, but a heterogeneous syndrome with multiple different causes that may require a range of preventative actions.[1,2] It can also be difficult to determine with currently available diagnostic tests as to whether the situation is one of risk and prevention, or whether in fact kidney injury has already occurred. Despite this, the potential value of AKI prevention is significant when the high morbidity, mortality, and health care resource utilization associated with AKI are considered.[3] The epidemiology of AKI in the ICU and identification of patients at risk have been discussed in Chapters 6 and 7, so this chapter will provide an overview of interventions to prevent AKI in the ICU, with common risk factors for AKI in critically ill patients summarized in **Table 8.1**.[4]

PREVENTATIVE STRATEGIES FOR PEOPLE AT HIGH RISK OF ACUTE KIDNEY INJURY IN THE INTENSIVE CARE UNIT

International guidelines that encompass AKI prevention include those from the European Society of Intensive Care Medicine (ESICM) in 2010,[5] their update in 2017,[6] the 2010 consensus guidelines on behalf of the American Thoracic Society, European Respiratory Society, ESICM, the Society of Critical Care Medicine,[7] and the 2012 Kidney Disease Improving Global Outcomes (KDIGO) clinical practice guidelines.[8,9]

Volume Expansion and Choice of Intravenous Fluid

Volume expansion to restore circulating volume or correct hypovolemia is an obvious step to prevent AKI, but most would regard this as a basic element of care of the critically ill patient. Furthermore, goal-directed therapy including central venous pressure (CVP) monitoring or protocolized fluid resuscitation without CVP use has been shown to be no more effective than usual care in reducing AKI incidence, at least in sepsis.[10] Restricting fluid volumes has also been suggested as a strategy to improve outcomes, although evidence in this area is incomplete.[11] In people with AKI, there is a strong association between excess fluid

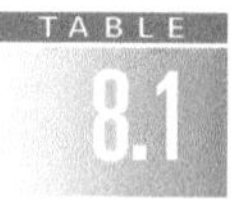

TABLE 8.1 Thirteen Risk Factors for the Development of AKI in Critically Ill Patients, Identified by Meta-analysis of 31 Studies Including 504,545 Patients

Patient-related factors
Older age
Higher baseline creatinine/CKD
Diabetes mellitus
Heart failure
Hypertension
Situational risk factors
Presence of sepsis/SIRS
Higher severity of disease scores
Use of vasopressors/inotropes
Use of "nephrotoxic" drugs
High-risk surgery
Emergency surgery
Use of IABP in cardiothoracic patients
Longer time in cardiopulmonary bypass pump in cardiothoracic patients

Nephrotoxic drugs were defined as any of: intravenous contrast, aminoglycosides, amphotericin B, vancomycin, nonsteroidal anti-inflammatory drugs, angiotensin-converting enzyme inhibitors, and angiotensin receptor blockers. Severity of disease was measured by different severity scores such as the acute physiologic and chronic health evaluation (APACHE) or the injury severity score (ISS).

AKI, acute kidney injury; CKD, chronic kidney disease; IABP, intra-aortic balloon pump; SIRS, systemic inflammatory response syndrome.

From Cartin-Ceba R, Kashiouris M, Plataki M, et al. Risk factors for development of acute kidney injury in critically ill patients: a systematic review and meta-analysis of observational studies. *Crit Care Res Pract.* 2012;2012:691013.

accumulation (defined as >10% increase in body weight relative to baseline) and increased mortality,[12] and a randomized parallel group feasibility trial has suggested that a restrictive volume replacement protocol may result in lower rates of AKI.[13] These results are also supported by the Fluids and Catheters Treatment Trial (FACTT), in which less kidney replacement therapy (KRT) was needed in patients with acute lung injury who received a conservative fluid management regime, although mortality was not different between groups.[14] However, in surgical patients, a restrictive fluid administration regime may increase AKI.[15] Further clarification is therefore required before definite conclusions can be drawn, and it is also possible that the impact of restrictive volume replacement may differ depending on the clinical setting. In the meantime, a judicious and individualized approach to fluid resuscitation is advisable, avoiding excessive fluid accumulation when possible (e.g., aiming for <10% increase in body weight because of fluid accumulation).

Choice of fluid may also be important in terms of AKI prevention; although also covered in Chapter 10, we will touch on this briefly here. Crystalloids are generally preferred to colloids for resuscitation, because of the lack of major benefit and increased costs of the latter. Additionally, a number of large randomized controlled trials (RCTs) have shown an increased risk of AKI and the need for KRT with the use of starches,[16-18] which have now largely been abandoned. There has also been extensive debate as to whether choice of crystalloid can influence the risk of AKI, specifically as to whether balanced solutions (Ringer's lactate, Hartmann's solution, Plasma-Lyte) confer benefit over normal (0.9%) saline. A number of observational studies have reported associations between normal saline and an increased risk of AKI, and the physiologic effects of chloride-rich, nonbuffered solutions that include hyperchloremic metabolic acidosis, reduced renal blood flow, and renal vasoconstriction could plausibly contribute to AKI.[19] Recent randomized trials have also addressed this question, but without providing a definitive answer. The SPLIT trial was a double-blind, cluster randomized, crossover trial that compared 0.9% saline and a balanced crystalloid solution (Plasma-Lyte 148) in 2,278 patients across four ICUs in New Zealand.[20] Participating ICUs were assigned a masked study fluid, either saline or a buffered crystalloid, for alternating 7-week treatment blocks over the 28 weeks of the study. There was no difference in the primary outcome of proportion of patients who developed AKI, nor in KRT rates or mortality. In contrast, the SMART trial (Isotonic Solutions and Major Adverse Renal Events Trial) did show benefit with balanced crystalloids.[21] SMART was a single-center, pragmatic trial of saline versus balanced crystalloids (Ringer's lactate or Plasma-Lyte A) in 15,802 adult ICU patients, which had a similar cluster-randomized multiple crossover design to SPLIT, with ICUs alternating between fluid types from month to month. The primary outcome of Major Adverse Kidney Events at 30 days (MAKE30) was seen in 14.3% of the balanced crystalloid group and 15.4% of the saline group (odds ratio, 0.90; 95% confidence interval [CI], 0.82-0.99; $p = 0.04$). MAKE30, a composite endpoint, was defined as mortality, new receipt of KRT, or persistent kidney dysfunction (final inpatient creatinine value of >200% baseline). However, when focusing on the question of AKI prevention, secondary endpoint analyses showed no difference between rates of AKI stage 2/3, highest serum creatinine, change from baseline to highest creatinine, or persistent kidney dysfunction between groups. KRT (as a single outcome measure) was delivered to 2.5% of the balanced crystalloid group versus 2.9% saline group, $p = 0.08$. Similar findings were seen in the SALT-ED trial, conducted at the same center with a similar design to SMART but in noncritically ill patients.[22] So while the SMART trial suggests benefit of balanced crystalloids overall, neither the SPLIT nor the SMART trials have demonstrated that their use prevents AKI in the ICU.

Prevention of Contrast-Associated Acute Kidney injury

Contrast-associated AKI (CA-AKI) is discussed in detail in Chapter 44, but the mainstay of CA-AKI prevention is prehydration in those at increased risk. Although performed outside of ICU, the well-conducted PRESERVE trial showed definitively that in patients at high risk of CA-AKI undergoing angiography, bicarbonate was not superior to normal saline in preventing a combined endpoint of death, the need for dialysis or a persistent increase of 50% or more from baseline in the serum creatinine level at 90 days, or in reducing rates of CA-AKI.[23] In addition, PRESERVE also demonstrated that *N*-acetylcysteine was ineffective. Smaller trials conducted in critically ill patients are consistent with these findings.[24,25]

Therefore, the administration of isotonic crystalloids to patients receiving intravascular contrast media should be considered when patients are hypovolemic or if they are particularly at high risk for CA-AKI (in particular with preexisting CKD, e.g., estimated glomerular filtration rate [eGFR] <30 mL/min/1.73 m^2); however, fluids should not be given if the patient is at risk of fluid overload. There is no role for intravenous bicarbonate or *N*-acetylcysteine. Minimizing contrast volume in high-risk patients is also important, particularly for intra-arterial contrast administration.

Blood Pressure and Vasopressors

Vasoactive medications and the management of septic shock are reviewed in Chapters 2, 13, and 36 and will not be discussed here. Nevertheless, interventions around intraoperative blood pressure may also be effective for AKI prevention. The INPRESS trial randomized 298 people deemed at higher risk of postoperative AKI to either the maintenance of a systolic blood pressure (SBP) within 10% of the patient's preoperative value intraoperatively and for 4 hours postoperatively, or standard management (treating SBP if <80 mm Hg or <40% from the preoperative value, initially with ephedrine boluses).[26] Intra-arterial monitoring and an infusion of norepinephrine were used in the intervention arm to achieve target SBP. Postoperative organ dysfunction was reduced with the intervention, and of particular interest kidney dysfunction occurred in 32.7% of the intervention group versus 49% of the controls ($p = 0.01$), equating to a number needed to treat to prevent one episode of kidney dysfunction of only 7.

Care Bundles and a Systematic Approach to Supportive Acute Kidney Injury Care

Outside of the ICU, variation in the quality of AKI care is common and linked to adverse outcomes.[27] In pediatric populations, a quality improvement program (NINJA) has been shown to sustainably reduce rates of AKI by quantifying exposures to nephrotoxic medication and highlighting these to the relevant clinical teams.[28-31] A number of other studies have evaluated complex interventions applied across entire hospitals, which have included elements of AKI prevention as well as improved delivery of AKI care.[32-36] For example, the ICE-AKI study tested an electronic clinical prediction rule (prevention) and an AKI e-alert (detection) that were both combined with care bundles in a controlled before-after study across two UK hospitals. Results showed a small reduction in the incidence of hospital-acquired AKI (odds ratio 0.99, 95% CI 0.98-1.00, $p = 0.049$), as well as lower mortality in those with hospital-acquired AKI and those identified as higher risk by the AKI prediction rule.[36] Improved outcomes, including reductions in AKI incidence, have been reported with various quality improvement projects,[33,35] and the introduction of an AKI computer decision support system across the ward and ICU areas of 14 US hospitals was associated with reduced mortality, lower KRT rates, and a shorter hospital length of stay.[37] However, these studies had before-after designs that cannot completely exclude effects of temporal trends on outcomes (i.e., changes that would have happened anyway). The Tackling AKI study was a pragmatic, multicenter cluster-randomized trial that employed a stepped-wedge design that did allow separation of temporal effects from those because of the intervention. The trial tested a complex intervention consisting of e-alerts, a care bundle, and an education program introduced across five UK hospitals and included 24,059 AKI episodes. The intervention did not alter the primary outcome of 30-day mortality but did result in improvements in the delivery of AKI care, better AKI detection, and reductions in AKI duration and hospital length of stay.[34] In a formal cost-effectiveness analysis, the latter resulted in significant savings to the health care system (manuscript under review). Conversely, a single-center randomized trial of e-alerts that were introduced in isolation did not impact on delivery of care or patient outcomes.[38]

More specific to ICU settings, two single-center randomized trials have evaluated the impact of the early application of a care bundle based on KDIGO recommendations for management/prevention of AKI in the early postoperative period.[39,40] Both studies had a similar design in that patients were eligible for randomization only if an AKI biomarker (Nephrocheck, urinary tissue inhibitor of metalloproteinase 2 [TIMP-2] × insulin-like growth factor binding protein 7 [IGFBP-7]) was elevated in the immediate postoperative period. Details of the care bundles used in each study are shown in **Table 8.2.** The PREV-AKI trial randomized 276 patients (requiring 882 to be screened) following cardiac surgery and reported lower rates of AKI within 72 hours in the care bundle group (55% vs 72%, $p = 0.004$). The rates of AKI stage 2/3 were also significantly lower (30% vs 45%, $p = 0.009$). The high rates of AKI seen in both groups were notable, and there was no difference between groups in other outcomes, including mortality. A larger, multicenter study to confirm these findings and examine effects of the intervention on harder outcomes is now underway (ClinicalTrials.gov Identifier: NCT03244514). The BigpAK trial randomized 121 patients after major abdominal surgery to standard care or AKI preventative care bundle. Although rates of AKI (all stages), the primary outcome, were not significantly lower in the intervention group (32% vs 48%, $p = 0.07$), rates of AKI stage 2/3 were (7% vs 20%, $p = 0.04$). There were also reductions in ICU and hospital length of stay. Both studies had weaknesses, in that they were single center, were unblinded, and the primary endpoint was the KDIGO definition of AKI (i.e., an outcome defined using urine output and serum creatinine, rather than harder clinical endpoints). Taken together,

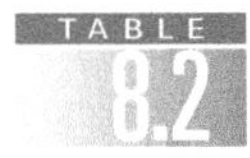

TABLE 8.2 Details of the Care Bundles That Were Used in PREV-AKI and BigpAK Trials

PREV-AKI Trial	BigpAK Trial
• Avoidance of nephrotoxic agents • Discontinuation of ACE inhibitors and ARBs for the first 48 hr after surgery • Close monitoring of serum creatinine and urinary output • Avoidance of hyperglycemia for the first 72 hr after surgery • Consideration of alternatives to radiocontrast • Close hemodynamic monitoring by using a PICCO catheter with an optimization of the volume status and hemodynamic parameters according to prespecified algorithm: • SVV <11 (otherwise therapy with 500-1,000 mL crystalloids), CI > 3 L/min/m² (otherwise therapy with dobutamine or epinephrine), MAP > 65 mm Hg (otherwise therapy with norepinephrine)	• Nephrology consult • MAP > 65 mm Hg • Take CVP measurement, perform dynamic test of volume responsiveness, and then prescribe fluid administration over next 0–3 hr. • Repeat CVP measurement then prescribe fluid administration over hours 4–6. • Repeat Nephrocheck after 12 hr.

ACE, angiotensin-converting enzyme; ARB, angiotensin receptor blocker; CI, confidence interval; CVP, central venous pressure; MAP, mean arterial pressure; PICCO, pulse contour cardiac output; SVV, stroke volume variation.

From Meersch M, Schmidt C, Hoffmeier A, et al. Prevention of cardiac surgery-associated AKI by implementing the KDIGO guidelines in high risk patients identified by biomarkers: the PrevAKI randomized controlled trial. *Intensive Care Med.* 2017;43(11):1551-1561; Gocze I, Jauch D, Gotz M, et al. Biomarker-guided intervention to prevent acute kidney injury after major surgery: the prospective randomized BigpAK study. *Ann Surg.* 2018;267(6):1013-1020.

these data do suggest that attention to the details of basic elements of AKI care and prevention is worthwhile. Furthermore, the approach of using a novel biomarker to enhance risk assessment followed by early application of an intervention should be noted—we can hypothesize that this approach may result in more successful trials in the future, particularly if a biomarker that indicates a process relevant to the mechanism of action of the intervention can be used to enrich the study population.

Ineffective Interventions

Unfortunately, there is a relatively long list of interventions that have been shown not to be effective for the prevention of AKI, as summarized in **Table 8.3**.

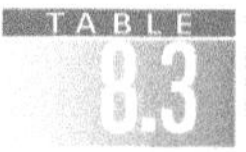

TABLE 8.3 Interventions That Have Been Shown Not to Be Effective to Reduce AKI in a Critical Care or Perioperative Setting

Ineffective Intervention	Setting(s) Tested	Proposed Mechanism(s) of Action
Furosemide	Cardiac surgery[43]	Prevention of tubular obstruction, increase renal blood flow, reduce medullary oxygen consumption, reduce venous congestion
Dopamine	Postoperative (cardiac, vascular, other), contrast, nephrotoxic medications, critically ill patients[44]	Vasodilator, prevents selective renal vasoconstriction, promotes natriuresis
Fenoldopam	Cardiac surgery, critically ill patients[45,46]	Dopamine A1 receptor agonist, renal vasodilation, promotes natriuresis
Levosimendan	Cardiac surgery, critically ill, sepsis[47-49]	Calcium sensitizer, vasodilator, anti-inflammatory effects
Erythropoietin	Cardiac surgery, contrast, critically ill patients[50]	Activation of EPO receptors reducing apoptosis, increased oxygen delivery
Intravenous selenium	Critically ill patients[51]	Reduced oxidative stress
RIPC	Cardiac surgery[52,53]	Protection of organs against ischemic injury after nonlethal ischemia to arm/leg, mechanisms not understood
Aspirin/ clonidine	Noncardiac surgery[54]	Aspirin: reduces platelet aggregation and microembolization, potentially improving GFR at a time of poor kidney perfusion, reduces urinary thromboxane, a potent vasoconstrictor Clonidine: centrally acting α2-adrenergic agonist, reduces sympathetic tone, anti-inflammatory effects

All pharmacologic except RIPC.
AKI, acute kidney injury; EPO, erythropoietin; GFR, glomerular filtration rate; RIPC, remote ischemic preconditioning.

Natriuretic peptides have been postulated to prevent AKI as they cause afferent vasodilation and efferent vasoconstriction, thereby increasing GFR and leading to natriuresis. They are not included in Table 8.3 because a number of studies that encompass cardiac surgery, CA-AKI, abdominal aortic surgery, heart failure, and liver resection have suggested that low-dose atrial natriuretic peptide (ANP) can reduce the incidence of AKI in these settings. It is not strictly accurate to state that they have been shown to be ineffective. However, the evidence is weak as most of these studies have small sample sizes and are of low methodologic quality; in addition, no studies have looked at AKI prevention in critically ill patients. Therefore, despite the overall trend toward suggested benefit, current evidence is not strong enough to support the use of ANP for the prevention of AKI.[41] Similarly, a number of studies and meta-analyses have suggested that statins may prevent CA-AKI. However, these studies are all conducted outside of the ICU and many studied patients with acute coronary syndromes. A recent secondary analysis of an RCT in critically ill patients with acute respiratory distress syndrome (ARDS) suggested no protective effect of statins in an ICU setting.[42]

SUMMARY AND CONCLUSIONS

The high incidence of AKI in critically ill patients, coupled with its strong association with increased mortality, greater health care resource utilization, and longer-term complications, makes a strong case for AKI prevention. However, this is not without challenges. While the common risk factors and clinical scenarios in which AKI occurs are clear, further work is required to build upon existing evidence to further develop, validate, and translate more sophisticated risk prediction for individual patients. While many of the pharmacologic agents tested to date have not shown benefit, careful attention to intravenous fluid administration, maintenance of intraoperative blood pressure, and systematic application of supportive elements of care are measures that can be taken currently to reduce AKI.

References

1. Hoste EA, Bagshaw SM, Bellomo R, et al. Epidemiology of acute kidney injury in critically ill patients: the multinational AKI-EPI study. *Intensive Care Med.* 2015;41(8):1411-1423.
2. Uchino S, Kellum JA, Bellomo R, et al. Acute renal failure in critically ill patients: a multinational, multicenter study. *JAMA.* 2005;294(7):813-818.
3. Hoste EAJ, Kellum JA, Selby NM, et al. Global epidemiology and outcomes of acute kidney injury. *Nat Rev Nephrol.* 2018;14(10):607-625.
4. Cartin-Ceba R, Kashiouris M, Plataki M, et al. Risk factors for development of acute kidney injury in critically ill patients: a systematic review and meta-analysis of observational studies. *Crit Care Res Pract.* 2012;2012:691013.
5. Joannidis M, Druml W, Forni LG, et al. Prevention of acute kidney injury and protection of renal function in the intensive care unit. Expert opinion of the Working Group for Nephrology, ESICM. *Intensive Care Med.* 2010;36(3):392-411.
6. Joannidis M, Druml W, Forni LG, et al. Prevention of acute kidney injury and protection of renal function in the intensive care unit: update 2017: expert opinion of the Working Group on Prevention, AKI section, European Society of Intensive Care Medicine. *Intensive Care Med.* 2017;43(6):730-749.
7. Brochard L, Abroug F, Brenner M, et al. An official ATS/ERS/ESICM/SCCM/SRLF statement: prevention and management of acute renal failure in the ICU patient: an international consensus conference in intensive care medicine. *Am J Respir Crit Care Med.* 2010;181(10):1128-1155.
8. Kidney Disease: Improving Global Outcomes (KDIGO) Acute Kidney Injury Work Group. KDIGO clinical practice guideline for acute kidney injury. *Kidney Int.* 2012;2(suppl 1):1-138.
9. Ostermann M, Bellomo R, Burdmann EA, et al. Controversies in acute kidney injury: conclusions from a Kidney Disease: Improving Global Outcomes (KDIGO) Conference. *Kidney Int.* 2020;98(2):294-309.
10. Kellum JA, Chawla LS, Keener C, et al. The effects of alternative resuscitation strategies on acute kidney injury in patients with septic shock. *Am J Respir Crit Care Med.* 2016;193(3):281-287.

11. Meyhoff TS, Moller MH, Hjortrup PB, et al. Lower vs. higher fluid volumes in sepsis-protocol for a systematic review with meta-analysis. *Acta Anaesthesiol Scand.* 2017;61(8):942-951.
12. Bouchard J, Soroko SB, Chertow GM, et al. Fluid accumulation, survival and recovery of kidney function in critically ill patients with acute kidney injury. *Kidney Int.* 2009;76(4):422-427.
13. Hjortrup PB, Haase N, Bundgaard H, et al. Restricting volumes of resuscitation fluid in adults with septic shock after initial management: the CLASSIC randomised, parallel-group, multicentre feasibility trial. *Intensive Care Med.* 2016;42(11):1695-1705.
14. National Heart Lung Blood Institute Acute Respiratory Distress Syndrome Clinical Trials Network, Wiedemann HP, Wheeler AP, et al. Comparison of two fluid-management strategies in acute lung injury. *N Engl J Med.* 2006;354(24):2564-2575.
15. Myre K, Rostrup M, Buanes T, et al. Plasma catecholamines and haemodynamic changes during pneumoperitoneum. *Acta Anaesthesiol Scand.* 1998;42(3):343-347.
16. Brunkhorst FM, Engel C, Bloos F, et al. Intensive insulin therapy and pentastarch resuscitation in severe sepsis. *N Engl J Med.* 2008;358(2):125-139.
17. Myburgh JA, Finfer S, Bellomo R, et al. Hydroxyethyl starch or saline for fluid resuscitation in intensive care. *N Engl J Med.* 2012;367(20):1901-1911.
18. Perner A, Haase N, Guttormsen AB, et al. Hydroxyethyl starch 130/0.42 versus Ringer's acetate in severe sepsis. *N Engl J Med.* 2012;367(2):124-134.
19. Semler MW, Rice TW. Sepsis resuscitation: fluid choice and dose. *Clin Chest Med.* 2016;37(2):241-250.
20. Young P, Bailey M, Beasley R, et al. Effect of a buffered crystalloid solution vs saline on acute kidney injury among patients in the intensive care unit: the SPLIT randomized clinical trial. *JAMA.* 2015;314(16):1701-1710.
21. Semler MW, Self WH, Wanderer JP, et al. Balanced crystalloids versus saline in critically ill adults. *N Engl J Med.* 2018;378(9):829-839.
22. Self WH, Semler MW, Wanderer JP, et al. Balanced crystalloids versus saline in noncritically ill adults. *N Engl J Med.* 2018;378(9):819-828.
23. Weisbord SD, Gallagher M, Jneid H, et al. Outcomes after angiography with sodium bicarbonate and acetylcysteine. *N Engl J Med.* 2018;378(7):603-614.
24. Valette X, Desmeulles I, Savary B, et al. Sodium bicarbonate versus sodium chloride for preventing contrast-associated acute kidney injury in critically ill patients: a randomized controlled trial. *Crit Care Med.* 2017;45(4):637-644.
25. Palli E, Makris D, Papanikolaou J, et al. The impact of N-acetylcysteine and ascorbic acid in contrast-induced nephropathy in critical care patients: an open-label randomized controlled study. *Crit Care.* 2017;21(1):269.
26. Futier E, Lefrant JY, Guinot PG, et al. Effect of individualized vs standard blood pressure management strategies on postoperative organ dysfunction among high-risk patients undergoing major surgery: a randomized clinical trial. *JAMA.* 2017;318(14):1346-1357.
27. NCEPOD. Acute kidney injury: adding insult to injury. https://www.ncepod.org.uk/2009report1/Downloads/AKI_report.pdf.
28. Goldstein SL, Kirkendall E, Nguyen H, et al. Electronic health record identification of nephrotoxin exposure and associated acute kidney injury. *Pediatrics.* 2013;132(3):e756-e767.
29. Goldstein SL, Mottes T, Simpson K, et al. A sustained quality improvement program reduces nephrotoxic medication-associated acute kidney injury. *Kidney Int.* 2016;90(1):212-221.
30. Goldstein SL, Dahale D, Kirkendall ES, et al. A prospective multi-center quality improvement initiative (NINJA) indicates a reduction in nephrotoxic acute kidney injury in hospitalized children. *Kidney Int.* 2020;97(3):580-588.
31. Bell S, Selby NM, Bagshaw SM. Danger in the jungle: sensible care to reduce avoidable acute kidney injury in hospitalized children. *Kidney Int.* 2020;97(3):458-460.
32. Chandrasekar T, Sharma A, Tennent L, et al. A whole system approach to improving mortality associated with acute kidney injury. *QJM.* 2017;110:657-666.
33. Ebah L, Hanumapura P, Waring D, et al. A multifaceted quality improvement programme to improve acute kidney injury care and outcomes in a large teaching hospital. *BMJ Qual Improv Rep.* 2017;6(1):u219176.w7476.
34. Selby NM, Casula A, Lamming L, et al. An organizational-level program of intervention for AKI: a pragmatic stepped wedge cluster randomized trial. *J Am Soc Nephrol.* 2019;30(3):505-515.
35. Sykes L, Sinha S, Hegarty J, et al. Reducing acute kidney injury incidence and progression in a large teaching hospital. *BMJ Open Qual.* 2018;7(4):e000308.
36. Hodgson LE, Roderick PJ, Venn RM, et al. The ICE-AKI study: impact analysis of a clinical prediction rule and electronic AKI alert in general medical patients. *PLoS One.* 2018;13(8):e0200584.
37. Al-Jaghbeer M, Dealmeida D, Bilderback A, et al. Clinical decision support for in-hospital AKI. *J Am Soc Nephrol.* 2018;29(2):654-660.
38. Wilson FP, Shashaty M, Testani J, et al. Automated, electronic alerts for acute kidney injury: a single-blind, parallel-group, randomised controlled trial. *Lancet.* 2015;385(9981):1966-1974.

39. Gocze I, Jauch D, Gotz M, et al. Biomarker-guided intervention to prevent acute kidney injury after major surgery: the prospective randomized BigpAK study. *Ann Surg.* 2018;267(6):1013-1020.
40. Meersch M, Schmidt C, Hoffmeier A, et al. Prevention of cardiac surgery-associated AKI by implementing the KDIGO guidelines in high risk patients identified by biomarkers: the PrevAKI randomized controlled trial. *Intensive Care Med.* 2017;43(11):1551-1561.
41. Yamada H, Doi K, Tsukamoto T, et al. Low-dose atrial natriuretic peptide for prevention or treatment of acute kidney injury: a systematic review and meta-analysis. *Crit Care.* 2019;23(1):41.
42. Hsu RK, Truwit JD, Matthay MA, et al. Effect of rosuvastatin on acute kidney injury in sepsis-associated acute respiratory distress syndrome. *Can J Kidney Health Dis.* 2018;5. doi:10.1177/2054358118789158
43. Lassnigg A, Donner E, Grubhofer G, et al. Lack of renoprotective effects of dopamine and furosemide during cardiac surgery. *J Am Soc Nephrol.* 2000;11(1):97-104.
44. Friedrich JO, Adhikari N, Herridge MS, et al. Meta-analysis: low-dose dopamine increases urine output but does not prevent renal dysfunction or death. *Ann Intern Med.* 2005;142(7):510-524.
45. Gillies MA, Kakar V, Parker RJ, et al. Fenoldopam to prevent acute kidney injury after major surgery—a systematic review and meta-analysis. *Crit Care.* 2015;19:449.
46. Bove T, Zangrillo A, Guarracino F, et al. Effect of fenoldopam on use of renal replacement therapy among patients with acute kidney injury after cardiac surgery: a randomized clinical trial. *JAMA.* 2014;312(21):2244-2253.
47. Gordon AC, Perkins GD, Singer M, et al. Levosimendan for the prevention of acute organ dysfunction in sepsis. *N Engl J Med.* 2016;375(17):1638-1648.
48. Landoni G, Lomivorotov VV, Alvaro G, et al. Levosimendan for hemodynamic support after cardiac surgery. *N Engl J Med.* 2017;376(21):2021-2031.
49. Mehta RH, Leimberger JD, van Diepen S, et al. Levosimendan in patients with left ventricular dysfunction undergoing cardiac surgery. *N Engl J Med.* 2017;376(21):2032-2042.
50. Elliott S, Tomita D, Endre Z. Erythropoiesis stimulating agents and reno-protection: a meta-analysis. *BMC Nephrol.* 2017;18(1):14.
51. Bloos F, Trips E, Nierhaus A, et al. Effect of sodium selenite administration and procalcitonin-guided therapy on mortality in patients with severe sepsis or septic shock: a randomized clinical trial. *JAMA Intern Med.* 2016;176(9):1266-1276.
52. Xie J, Zhang X, Xu J, et al. Effect of remote ischemic preconditioning on outcomes in adult cardiac surgery: a systematic review and meta-analysis of randomized controlled studies. *Anesth Analg.* 2018;127(1):30-38.
53. Hausenloy DJ, Candilio L, Evans R, et al. Remote ischemic preconditioning and outcomes of cardiac surgery. *N Engl J Med.* 2015;373(15):1408-1417.
54. Garg AX, Kurz A, Sessler DI, et al. Perioperative aspirin and clonidine and risk of acute kidney injury: a randomized clinical trial. *JAMA.* 2014;312(21):2254-2264.

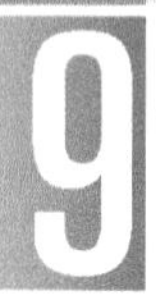

9 Treatment of Acute Kidney Injury

Tanima Arora and Francis Perry Wilson

Acute kidney injury (AKI) is common in the intensive care unit (ICU), with some studies estimating a prevalence of nearly 50%.[1] ICU and inpatient mortality are substantially higher in those with AKI, suggesting that efforts to modify or reverse the injury may lead to substantial improvements in outcome.[2,3] However, to date, no single therapy has been shown to be effective for the treatment of AKI.

ACUTE KIDNEY INJURY IS A HETEROGENEOUS DISEASE

AKI is a syndrome defined by an increase in serum creatinine or a fall in urine output.[4] These changes occur in a variety of pathophysiologic settings including hemodynamic changes, intrinsic kidney injury, inflammation, ischemia, and obstruction (as outlined in Chapter 5). As such, it is not surprising that no single therapy has been shown to be effective at modifying the course of AKI in all clinical scenarios. As an example, the relief of obstructive AKI in the setting of benign prostatic hypertrophy by the placement of a Foley catheter is curative, but this intervention is unlikely to benefit the patient with septic AKI or acute lithium toxicity. The guiding principle for AKI treatment is individualization.

UNIVERSAL TREATMENT MEASURES

Although there is no single treatment that will modify the course of AKI from diffuse etiologies, there is broad scientific consensus that certain universal measures are likely to be beneficial. These include maintenance of kidney perfusion, avoidance of nephrotoxic insults, and appropriate medication dosing.

MAINTENANCE OF KIDNEY PERFUSION

Blood flow through the kidney serves two purposes. First, the blood flow to the kidneys forms the substrate upon which glomerular filtration and tubular modification of the glomerular ultrafiltrate operate. Without this substrate, the glomerular filtration rate (GFR) must necessarily fall. Second, blood flow provides oxygen and removes waste products from the highly metabolically active renal tubules. These cells are located in a hostile environment, with very low oxygen tension and high osmolarity with the potential for large osmolar shifts.[5] It may not be surprising then that tubular epithelial cells often undergo apoptosis and necrosis when systemic hemodynamics are not severe enough to cause diffuse cell damage elsewhere in the body.[6]

AVOIDANCE OF NEPHROTOXIC INSULTS

Although common sense would dictate that further exposure to nephrotoxic agents is counterproductive in the setting of AKI, a careful assessment of the risks and benefits is warranted, lest *renalism*—the sacrifice of good care for fear of worsening kidney function—worsens patient outcomes.[7]

There is perhaps no place where this mentality is clearer than in the use of iodinated contrast. As Cashion and Weisbord point out in Chapter 44, there is substantial debate regarding the nephrotoxicity of current contrast agents in the setting of computed tomography (CT) scans.[8] But even assuming there is some risk of kidney injury, the information gleaned from a necessary CT scan may often outweigh the risk of worsening kidney function. Once again, the watchword is individualization. A careful assessment of the risks and benefits of potentially nephrotoxic agents is key. The development of the systematic screening program called Nephrotoxic Injury Negated by Just-in-Time Action (NINJA), recommending the daily assessment of serum creatinine, has also been implemented for use in hospitalized children with a high risk of nephrotoxic medication–associated AKI in an attempt to counteract the long-term negative outcomes associated with nephrotoxic exposure.[9] Stoops et al demonstrated a reduction of nephrotoxin exposure by 42% and rate of AKI by 78% in their study, applying the NINJA surveillance system to an ICU setting, thus highlighting the efficacy of systematic surveillance of nephrotoxin exposure as an effective method to prevent episodes of AKI.[10]

APPROPRIATE DOSING OF MEDICATION

Many medications are excreted by the kidney and thus may reach supratherapeutic concentrations in the setting of AKI. Even medications that are not directly nephrotoxic, but may lead to other systemic adverse events, must be appropriately dosed when GFR declines. However, *how* to dose-adjust medications in the setting of AKI is somewhat difficult (as discussed in Chapter 26).

Most patients with AKI will not be in steady state with regard to serum creatinine, meaning that an estimate of GFR is not possible using traditional estimating equations, such as the Cockroft-Gault (most commonly used by clinical pharmacists) or Chronic Kidney Disease Epidemiology Collaboration (CKD-EPI) equations.[11] Although equations that attempt to estimate GFR in the setting of dynamic changes in creatinine (e.g., the Jelliffe equation) exist, they have not been uniformly introduced into clinical practice.[12]

Redosing medications must take into account the therapeutic window of the particular medication. Medications with very limited or absent toxicity in high doses do not need to be as aggressively titrated as those with narrow therapeutic indexes. Medications with a low toxicity threshold, such as vancomycin and the aminoglycosides, are best dosed via direct measurement of plasma levels as opposed to estimates of clearance based on serum creatinine or other markers.

INDIVIDUALIZED TREATMENT MEASURES

The above considerations are relevant for essentially all patients with AKI, but the downstream consequences of AKI are key targets for therapy. These include volume overload, electrolyte and acid/base derangement, and uremia.

VOLUME MANAGEMENT

Volume overload is the most common reason for the initiation of dialysis in hospitalized patients with AKI.[13] Hypervolemia has been associated with substantially worse inpatient outcomes, even when adjusting for comorbid disease, suggesting causative links between excessive third spacing of fluids, ventilator-dependent respiratory failure, and poor cardiac function exist.[14] Additionally, patients with severe illness and AKI often have high obligate intake in the form of intravenous medications and hyperalimentation. Without adequate kidney function to excrete this volume load, the clinical course may rapidly decline.

The use of diuretics is specifically *not* advocated by the Kidney Disease Improving Global Outcomes (KDIGO) for the treatment of AKI (as discussed in Chapter 12).[4] However, in the setting of volume overload where an increase in urine output may reduce the risk of intubation or dialysis for volume overload, a trial of diuretics is reasonable. Response to diuretic challenge has been formalized as the "furosemide stress test"—a validated treatment paradigm that identifies patients with a higher likelihood of treatment recovery.[15]

Several algorithms exist to guide choice of diuretics in the setting of volume overload, but broadly two main principles apply. First, the dose chosen should be appropriate for the degree of kidney dysfunction. Second, sequential tubular blockade (e.g., by the combination of loop and thiazide-type diuretics) may be reasonable *after* maximal dosing of a single diuretic class has been achieved. This recommendation is on the basis of several studies that suggest that adding thiazide to loop diuretics before the latter have been titrated appropriately may in fact worsen clinical outcomes.[16]

There are several risks to aggressive diuretic administration. The first is overly exuberant urine output resulting in volume depletion. There is little evidence that this is a common occurrence, and should this occur the treatment (intravenous fluids) is obvious and readily available. Second, and more concerning, diuretics increase a host of neurohormonal mediators via their effect on tubuloglomerular feedback, which may worsen cardiac function.[17] Finally, the unique toxicities of high-dose diuretics (such as ototoxicity in the case of loop diuretics) are worth consideration, but we note that studies demonstrating the ototoxicity of diuretics used markedly higher doses than are commonly used today.[18]

ELECTROLYTE MANAGEMENT

Electrolyte management is a central component of critical care and nephrology, as multiple processes perturb electrolyte concentrations in the critically ill. Details on the mechanisms of electrolyte abnormalities and their appropriate treatment are described in Chapters 19 to 24, but several issues regarding electrolyte management in the setting of AKI bear mentioning.

Although hyperkalemia is a common complication of AKI (as outlined in Chapter 21), hypokalemia is seen in up to 10% of patients with AKI and is often the result of substantial total body potassium depletion. Hypokalemia has several relevant clinical consequences for the critically ill patient; it may prolong ventilation, worsen ammoniagenesis, and precipitate arrhythmias. As such hypokalemia should be treated aggressively in most cases even in the setting of ongoing AKI. An exception to this rule is in the case of anticipated large shifts of potassium from the intracellular to extracellular space (such as in the case of tumor lysis syndrome or rhabdomyolysis), in which case more caution is advised.

As discussed in Chapter 22, hypocalcemia can generally be treated with intravenous (IV) calcium supplementation, but in the case of AKI when hyperphosphatemia is present, the increased calcium load can lead to metastatic calcification and should be avoided. When symptomatic hypocalcemia coexists with severe hyperphosphatemia, the appropriate ultimate therapy is usually dialysis, although IV calcium can be administered to temporize in urgent or emergent situations.

UREA MANAGEMENT

Uremia is a clinical diagnosis, but azotemia, an elevated blood urea nitrogen (BUN), is a reasonable proxy. Critically ill patients often display altered sensoria, diminished levels of consciousness, confusion, and delirium.[19] In the setting of an elevated BUN, distinguishing uremia—which would necessitate dialysis—from benign azotemia can be challenging. Few clinical signs provide objective evidence of uremia, but an otherwise unexplained pericardial effusion should certainly prompt kidney replacement therapy (KRT) in the proper clinical setting.

To avoid potentially unnecessary dialysis, attempting to limit the rise of BUN during AKI is worthwhile. As such, a reduction in the use of catabolic steroids and hyperalimentation (both of which provide "protein loads" as a substrate for urea generation) may be warranted. If this is not clinically feasible, providers should recognize the possibility that an elevated BUN is not necessarily evidence for uremia.

ACUTE KIDNEY INJURY CARE BUNDLES

The concept of an AKI "care bundle" has been proposed as a tool to improve the quality of care of patients with AKI.[20] A care bundle is defined as a method of improving processes of care and patient outcomes: a small, straightforward set of evidence-based practices, treatments, and/or interventions for a defined patient segment population and care setting that, when implemented collectively, significantly improves the reliability of care and patient outcomes beyond that expected when implemented individually.[21] An AKI care bundle is usually not a single intervention, but rather a number of different elements (usually between three and six) that are delivered together as a complex intervention.[22] An example of a care bundle developed by Kolhe et al in 2015 included elements such as fluid assessment, urinalysis, diagnosis of the cause of AKI, ordering investigations, initiating treatment, and referral.[23] A list of the specific elements used in the design of previously studied AKI care bundles is shown in **Table 9.1**.[22] Such care bundles aim to change clinician behaviors and improve delivery of care.[22] Recent data suggested that implementation of specifically designed AKI care bundles can improve processes, lead to more efficient resource use, and potentially improve outcomes.[23,24] However, it may be challenging to design and implement a care bundle for AKI because of heterogeneity of AKI patients, range of clinical settings in acute care, coexisting life-threatening conditions, and uncertainty in the evidence base for how to optimally dose and manage AKI.[25]

KIDNEY REPLACEMENT THERAPY

Management of AKI requires meticulous attention to fluid, acid-base, and electrolyte balance as well as removal of uremic toxins. The above sections detailed individual steps that can be taken to control these factors, but when they present in aggregate, KRT may be the only appropriate solution. For example, nonanion gap metabolic acidosis can be treated with intravenous solutions containing bicarbonate, but in the setting of concomitant volume overload, this is impractical. As discussed in Chapter 31, the decision to initiate KRT then is rarely determined by a single factor (though in emergency situations like life-threatening hyperkalemia, this can be the case) but by a constellation of metabolic derangements that cannot be mutually addressed in the absence of KRT. A "furosemide stress test" can be considered when deciding to start KRT, with nonresponders (those who produce less than 200 mL of urine after a bolus of 1 mg/kg furosemide if furosemide naïve or 1.5 mg/kg if previously exposed to furosemide) predicting a progression to more severe AKI and thus adding weight to the case for KRT initiation.[26]

TABLE 9.1 AKI Care Bundles, Showing Elements Used in Design and Outcomes Observed

Study	Setting	Study Size, Duration, and Design	CB Content	Implementation Approach	Outcomes
Forde et al[37] (2012)	30 bed surgical ward, followed by roll-out to surgical wards and MAU	Initial 6 wk implementation followed by 2 × 2-mo roll-out periods. Before and after implementation comparison. Sample size not reported	5 elements: medication review; manage hypotension; fluid balance; urinalysis; exclude obstruction	Education across the MDT, adapting approach to feedback, measurement of CB usage	In the postimplementation phase, 100% AKI recognition, 80% CB completion in 67% of AKI cases. No process measures or patient outcomes were reported
Tsui et al[24] (2014)	MAU	100 patients, before and after implementation comparison (6 and 4 wk periods, respectively)	11 elements: record baseline creatinine, assess fluid status, urinalysis, medication review (2 elements); urine protein-creatinine ratio; monitor urine output; kidney US; 3 referral elements	Education to junior doctors and at divisional meetings. Advertising posters in MAU	Improvements in the following: documentation of baseline creatinine (52.7%-83%, $p < 0.001$), assessment of fluid status (58.2%-81%, $p < 0.001$), urinalysis (41.8%-92%, $p < 0.001$), nephrotoxic drugs stopped (18.5%-85.7%, $p < 0.001$), kidney dose adjustments (18.5%-83.3%, $p < 0.001$), fluid balance monitoring (10.9%-67.9%, $p < 0.001$), urine protein-creatinine ratio (0.62%, $p < 0.001$), and kidney US (7.27%-75%, $p < 0.001$). Possible reduction in HDU utilization and KRT in ICU but event rates in this sample size were small

Joslin et al[38] (2015)	Hospital wide	192 patients, before (2011) and after (2013) comparison, data collection periods were 7 d	8 elements: patient assessment; fluid therapy; manage hyperkalemia; urinalysis; medication reviews; repeat serum creatinine; kidney US; fluid balance charting	Hospital-wide publicity campaign; AKI audit results presented at educational and induction meetings	Between 2011 and 2013, there were significant improvements in: AKI recognition (59% vs 75%, $p < 0.001$); assessment of fluid status (37% vs 65%, $p < 0.001$); completion of fluid balance chart (32% vs 45%, $p = 0.002$); discontinuation of nephrotoxic medications (27% vs 61%, $p < 0.001$); AKI inclusion in discharge summary (38% vs 55%, p value not presented). No significant improvement in three other measures was observed. Mortality rates were between 12% and 10% pre- and post-CB.

(*continued*)

TABLE 9.1 AKI Care Bundles, Showing Elements Used in Design and Outcomes Observed (*continued*)

Study	Setting	Study Size, Duration, and Design	CB Content	Implementation Approach	Outcomes
Kolhe et al[23] (2015)	Hospital wide	2,297 patients; 306 had CB completion within 24 hr of AKI. Retrospective observational study	6 elements; fluid assessment; urinalysis; diagnose cause of AKI; order investigations; initiate treatment; referral	CB linked to electronic alert. Education to junior doctors and at divisional meetings. Advertising posters in wards	Lower mortality with CB completion (18% vs 23.1%, $p = 0.0046$), lower progression to higher AKI stages (3.9% vs 8.1%, $p = 0.01$). Differences maintained in logistic regression analysis. Process measures not collected, although data on proportions of patients who received individual elements of CB are presented
Tsui et al[24] (2014)	Hospital wide	3,518 patients; analysis of 939 with CB and 1,823 without. Retrospective propensity score case-control analysis	As above	As above	Mortality lower (20.4% vs 24.4%, $p = 0.017$) and AKI progression lower (4.2% vs 6.7%, $p = 0.02$) in those with CB completion. Differences maintained in logistic regression analysis. Process measures not collected

AKI, acute kidney injury; CB, care bundle; HDU, high-dependency unit; ICU, intensive care unit; MAU, medical admissions unit; MDT, multidisciplinary team; KRT, kidney replacement therapy; US, ultrasound.

KDIGO guidelines state that KRT should be initiated emergently when life-threatening changes in fluid, electrolyte, and acid-base balance exist, but clinical decision-making may take precedence in nonlife-threatening instances, where KRT may be delayed.[27] However, many randomized controlled trials that have compared strategies of early versus delayed initiation of KRT have yielded conflicting results.[28-30] A meta-analysis of 11 randomized trials showed no difference between early and late initiation on the risk of dialysis dependence, length of ICU stay, or recovery of renal function.[31]

As Ramakrishnan and Vijayan review in Chapter 32, a wide array of modalities are available for KRT, including intermittent hemodialysis (IHD), peritoneal dialysis (PD), continuous kidney replacement therapy (CKRT), and hybrid therapies such as sustained low-efficacy hemodialysis (SLED). Optimal choice of dialysis modality and dosage, based on individual indications, is important for the efficacious management of AKI (**Figure 9.1**). KDIGO suggests the use of IHD and CKRT as complementary therapies for the management of patients with AKI; however, some studies have shown CKRT to be more advantageous than IHD.[32] There is superior management of volume overload and nutritional requirements because of more consistent net salt and water removal in hemodynamically unstable patients.[33] In addition, enhanced clearance of inflammatory mediators, alongside better preservation of cerebral perfusion in patients with acute brain injury and fulminant hepatic failure, is seen with CKRT.[34]

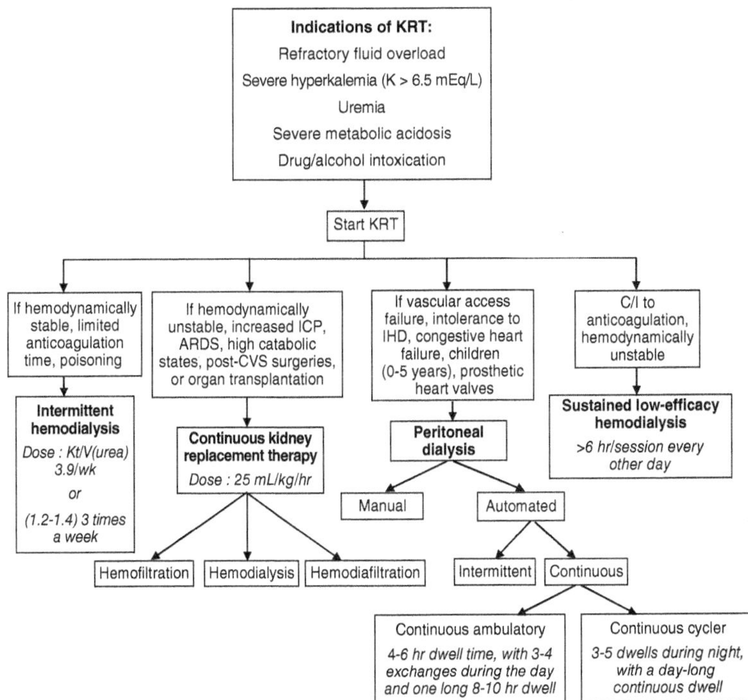

FIGURE 9.1: Indications, types, and dosages in KRT for the management of AKI. AKI, acute kidney injury; ARDS, acute respiratory distress syndrome; CVS, cardio-vascular surgery; ICP, intracranial pressure; IHD, intermittent hemodialysis; KRT, kidney replacement therapy.

A vascular access must be obtained for the use of KRT in AKI (explained in Chapter 29). The suggested lengths of the catheter used are based on the site of insertion as follows: right internal jugular vein 15 cm, left internal jugular vein 20 cm, femoral vein 25 cm. Whenever possible, ultrasound guidance for catheter insertion should be employed. The most common complications associated with the use of KRT in the management of AKI are fluid volume deficiency because of excessive ultrafiltration without adequate volume replacement, electrolyte abnormalities (e.g., low phosphorus, low magnesium, low potassium), hypothermia, air embolus, and filter clotting.

NOVEL THERAPIES

In light of the expanding research in the domain of AKI treatment, many novel therapies have been studied and clinical trials have been conducted to improve outcomes for patients with AKI. Kyung Jo et al, in their 2007 review,[35] highlight some of the therapies that have recently been implemented in the care of AKI. These include antiapoptotic/necrotic agents, free radical scavengers, antisepsis agents such as ethyl pyruvate, growth factors such as recombinant erythropoietin (EPO) and hepatocyte growth factor, vasodilators, and anti-inflammatory drugs such as sphingosine-1-phosphate analogs, $\alpha 2$ agonists, inducible nitric oxide (NO) synthase inhibitors, and fibrates. Likewise, Kaushal and Shah[36] also elaborate on these therapies and introduce the use of α-melanocyte-stimulating hormone, small interfering ribonucleic acid (RNA) proteins, bone morphogenetic family of proteins, mesenchymal stem cells, RenalGuard Therapy (a closed-loop fluid management system), alkaline phosphatase, catalytic iron, renal cell therapy, and bioartificial renal epithelial cell system therapy. Implementation of such new therapies to prevent or treat AKI requires further research and collaborative efforts from academic institutions, private industry, and the federal governments and the conduct of well-designed clinical trials.

ACKNOWLEDGMENT

Dr. Wilson is supported by grants R01DK113191 and P30DK079210.

References

1. Joannidis M, Metnitz B, Bauer P, et al. Acute kidney injury in critically ill patients classified by AKIN versus RIFLE using the SAPS 3 database. *Intensive Care Med.* 2009;35(10):1692-1702.
2. Bagshaw SM, Uchino S, Kellum JA, et al. Association between renal replacement therapy in critically ill patients with severe acute kidney injury and mortality. *J Crit Care.* 2013;28(6):1011-1018.
3. Coca SG, Singanamala S, Parikh CR. Chronic kidney disease after acute kidney injury: a systematic review and meta-analysis. *Kidney Int.* 2012;81(5):442-448.
4. Kidney Disease: Improving Global Outcomes (KDIGO) Acute Kidney Injury Work Group. KDIGO clinical practice guideline for acute kidney injury. *Kidney Int.* 2012;2(suppl):1-138.
5. Epstein FH. Oxygen and renal metabolism. *Kidney Int.* 1997;51(2):381-385.
6. Devarajan P. Update on mechanisms of ischemic acute kidney injury. *J Am Soc Nephrol.* 2006;17(6):1503-1520.
7. Chertow GM, Normand S-LT, McNeil BJ. "Renalism": inappropriately low rates of coronary angiography in elderly individuals with renal insufficiency. *J Am Soc Nephrol.* 2004;15(9):2462-2468.
8. Wilhelm-Leen E, Montez-Rath ME, Chertow G. Estimating the risk of radiocontrast-associated nephropathy. *J Am Soc Nephrol.* 2017;28(2):653-659.
9. Goldstein SL, Kirkendall E, Nguyen H, et al. Electronic health record identification of nephrotoxin exposure and associated acute kidney injury. *Pediatrics.* 2013;132(3):e756-e767.
10. Stoops C, Stone S, Evans E, et al. Baby NINJA (Nephrotoxic Injury Negated by Just-in-Time Action): reduction of nephrotoxic medication-associated acute kidney injury in the neonatal intensive care unit. *J Pediatr.* 2019;215:223-228.e6.

11. Nielsen AL, Henriksen DP, Marinakis C, et al. Drug dosing in patients with renal insufficiency in a hospital setting using electronic prescribing and automated reporting of estimated glomerular filtration rate. *Basic Clin Pharmacol Toxicol.* 2014;114(5):407-413.
12. Bouchard J, Macedo E, Soroko S, et al. Comparison of methods for estimating glomerular filtration rate in critically ill patients with acute kidney injury. *Nephrol Dial Transplant.* 2009;25(1):102-107.
13. Bagshaw SM, Wald R, Barton J, et al. Clinical factors associated with initiation of renal replacement therapy in critically ill patients with acute kidney injury—a prospective multicenter observational study. *J Crit Care.* 2012;27(3):268-275.
14. Teixeira C, Garzotto F, Piccinni P, et al. Fluid balance and urine volume are independent predictors of mortality in acute kidney injury. *Crit Care.* 2013;17(1):R14.
15. Koyner JL, Davison DL, Brasha-Mitchell E, et al. Furosemide stress test and biomarkers for the prediction of AKI severity. *J Am Soc Nephrol.* 2015;26(8):2023-2031.
16. Brisco-Bacik MA, ter Maaten JM, Houser SR, et al. Outcomes associated with a strategy of adjuvant metolazone or high-dose loop diuretics in acute decompensated heart failure: a propensity analysis. *J Am Heart Assoc.* 2018;7(18):e009149.
17. Francis GS, Goldsmith SR, Levine TB, Olivari MT, Cohn JN. The neurohumoral axis in congestive heart failure. *Ann Intern Med.* 1984;101(3):370-377.
18. Rybak L. Ototoxicity of loop diuretics. *Otolaryngol Clin North Am.* 1993;26(5):829-844.
19. Ouimet S, Kavanagh BP, Gottfried SB, Skrobik Y. Incidence, risk factors and consequences of ICU delirium. *Intensive Care Med.* 2007;33(1):66-73.
20. Hoste EAJ, De Corte W. Implementing the kidney disease: improving global outcomes/acute kidney injury guidelines in ICU patients. *Curr Opin Crit Care.* 2013;19(6):544-553.
21. Resar R, Griffin FA, Haraden C, Nolan TW. *Using Care Bundles to Improve Health Care Quality.* IHI Innovation Series white paper. Institute for Healthcare Improvement; 2012.
22. Selby NM, Kolhe NV. Care bundles for acute kidney injury: do they work? *Nephron.* 2016;134(3):195-199.
23. Kolhe NV, Staples D, Reilly T, et al. Impact of compliance with a care bundle on acute kidney injury outcomes: a prospective observational study. *PLoS One.* 2015;10(7):e0132279-e0132279.
24. Tsui A, Rajani C, Doshi R, et al. Improving recognition and management of acute kidney injury. *Acute Med.* 2014;13(3):108-112.
25. Bagshaw SM. Acute kidney injury care bundles. *Nephron.* 2015;131(4):247-251.
26. Chawla LS, Davison DL, Brasha-Mitchell E, et al. Development and standardization of a furosemide stress test to predict the severity of acute kidney injury. *Crit Care.* 2013;17(5):R207.
27. Palevsky PM, Liu KD, Brophy PD, et al. KDOQI US commentary on the 2012 KDIGO clinical practice guideline for acute kidney injury. *Am J Kidney Dis.* 2013;61(5):649-672.
28. Gaudry S, Hajage D, Schortgen F, et al. Initiation strategies for renal-replacement therapy in the intensive care unit. *N Engl J Med.* 2016;375(2):122-133.
29. Jamale TE, Hase NK, Kulkarni M, et al. Earlier-start versus usual-start dialysis in patients with community-acquired acute kidney injury: a randomized controlled trial. *Am J Kidney Dis.* 2013;62(6):1116-1121.
30. Wald R, Adhikari NKJ, Smith OM, et al. Comparison of standard and accelerated initiation of renal replacement therapy in acute kidney injury. *Kidney Int.* 2015;88(4):897-904.
31. Besen BAMP, Romano TG, Mendes PV, et al. Early versus late initiation of renal replacement therapy in critically ill patients: systematic review and meta-analysis. *J Intensive Care Med.* 2019;34(9):714–722.
32. Augustine JJ, Sandy D, Seifert TH, Paganini EP. A randomized controlled trial comparing intermittent with continuous dialysis in patients with ARF. *Am J Kidney Dis.* 2004;44(6): 1000-1007.
33. Bouchard J, Soroko SB, Chertow GM, et al. Fluid accumulation, survival and recovery of kidney function in critically ill patients with acute kidney injury. *Kidney Int.* 2009;76(4):422-427.
34. Davenport A, Will EJ, Davison AM. Continuous vs. intermittent forms of haemofiltration and/or dialysis in the management of acute renal failure in patients with defective cerebral autoregulation at risk of cerebral oedema. *Contrib Nephrol.* 1991;93:225-233.
35. Jo SK, Rosner MH, Okusa MD. Pharmacologic treatment of acute kidney injury: why drugs haven't worked and what is on the horizon. *Clin J Am Soc Nephrol.* 2007;2(2):356-365.
36. Kaushal GP, Shah SV. Challenges and advances in the treatment of AKI. *J Am Soc Nephrol.* 2014;25(5):877-883.
37. Forde C, McCaughan J, Leonard L. Acute kidney injury: it's as easy as ABCDE. *BMJ Qual Improv Rep.* 2012;1(1):u200370.w326.
38. Joslin J, Wilson H, Zubli D, et al. Recognition and management of acute kidney injury in hospitalised patients can be partially improved with the use of a care bundle. *Clin Med (Lond).* 2015;15(5):431-436.

SECTION III

Drugs and Blood Products in the Intensive Care Unit Setting

10 Resuscitation Fluids: Which One, How Much, and How to Assess

Anna Gaddy, Sai Sudha Mannemuddhu, Priti Meena, and Joel M. Topf

INTRODUCTION

Increasingly, intensivists and nephrologists are treating intravenous (IV) fluids like drugs. That means individualizing the type and dose of fluids for each patient. The days of 100 mL/hr of normal saline for every patient in the intensive care unit (ICU) are over. The 21st century has been marked by three fundamental questions regarding resuscitation fluids in the ICU:

1. Crystalloids or colloids: which is better?
2. Within crystalloids, are balanced solutions better than isotonic saline?
3. How much IV fluids should we be giving patients?

After a brief overview of the role IV fluids play in the ICU, each of these questions will be summarized, looking at the major trials that have attempted to answer these questions.

THE ROLE OF INTRAVENOUS FLUIDS IN THE INTENSIVE CARE UNIT

IV fluids are given to just about every patient in the ICU. They are used to carry medications, bypassing the gastrointestinal (GI) tract that is often unreliable in critically ill patients. They are used to adjust serum tonicity in dysnatremia and providing nutrition, and they have a central role in the treatment of shock and sepsis. (See **Table 10.1**).

IV fluids come in various compositions designed to achieve various goals (**Table 10.2**). The standard teaching of IV fluids divides the body water into three

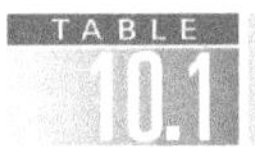

TABLE 10.1 Role of Intravenous Fluids

Role of Intravenous Fluids
Treatment of sepsis
Increase in blood pressure
Replace fluid losses
Change osmolality (up or down)
As a carrier fluid for other medicines and electrolytes
Nutrition
Increasing urine output

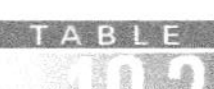

TABLE 10.2 Compositions of Various Intravenous Fluids

IV Fluid	Na	K	Ca	Cl	Alkali	Glucose	Osmolality	Albumin	HES
	mmol/L					g/L	mOsm/kg	g/L	
Normal Composition of Human Plasma									
Plasma	135-145	3.5-5.1	2.1-2.55	98-107	22-29 HCO_3	0.007-0.0105	275-295	35-50	
Dextrose Solutions[1]									
D5 water	–	–	–	–	–	50[a]	252	–	–
Crystalloid Solutions[2]									
0.9% saline	154	–	–	154	–	–	308	–	–
0.45% saline	77	–	–	77	–	–	154	–	–
3% saline	513	–	–	513	–	–	1,026	–	–
D5 0.9% saline	154	–	–	154	–	50[a]	560	–	–
Ringer's lactate	130	4	3	109	28 Lactate	–	272	–	–
Plasma-Lyte A	140	5	–	98	27 Acetate	–	294	–	–
Colloid Solutions[3]									
Albumin 5%	154	–	–	154	–	–	308	50	–
Albumin 25%	154	–	–	154	–	–	1,500[2]	250	–
HES (6%)	154	–	–	154	–	–	310	–	60

HES, hydroxyethyl starch; IV, intravenous.

[a]Dextrose solutions actually contain glucose monohydrate (molecular weight [MW] 198) rather than dextrose (MW 180).

1. Dextrose solutions: These fluids are mostly like free water. The classic physiologic teaching has two-thirds of the water in dextrose solutions moving into the intracellular compartment and one-third distributed between the interstitial and plasma compartments at a 3:1 ratio, so that for every liter of D5W, roughly 660 mL moves to the intracellular compartment, 250 mL into the interstitial compartment, and only 80 mL remains in the plasma compartment. They are good for treating hypernatremia and hypoglycemia. When dextrose solutions are used as maintenance fluid, patients are at risk for hyponatremia.[3] They can be mixed with crystalloids, but in terms of fluid distribution, the crystalloid component determines where the volume ends up. So D5 0.9% NaCl distributes like 0.9% NaCl, not D5W.
2. Crystalloid solutions: These are aqueous solutions of mineral salts and other small, water-soluble molecules. In the classic description of crystalloid fluid distribution, they deliver volume solely to the extracellular compartments, with 75% going to the interstitial compartment and 25% going to the plasma compartment. Crystalloids can further be categorized as saline solutions or balanced solutions. Saline solutions are made of water and sodium chloride, whereas balanced solutions have numerous ingredients in an attempt to mirror the content and concentrations found in human plasma.
3. Colloid solutions: These are fluids with large, osmotically active particles that are intended to be trapped in the plasma compartment. The prototypical colloid solution is albumin. Synthetic colloids, like HES, are intended to have the same benefits as albumin but are less expensive.

compartments: intracellular, interstitial, and the plasma compartment. This model was used to divide IV fluids into three broad categories of fluids.

The classic physiology of IV fluids described depends largely on Starling equation, which states that movement of fluids is driven by hydrostatic capillary pressure and interstitial protein osmotic pressure, counteracted by plasma protein osmotic pressure and interstitial pressure.[4] (See **Figure 10.1**). This classical view of capillary physiology has been challenged by in vitro and in vivo observations. One of the central aspects of the model is the movement of interstitial fluid back into the capillary at the venous end of the capillary bed. Contemporary studies do not show fluid moving back into the vasculature. Without this movement back into the capillary, traditional Starling values result in fluid movement from the plasma to the interstitium that is 5- to 10-fold higher than lymph flow. This cannot be, so Starling's equation needs an adjustment to decrease flow from the capillaries to match the lymph flow draining them. The adjustment comes in the form of an additional osmotic barrier beyond the endothelial cells. The capillaries are lined with a 2-µm-thick endothelial glycocalyx layer (EGL). This layer decreases the flow from the plasma to the interstitial compartment. The EGL and its transport characteristics change in response to sepsis, surgery, trauma, and hypotension.[5]

The recognition of these changes in Starling equation can be used to explain one of the recurring observations regarding the use of colloids versus crystalloid solutions. Colloids should be trapped in the plasma space, whereas roughly only a quarter of isotonic saline solution should remain in the plasma. But instead of the expected 1:4 or 1:5 ratio of albumin to isotonic saline required to get equivalent plasma expansion, blinded studies only showed a 1:1.4 ratio.[6] Similarly, in a 2001 study of perioperative patients given 1.3 L of isotonic albumin or hydroxyethyl starch (HES), only 40% of the volume remained in the plasma compartment 30 minutes after the infusion.[7] Additionally, the revised Starling equation showed that even highly concentrated albumin infusions (25% albumin) will not be effective at drawing fluid from the interstitial compartment and restore that to the plasma compartment. There is some disagreement on these points.[8]

THE QUESTIONS

Crystalloids or Colloids: Which Is a Better Solution?

Traditional fluid physiology indicates that colloids should remain in the vascular space better than crystalloids so they should be much better at volume resuscitation. However, in 1998, a Cochrane systematic review and meta-analysis showed a higher mortality rate with the use of albumin compared to saline.[9] This analysis led to the SAFE trial, a randomized controlled trial (RCT) of saline versus albumin that revealed no difference in 28-day mortality.[6]

Albumin

Albumin is the main protein constituent of human plasma, and it constitutes approximately 80% of normal colloid oncotic pressure. It is commercially available as a slightly hypo-oncotic 4% solution, iso-oncotic 5% solution, and hyperoncotic 20% and 25% solution. Normally, transcapillary leakage rate of albumin is 5% per hour; however, this rate was 40% in 30 minutes in a trial of perioperative patients.[7,10]

The SAFE trial, a randomized, multicenter, double-blind trial involving 6,997 patients, found no difference in patient survival between 4% albumin and 0.9% normal saline (NS) in critically ill patients. During the initial 4 days, the overall

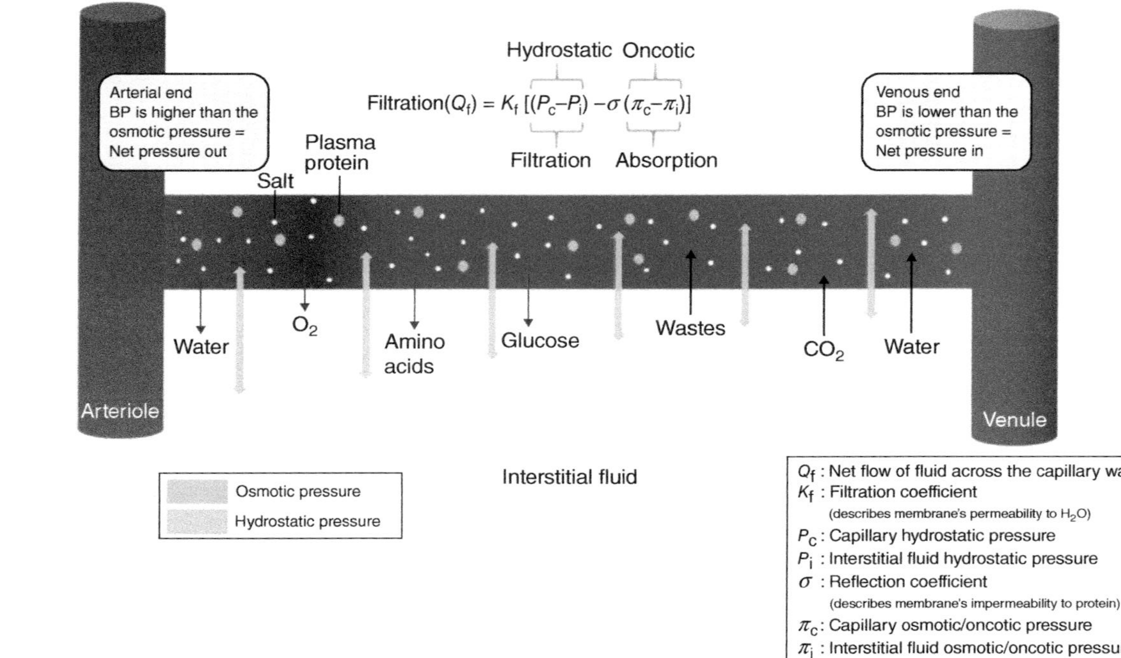

FIGURE 10.1: Exchange across the capillary bed and Starling forces. Exchange at the capillary beds is primarily as a result of net osmotic (oncotic) and hydrostatic (blood) pressures. BP, blood pressure.

ratio of volume of albumin to the volume of saline was approximately 1:1.4. After those first days there was no difference in the volume of fluids administered between the groups. Of note, the study did have two important findings in subgroup analysis:

1. Trauma patients had a worse outcome with 4% albumin.
2. Septic patients had a trend toward improved survival with albumin.

The trauma patients that drove the adverse finding for albumin were specifically patients with traumatic brain injury. A subsequent post hoc analysis of SAFE confirmed increased mortality with albumin in patients with traumatic brain injury.[11]

In the Albumin Italian Outcome Sepsis (ALBIOS) open-label randomized trial, patients were randomized to a protocol of daily infusions of 60 g of albumin (in the form of 300 mL of 20% albumin solutions) in order to keep the serum albumin above 3 g/dL. Both groups received crystalloid infusions as clinically indicated. The albumin group had higher mean arterial pressures, lower net fluid balance, but no difference in mortality, total volume of fluid administered, incidence of acute kidney injury (AKI), or need for dialysis.[12]

Surviving Sepsis Campaign recommended the use of albumin for initial resuscitation and subsequent volume replacement only in patients with sepsis and septic shock requiring high volumes of crystalloid solutions. The guidelines describe the albumin recommendation as "weak" supported by low-quality evidence.[13]

There is a lack of evidence to suggest a beneficial role of albumin use in patients with burns, trauma, and malnutrition.[14]

In an observational study of colloids, hyperoncotic albumin (20%-25% albumin) was associated with more kidney events (doubling of serum creatinine or need for dialysis) (odds ratio [OR] 5.99 [2.75-13.08]) and increased ICU mortality (OR 2.79 [1.42-5.47]) in a propensity-matched sample when compared to crystalloids. Albumin with lower osmolality (as used in SAFE) did not show this signal. A possible explanation is that increased capillary oncotic pressure from the infused albumin slows filtration at the glomerulus.[15]

In cirrhosis, albumin is used for a number of indications. This is covered in Chapter 42.

Hydroxyethyl Starch (HES)

HES is a glucose polymer with hydroxyethyl substitutions at some of the carbons. Its molecular weight varies from 70 to 670 kDa.[2]

The use of HES for resuscitation in critically ill patients has been examined in multiple randomized trials and meta-analyses.[16] The three most important trials are CHEST, 6S, and CRYSTAL.[17,18]

- CHEST randomized 7,000 ICU patients to either 6% HES (130/0.4) or NS. There was no difference in 90-day mortality. However, a higher number of patients in the HES group were treated with kidney replacement therapy (KRT). Post hoc analysis found a dose-response increase in the risk of AKI with HES compared to saline.
- In 6S, 804 patients were randomized to HES (130/0.4) or Ringer's acetate. The HES group had increased mortality at 90 days and was more likely to require KRT.
- CRYSTAL had a different question and study design. It did not test a specific colloid, but each participating institution used their colloid of choice. They

randomized 2,857 patients. The experimental group included gelatins, albumin, dextrans, and HES solutions. Additionally, this trial included the entire resuscitation period, whereas the other studies had a delay in starting the study fluids (6S: 14 hours, CHEST: 12 hours) so the intervention did not include the initial resuscitation. CRYSTAL failed to show a mortality benefit at 28 days (the primary outcome), but colloids did show improved mortality at 90 days. There was no signal of increased AKI.[19]

The AKI from HES is believed to be due to osmotic nephrosis, with vacuolization and swelling of the proximal tubule.[20] Other adverse effects from HES include coagulopathy and rare allergic reactions.[21]

Given the adverse events, increased AKI, and a lack of clear clinical benefit, the Kidney Disease Improving Global Outcomes (KDIGO) AKI guidelines recommend against using synthetic colloids for volume resuscitation.[22]

Therefore, given the current data, the answer to the first question, "Crystalloids or Colloids: Which is a better solution?," *appears to be crystalloids.* (**Table 10.3**) summarizes important clinical trials comparing colloids and crystalloids.

Within Crystalloids, Are Balanced Solutions Better Than Isotonic Saline?

Balanced Solutions

As seen from Table 10.2, NS, though isotonic, differs greatly from the electrolyte composition of plasma. Every liter of NS delivers around 50 mmol more chloride than a liter of plasma. This chloride is core to the central concern regarding saline. The increased chloride gets filtered at the glomerulus, overwhelms proximal tubule reabsorption, and trips salt detectors in the macula densa of the thick ascending loop of Henle. These salt detectors are part of the tubular glomerular feedback system and, when activated, cause mesangial contraction and vasoconstriction of the afferent arteriole, decreasing both renal blood flow and glomerular filtration rate (GFR).[23]

In denervated dog kidneys, chloride-containing fluids lowered renal blood flow and GFR compared to nonchloride fluids. Sodium-containing fluids did not have this effect.[24] In healthy volunteers, time to micturition was longer with large volumes (50 mL/kg) of saline than with lactated Ringers (LR).[25] Looking at patients, a propensity-matched, retrospective analysis of 22,851 noncardiac surgical patients found a chloride level greater than 110 to be associated with longer length of stay and increased mortality.[26] High-chloride fluids used in resuscitation were similarly associated with worse outcomes in SIRS.[27] A double-blind RCT of saline versus balanced solutions in major abdominal surgery had to be stopped after 60 patients (of a planned 240) because of a safety signal; 97% of saline patients, compared with only 67% of balanced solution patients, required vasopressors.[28] The potential for AKI from high-chloride fluids became very apparent after Yunos et al published their prospective, open-label, sequential period study of 760 patients. Patients during the low-chloride period (largely balanced solutions) had an OR of KRT of 0.52.[29]

Following the data of Yunos et al, in 2015 the SPLIT trial became the first, major, randomized, double-blind, head-to-head comparison of balanced solution (Plasma-Lyte in this case) versus saline in a group of ICU patients in New Zealand.[30] There was no significant difference in rates of AKI between groups treated with NS versus Plasma-Lyte, nor was there a significant difference in need for KRT or mortality. It is worth noting that a large proportion of patients in this study were postsurgical patients and that the median volume of fluid administered was 2 L.

TABLE 10.3 Clinical Trials Comparing Colloids and Crystalloids

Trial	Type	*N*	Treatment Arms	Primary Outcomes and Results
SAFE study[11]	Multicenter RCT in ICU	6,997	3,497: 4% albumin 3,500: NS	All-cause mortality within 28 d: albumin vs NS: 20% vs 21%, $p = 0.87$
Cooper et al[40]	Single-center RCT. Hypotension and TBI	229	114: 7.5% saline 115: RL	No significant difference between the groups in favorable outcomes (moderate disability and good outcome survivors) (risk ratio, 0.99; 95% CI, 0.76-1.30; $p = 0.96$) or in any other measure of postinjury neurologic function
Bulger et al[41]	Multicenter. Three group RCTs (US and Canada)		7.5% saline/6% dextran 70 7.5% saline NS	6-mo neurologic outcome: no difference among groups Severe TBI: hypertonic saline/dextran vs NS: 53.7% vs 51.5%; hypertonic saline vs NS: 54.3% vs 51.5%
Yunos et al[29]	Prospective, open-label, sequential period pilot study	1,533	760: Cl-rich fluids (NS, 4% succinylated gelatin, or 4% albumin) 773: Cl poor (Hartmann solution), a balanced solution (Plasma-Lyte), and Cl-poor 20% albumin	Cl-rich vs Cl-restrictive Mean change in serum creatinine level: 22.6 vs 14.8 μmol/L, $p = 0.03$ The incidence of injury and failure class of RIFLE-defined AKI: 14% vs 8.4%, $p < 0.001$ Use of KRT was 10% vs 6.3%, $p = 0.005$

(*continued*)

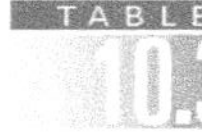

TABLE 10.3 Clinical Trials Comparing Colloids and Crystalloids (*continued*)

Trial	Type	*N*	Treatment Arms	Primary Outcomes and Results
CRIS[19]	Multicenter RCT. Sepsis, trauma, or hypovolemic shock without sepsis or trauma. 57 ICUs	2,857	1,414: Colloids (gelatins, dextrans, HES, or 4% or 20% of albumin) 1,443: Crystalloids: isotonic or hypertonic saline or RL	All-cause mortality within 28 d: colloids vs crystalloids: 25.4% vs 27%, $p = 0.26$
ALBIOS[12]	Multicenter sepsis study. 100 ICUs	1,818	895: 20% albumin + crystalloid 900: Crystalloid	All-cause mortality at 28 d: 31.8% in albumin vs 32%, $p = 0.94$
SPLIT[30]	Multicenter RCT. New Zealand	2,278	1,152: buffered crystalloid 1,110: NS	Buffered crystalloid vs NS AKI within 90 d: 9.6% vs 9.2%, $p = 0.77$ KRT: 3.3% vs 3.4%, $p = 0.91$
Pfortmueller et al[28]	Single-center RCT (Austria)	60	30: NS 30: balanced crystalloids	Need for vasopressors during hospitalization: NS vs balanced crystalloid: 97% vs 67%, $p = 0.033$. Terminated because of safety issues

AKI, acute kidney injury; CI, confidence interval; HES, hydroxyethyl starch; ICU, intensive care unit; NS, normal saline; RCT, randomized controlled trial; RL, Ringer's lactate; KRT, kidney replacement therapy; TBI, traumatic brain injury.

A follow-up study, SPLIT-Plus, is underway to evaluate 90-day mortality between saline and Plasma-Lyte in critically ill patients. Generalizability of these results is most likely sound despite minor differences in composition of parenteral fluids around the world. In 2018, the Smart Trial assigned nearly 16,000 critically ill patients to receive NS or balanced solutions.[31] Patients who received balanced solutions had less major adverse kidney events at 30 days (composite of death, persistent kidney dysfunction, or need for KRT). The median volume of fluid administered in either group was only around 1 L. Subgroup analyses revealed more marked benefit from balanced solutions in patients with sepsis. These findings were echoed by the 2018 SALT-ED trial, which found patients treated with balanced crystalloid in the emergency department had significantly less adverse kidney events than those treated with NS.[32]

Despite these findings, saline remains a popular fluid for resuscitation. Part of this is the inertia of "this is how we always did it" and part of this is likely due to beliefs about balanced solutions, some of which do not hold up to scrutiny:

- **Can you use LR in patients with liver failure? Probably not.** Lactate is converted to pyruvate in the liver, generating a bicarbonate ion. In liver failure, it is presumed this is inhibited and LR is generally contraindicated in cirrhosis and liver failure.[33]
- **Can LR cause lactic acidosis? No.** The lactate in LR is sodium lactate, not lactic acid, so it cannot cause lactic acidosis. It can, however, increase the serum lactate, so some caution should be used when using lactate to judge the adequacy of resuscitation.[34]
- **Is LR contraindicated in hyperkalemia? No.** LR has 4 mmol/L of potassium, so diluting plasma with a normal potassium should not raise the serum potassium. Additionally, because NS causes a nonanion gap metabolic acidosis, this may cause movement of potassium from inside to outside of the cell. In studies of LR versus NS following kidney transplant, there was less hyperkalemia with LR.[35,36]
- **Can you run LR with a blood transfusion? No.** Blood transfusions use citrate anticoagulation to prevent clotting. The calcium in LR is the antidote to citrate and could inadvertently cause the blood to clot.

Isotonic Saline

Though the data seem to be tipping toward balanced solutions over normal saline, there are some situations where NS is superior to balanced solutions. Metabolic alkalosis is one. Most cases of metabolic alkalosis are due to a chloride deficiency, so the high-chloride content of NS makes it a good match for this condition.[37] Neurosurgery and traumatic brain injury are another area where caution should be used with balanced solutions. Though LR is nearly iso-osmolar, the lactate is not an effective osmole, so the fluid is slightly hypotonic. This means it can cause a shift of fluid into the brain and increase intracranial pressure.[38,39]

Lastly, NS is preferred in situations where LR is contraindicated such as liver failure and hypercalcemia.

Hypertonic Saline

There are some specific scenarios in which hypertonic saline has been suggested as a resuscitation fluid. One scenario is traumatic brain injury with the aim of decreasing cerebral edema. Cooper et al used this to successfully increase serum tonicity but did not improve mortality or neurologic outcomes.[40] An attempt to use 7.5% saline in prehospital patients with trauma was stopped early because of futility and safety concerns.[41] The HYPERS2S trial, which randomized patients in septic shock to resuscitation with either 0.9% or 3% saline, did not show a survival benefit with hypertonic saline and it was terminated early because of increased mortality in the hypertonic saline arm.[42] Some heart failure researchers have used hypertonic saline in conjunction with loop diuretics to treat refractory acute decompensated heart failure with some efficacy.[43]

And so given the current data, the answer to the second question, "Saline or balanced solutions: Which is a better solution?," *in most cases, appears to be balanced solutions.*

How Should We Dose Resuscitation Fluids?

Beyond determining which type of fluid, the dose of fluids is important. In 2001, the Rivers trial on early goal-directed therapy (EGDT) showed a dramatic improvement in mortality for patients presenting with severe sepsis and influenced international guidelines and sepsis treatment for over a decade.[44] Patients received an average of 5 L of fluid over the first 6 hours. Current Surviving Sepsis guidelines recommend an initial bolus of 30 mL/kg to be followed by additional fluid to maintain and improve perfusion.[13]

Enthusiasm for EGDT has waned as three large, multicenter trials failed to reproduce the results of the Rivers trial. (See **Table 10.4**). Although the three multicenter trials of EGDT did not show improved outcomes, they also did not show harm. However, when EGDT for sepsis was studied in low-resource Zambia,[45] there was a profound increase in mortality, 33% usual care and 48% with EGDT.

The study of Andrews et al is not the only data to call into question the safety and wisdom of large-volume resuscitation. The FEAST trial[46] compared initial resuscitation strategies in African children with sepsis (largely because of malaria). Similar to SAFE, there was no difference between albumin and saline boluses, but *both were significantly worse than no bolus at all.* So despite the questionable generalizability of using septic children in Africa, this remains the only explicit RCT of the use of a bolus for the initial management of septic shock.

To try to understand the contradictions and unintuitive findings of the above trials, multiple trials have evaluated liberal versus restrictive use of fluids in various settings.

The CLASSIC study was a single-center trial of 153 patients that randomized patients to restricted versus liberal fluid protocol in septic patients. There was a separation of 1.2 L of resuscitation fluid at 5 days and 1.4 L at the end of the ICU stay. There was no difference in outcomes or adverse events between the two groups, although the study was not powered for this finding. Of interest to readers of this handbook, there was *less* worsening of AKI in the restricted protocol arm.[47]

A retrospective review of sepsis treatment in New York looked at the time to completion of a three-part sepsis bundle: antibiotics, measurement of lactate, and receiving bolus fluids. The time to completion of the bundle was critical to patient survival, but this was entirely dependent on the time to antibiotics. Time to completion of the fluid bolus was irrelevant.[48]

The Acute Respiratory Distress Syndrome (ARDS) trial[49] in 2006 compared a conservative versus liberal fluid strategy in acute lung injury. The net fluid balance in the conservative strategy was −136 mL compared to +6,992 mL with the liberal strategy. Although there was no difference in 60-day mortality, the primary outcome, the use of a conservative strategy, improved lung function, shortened the duration of mechanical ventilation, and decreased intensive care stay without increasing shock.

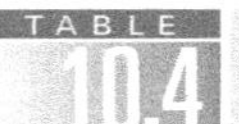

TABLE 10.4 Trials Comparing EGDT in Septic Shock

Trial	Type	*N*	Treatment Arms	Primary Outcomes and Results
Rivers et al[44]	Single-center prospective RCT	263	130 EGDT 133 standard therapy (usual care)	In-hospital mortality: lower in EGDT 30.5% vs 46.5% in standard, $p = 0.009$. All-cause mortality at 28 and 60 d: 33.3% vs 49.2, $p = 0.01$ and 44.3% vs 56.9%, $p = 0.03$, respectively
ProCESS et al[60]	Multicenter RCT (31 US centers)	1,341	439 EGDT 446 PSC 456 usual care	In-hospital mortality at 60 d: protocol-based EGDT group (21.0%) vs protocol-based standard therapy group (18.2%) vs usual care group (18.9%) No significant differences in 90-d mortality, 1-yr mortality, or the need for organ support No significant benefit of the mandated use of central venous catheterization and central hemodynamic monitoring in all patients
ARISE et al[61]	Multicenter RCT (51 Australasia centers)	1,600	796 EGDT 804 usual care group	All-cause mortality within 90 d: EGDT did not reduce all-cause mortality at 90 d (rates of death of 18.6% EGDT vs 18.8% usual care)
ProMISe[62]	Multicenter RCT (56 England hospitals)	1,260	630 EGDT 630 usual care	All-cause mortality at 90 d: EGDT 29.2% vs 29.5%. EGDT increased costs with no significant difference in primary or secondary outcomes
Andrews et al[45]	Single center Zambia	212	107 EGDT 105 usual care	In-hospital mortality: EGDT 48.1% vs 33% Most of the patients were positive for HIV

CVP, central venous pressure; EGDT, early goal-directed therapy; Hct, hematocrit; HIV, human immunodeficiency virus; MAP, mean arterial pressure; pRBC, packed red blood cell; PSC, protocol-based standard care; RCT, randomized controlled trial.

EGDT: In the first 6 hours (1) a 500 mL of crystalloid bolus every 30 minutes to maintain CVP 8 to 12 mm Hg; (2) vasodilators and vasoconstrictors to maintain MAP of 65 to 90 mm Hg; (3) pRBC to maintain venous saturation >70 mm Hg, to achieve Hct >30; (4) after the above measures if venous saturation is <70 mm Hg, dobutamine is started.

PSC: a set of 6-hr resuscitation instructions, but the components were less aggressive than those used for protocol-based EGDT, based on noninvasive monitoring.

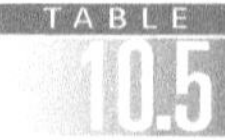

Strategies to Decrease the Volume Load in the Intensive Care Unit

Decrease or eliminate use of maintenance and replacement fluids
Decreasing the tonicity of fluids (use half-NS or dextrose fluids when possible)
Use a small volume of carrier fluids with intravenous medications
Use enteral medications and nutrition as often and as soon as possible

NS, normal saline.

Acute pancreatitis (AP) is another area where fluid resuscitation is the cornerstone of management as it provides macro- and microcirculatory support and prevents pancreatic necrosis. Until recently, aggressive fluid therapy was considered the basis of treatment; however, retrospective studies show that aggressive fluid resuscitation (≥33% of the total volume in 72 hours of infusion performed in the first 24 hours) results in higher mortality and higher SIRS scores.[50] Permissive hypovolemia in a study of burn patients with 20% or more body surface area (BSA) was safe and reduced multiple-organ dysfunction scores in a pilot study of 24 patients.[51]

But enthusiasm for conservative fluid approaches should be cautious. In an international, randomized, partially blinded trial of liberal versus conservative fluid strategies for high-risk patients undergoing major abdominal surgery, there was a 50% increase in AKI and a trebling of KRT for AKI.[52] The important trials examining EGDT in septic shock are shown in Table 10.4.

So a safe conclusion should be to give fluid when it is necessary, but not too much, and only enough. Strategies to decrease fluid buildup in ICUs are shown in **Table 10.5**.

RATING FLUID RESPONSE

With recognition that giving excess fluid is harmful to patients, it becomes obvious that patients should only be given fluids when it improves hemodynamics; this is termed fluid responsive. An operative definition of fluid responsiveness is an increase of stroke volume by at least 10% following a fluid bolus.[53] Currently, there is not a consensus method to predict fluid responsiveness. Methods to assess fluid response can be divided into static or dynamic techniques, see (**Table 10.6**).[54] Discussing the merits of each technique is beyond the scope of this chapter and readers are directed to Chapter 1. Numerous studies and meta-analyses have questioned the utility of central venous pressure (CVP), which is affected by thoracic, pericardial, and abdominal pressures, RV compliance as well as tricuspid valve competence. Also, there are no clear cut-off values. Rivers et al used a target CVP range of 8 to 12 mm Hg. The majority of patients are fluid responsive when CVP is less than 8 mm Hg, and only a few patients respond when the CVP is more than 12 mm Hg.[44]

Dynamic indices like pulse pressure and stroke volume variation may have a better role in assessing fluid responsiveness.[55] Assessment of respiratory variation in inferior vena cava (IVC) diameter is a noninvasive, quick, and reliable method to predict fluid responsiveness. With positive pressure ventilation, the IVC diameter expands at the end of inspiration compared to the end of expiration; when expressed as a percentage, it predicts response to a fluid bolus. In patients on positive pressure ventilation, values greater than 18% predicted fluid responsiveness.[56]

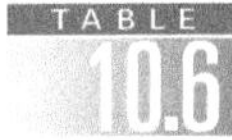

Parameters for Evaluation of Volume Responsiveness

Static Techniques	Dynamic Techniques	Techniques Based on Real or Virtual Fluid Challenge
CVP	Pulse pressure variation	PLR test
IVC diameter	Stroke volume variation	Fluid bolus
Inferior vein collapsibility	Plethysmographic variability index	
End-diastolic volume		
Corrected flow time		

CVP, central venous pressure; IVC, inferior vena cava; PLR, passive leg raise.

A meta-analysis highlighted a beneficial role of assessing respiratory variation in IVC by point-of-care ultrasonography with a pooled sensitivity and specificity of 76% and 86%, respectively.[57] The same technique can be used in patients not on positive pressure ventilation, but there is less consensus on its efficacy.[58]

The passive leg raise (PLR) test is among the most promising of these techniques. PLR requires the use of ultrasound in the apical five-chamber view with a pulsed-wave Doppler sample to measure the velocity-time integral (VTI), which assesses variations in stroke volume. After measurements of VTI are performed in a semirecumbent position with the trunk at 30 degrees and legs in a horizontal position, the legs are elevated to 45 degrees and the trunk of the patient placed flat and a second set of measurements are made. Douglas et al demonstrated the effectiveness of PLR in an RCT of septic patients. In the intervention arm, patients who develop hypotension had their management guided by PLR. If the patient was deemed fluid responsive and VTI increased by more than 10%, crystalloid fluids were given. If the patient was not determined to be fluid responsive, vasopressors were started or increased. A total of 124 patients were analyzed from 13 sites. The intervention lowered fluid balance 1.4 L at 72 hours (primary outcome). Additionally, the intervention group had less need for KRT (5.1% vs 17.5%, $p = 0.04$) and mechanical ventilation (17.7% vs 34.1%, $p = 0.04$).[59] Further studies and meta-analyses involving larger, more diverse populations are warranted to see if these results are robust.

References

1. Tietz NW, ed. *Clinical Guide to Laboratory Tests.* W.B. Saunders Company; 1990.
2. Roberts JS, Bratton SL. Colloid volume expanders. *Drugs.* 1998;55(5):621-630.
3. McNab S, Ware RS, Neville KA, et al. Isotonic versus hypotonic solutions for maintenance intravenous fluid administration in children. *Cochrane Database Syst Rev.* 2014;(12):CD009457.
4. Levick JR. Revision of the Starling principle: new views of tissue fluid balance. *J Physiol.* 2004;557(3):704. doi:10.1113/jphysiol.2004.066118
5. Woodcock TE, Woodcock TM. Revised Starling equation and the glycocalyx model of transvascular fluid exchange: an improved paradigm for prescribing intravenous fluid therapy. *Br J Anaesth.* 2012;108(3):384-394.
6. Finfer S, Bellomo R, Boyce N, et al. A comparison of albumin and saline for fluid resuscitation in the intensive care unit. *N Engl J Med.* 2004;350(22):2247-2256.
7. Rehm M, Haller M, Orth V, et al. Changes in blood volume and hematocrit during acute preoperative volume loading with 5% albumin or 6% hetastarch solutions in patients before radical hysterectomy. *Anesthesiology.* 2001;95(4):849-856.
8. Hahn RG, Dull RO, Zdolsek J. The Extended Starling principle needs clinical validation. *Acta Anaesthesiol Scand.* 2020;64(7). doi:10.1111/aas.13593

9. Cochrane Injuries Group Albumin Reviewers. Human albumin administration in critically ill patients: systematic review of randomised controlled trials. *BMJ.* 1998;317(7153):235-240.
10. Fleck A, Raines G, Hawker F, et al. Increased vascular permeability: a major cause of hypoalbuminaemia in disease and injury. *Lancet.* 1985;1(8432):781-784.
11. SAFE Study Investigators, Australian and New Zealand Intensive Care Society Clinical Trials Group, Australian Red Cross Blood Service, et al. Saline or albumin for fluid resuscitation in patients with traumatic brain injury. *N Engl J Med.* 2007;357(9):874-884.
12. Caironi P, Tognoni G, Masson S, et al. Albumin replacement in patients with severe sepsis or septic shock. *N Engl J Med.* 2014;370(15):1412-1421.
13. Rhodes A, Evans LE, Alhazzani W, et al. Surviving sepsis campaign: international guidelines for management of sepsis and septic shock: 2016. *Intensive Care Med.* 2017;43(3):304-377.
14. Vincent J-L, Russell JA, Jacob M, et al. Albumin administration in the acutely ill: what is new and where next? *Crit Care.* 2014;18(4):231.
15. Schortgen F, Girou E, Deye N, et al. The risk associated with hyperoncotic colloids in patients with shock. *Intensive Care Med.* 2008;34(12):2157-2168.
16. Bagshaw SM, Chawla LS. Hydroxyethyl starch for fluid resuscitation in critically ill patients. *Can J Anaesth.* 2013;60(7):709-713.
17. Myburgh JA, Finfer S, Bellomo R, et al. Hydroxyethyl starch or saline for fluid resuscitation in intensive care. *N Engl J Med.* 2012;367(20):1901-1911.
18. Perner A, Haase N, Guttormsen AB, et al. Hydroxyethyl starch 130/0.42 versus Ringer's acetate in severe sepsis. *N Engl J Med.* 2012;367(2):124-134.
19. Annane D, Siami S, Jaber S, et al. Effects of fluid resuscitation with colloids vs crystalloids on mortality in critically ill patients presenting with hypovolemic shock: the CRISTAL randomized trial. *JAMA.* 2013;310(17):1809-1817.
20. Dickenmann M, Oettl T, Mihatsch MJ. Osmotic nephrosis: acute kidney injury with accumulation of proximal tubular lysosomes due to administration of exogenous solutes. *Am J Kidney Dis.* 2008;51(3):491-503.
21. Kozek-Langenecker SA, Scharbert G. Effects of hydroxyethyl starches on hemostasis. *Transfus Altern Transfus Med.* 2007;9(3):173-181.
22. KDIGO. Guidelines. https://kdigo.org/guidelines/
23. Peti-Peterdi J, Harris RC. Macula densa sensing and signaling mechanisms of renin release. *J Am Soc Nephrol.* 2010;21(7):1093-1096.
24. Wilcox CS. Regulation of renal blood flow by plasma chloride. *J Clin Invest.* 1983;71(3):726-735.
25. Williams EL, Hildebrand KL, McCormick SA, et al. The effect of intravenous lactated Ringer's solution versus 0.9% sodium chloride solution on serum osmolality in human volunteers. *Anesth Analg.* 1999;88(5):999-1003.
26. McCluskey SA, Karkouti K, Wijeysundera D, et al. Hyperchloremia after noncardiac surgery is independently associated with increased morbidity and mortality: a propensity-matched cohort study. *Anesth Analg.* 2013;117(2):412-421.
27. Shaw AD, Raghunathan K, Peyerl FW, et al. Association between intravenous chloride load during resuscitation and in-hospital mortality among patients with SIRS. *Intensive Care Med.* 2014;40(12):1897-1905.
28. Pfortmueller CA, Funk G-C, Reiterer C, et al. Normal saline versus a balanced crystalloid for goal-directed perioperative fluid therapy in major abdominal surgery: a double-blind randomised controlled study. *Br J Anaesth.* 2018;120(2):274-283.
29. Yunos NM, Bellomo R, Hegarty C, et al. Association between a chloride-liberal vs chloride-restrictive intravenous fluid administration strategy and kidney injury in critically ill adults. *JAMA.* 2012;308(15):1566-1572.
30. Young P, Bailey M, Beasley R, et al. Effect of a buffered crystalloid solution vs saline on acute kidney injury among patients in the intensive care unit: the SPLIT randomized clinical trial. *JAMA.* 2015;314(16):1701-1710.
31. Semler MW, Self WH, Wanderer JP, et al. Balanced crystalloids versus saline in critically ill adults. *N Engl J Med.* 2018;378(9):829-839.
32. Self WH, Semler MW, Wanderer JP, et al. Balanced crystalloids versus saline in noncritically ill adults. *N Engl J Med.* 2018;378(9):819-828.
33. Singh S, Davis D. Ringer's lactate. In: *StatPearls.* StatPearls Publishing; 2019.
34. Zitek T, Skaggs ZD, Rahbar A, et al. Does intravenous lactated Ringer's solution raise serum lactate? *J Emerg Med.* 2018;55(3):313-318.
35. O'Malley CMN, Frumento RJ, Hardy MA, et al. A randomized, double-blind comparison of lactated Ringer's solution and 0.9% NaCl during renal transplantation. *Anesth Analg.* 2005;100(5):1518-1524, table of contents.
36. Khajavi MR, Etezadi F, Moharari RS, et al. Effects of normal saline vs. lactated Ringer's during renal transplantation. *Ren Fail.* 2008;30(5):535-539.

37. Luke RG, Galla JH. It is chloride depletion alkalosis, not contraction alkalosis. *J Am Soc Nephrol.* 2012;23(2):204-207.
38. Alvis-Miranda HR, Castellar-Leones SM, Moscote-Salazar LR. Intravenous fluid therapy in traumatic brain injury and decompressive craniectomy. *Bull Emerg Trauma.* 2014;2(1):3-14.
39. Tommasino C, Moore S, Todd MM. Cerebral effects of isovolemic hemodilution with crystalloid or colloid solutions. *Crit Care Med.* 1988;16(9):862-868.
40. Cooper DJ, Myles PS, McDermott FT, et al. Prehospital hypertonic saline resuscitation of patients with hypotension and severe traumatic brain injury: a randomized controlled trial. *JAMA.* 2004;291(11):1350-1357.
41. Bulger EM, May S, Brasel KJ, et al. Out-of-hospital hypertonic resuscitation following severe traumatic brain injury: a randomized controlled trial. *JAMA.* 2010;304(13):1455-1464.
42. Asfar P, Schortgen F, Boisramé-Helms J, et al. Hyperoxia and hypertonic saline in patients with septic shock (HYPERS2S): a two-by-two factorial, multicentre, randomised, clinical trial. *Lancet Respir Med.* 2017;5(3):180-190.
43. Paterna S, Di Pasquale P, Parrinello G, et al. Effects of high-dose furosemide and small-volume hypertonic saline solution infusion in comparison with a high dose of furosemide as a bolus, in refractory congestive heart failure. *Eur J Heart Fail.* 2000;2(3):305-313. doi:10.1016/s1388-9842(00)00094-5
44. Rivers E, Nguyen B, Havstad S, et al. Early goal-directed therapy in the treatment of severe sepsis and septic shock. *N Engl J Med.* 2001;345(19):1368-1377.
45. Andrews B, Semler MW, Muchemwa L, et al. Effect of an early resuscitation protocol on in-hospital mortality among adults with sepsis and hypotension: a randomized clinical trial. *JAMA.* 2017;318(13):1233-1240.
46. Maitland K, Kiguli S, Opoka RO, et al. Mortality after fluid bolus in African children with severe infection. *N Engl J Med.* 2011;364(26):2483-2495.
47. Hjortrup PB, Haase N, Bundgaard H, et al. Restricting volumes of resuscitation fluid in adults with septic shock after initial management: the CLASSIC randomised, parallel-group, multicentre feasibility trial. *Intensive Care Med.* 2016;42(11):1695-1705.
48. Seymour CW, Gesten F, Prescott HC, et al. Time to treatment and mortality during mandated emergency care for sepsis. *N Engl J Med.* 2017;376(23):2235-2244.
49. National Heart, Lung, and Blood Institute Acute Respiratory Distress Syndrome (ARDS) Clinical Trials Network, Wiedemann HP, Wheeler AP, et al. Comparison of two fluid-management strategies in acute lung injury. *N Engl J Med.* 2006;354(24):2564-2575.
50. Aggarwal A, Manrai M, Kochhar R. Fluid resuscitation in acute pancreatitis. *World J Gastroenterol.* 2014;20(48):18092-18103.
51. Arlati S, Storti E, Pradella V, et al. Decreased fluid volume to reduce organ damage: a new approach to burn shock resuscitation? A preliminary study. *Resuscitation.* 2007;72(3):371-378.
52. Myles PS, Bellomo R, Corcoran T, et al. Restrictive versus liberal fluid therapy for major abdominal surgery. *N Engl J Med.* 2018;378(24):2263-2274.
53. Marik PE, Lemson J. Fluid responsiveness: an evolution of our understanding. *Br J Anaesth.* 2014;112(4):617-620.
54. Monnet X, Marik PE, Teboul J-L. Prediction of fluid responsiveness: an update. *Ann Intensive Care.* 2016;6(1):111.
55. Suehiro K, Rinka H, Ishikawa J, et al. Stroke volume variation as a predictor of fluid responsiveness in patients undergoing airway pressure release ventilation. *Anaesth Intensive Care.* 2012;40(5):767-772.
56. Barbier C, Loubières Y, Schmit C, et al. Respiratory changes in inferior vena cava diameter are helpful in predicting fluid responsiveness in ventilated septic patients. *Intensive Care Med.* 2004;30(9):1740-1746.
57. Zhang Z, Xu X, Ye S, et al. Ultrasonographic measurement of the respiratory variation in the inferior vena cava diameter is predictive of fluid responsiveness in critically ill patients: systematic review and meta-analysis. *Ultrasound Med Biol.* 2014;40(5):845-853.
58. Muller L, Bobbia X, Toumi M, et al. Respiratory variations of inferior vena cava diameter to predict fluid responsiveness in spontaneously breathing patients with acute circulatory failure: need for a cautious use. *Crit Care.* 2012;16(5):R188.
59. Douglas IS, Alapat PM, Corl KA, et al. Fluid response evaluation in sepsis hypotension and shock: a randomized clinical trial. *Chest.* 2020;58(4):1431-1445. doi:10.1016/j.chest.2020.04.025
60. ProCESS Investigators, Yealy DM, Kellum JA, et al. A randomized trial of protocol-based care for early septic shock. *N Engl J Med.* 2014;370(18):1683-1693.
61. ARISE Investigators, ANZICS Clinical Trials Group, Peake SL, et al. Goal-directed resuscitation for patients with early septic shock. *N Engl J Med.* 2014;371(16):1496-1506.
62. Mouncey PR, Osborn TM, Power GS, et al. Trial of early, goal-directed resuscitation for septic shock. *N Engl J Med.* 2015;372(14):1301-1311.

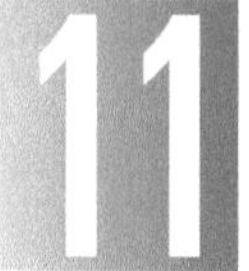

Transfusion Medicine in the Intensive Care Unit

Benjamin R. Griffin, Nathan J. Clendenen, John S. Kim, and Sarah Faubel

ANEMIA IN CRITICALLY ILL PATIENTS

Introduction

Anemia, defined as hemoglobin less than 13 g/dL in men and less than 12 g/dL in women, is a common complication in critically ill patients that is associated with increased morbidity and mortality. Nearly two-thirds of patients admitted to the intensive care unit (ICU) have anemia at the time of admission, and 97% of ICU patients develop anemia within 1 week.[1] Anemia in critically ill patients is associated with poor outcomes, including acute kidney injury (AKI), prolonged mechanical ventilation,[2] myocardial infarction,[3] and death.[4] Anemia at hospital admission or prior to cardiac surgery is also a predictor of both the incidence and severity of AKI.[1]

Anemia may contribute to poor outcomes by reducing oxygen carrying capacity in the blood and thereby decrease oxygen delivery to peripheral tissues. Packed red blood cells (pRBCs) in the past were transfused liberally to a goal of greater than 10 g/dL in an effort to improve oxygen delivery; however, prospective trials in ICU patients failed to show a survival benefit.[5,6] Furthermore, transfusions themselves are known to cause complications ranging from mild febrile reactions to life-threatening conditions, such as transfusion-related acute lung injury (TRALI) or anaphylaxis.[7] As a result, a "restrictive" strategy of transfusion is recommended in the majority of the critically ill population.[8] Despite the change in strategy, the United States still transfuses 15 million units of pRBCs annually, and 85 million units are transfused worldwide,[9] underscoring the necessity of recognizing the causes of anemia, indications for transfusion, and possible adverse effects of pRBC transfusion. In this section, we review the causes of anemia in the ICU, indications for pRBC transfusion, and potential complications of transfusions.

Causes of Anemia in Intensive Care Unit Patients

The cause of anemia in an ICU patient is often multifactorial. Even in those without active bleeding (i.e., postsurgical bleeding or gastrointestinal [GI] bleeding), blood loss due to frequent phlebotomy is nearly universal.[10] In addition, bone marrow production of RBCs is often suppressed in the setting of inflammation.[11] Finally, coagulopathy related to endogenous factors, such as sepsis, or exogenous factors, such as the use of extracorporeal membrane oxygenation (ECMO) or ventricular assist devices (VADs), frequently causes hemolysis in this population[1,12] (for further discussion of VADs and ECMO, see Chapters 35 and 41, respectively). RBC loss or destruction, coupled with the inability to efficiently make new RBCs, are the key reasons for the near-universal anemia observed in the critically ill population.

Anemia Associated With Acute Kidney Injury, End-Stage Kidney Disease, and Kidney Replacement Therapy

Anemia is common in the setting of kidney disease. In AKI, anemia is both a risk factor for disease[13] and a predictor of poor patient outcomes.[14]

Patients with AKI requiring continuous kidney replacement therapy (CKRT) may have even higher rates of anemia owing to clotting of the hemofilters during the procedure,[15] although the impact of anemia on recovery of kidney function in this population is uncertain.[16]

In patients with chronic kidney disease (CKD) or end-stage kidney disease (ESKD), anemia is common owing to the lack of erythropoietin. In the inpatient setting, this can further exacerbate bone marrow suppression, seen in the setting of inflammation. Resistance to erythropoietin-stimulating agents (ESAs) also often occurs in the setting of inflammation, which can lead to further decreases in hemoglobin in ESRD patients.[17] As in AKI, anemic patients with CKD and ESRD are at higher risk for poor outcomes.[18] Common causes of anemia are summarized in **Table 11.1**.

Indications for Blood Transfusions

Current data support the use of a restrictive strategy in most patients with anemia, defined as a transfusion threshold of 7 g/dL. A recent Cochrane review of 31 trials involving 12,587 patients from a variety of inpatient settings found no significant difference in 30-day mortality with a restrictive strategy (relative risk [RR] = 0.97) as opposed to a liberal strategy, with a reduction in the risk of RBC transfusion of 43% (RR = 0.57).[19] Studies in the ICU population show similar results.

The Transfusion Requirements in Critical Care (TRICC) trial randomized 838 critically ill patients to a transfusion threshold of 7 versus 10 g/dL and showed no difference in 30-day mortality.[5] The TRICC study was followed by the Transfusion Strategies for Acute Upper Gastrointestinal Bleeding trial,[20] the Transfusion Requirements in Septic Shock (TRISS) trial,[21] and the Transfusion Requirements in

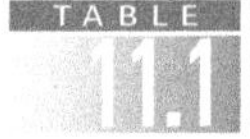

TABLE 11.1 Causes of Anemia in Critically Ill Patients

Blood Loss	**Phlebotomy Gastrointestinal Bleeding Surgery**
Impaired RBC production	Bone marrow suppression Inflammation Medications Sepsis Iron deficiency/inaccessibility Folate or B12 deficiency
Hemolysis	Ventricular assist devices (VADs) Continuous kidney replacement therapy (CKRT) Extracorporeal membrane oxygenation (ECMO) Medical conditions associated with hemolytic anemia (e.g., thrombotic microangiopathy [TMA], drug reactions)
Kidney associated	Reduced erythropoietin production Anemia at baseline (CKD, ESKD) Impaired iron homeostasis

CKD, chronic kidney disease; ESKD, end-stage kidney disease; RBC, red blood cell.

Cardiac Surgery (TRICS) III trial,[22] which studied restrictive versus liberal strategies in GI bleeding, sepsis, and postcardiac surgery, respectively, and in all three, there were no differences in 30-day mortality between the two groups. Preoperative anemia is a well-established risk factor for cardiac surgery–associated AKI (CSA-AKI),[23] although, in the TRICS III trial, the rates of AKI were identical in the restrictive and conservative transfusion groups.[22,24,25] Ambiguity remains regarding transfusion thresholds in acute myocardial infarction because of a lack of large randomized trials within this group,[26,27] and guidelines such as those by the AABB (formerly American Association of Blood Banks) do not recommend for or against liberal or restrictive thresholds in this patient population.[8]

Transfusion thresholds have not been specifically evaluated in hospitalized patients with CKD or ESRD, although these patients were not excluded from the studies mentioned earlier. In patients who are or may be eligible for organ transplantation in the future, current guidelines suggest avoiding pRBCs when possible to minimize the risk of allosensitization.[28] When acute correction of hemoglobin is needed, such as during hemorrhage, myocardial infarction, or prior to surgery, a goal of 7 g/dL is recommended. However, in nonurgent and nonacute anemia, transfusion should not be based on a threshold, but rather on the presence of clinical symptoms.[28]

ESAs have not been shown to be effective in preventing the need for pRBC transfusions in critically ill patients. In the largest randomized study of ESA use to date,[29] 1,460 patients were given epoetin alfa 40,000 U (EPO) or placebo weekly. There were no differences in the mean number of pRBCs transfused, and there were higher rates of serious thrombotic events in the EPO group. A subgroup analysis of trauma patients showed lower mortality with EPO, although the mechanism did not seem to be related to fewer transfusions or higher hemoglobin levels. Adding intravenous iron to erythropoietin does not reduce pRBC requirements[30] and may worsen infectious complications,[31] although human data are unclear.[32] More recent studies have focused on the pleiotropic effects of erythropoietin in regulating inflammation, apoptosis, and immune function; however, whether there are benefits to ESA use in critically ill patients remains unclear.[33-36]

Packed Red Blood Cell Preparation

pRBCs are made through centrifugation or apheresis of whole blood. A single unit is approximately 350 mL in volume and has a hematocrit of 60% to 80%. Each unit contains approximately 250 mg of iron. An anticoagulant, usually citrate, is added, which allows for storage up to 35 days.[37] However, transfusion-related adverse events may increase with longer pRBC storage times.[38]

pRBCs can be further treated depending on the clinical situation. Leukoreduced pRBCs have had most of their white blood cells (WBCs) removed, which may reduce the risk of febrile transfusion reactions, prevent alloimmunization to major histocompatibility complex (MHC) donor antigens, and reduce the risk of cytomegalovirus (CMV) transmission. pRBCs are irradiated to remove (or destroy) all remaining leukocytes and are used to prevent transfusion-associated graft-versus-host disease (GVHD). Washed pRBCs are cleaned using saline to remove proteins, reducing the risk of allergic reaction. The washing process also reduces the extracellular potassium concentration, which is especially notable in irradiated pRBCs.[39,40] pRBCs must be used within 24 hours of washing.[41]

Complications

Transfusions of pRBCs carry numerous risks, which range from trivial to life-threatening.

A summary of common complications is given in **Table 11.2.**

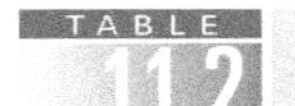

Potential Complications of Packed Red Blood Cell Transfusions

Complication	Frequency (per Patient)	Signs/Symptoms	Cause	Treatment
Febrile reaction	1:10-100	A temperature increase of ≥1°C within 2 hr of transfusion	Anti-WBC antibodies	Premedicate with acetaminophen Use leukoreduced pRBCs
Allergic (urticarial) reaction	1:30-100	Urticaria, pruritis	Occurs due to antibody to donor plasma proteins	Antihistamines
Anaphylaxis	1:20,000-50,000	Angioedema, hypotension, bronchospasm	Antibody to plasma proteins	Antihistamines, corticosteroids, epinephrine
TRALI	1:12,000	Hypoxemia, hypotension, bilateral pulmonary edema, transient leukopenia, and fever within 6 hr of transfusion	HLA or neutrophil antibodies in donor product	Supportive care
TACO	1:100	New onset or exacerbation of acute respiratory distress (dyspnea, orthopnea, count) 3-6 hr after transfusion	↑ CVP, left heart failure, positive fluid balance, pulmonary edema on chest x-ray. Risk factors include cardiac or kidney dysfunction, female gender, age> 60 yr, severe anemia with volume expansion, positive fluid balance, transfusion of multiple products	Stop all transfusions Supplemental oxygen Diuretics

(*continued*)

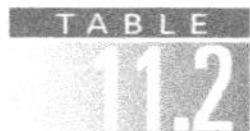

TABLE 11.2 Potential Complications of Packed Red Blood Cell Transfusions (*continued*)

Complication	Frequency (per Patient)	Signs/Symptoms	Cause	Treatment
HIV or hepatitis C infection	>1:1,000,000	Seropositivity following transfusion	Presence of virus in transfused blood	Appropriate treatment of HIV or hepatitis C
Acute hemolytic transfusion reaction	1:76,000	Chills, fever, hypotension, hemoglobinuria, kidney failure, back pain, DIC	Preformed antibodies to incompatible product	IV fluids Pressors if needed Treat DIC
Electrolyte abnormalities	Variable	Hypocalcemia, hypomagnesemia, hyperkalemia	Citrate anticoagulation binds calcium and magnesium, especially in massive transfusion protocols. RBC lysis during storage can cause hyperkalemia	Supportive

CVP, central venous pressure; DIC, disseminated intravascular coagulation; HIV, human immunodeficiency virus; HLA, human leukocyte antigen; IV, intravenous; pRBC, packed red blood cell; TACO, transfusion-associated circulatory overload; TRALI, transfusion-related acute lung injury; WBC, white blood cell.

THROMBOCYTOPENIA IN CRITICALLY ILL PATIENTS

Thrombocytopenia is common in critically ill patients in the ICU, with prevalence rates ranging from 15% to 55%.[42-44] A large number of these studies have further shown that thrombocytopenia in the ICU is associated with increased mortality and that mortality increases along with the degree of thrombocytopenia.[45,46] Risk factors for the development of thrombocytopenia include sepsis, liver dysfunction, and the use of a number of pharmacologic agents, including heparin, phenytoin, piperacillin, vancomycin, and imipenem.[47,48] The effect of thrombocytopenia on mortality rates persists even when adjusting for factors such as severity of illness, demographics, and comorbid conditions. Like anemia, most cases of thrombocytopenia are multifactorial. Etiologies of thrombocytopenia can be broadly categorized into decreased production, sequestration, and destruction or consumption.[49]

Thrombocytopenia may be a risk factor for AKI, which has been demonstrated in patients following cardiac surgery requiring cardiopulmonary bypass.[50] Patients requiring CKRT have been shown to have increased rates of thrombocytopenia. The mechanism is unclear, but may be related to a combination of machine factors, including shear stress and platelet-membrane interactions, underlying processes such as Thrombotic Thrombocytopenic Purpura (TTP) or endothelial cell dysfunction, or bone marrow suppression in the setting of inflammation and critical illness.[51] As in other types of thrombocytopenia, CKRT-associated thrombocytopenia is associated with increased mortality.[52] The impact of thrombocytopenia in patients with CKD or ESRD has not been well investigated.

Indications for Transfusions

The major indications for platelet transfusion include treatment or prevention of bleeding in the setting of thrombocytopenia or impaired platelet function. The 2015 AABB guidelines give the following recommendations for platelet transfusions:

- Hospitalized patients with 10×10^9 cells/L or less should be transfused to prevent spontaneous bleeding.
- Patients undergoing central catheter placement should be transfused to a goal of greater than 20×10^9 cells/L.
- Patients undergoing lumbar puncture or elective non-neuraxial surgery should be transfused to a goal of 50×10^9 cells/L or more.
- AABB recommends against prophylactic platelet transfusions in patients without thrombocytopenia undergoing cardiopulmonary bypass surgery, unless there is evidence of platelet dysfunction.
- In the case of kidney biopsy, the threshold at which a biopsy can be safely performed is unclear. Many nephrologists will not perform a biopsy if platelets are less than $100 \times 10^3/\mu L$, although specific data are lacking.[53]

Risks of Platelet Transfusion

The complications of platelet transfusions are similar to those seen in pRBC transfusions and include febrile reactions, TRALI, GVHD, hemolysis, and anaphylaxis. However, platelet transfusions are associated with higher rates of bacterial contamination than pRBCs, likely due to the fact that platelets are stored at room temperature to preserve function.[54] In addition, platelet transfusions carry risk for post-transfusion thrombocytopenia (PTP), a condition that primarily affects female patients who lack human platelet antigen 1a with sensitization through prior platelet transfusions.[2] PTP is rare, but presents with severe thrombocytopenia and is fatal in 10% to 20% of cases.

Plasma and Cryoprecipitate Content

Fresh-frozen plasma (FFP) and cryoprecipitate are allogeneic blood products used to treat deficiencies in the amount or function of coagulation system proteins. Plasma is the acellular liquid fraction of whole blood that contains circulating proteins that remain after centrifugation of anticoagulated whole blood. Cryoprecipitate is produced from FFP by slowly thawing the plasma, collecting the supernatant, and precipitating the suspended proteins with centrifugation. This process enriches the level of factor VIII, factor XIII, and fibrinogen in cryoprecipitate compared to FFP. Each pooled cryoprecipitate unit is derived from five separate donors. Both FFP and cryoprecipitate contain plasma proteins important in hemostasis, which can be transfused to restore deficiencies in the coagulation system.

Indications for Use of Plasma and Cryoprecipitate

The most common indications for the administration of FFP are to restore coagulation protein levels depleted by bleeding after trauma or surgery, reverse acquired dysfunction in coagulation proteins, and prevent bleeding associated with invasive procedures. Current guidelines recommend transfusing FFP into patients requiring massive transfusion (defined as transfusion of 10 or more units of RBCs within 24 hours) and for those treated with warfarin complicated by intracranial hemorrhage. Although high-quality evidence is lacking, FFP transfusion is appropriate when the risk of harm from bleeding exceeds the risk of transfusion. Common clinical practice includes transfusing FFP to target a specific international normalized ratio (INR) prior to line insertion and restoring acquired coagulation system dysfunction owing to exposure to foreign surfaces in extracorporeal circuits necessary for cardiopulmonary bypass, ECMO, or CKRT.

The majority of national guidelines recommend transfusing cryoprecipitate for patients with hypofibrinogenemia and evidence of clinical bleeding when the fibrinogen level falls below 100 mg/dL.[54] Fibrinogen replacement is indicated as part of a massive transfusion protocol or in the setting of hypofibrinogenemia with active bleeding or disseminated intravascular coagulation (DIC). Expert consensus and guidelines recommend transfusing plasma in a 1:1:1 ratio with RBC and platelet transfusions, and fibrinogen replacement should be guided by laboratory testing with a treatment threshold below 100 mg/dL in the massive transfusion protocol.

Risks

The most common complications following FFP or cryoprecipitate transfusion are TRALI, transfusion-associated circulatory overload (TACO), and anaphylaxis. Acquiring an infection after transfusion is rare, with less than 1 per 2 million transfusions, and includes pathogen transmission and transfusion-associated sepsis. Citrate toxicity is another rare complication resulting in hypocalcemia that responds to intravenous calcium replacement.

Transfusion-Related Acute Lung Injury

TRALI is defined as acute respiratory failure within 6 hours of a blood transfusion without evidence of circulatory overload and has an incidence of 0.1%. Diagnostic specificity is difficult in practice and relies on the new onset of symptoms and the temporal relationship to blood transfusion. Two detailed guidelines provide recommendations for accurate diagnosis,[2,3] which remains a challenge in clinical practice leading to under reporting of the incidence of TRALI. FFP transfusion has the highest rate of TRALI compared to all the allogeneic blood products, and a key inciting factor is the presence of anti-WBC antibodies in the donor. These antibodies are more common in multiparous women, which led to national policy changes to collect only FFP from males or from women without anti-WBC antibodies. These changes in transfusion practice led to a sharp reduction in mortality because as a result of TRALI, no targeted interventions exist for TRALI and management relies on providing supportive care. Specifically, clinicians should immediately stop a transfusion suspected of causing harm and assess the patient for signs of respiratory failure and circulatory overload. Patients may report symptoms such as dyspnea or chest tightness accompanied by an increased respiratory rate, wheezing, or increased oxygen requirements. When severe, patients may require urgent respiratory support with mechanical ventilation or, possibly, veno venous ECMO.

Transfusion-Associated Circulatory Overload

TACO is the most common cause of death due to transfusion and is defined as acute respiratory distress within 6 hours of a blood transfusion with evidence of left heart failure and pulmonary edema with an incidence between 1% and 2%. Key risk factors for TACO include cardiac failure, acute CKD and CKD, and hypertension. A key diagnostic feature that distinguishes TACO from TRALI is the rapid response to diuretic therapy. Therefore, in the setting of a suspected transfusion reaction, the benefit of a therapeutic trial of diuretic therapy exceeds the potential harm of unnecessary diuresis and should be considered early in the management of a transfusion reaction.

Citrate Toxicity

Citrate toxicity is an uncommon transfusion complication, resulting in clinically significant hypocalcemia, most often during massive transfusion. Citrate is the primary anticoagulant used in preparing blood products and works by chelating calcium. Citrate is rapidly metabolized by the liver in patients with normal hepatic function, but during massive transfusion, citrate levels may exceed the metabolic capacity of a patient's liver, leading to reduced cardiac function and hypotension by decreased cardiac output and reduced vascular tone. Patients with hepatic failure are at increased risk of citrate toxicity, especially during liver transplantation, which includes an anhepatic phase that prevents all citrate metabolism. Citrate toxicity results in a characteristic prolongation of the QT interval measured by electrocardiogram. This may be associated with hypotension due to a decrease in vascular tone and myocardial contractility. Citrate toxicity responds rapidly to calcium supplementation with intravenous calcium chloride.

Coagulation Factor Concentrates

Coagulation factor concentrates are virally inactivated forms of plasma-derived or recombinant proteins indicated for restoring coagulation system function for inherited or acquired factor deficiencies. Acquired coagulation disorders include warfarin treatment, hypofibrinogenemia, and heparin resistance. Prothrombin complex concentrates (PCCs) contain coagulation factors II, VII, IX, and X, with a variable amount of factor VII, which determines whether the PCC is considered a three- or four-factor concentrate. Fibrinogen concentrate is also isolated from plasma, pathogen inactivated, and lyophilized to allow for rapid reconstitution and administration. Fibrinogen concentrate is indicated for the treatment of bleeding when fibrinogen levels are below 100 mg/dL. Coagulation factor concentrates are highly effective for targeting specific deficiencies in the coagulation system with a favorable safety profile.

Massive Transfusion Protocol

Massive transfusion protocols vary by institution, but a consensus statement by experts agreed that a standardized protocol targeting a transfusion ratio approximating whole blood (1:1:1, FFP:platelets:RBC) is ideal.[4] Initiating a massive transfusion protocol notifies the blood bank of a patient's ongoing transfusion requirements and avoids delays in treatment, which may otherwise be fatal. Key evidence in support of a 1:1:1 transfusion ratio in severe trauma is from the PROPPR (Pragmatic Randomized Optimal Platelet and Plasma Ratios) clinical trial, demonstrating that exsanguination was less common and that hemostasis was more common compared to a 1:1:2 ratio with more RBC transfusions.[5] Although the trial did not demonstrate an overall mortality benefit, a 1:1:1 transfusion ratio is accepted as the standard of care, given the established benefits of reducing coagulopathy associated with severe injuries.

Assay-Directed Management of Hemostasis

Management of hemostasis has traditionally been directed by conventional coagulation assays (CCAs) such as prothrombin time (PT) with INR, partial thromboplastin time (PTT), platelet count, and fibrinogen concentration. The PT and PTT assays indicate the time to fibrin formation through either the extrinsic or intrinsic pathways.

Recently, viscoelastic hemostatic assays (VHAs) are emerging in the management of hemostasis and massive transfusion in critical care, surgery, cardiopulmonary bypass, and trauma. The two most commonly used VHAs include thromboelastography (TEG) (Haemonetics Corp., Niles, IN) and rotational thromboelastometry (ROTEM; TEM International, GmbH, Munich, Germany). These VHAs characterize the life span of clot formation from the initiation of fibrin cross-link formation through clot breakdown and fibrinolysis. A recent randomized controlled trial (RCT) demonstrated improved survival with reduced platelet and plasma transfusions when massive transfusion is guided by TEG versus CCA in patients after trauma; however, no difference in AKI rates was seen.[55] In addition to a body of literature supporting the use of VHA in cardiac surgery with cardiopulmonary bypass, such RCTs continue to mount evidence for their efficacy and benefit in trauma and other more generalizable circumstances.[56-58] A Cochrane review of 17 studies comparing VHA-directed management of blood product transfusion to CCA demonstrated a 54% reduced risk of dialysis-dependent kidney failure.[57] VHAs such as TEG and ROTEM may have potential utility in the management of coagulopathy associated with critical kidney disease.

Management algorithms are described in the literature for both TEG and ROTEM. The selection of hemostatic products for replacement in coagulopathic patients is founded in the interpretation of these VHAs in the context of the cell-based model of hemostasis (summarized in **Table 11.3** and **Table 11.4**). The cell-based model describes clot formation as overlapping stages (rather than a cascade) from initiation, amplification, propagation, and through fibrinolysis.[59,60]

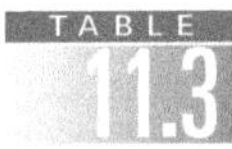

TEG-Directed Management of Hemostasis via the Cell-Based Model

VHA Derangement	Hemostatic State	Recommended Intervention
Short *R time* (TEG) or short *clot formation time* (ROTEM)	Hypercoagulability	Consider systemic anticoagulation, if indicated or at risk for thrombosis
Prolonged *R time* (TEG) or prolonged *clot formation time* (ROTEM)	Coagulopathy secondary to low clotting factors	FFP transfusion
Low *angle* (TEG or ROTEM)	Coagulopathy secondary to low clotting factors (especially fibrinogen)	FFP or cryoprecipitate transfusion (if serum fibrinogen concentration is low)
Low *MA* (TEG) or low *maximum clot firmness* (ROTEM)	Platelet dysfunction or thrombocytopenia	Platelet transfusion
High *MA* (TEG) or high *maximum clot firmness* (ROTEM)	Hypercoagulability	Consider systemic anticoagulation or antiplatelet therapy, if indicated or at risk for thrombosis
High *LY30* (TEG) or high *maximum lysis* (ROTEM)	Fibrinolysis	Consider antifibrinolytic infusion, if indicated and at risk for bleeding

FFP, fresh-frozen plasma; ROTEM, rotational thromboelastometry; TEG, thromboelastography;

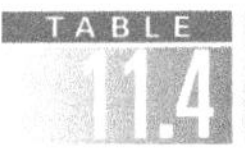

Reported Indications and Potential Uses for VHA Assessment

Reported Indications for Use of VHA	Potential Uses for VHA Assessment
Product replacement selection: • Massive transfusion and trauma • Active hemorrhage Product replacement selection in bleeding patients or patients at risk for bleeding after: • Cardiac surgery with cardiopulmonary bypass • Orthopedic surgery • Solid organ transplantation Monitoring of systemic anticoagulation: • Patients at risk for thrombosis • Treatment of active thrombosis (pulmonary or venous thromboembolism) • Patients requiring systemic anticoagulation for mechanical cardiopulmonary circulatory support (ECMO or ventricular assist device)	Product replacement selection for treatment of coagulopathies in patients at risk for bleeding: • Prior to procedures (e.g., kidney biopsy) • Following procedure with refractory bleeding • Evaluation of potential clotting factor loss from excessive peritoneal dialysis catheter output • Evaluation of kidney disease–associated platelet dysfunction Monitoring of systemic anticoagulation: • During extracorporeal kidney replacement therapies

ECMO, extracorporeal membrane oxygenation; VHA, viscoelastic hemostatic assay.

Clot initiation (*R time* on the TEG) occurs as tissue factor activates and forms a complex with factor VIIa, which, in turn, activates other coagulation factors. Clot amplification (*K time* and *angle*) occurs as platelets, and cofactors are activated in preparation for a large thrombin burst. Clot propagation occurs as the platelets are activated and thrombin is generated on the platelet surface, which, in turn, induces fibrinogen conversion to fibrin to stabilize the clot (*MA* of the TEG). Fibrinolysis is demonstrated by the *LY30* of the TEG.[61,62]

References

1. Rawal G, Kumar R, Yadav S, et al. Anemia in intensive care: a review of current concepts. *J Crit Care Med (Targu Mures)*. 2016;2(3):109-114.
2. Karkouti K, Wijeysundera DN, Yau TM, et al. Acute kidney injury after cardiac surgery: focus on modifiable risk factors. *Circulation*. 2009;119(4):495-502.
3. Rasmussen L, Christensen S, Lenler-Petersen P, et al. Anemia and 90-day mortality in COPD patients requiring invasive mechanical ventilation. *Clin Epidemiol*. 2010;3:1-5.
4. Ducrocq G, Puymirat E, Steg PG, et al. Blood transfusion, bleeding, anemia, and survival in patients with acute myocardial infarction: FAST-MI registry. *Am Heart J*. 2015;170(4):726.e722-734.e722.
5. Vincent JL, Baron JF, Reinhart K, et al. Anemia and blood transfusion in critically ill patients. *JAMA*. 2002;288(12):1499-1507.
6. Hebert PC, Wells G, Blajchman MA, et al. A multicenter, randomized, controlled clinical trial of transfusion requirements in critical care. Transfusion Requirements in Critical Care Investigators, Canadian Critical Care Trials Group. *N Engl J Med*. 1999;340(6):409-417.
7. Afshar M, Netzer G. Update in critical care for the nephrologist: transfusion in nonhemorrhaging critically ill patients. *Adv Chronic Kidney Dis*. 2013;20(1):30-38.
8. Delaney M, Wendel S, Bercovitz RS, et al. Transfusion reactions: prevention, diagnosis, and treatment. *Lancet*. 2016;388(10061):2825-2836.
9. Carson JL, Guyatt G, Heddle NM, et al. Clinical practice guidelines from the AABB: red blood cell transfusion thresholds and storage. *JAMA*. 2016;316(19):2025-2035.
10. Harder L, Boshkov L. The optimal hematocrit. *Crit Care Clin*. 2010;26(2):335-354.
11. Koch CG, Li L, Sun Z, et al. Hospital-acquired anemia: prevalence, outcomes, and healthcare implications. *J Hosp Med*. 2013;8(9):506-512.
12. Weiss G, Ganz T, Goodnough LT. Anemia of inflammation. *Blood*. 2019;133(1):40-50.
13. Jenq CC, Tsai FC, Tsai TY, et al. Effect of anemia on prognosis in patients on extracorporeal membrane oxygenation. *Artif Organs*. 2018;42(7):705-713.
14. Shema-Didi L, Ore L, Geron R, et al. Is anemia at hospital admission associated with in-hospital acute kidney injury occurrence? *Nephron Clin Pract*. 2010;115(2):c168-c176.
15. du Cheyron D, Parienti JJ, Fekih-Hassen M, et al. Impact of anemia on outcome in critically ill patients with severe acute renal failure. *Intensive Care Med*. 2005;31(11):1529-1536.
16. Himmelfarb J. Continuous renal replacement therapy in the treatment of acute renal failure: critical assessment is required. *Clin J Am Soc Nephrol*. 2007;2(2):385-389.
17. Hu SL, Said FR, Epstein D, et al. The impact of anemia on renal recovery and survival in acute kidney injury. *Clin Nephrol*. 2013;79(3):221-228.
18. Jelkmann I, Jelkmann W. Impact of erythropoietin on intensive care unit patients. *Transfus Med Hemother*. 2013;40(5):310-318.
19. Garlo K, Williams D, Lucas L, et al. Severity of anemia predicts hospital length of stay but not readmission in patients with chronic kidney disease: a retrospective cohort study. *Medicine (Baltimore)*. 2015;94(25):e964.
20. Carson JL, Stanworth SJ, Roubinian N, et al. Transfusion thresholds and other strategies for guiding allogeneic red blood cell transfusion. *Cochrane Database Syst Rev*. 2016;10(10):CD002042.
21. Villanueva C, Colomo A, Bosch A, et al. Transfusion strategies for acute upper gastrointestinal bleeding. *N Engl J Med*. 2013;368(1):11-21.
22. Holst LB, Haase N, Wetterslev J, et al. Lower versus higher hemoglobin threshold for transfusion in septic shock. *N Engl J Med*. 2014;371(15):1381-1391.
23. Mazer CD, Whitlock RP, Fergusson DA, et al. Restrictive or liberal red-cell transfusion for cardiac surgery. *N Engl J Med*. 2017;377(22):2133-2144.
24. Kulier A, Levin J, Moser R, et al. Impact of preoperative anemia on outcome in patients undergoing coronary artery bypass graft surgery. *Circulation*. 2007;116(5):471-479.
25. Karkouti K. Transfusion and risk of acute kidney injury in cardiac surgery. *Br J Anaesth*. 2012;109 suppl 1:i29-i38.

26. Thiele RH, Isbell JM, Rosner MH. AKI associated with cardiac surgery. *Clin J Am Soc Nephrol.* 2015;10(3):500-514.
27. Cooper HA, Rao SV, Greenberg MD, et al. Conservative versus liberal red cell transfusion in acute myocardial infarction (the CRIT Randomized Pilot Study). *Am J Cardiol.* 2011;108(8):1108-1111.
28. Carson JL, Brooks MM, Abbott JD, et al. Liberal versus restrictive transfusion thresholds for patients with symptomatic coronary artery disease. *Am Heart J.* 2013;165(6):964.e961-971.e961.
29. Chapter 4: Red cell transfusion to treat anemia in CKD. *Kidney Int Suppl (2011).* 2012;2(4):311-316.
30. Corwin HL, Gettinger A, Fabian TC, et al. Efficacy and safety of epoetin alfa in critically ill patients. *N Engl J Med.* 2007;357(10):965-976.
31. Shah A, Roy NB, McKechnie S, et al. Iron supplementation to treat anaemia in adult critical care patients: a systematic review and meta-analysis. *Crit Care.* 2016;20(1):306.
32. Zager RA, Johnson AC, Hanson SY. Parenteral iron therapy exacerbates experimental sepsis. *Kidney Int.* 2004;65(6):2108-2112.
33. Maynor L, Brophy DF. Risk of infection with intravenous iron therapy. *Ann Pharmacother.* 2007;41(9):1476-1480.
34. de Seigneux S, Ponte B, Weiss L, et al. Epoetin administrated after cardiac surgery: effects on renal function and inflammation in a randomized controlled study. *BMC Nephrol.* 2012;13:132.
35. Nichol A, French C, Little L, et al. Erythropoietin in traumatic brain injury (EPO-TBI): a double-blind randomised controlled trial. *Lancet.* 2015;386(10012):2499-2506.
36. Litton E, Latham P, Inman J, et al. Safety and efficacy of erythropoiesis-stimulating agents in critically ill patients admitted to the intensive care unit: a systematic review and meta-analysis. *Intensive Care Med.* 2019;45(9):1190-1199.
37. Singer M, Deutschman CS, Seymour CW, et al. The third international consensus definitions for sepsis and septic shock (Sepsis-3). *JAMA.* 2016;315(8):801-810.
38. Basu D, Kulkarni R. Overview of blood components and their preparation. *Indian J Anaesth.* 2014;58(5):529-537.
39. Yoshida T, Prudent M, D'Alessandro A. Red blood cell storage lesion: causes and potential clinical consequences. *Blood Transfus.* 2019;17(1):27-52.
40. Raza S, Ali Baig M, Chang C, et al. A prospective study on red blood cell transfusion related hyperkalemia in critically ill patients. *J Clin Med Res.* 2015;7(6):417-421.
41. Bansal I, Calhoun BW, Joseph C, et al. A comparative study of reducing the extracellular potassium concentration in red blood cells by washing and by reduction of additive solution. *Transfusion.* 2007;47(2):248-250.
42. Lannan KL, Sahler J, Spinelli SL, et al. Transfusion immunomodulation—the case for leukoreduced and (perhaps) washed transfusions. *Blood Cells Mol Dis.* 2013;50(1):61-68.
43. Crowther MA, Cook DJ, Meade MO, et al. Thrombocytopenia in medical-surgical critically ill patients: prevalence, incidence, and risk factors. *J Crit Care.* 2005;20(4):348-353.
44. Akca S, Haji-Michael P, de Mendonca A, et al. Time course of platelet counts in critically ill patients. *Crit Care Med.* 2002;30(4):753-756.
45. Vanderschueren S, De Weerdt A, Malbrain M, et al. Thrombocytopenia and prognosis in intensive care. *Crit Care Med.* 2000;28(6):1871-1876.
46. Venkata C, Kashyap R, Farmer JC, et al. Thrombocytopenia in adult patients with sepsis: incidence, risk factors, and its association with clinical outcome. *J Intensive Care.* 2013;1(1):9.
47. Moreau D, Timsit JF, Vesin A, et al. Platelet count decline: an early prognostic marker in critically ill patients with prolonged ICU stays. *Chest.* 2007;131(6):1735-1741.
48. Hanes SD, Quarles DA, Boucher BA. Incidence and risk factors of thrombocytopenia in critically ill trauma patients. *Ann Pharmacother.* 1997;31(3):285-289.
49. Bonfiglio MF, Traeger SM, Kier KL, et al. Thrombocytopenia in intensive care patients: a comprehensive analysis of risk factors in 314 patients. *Ann Pharmacother.* 1995;29(9):835-842.
50. Zarychanski R, Houston DS. Assessing thrombocytopenia in the intensive care unit: the past, present, and future. *Hematology Am Soc Hematol Educ Program.* 2017;2017(1):660-666.
51. Griffin BR, Bronsert M, Reece TB, et al. Thrombocytopenia after cardiopulmonary bypass is associated with increased morbidity and mortality. *Ann Thorac Surg.* 2019;110:50-57.
52. Guru PK, Singh TD, Akhoundi A, et al. Association of thrombocytopenia and mortality in critically ill patients on continuous renal replacement therapy. *Nephron.* 2016;133(3):175-182.
53. Griffin BR, Jovanovich A, You Z, et al. Effects of baseline thrombocytopenia and platelet decrease following renal replacement therapy initiation in patients with severe acute kidney injury. *Crit Care Med.* 2019;47(4):e325-e331.
54. Brachemi S, Bollee G. Renal biopsy practice: what is the gold standard? *World J Nephrol.* 2014;3(4):287-294.

55. Gonzalez E, Moore EE, Moore HB, et al. Goal-directed hemostatic resuscitation of trauma-induced coagulopathy: a pragmatic randomized clinical trial comparing a viscoelastic assay to conventional coagulation assays. *Ann Surg.* 2016;263:1051-1059.
56. Fahrendorff M, Oliveri RS, Johansson PI. The use of viscoelastic haemostatic assays in goal-directing treatment with allogeneic blood products—a systematic review and meta-analysis. *Scand J Trauma Resusc Emerg Med.* 2017;25:39.
57. Wikkelsø A, Wetterslev J, Møller AM, et al. Thromboelastography (TEG) or thromboelastometry (ROTEM) to monitor haemostatic treatment versus usual care in adults or children with bleeding. *Cochrane Database Syst Rev.* 2016;CD007871.
58. Whiting D, DiNardo JA. TEG and ROTEM: technology and clinical applications. *Am J Hematol.* 2014;89:228-232.
59. Hoffman M, Monroe DM. A cell-based model of hemostasis. *Thromb Haemost.* 2001;85:958-965.
60. Wisler JW, Becker RC. Oral factor Xa inhibitors for the long-term management of ACS. *Nat Rev Cardiol.* 2012;9:392-401.
61. Johansson PI, Stissing T, Bochsen L, et al. Thromboelastography and thromboelastometry in assessing coagulopathy in trauma. *Scand J Trauma Resusc Emerg Med.* 2009;17:45.
62. Ho KM, Pavey W. Applying the cell-based coagulation model in the management of critical bleeding. *Anaesth Intensive Care.* 2017;45:166-176.

Suggested Readings

Gameiro J, Lopes JA. Complete blood count in acute kidney injury prediction: a narrative review. *Ann Intensive Care.* 2019;9(1):87.

Hawkins J, Aster RH, Curtis BR. Post-transfusion purpura: current perspectives. *J Blood Med.* 2019;10:405-415.

Jacobs MR, Smith D, Heaton WA, et al; Group PGDS. Detection of bacterial contamination in prestorage culture-negative apheresis platelets on day of issue with the Pan Genera Detection test. *Transfusion.* 2011;51(12):2573-2582.

12

Diuretics and Acute Kidney Injury

Anam Tariq and Blaithin A. McMahon

INTRODUCTION

Optimizing fluid status is fundamental in critical care but is challenging to achieve, especially in patients receiving vasoactive medications. Almost half of all intensive care admissions are prescribed diuretics.[1-4] Although diuretics have many uses, for the purpose of this chapter we discuss diuretic classification, pharmacology, the role of diuretics in the treatment of extracellular fluid (ECF) expansion, and their current utility in acute kidney injury (AKI).

CLASSIFICATION

Diuretics are normally classified according to their site and mechanism of action along the nephron. Currently, there are three common categories of diuretics used in the intensive care unit (ICU): loop diuretics, thiazide diuretics (and thiazide-like diuretics), and potassium-sparing diuretics (including mineralocorticoid receptor antagonists) (**Table 12.1**).

PHARMACOLOGY

Loop Diuretics

Loop diuretics (e.g., furosemide, bumetanide, torsemide, and ethacrynic acid) exert their natriuretic effect in the nephron by inhibiting the Na-K-2Cl (NKCC2) cotransporter in the apical membrane of the ascending loop of Henle (LOH) to decrease sodium transport.[1-5] Furosemide is absorbed quickly after oral administration with peak concentrations within 0.5 to 2 hours. Loop diuretics are organic anions that are poorly lipid soluble, and highly bound (>95%) to serum albumin, thus limiting their filtration at the glomerulus.[6,7] There is great variability in the bioavailability of all types of loop diuretics: furosemide (40%-60%), bumetanide (80%), or torsemide (>91%).[4,7,8] To gain access to the peritubular region, loop diuretics must be secreted across the proximal tubule via organic anion transporters (OATs) 1 and 3 on the basolateral membrane.[7] Once secreted into the tubular fluid on the luminal side, a loop diuretic binds to the NKCC2 cotransporter at the thick ascending limb (TAL) of the LOH.

The choice of loop diuretic is important because the half-life is significantly different among loop diuretics and longer for torsemide compared to bumetanide and furosemide (Table 12.1). This has led many clinicians to use an IV infusion of furosemide over bolus administrations.[7-10] The Diuretic Optimization Strategies Evaluation (DOSE) trial attempted to answer the question of whether more aggressive decongestion can improve acute heart failure outcomes. The trial examined outcomes between high- versus low-dose furosemide treatment

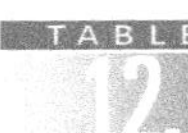

TABLE 12.1 Pharmacokinetics and Use of Diuretics in the Management of Volume Overload, Oliguria, and AKI Status in the ICU

Type	**Loop Diuretic**			**Thiazide Diuretic**			**K+ Sparing Diuretic**		
Diuretic name	Furosemide	Bumetanide	Torsemide	Hydrochlorothiazide	Chlorthalidone	Metolazone	Amiloride	Triamterene	Spironolactone
Mechanism of action	Inhibition of Na-K+-2Cl cotransporter (NKCC2)			Inhibition of NaCl cotransporter (NCC)			Inhibition of sodium channels (ENAC)		Mineralocorticoid receptor antagonists
Site of action	LOH			DCT			CD		
Oral dose administration range, mg	20-80	0.5-2	5-20	12.5-50	12.5-50	2.5-10	5-10	50	25-50
Equipotent doses, mg	40	1	15-20	25	12.5	2.5	–	–	–
IV administration range, mg	Bolus 20-600 mg or continuous 5-30 mg/hr	Bolus 0.5-10 mg	Bolus 5-200	250-500	–	–	–	–	–
$t_{1/2}$, hr, normal kidney function	0.5-2	1	3-4	6-15	40-60	14-20	6-26	1-2	1.5

$t_{1/2}$, hr, kidney dysfunction	2.8	1.6	4-5	Extended	Extended	Extended	100	Extended	Extended
Sulfa cross-reactivity	Sulfur-containing organic molecule	Sulfur-containing organic molecule	Sulfur-containing organic molecule	Sulfur-containing organic molecule	Sulfur-containing organic molecule	Sulfur-containing organic molecule[a]			
Metabolism	100% kidney	50% liver 50% kidney	80% in liver	– Excretion: urine (10%-15%) (oral), 96% (IV) as unchanged drug	– Excretion: urine (unchanged)	– Excretion: urine (80%)	Substrate of OCT Excretion: urine (~50%; as unchanged drug)	– Excretion: urine (21% to <50%; primarily as metabolites)	– Excretion: urine (primarily as metabolites)

Data are presented as single reported values or range of reported values.

AKI, acute kidney injury; CD, collecting duct; DCT, distal convoluted tubule; ICU, intensive care unit; IV, intravenous; LOH, loop of Henle; OCT, organic cation transporter 2; PCT, proximal convoluted tubule.

[a]Absorption may be decreased in congestive heart failure.

and continuous infusion versus every-12-hour bolus furosemide administration. The high-dose group (e.g., total daily IV furosemide dose 2.5 times their total daily oral loop diuretic dose in furosemide equivalents) had a nonsignificant improvement in patients' global assessment of symptoms (co-primary end point, $p = 0.06$) and greater diuresis without a change in kidney function. Interestingly, even though the high-dose group had more AKI (23% compared to 14% in the low dose group, $p = 0.04$), the effects were transient, resolving before 60 days and without a change in overall survival. Important adverse effects of high-dose diuretics include hypovolemia,[11] electrolyte imbalances,[12,13] hyperuricemia, hyperglycemia, tinnitus, and deafness.[14]

Thiazide Diuretics

Similar to loop diuretics, thiazide diuretics are organic anions. Examples include chlorthalidone, hydrochlorothiazide, metolazone, and chlorothiazide. Thiazides exert their effect by blocking the NaCl cotransporter (NCC) along the distal convoluted tubule (DCT) to promote natriuresis. Thiazides are particularly effective in correcting loop diuretic resistance in patients with severe congestion.[15-17] Pharmacologic properties of thiazide diuretics are highlighted in Table 12.1. Thiazides normally have 50% or more bioavailability, with metolazone having a bioavailability of 70%.[15] Half-lives of thiazides are prolonged in AKI and chronic kidney disease (CKD). The most common adverse effects associated with the thiazide diuretics include skin rashes, interstitial nephritis, gout, alkalosis, pancreatitis, volume depletion, hypokalemia, hyponatremia, hypomagnesemia, hypercholesterolemia, hypertriglyceridemia, hyperglycemia, and azotemia. Limited observational data suggest an increased risk of hyponatremia and hypokalemia when thiazides are used in combination with loop diuretics.[18]

K+ Sparing Diuretics

This class of diuretics includes triamterene, amiloride, and spironolactone.[19-22] Spironolactone (and eplerenone) acts as an aldosterone antagonist, so the diuretic effect occurs distal in the nephron, potentially limiting their natriuresis effect. As such, they are often paired with other diuretics in order to increase sodium elimination. Where these agents excel is in patients with hypervolemia from heart failure or end-stage liver disease where they limit the adverse circulatory effects of aldosterone and improve patient outcomes.[23-25] The oral bioavailability of these medications is 50% or more, and the half-life is anywhere from 1.5 to 26 hours. Commonly reported side effects include hyperkalemia, worsening renal function (WRF), hypersensitivity, metabolic acidosis, or gynecomastia. For this reason, they should be used with caution in patients with an active AKI.

Others

Mannitol is an osmotic diuretic that impairs the ability to concentrate urine by inhibiting sodium and water reabsorption in both the proximal tubule as well as the LOH.[26] Mannitol infusion is most commonly used in the treatment of intracranial hypertension following traumatic brain injury in the neurocritical care setting; it is therefore not primarily employed as a diuretic for volume overload. However, when used in any clinical setting, its water diuresis can lead to an increase in plasma osmolality and induce volume expansion/overload and dysnatremias.[27,28] Carbonic anhydrase inhibitors are a separate class of weak diuretics that inhibit sodium bicarbonate reabsorption in the proximal tubules and promote water and bicarbonate loss in the urine. These agents are frequently used in the treatment of both metabolic alkalosis and glaucoma. Acetazolamide was studied in the setting of patients requiring mechanical ventilation because of chronic obstructive pulmonary disease and the aforementioned metabolic alkalosis. In this study, 500 to 1000 mg twice a day led to lower serum bicarbonate levels and fewer days with metabolic alkalosis compared to placebo. Unfortunately, there was no significant difference in the duration of mechanical ventilation; however, given the changes in metabolic parameters, there may still be a role for these agents in this specific patient population.[29]

DIURETIC USE FOR THE MANAGEMENT OF GENERALIZED EDEMA

Loop diuretics remain the initial choice of therapy to alleviate fluid overload that may result from edematous states. However, many factors influence the efficacy of loop diuretics in critically ill patients in the ICU, including age, body weight, mean arterial pressure, hypoalbuminemia, severity of AKI, metabolic acidosis, hypokalemia, nonsteroidal anti-inflammatory drugs (NSAIDs), cephalosporins, and premorbid diuretic naivety.[14,30-34] These are important factors when considering the initial starting dose of loop diuretics, but very little guidance exists in the literature on this topic. All loop diuretics produce similar responses when given in equipotent doses. In the setting of normal kidney function, 40 mg of furosemide is approximately equal to 1 mg of bumetanide and 20 mg of torsemide. Typically, the recommendation is to "double the dose" of loop diuretic until a "threshold" dose of diuretic is reached. Below this threshold plasma concentration, there is no significant natriuresis and above it the response rises rapidly. At higher concentrations, a "ceiling" or plateau concentration is reached such that with increasingly higher plasma concentrations of diuretic, there is no further natriuresis.[35] For the initial starting dose of loop diuretic, in a naive patient with preserved kidney function, a dose of 40 mg of intravenous furosemide (or equivalents) is an appropriate starting point. However, in settings of prior exposure to loop diuretics, reduced blood flow to the kidneys, enhanced sodium reabsorption (renin-angiotensin activation), or decreased glomerular filtration rate (GFR), higher doses will likely be needed to achieve diuresis. In these situations, clinicians can consider starting by doubling the home dose of diuretic or base dosing on the patient's weight (e.g., 1 mg/kg for diuretic-naive patients or 1.5 mg/kg for nondiuretic-naive patients). Table 12.1 describes the range of doses and equivalent doses (in both oral and parental forms) across the spectrum of diuretics. Over time, with effective natriuresis, the efficacy of diuretics can wane as ECF space declines, an effect often referred to as the "braking phenomenon" whereby the nephron avidly reabsorbs sodium and is equal to dietary NaCl intake.[14,36] Many factors account for these changes, but remodeling and adaptive changes (hypertrophy and hyperplasia) in the distal nephron play a significant role, specifically leading to an increased reabsorption of sodium and blunting the natriuretic effect.[16,37-39] The addition of a thiazide or thiazide-like drug can help to treat this type of adaptation by blocking NaCl absorption along the distal nephron and can improve diuretic resistance and restore diuretic efficacy.[14,40,41] Other mechanisms of diuretic resistance include (a) poor diuretic delivery to kidney (e.g., hypoalbuminemia, dose too low or too infrequent and poor absorption), (b) reduced diuretic secretion (because of decreased kidney perfusion in the setting of heart failure or vasoconstriction within the kidney in the setting of end-stage liver disease or competitive inhibition of OATs by uremic toxics [such as cresol and indoxyl sulfate], which are increased in the setting of decreased glomerular filtration) or decreased functional kidney mass, and (c) insufficient kidney response (because of CKD, activation of renin-angiotensin-aldosterone system [RAAS], use of NSAIDs, and excessive sodium intake).[15]

Strategies to improve diuretic resistance despite maximum doses of loop diuretic include changing from one loop diuretic to another member of the same class. As the bioavailability of loop agents is highly variable, with oral furosemide having notoriously heterogenous availability, some have reported success after switching from furosemide to bumetanide or torsemide.[42] Other strategies include changing to a continuous infusion versus bolus or the coadministration with thiazides or potassium-sparing diuretics.

While there are some data to suggest that the coadministration of intravenous albumin with diuretics may augment the diuretic response in the setting of cirrhosis or nephrotic syndrome, a systematic review demonstrated that there was only marginal increase in sodium excretion and urine output using this technique.[15,17,43] Finally, sequential nephron blockade with use of a combination types of diuretics effecting the proximal convoluted tubule (PCT), DCT, and collecting duct (CD) can cumulatively result in an additive or synergistic diuretic response when compared to monotherapy. While theoretically different mechanisms of diuresis (e.g. RAAS blockade or inhibiting specific electrolyte transporters) should improve urine output, the comparative efficacies of exact diuretic combinations are not well known.

LOOP DIURETICS AND ACUTE KIDNEY INJURY OUTCOME

Diuretics are ineffective in the prevention and treatment of AKI (**Table 12.2**).[17,22,30,44–49] Some studies comparing loop diuretics to no diuretic therapy in patients undergoing either cardiac angiography or cardiac surgery did not prevent AKI.[44,45] However, newer studies have shown there might be a benefit of loop diuretics when used with hydration fluid to prevent contrast-associated AKI (CA-AKI). Induced Diuresis With Matched Hydration Compared to Standard Hydration for Contrast Induced Nephropathy Prevention (MYTHOS) study trial compared IV hydration alone or with hydration plus 0.5 mg/kg of IV furosemide after a coronary procedure.[46] The furosemide group displayed lower AKI rate (4.6% in the fluid with matched hydration group, vs 18% in the control group, $p = 0.005$). The use of matched hydrated protocols (every mL of urine produced matched with mL of hydration fluid) such as that used in the AKIGUARD (Acute Kidney Injury GUARding Device) trial also showed promising results but has yet to be recommended for use in the absence of multicenter randomized controlled trials (RCTs).[50]

Other forms of AKI do not support the use of diuretics in AKI therapeutics. Additionally, furosemide administration in patients undergoing kidney replacement therapy (KRT) does not improve the overall rate of kidney recovery.[48] Older studies have reported that diuretic use is significantly associated with higher hospital mortality among critically ill patients with AKI.[51] Cumulative IV dosing, from 1.5 to 3 mg/hr, of diuretics in postsurgical patients was predictive of mortality, and the higher the dose, the more the associated hypotension during KRT.[45] In patients undergoing cardiac surgery, furosemide did not have notable differences in kidney dysfunction when used before or during surgery.[22] RCTs and meta-analyses involving use of diuretics also showed improvement in urine output without improvement in patient-centered outcomes such as duration of KRT, hospitalization, or mortality.[47,52]

Despite the lack of effect of furosemide in the prevention, treatment, and recovery of AKI, more recent studies suggest a beneficial effects of loop diuretics, particularly in maintaining fluid balance in critically ill patients with AKI. Post

TABLE 12.2 Summary of Studies Associated With Diuretics and Clinical Outcomes

Study, Ref.	Study Year	*N*	Study Design	Study Population	Diuretic Type	Median Dose	Duration	Outcome
Prevention								
Hager et al[44]	1996	121	RCT Intervention vs placebo	Post major thoraco-abdominal or vascular surgery	Furosemide	1 mg/hr	Continuous	No difference in patients in AKI rate treated with furosemide
Lassnigg et al[45]	2000	132	RCT Dopamine vs furosemide vs placebo	Patients with normal kidney function undergoing cardiac surgery	Furosemide	Total 50 mg (1.5-3 mL/hr)	Continuous	Continuous infusion of furosemide was associated with the highest risk of AKI
Mahesh et al[22]	2008	42	RCT Intervention vs saline	High-risk cardiac surgery patients	Furosemide	4 mg/hr	Continuous	No decrease in rate of AKI
Marenzi et al[46]	2012	170	MYTHOS RCT-induced diuresis with matched hydration compared to standard hydration	CKD patients undergoing coronary procedures	Furosemide	0.5 mg/kg	IV bolus	Furosemide-induced high urine output with matched hydration significantly reduced the risk of CA-AKI

(continued)

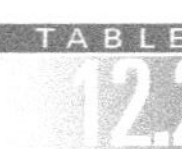

TABLE 12.2 Summary of Studies Associated With Diuretics and Clinical Outcomes (*continued*)

Study, Ref.	Study Year	*N*	Study Design	Study Population	Diuretic Type	Median Dose	Duration	Outcome
Usmiani et al[50]	2016	130	RCT Bicarbonate/isotonic saline/NAC/vitamin C vs high-volume forced diuresis with matched hydration	CKD patients undergoing coronary angiography	Furosemide	0.5 mg/kg	IV bolus	Forced diuresis with matched hydration had lowest incidence of CA-AKI (7% vs 25%, $p = 0.01$) and major adverse cardiac and cerebrovascular events at 1 year (7% vs 32%, $p < 0.01$)
Dormans and Gerlag[17]	1996	20	Prospective single arm, open label	Severe congestive heart failure (NYHA stage III-IV) with ≥5 kg weight gain and a proven diuretic resistance treated with furosemide × 2 wk	Furosemide HCTZ	250-4,000 mg daily 25-100 mg daily	Oral or IV 3-12 d	Mean creatinine clearance did not significantly decrease from 32.7 ± 22.5 to 27.6 ± 22.5 mL/min/1.73 m^2
Shilliday et al[47]	1997	92	RCT Torsemide vs furosemide vs placebo	AKI patients receiving dopamine, mannitol	Furosemide Torsemide	3 mg/kg	IV q6h for +21 d	No differences in need for KRT ($p = 0.87$), kidney recovery ($p = 0.56$), or mortality ($p = 0.24$)

van der Voort et al[48]	2009	71	RCT Interventions vs placebo	AKI patients requiring KRT	Furosemide	0.5 mg/kg/hr	Continuous infusion	Increase in urinary volume and sodium excretion but did not lead to a shorter duration of kidney failure or more frequent kidney recovery
Felker et al[30]	2011	308	RCT 1:1:1:1 Intravenous vs oral and low dose vs high dose	Outpatients with ADHF (furosemide or thiazide) × 1 mo	Furosemide	Equivalent to the patients' previous oral dose of 80 and 240 mg or a high dose (2.5 × previous oral dose)	1. IV bolus q12h 2. Continuous	Nonsignificant differences in patients' global assessment of symptoms or in the change in kidney function when diuretic therapy was administered by bolus as compared with continuous infusion or at a high dose as compared with a low dose
Recovery								
Mehta et al[51]	2002	552	Retrospective	ICU patients with AKI referred to nephrology	1. Furosemide 2. Bumetanide 3. Metolazone 4. HydroDiuril 5. Loop and thiazide	1. 80 mg (20-320) 2. 10 mg (2-29) 3. 10 mg (5-20)	Daily (for either dosing)	Increased mortality and nonrecovery of kidney function in AKI patients receiving diuretics No significant differences among patients taking single vs combination diuretics
Cantarovich et al[49]	2004	338	RCT Intervention (two types) vs placebo	AKI patients receiving KRT at enrolment	Furosemide	1. 25 mg/kg/d 2. 35 mg/kg/d	1. IV daily 2. Oral daily	No difference in mortality ($p = 0.36$), duration of KRT ($p = 0.21$), or kidney recovery ($p = 0.51$)

(*continued*)

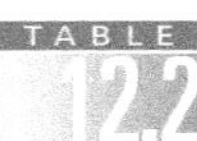

Summary of Studies Associated With Diuretics and Clinical Outcomes (*continued*)

Study, Ref.	Study Year	*N*	Study Design	Study Population	Diuretic Type	Median Dose	Duration	Outcome
Grams et al[53]	2011	306	Fluid and Catheter Treatment Trial (FACTT) RCT Conservative vs liberal fluid management strategy	Patients with ALI and AKI	Furosemide	1. 3-24 mg/hr 2. 20-160 mg	1. Continuous 2. Bolus	Post-AKI diuretic therapy was associated with 60-d patient survival
Wu et al[65]	2012	572	Prospective, observational multicenter	Postsurgical AKI patients receiving KRT	Diuretics	–	–	Higher 3-d accumulative diuretic dose predicts mortality. Higher diuretic doses are associated with hypotension and a lower intensity of dialysis
Teixeira et al[34]	2013	601	Secondary Analysis of Prospective Multicenter Cohort study NEFROlogia e Cura INTensiva (NEFROINT) Study	Patients with critical illness and AKI	Diuretics	–	1. Continuous 2. Bolus	Diuretic use was associated with better survival (adjusted HR 0.25, 95% CI: 0.12–0.52; $p < 0.001$)

ADHF, acute decompensated heart failure; AKI, acute kidney injury; ALI, acute lung injury; CI, confidence interval; CA-AKI, contrast-induced AKI; CKD, chronic kidney disease; HCTZ, hydrochlorothiazide; HR, hazard ratio; IV, intravenous; NAC, *N*-acetylcysteine; NYHA, New York Heart Association; RCT, randomized controlled trial; KRT, kidney replacement therapy.

hoc analysis of the multicenter FACTT (Fluid and Catheter Trial Therapy) trial showed that patients with AKI in the fluid-conservative group received more furosemide (80 vs 23 mg/d than those in the fluid-liberal group, $p < 0.001$). Additionally, those in the fluid conservative arm had less fluid accumulation compared to those in the fluid-liberal group, (0.9 vs 2.2 L/day, $p < 0.001$). Thus, in the setting of acute respiratory distress syndrome (ARDS), protocolized diuretic use as part of a fluid conservative strategy is associated with a protective effect on 60-day mortality even in the presence of positive fluid balance.[53] In a second study from a multicenter prospective cohort in ten Italian ICUs involving 601 critically ill patients, nonsurviving AKI patients had higher mean fluid balance (1.31 ± 1.24 vs 0.17 ± 0.72 L/d; $p < 0.001$) and lower mean urine volume (1.28 ± 0.90 vs 2.35 ± 0.98 L/d; $p < 0.001$) as compared to survivors. Proportion of ICU days in which diuretics were used as a surrogate for diuretic use and occurred over 1-10 ICU days. Diuretic use was associated with better survival in this population (adjusted hazard ratio [HR] 0.25, 95% confidence interval [CI]: 0.12-0.52; $p < 0.001$).[34] This supports the concept that a positive fluid balance has a detrimental effect on mortality of critically ill AKI patients.

DIURETIC USE IN HEART FAILURE

In the DOSE trial, mentioned earlier, twice-daily IV bolus versus continuous furosemide infusion and high-dose versus low-dose furosemide were compared, with no significant differences in the patient's global assessment of symptoms. However, there remains many advantages to using a continuous infusion of loop diuretic over IV bolus including lower peak plasma concentrations. These lower levels protect patients from ototoxicity, which is often temporary but can be permanent, and is an often overlooked complication of diuretic use in AKI. For the comparison of high- versus low-dose furosemide, WRF (defined as increase in plasma creatinine >0.3 mg/dL within 72 hours) occurred more frequently in the high-dose arm, although subsequent statistical analyses showed WRF was associated with improved rather than worse long-term clinical outcomes.[55] Further data have questioned the clinical significance of serum creatinine (SCr) rise during ADHF. Acute Kidney Injury Neutrophil Gelatinase-Associated Lipocalin (N-GAL) Evaluation of Symptomatic Heart Failure Study (AKINESIS) study of AKI biomarkers during ADHF has confirmed an overall lack of substantial kidney tubular injury in ADHF.[56,57]

Regarding the choice of loop diuretic for the management of ADHF, there are an increasing number of studies that have shown benefit of torsemide over furosemide in ADHF with improved ADHF outcomes. A systematic review and meta-analysis from 1996 through 2019 demonstrated 19 studies, where mean follow-up duration was 15 months and torsemide was associated with a lower risk of hospitalization among ADHF patients (10.6% vs 18.4%; odds ratio [OR] 0.72, 95% CI 0.51-1.03, $p = 0.07$, $I^2 = 18\%$; number needed to treat [NNT] = 23) compared with furosemide.[58] However, all-cause mortality was nonsignificant between torsemide and furosemide use.

DIURETIC USE IN PATIENTS WITH END-STAGE LIVER DISEASE

Diuretics such as loop diuretics and aldosterone antagonists are the mainstay of therapy for ascites and volume overload in patients with end-stage liver disease. Aldosterone antagonist use is superior to loop diuretics in the treatment of ascites, but loop diuretics do help augment the diuretic effects.[59] Spironolactone can be titrated every 7 days (in increments of 50 mg) with furosemide (40-160 mg/d, in 40 mg/d steps) provided kidney function and electrolytes are closely monitored.[60,61] The use of diuretics in patients with end-stage liver disease who are admitted to the ICU with AKI presents a challenging scenario. Diuretics can contribute to AKI in end-stage liver disease patients through hemodynamic mechanisms and should warrant a trial of discontinuation of diuretics together with volume expansion.[62]

USE OF FUROSEMIDE FOR THE ASSESSMENT OF TUBULAR INTEGRITY IN EARLY ACUTE KIDNEY INJURY

Furosemide-induced urine output can be used to assess the integrity of the kidney tubular function (furosemide stress test [FST]) in the setting of AKI and was formally described in a pilot study by Chawla et al in 2013.[63] In this study, 77 subjects (with early-stage AKI) were challenged with a one-time dose of IV furosemide (1 mg/kg for loop diuretic–naive patients and 1.5 mg/kg for those who had prior loop diuretic exposure) and assessed to predict progression to severe AKI (need for KRT or increased SCr to 3 times baseline or urine output <0.3 mL/kg/hr). This was an isovolemic challenge with every 1 mL of urine output replaced with 1 mL IV crystalloid (as per the discretion of the primary ICU team). This pilot study demonstrated that the 2-hour urine output (<200 mL) in response to a furosemide challenge was able to predict progression to Stage III AKI.[63]

Since publication of this initial pilot study, there have been several retrospective validations of this cutoff and the publication of the multicenter FST prospective study.[54,64] This 92 ICU patients multicenter study found similar operating characteristics for the FST with a urinary cutoff of 200 mL over the first 2 hours (sensitivity 73.9% and specificity 89.9%).[54] The incidence of hypotension was 9.8%, almost double that in the pilot study, suggesting that the FST should not be utilized in hypovolemic patients. There were no critical life-threatening events recorded in the multicenter study.

References

1. McCoy IE, Chertow GM, Chang TIH. Patterns of diuretic use in the intensive care unit. *PLoS One.* 2019;14:e0217911.
2. Grodin JL, Stevens SR, de Las Fuentes L, et al. Intensification of medication therapy for cardiorenal syndrome in acute decompensated heart failure. *J Card Fail.* 2016;22:26-32.
3. Ellison DH, Felker GM. Diuretic treatment in heart failure. *N Engl J Med.* 2017;377:1964-1975.
4. Ellison DH. Clinical pharmacology in diuretic use. *Clin J Am Soc Nephrol.* 2019;14:1248.
5. Wilcox CS, Mitch WE, Kelly RA, et al. Response of the kidney to furosemide. I. Effects of salt intake and renal compensation. *J Lab Clin Med.* 1983;102:450-458.
6. Shankar SS, Brater DC. Loop diuretics: from the Na-K-2Cl transporter to clinical use. *Am J Physiol Renal Physiol.* 2003;284:F11-F21.
7. Huang X, Mees ED, Vos P, et al. Everything we always wanted to know about furosemide but were afraid to ask. *Am J Physiol Renal Physiol.* 2016;310:F958-F971.
8. Brater DC, Chennavasin P, Day B, et al. Bumetanide and furosemide. *Clin Pharmacol Ther.* 1983;34:207-213.
9. Lesne M, Clerckx-Braun F, Duhoux P, et al. Pharmacokinetic study of torasemide in humans: an overview of its diuretic effect. *Int J Clin Pharmacol Ther Toxicol.* 1982;20:382-387.
10. Huang A, Luethi N, Martensson J, et al. Pharmacodynamics of intravenous furosemide bolus in critically ill patients. *Crit Care Resusc.* 2017;19:142-149.
11. Gottlieb SS, Brater DC, Thomas I, et al. BG9719 (CVT-124), an A1 adenosine receptor antagonist, protects against the decline in renal function observed with diuretic therapy. *Circulation.* 2002;105:1348-1353.
12. Klein L, O'Connor CM, Leimberger JD, et al. Lower serum sodium is associated with increased short-term mortality in hospitalized patients with worsening heart failure: results from the Outcomes of a Prospective Trial of Intravenous Milrinone for Exacerbations of Chronic Heart Failure (OPTIME-CHF) study. *Circulation.* 2005;111:2454-2460.

13. Cooper HA, Dries DL, Davis CE, et al. Diuretics and risk of arrhythmic death in patients with left ventricular dysfunction. *Circulation.* 1999;100:1311-1315.
14. Felker GM, O'Connor CM, Braunwald E, Heart failure clinical research network I. Loop diuretics in acute decompensated heart failure: necessary? Evil? A necessary evil? *Circ Heart Fail.* 2009;2:56-62.
15. Hoorn EJ, Ellison DH. Diuretic resistance. *Am J Kidney Dis.* 2017;69:136-142.
16. Ellison DH, Velazquez H, Wright FS. Adaptation of the distal convoluted tubule of the rat. Structural and functional effects of dietary salt intake and chronic diuretic infusion. *J Clin Invest.* 1989;83:113-126.
17. Dormans TP, Gerlag PG. Combination of high-dose furosemide and hydrochlorothiazide in the treatment of refractory congestive heart failure. *Eur Heart J.* 1996;17:1867-1874.
18. Jentzer JC, DeWald TA, Hernandez AF. Combination of loop diuretics with thiazide-type diuretics in heart failure. *J Am Coll Cardiol.* 2010;56(19):1527-1534.
19. Feria I, Pichardo I, Juarez P, et al. Therapeutic benefit of spironolactone in experimental chronic cyclosporine A nephrotoxicity. *Kidney Int.* 2003;63:43-52.
20. Mejia-Vilet JM, Ramirez V, Cruz C, et al. Renal ischemia-reperfusion injury is prevented by the mineralocorticoid receptor blocker spironolactone. *Am J Physiol Renal Physiol.* 2007;293:F78-F86.
21. Sanchez-Pozos K, Barrera-Chimal J, Garzon-Muvdi J, et al. Recovery from ischemic acute kidney injury by spironolactone administration. *Nephrol Dial Transplant.* 2012;27:3160-3169.
22. Mahesh B, Yim B, Robson D, et al. Does furosemide prevent renal dysfunction in high-risk cardiac surgical patients? Results of a double-blinded prospective randomised trial. *Eur J Cardiothorac Surg.* 2008;33:370-376.
23. Randomized Aldactone Evaluation Study. Effectiveness of spironolactone added to an angiotensin-converting enzyme inhibitor and a loop diuretic for severe chronic congestive heart failure (the Randomized Aldactone Evaluation Study [RALES]). *Am J Cardiol.* 1996;78(8):902-907.
24. Fogel MR, Sawhney VK, Neal EA, et al. Diuresis in the ascitic patient: a randomized controlled trial of three regimens. *J Clin Gastroenterol.* 1981;3 (Suppl 1):73-80.
25. Runyon BA, AASLD Practice Guidelines Committee. Management of adult patients with ascites due to cirrhosis: an update. *Hepatology.* 2009;49:2087-2107.
26. Mathisen O, Raeder M, Kiil F. Mechanism of osmotic diuresis. *Kidney Int.* 1981;19(3):431-437.
27. Gipstein RM, Boyle JD. Hypernatremia complicating prolonged mannitol diuresis. *N Engl J Med.* 1965;272:1116-1117.
28. Aviram A, Pfau A, Czaczkes JW, et al. Hyperosmolality with hyponatremia, caused by inappropriate administration of mannitol. *Am J Med.* 1967;42(4):648-650.
29. Faisy C, Meziani F, Planquette B, et al. Effect of acetazolamide vs placebo on duration of invasive mechanical ventilation among patients with chronic obstructive pulmonary disease: a randomized clinical trial. *JAMA.* 2016;315(5):480-488.
30. Felker GM, Lee KL, Bull DA, et al. Diuretic strategies in patients with acute decompensated heart failure. *N Engl J Med.* 2011;364:797-805.
31. Burckhardt G. Drug transport by organic anion transporters (OATs). *Pharmacol Ther.* 2012;136:106-130.
32. Wu W, Bush KT, Nigam SK. Key role for the organic anion transporters, OAT1 and OAT3, in the in vivo handling of uremic toxins and solutes. *Sci Rep.* 2017;7:4939.
33. Cemerikic D, Wilcox CS, Giebisch G. Intracellular potential and K+ activity in rat kidney proximal tubular cells in acidosis and K+ depletion. *J Membr Biol.* 1982;69:159-165.
34. Teixeira C, Garzotto F, Piccinni P, et al. Fluid balance and urine volume are independent predictors of mortality in acute kidney injury. *Crit Care.* 2013;17:R14.
35. Brater DC, Day B, Burdette A, et al. Bumetanide and furosemide in heart failure. *Kidney Int.* 1984;26(2):183-189.
36. Subramanya AR, Ellison DH. Distal convoluted tubule. *Clin J Am Soc Nephrol.* 2014;9:2147-2163.
37. Kaissling B, Stanton BA. Adaptation of distal tubule and collecting duct to increased sodium delivery. I. Ultrastructure. *Am J Physiol.* 1988;255:F1256-F1268.
38. Stanton BA, Kaissling B. Adaptation of distal tubule and collecting duct to increased Na delivery. II. Na+ and K+ transport. *Am J Physiol.* 1988;255:F1269-F1275.
39. Loon NR, Wilcox CS, Unwin RJ. Mechanism of impaired natriuretic response to furosemide during prolonged therapy. *Kidney Int.* 1989;36:682-689.
40. Marti C, Cole R, Kalogeropoulos A, et al. Medical therapy for acute decompensated heart failure: what recent clinical trials have taught us about diuretics and vasodilators. *Curr Heart Fail Rep.* 2012;9:1-7.
41. Hanberg JS, Tang WHW, Wilson FP, et al. An exploratory analysis of the competing effects of aggressive decongestion and high-dose loop diuretic therapy in the DOSE trial. *Int J Cardiol.* 2017;241:277-282.

42. Müller K, Gamba G, Jaquet F, et al. Torasemide vs. furosemide in primary care patients with chronic heart failure NYHA II to IV—efficacy and quality of life. *Eur J Heart Fail.* 2003;5(6):793-801.
43. Kitsios GD, Mascari P, Ettunsi DR, et al. Co-administration of furosemide with albumin for overcoming diuretic resistance in patients with hypoalbuminemia: a meta-analysis. *J Crit Care.* 2014;29(2):253-259.
44. Hager B, Betschart M, Krapf R. Effect of postoperative intravenous loop diuretic on renal function after major surgery. *Schweiz Med Wochenschr.* 1996;126:666-673.
45. Lassnigg A, Donner E, Grubhofer G, et al. Lack of renoprotective effects of dopamine and furosemide during cardiac surgery. *J Am Soc Nephrol.* 2000;11(1):97-104.
46. Marenzi G, Ferrari C, Marana I, et al. Prevention of contrast nephropathy by furosemide with matched hydration: the MYTHOS (induced diuresis with matched hydration compared to standard hydration for contrast induced nephropathy prevention) trial. *JACC Cardiovasc Interv.* 2012;5:90-97.
47. Shilliday IR, Quinn KJ, Allison ME. Loop diuretics in the management of acute renal failure: a prospective, double-blind, placebo-controlled, randomized study. *Nephrol Dial Transplant.* 1997;12:2592-2596.
48. van der Voort PH, Boerma EC, Koopmans M, et al. Furosemide does not improve renal recovery after hemofiltration for acute renal failure in critically ill patients: a double blind randomized controlled trial. *Crit Care Med.* 2009;37:533-538.
49. Cantarovich F, Rangoonwala B, Lorenz H, et al. High-dose furosemide for established ARF: a prospective, randomized, double-blind, placebo-controlled, multicenter trial. *Am J Kidney Dis.* 2004;44:402-409.
50. Usmiani T, Andreis A, Budano C, et al. AKIGUARD (Acute Kidney Injury GUARding Device) trial: in-hospital and one-year outcomes. *J Cardiovasc Med (Hagerstown).* 2016;17:530-537.
51. Mehta RL, Pascual MT, Soroko S, et al. Diuretics, mortality, and nonrecovery of renal function in acute renal failure. *JAMA.* 2002;288:2547-2553.
52. Bagshaw SM, Delaney A, Haase M, et al. Loop diuretics in the management of acute renal failure: a systematic review and meta-analysis. *Crit Care Resusc.* 2007;9:60-68.
53. Grams ME, Estrella MM, Coresh J, et al. Fluid balance, diuretic use, and mortality in acute kidney injury. *Clin J Am Soc Nephrol.* 2011;6:966-973.
54. Rewa OG, Bagshaw SM, Wang X, et al. The furosemide stress test for prediction of worsening acute kidney injury in critically ill patients: a multicenter, prospective, observational study. *J Crit Care.* 2019;52:109-114.
55. Metra M, Davison B, Bettari L, et al. Is worsening renal function an ominous prognostic sign in patients with acute heart failure? The role of congestion and its interaction with renal function. *Circ Heart Fail.* 2012;5:54-62.
56. Murray PT, Wettersten N, van Veldhuisen DJ, et al. Utility of urine neutrophil gelatinase-associated lipocalin for worsening renal function during hospitalization for acute heart failure: primary findings of the urine N-gal acute kidney injury N-gal evaluation of symptomatic heart failure study (AKINESIS). *J Card Fail.* 2019;25:654-665.
57. Wettersten N, Horiuchi Y, van Veldhuisen DJ, et al. Short-term prognostic implications of serum and urine neutrophil gelatinase-associated lipocalin in acute heart failure: findings from the AKINESIS study. *Eur J Heart Fail.* 2020;22:251-263.
58. Abraham B, Megaly M, Sous M, et al. Meta-analysis comparing torsemide versus furosemide in patients with heart failure. *Am J Cardiol.* 2020;125:92-99.
59. European Association for the Study of the Liver. EASL clinical practice guidelines on the management of ascites, spontaneous bacterial peritonitis, and hepatorenal syndrome in cirrhosis. *J Hepatol.* 2010;53:397-417.
60. Angeli P, Fasolato S, Mazza E, et al. Combined versus sequential diuretic treatment of ascites in non-azotaemic patients with cirrhosis: results of an open randomised clinical trial. *Gut.* 2010;59:98.
61. Santos J, Planas R, Pardo A, et al. Spironolactone alone or in combination with furosemide in the treatment of moderate ascites in nonazotemic cirrhosis. A randomized comparative study of efficacy and safety. *J Hepatol.* 2003;39:187-192.
62. Velez JCQ, Therapondos G, Juncos LA. Reappraising the spectrum of AKI and hepatorenal syndrome in patients with cirrhosis. *Nat Rev Nephrol.* 2020;16:137-155.
63. Chawla LS, Davison DL, Brasha-Mitchell E, et al. Development and standardization of a furosemide stress test to predict the severity of acute kidney injury. *Crit Care.* 2013;17:R207.
64. McMahon BA, Koyner JL, Novick T, et al. The prognostic value of the furosemide stress test in predicting delayed graft function following deceased donor kidney transplantation. *Biomarkers.* 2018;23:61-69.
65. Wu VC, Lai CF, Shiao CC, et al. Effect of diuretic use on 30-day postdialysis mortality in critically ill patients receiving acute dialysis. *PLoS One.* 2012;7:e30836.

13

Vasoactive Medications

Stephen Duff and Patrick T. Murray

INTRODUCTION

Vasoactive medications have been a standard component of critical care since the 1940s. They are used to correct shock states and maintain adequate end-organ perfusion. Despite their long history, there is often little evidence for the choice of agent. Vasoactive medications are generally divided into three classes: vasopressors, inotropes, and vasodilators.

VASOPRESSORS

Vasopressors are medications whose predominant action is to induce peripheral vasoconstriction and increase systemic vascular resistance (SVR). They are the key means of correcting vasoparesis in vasodilatory shock. The Surviving Sepsis Guidelines have recommended a mean arterial pressure (MAP) target of greater than or equal to 65 mm Hg. A large randomized controlled trial (RCT) comparing low (65-70 mm Hg) with high (80-85 mm Hg) MAP found no difference in the primary outcome of 28-day mortality.[1] However, a subgroup analysis indicated a possible reduction in acute kidney injury (AKI) rates among patients with chronic hypertension in the high MAP arm of the trial.

The 65 trial (n = 2,600) randomized patients older than 65 years with vasodilatory shock to permissive hypotension, a target MAP of 60 to 65 mm Hg, or usual care as directed by the treating physician.[2] There was a shorter duration of exposure to vasopressors in the intervention group with a median duration of 33 versus 38 hours in the usual care group (difference, −5.0; 95% confidence interval [CI], −7.8 to −2.2). The total vasopressor dose administered was also reduced (8.7 mg, 95% CI, −12.8 to −7.6 mg, norepinephrine equivalent).

There was a trend toward lower mortality in the hypotension group with 500 (41.0%) versus 544 (43.8%) deaths in the usual care arm ($p = 0.15$). This effect was statistically significant after multivariate adjustment with an adjusted odds ratio (OR) of 0.82 (95% CI, 0.68-0.98).

Data on mild-to-moderate AKI were not provided, but there was no difference in urine output or the incidence of kidney replacement therapy (KRT) between groups. An important limitation of the trial is that the MAP achieved in the permissive hypotension group was higher than targeted, with a median MAP of 67 mm Hg (interquartile range [IQR] 64.5-69.8) versus 72.6 mm Hg (69.4-76.5) in the usual care group. Thus, the study cannot establish whether there is benefit or harm in achieving an MAP target of 60 to 65 mm Hg. These data would support reducing vasopressor exposure in patients older than 65 years but do not contradict the Surviving Sepsis recommendation of an MAP target of greater than or equal to

65 mm Hg. The more pronounced mortality benefit in the chronic hypertension subgroup is surprising and requires further investigation in future studies.

Norepinephrine

Norepinephrine is an endogenous vasopressor released at end organs by postganglionic fibers of the sympathetic nervous system. Norepinephrine has the advantage over pure α-1-adrenergic agonists such as phenylephrine in that its β-1-adrenergic effects augment cardiac output (CO). The disadvantage of this is increased myocardial oxygen demand and risk of arrhythmias.

Norepinephrine is currently the first-line vasoactive medication recommended in septic shock as per the Surviving Sepsis Guidelines (see Chapter 36).[3] Clinically, it is administered as an infusion with a dose range of 0.05 to 0.5 μg/kg/min. Fluid resuscitation should first be completed to avoid masked hypovolemia and tissue hypoperfusion. A 30 mL/kg crystalloid fluid bolus and/or albumin is recommended in the Surviving Sepsis Guidelines. Early norepinephrine administration resulted in faster time to achieving target hemodynamic parameters in a recent phase II trial from Thailand.[4] Further large RCTs are required to determine whether early administration should become routine practice.

Epinephrine

Epinephrine is a naturally occurring catecholamine that is released by the sympathetic nervous system via the adrenal medulla. It acts on both α- and β-adrenoceptor(-s), with predominant β-1-adrenergic effects at low doses. At low doses, CO increases and β-2-adrenoceptor-mediated vasodilation can lead to a drop in SVR. However, at higher doses, potent α-1-adrenergic vasoconstriction causes a rise in SVR.

Epinephrine, delivered as a bolus, is the primary agent in the management of anaphylaxis (1 mg intramuscularly [IM] or 50-100 μg intravenously [IV]) and is a component of advanced cardiac life support (ACLS) cardiac arrest protocols (1 mg IV). It has a short half-life of approximately 2 minutes. An infusion (range 0.01-0.5 μg/kg/min) is an option for the management of post–coronary artery bypass grafting (CABG) low cardiac output state (LCOS) and as an alternative to norepinephrine in vasodilatory and mixed shock states. Epinephrine use is more prevalent in pediatric critical care units.

The **CAT study** (n = 280; see **Visual Abstract 13.1**) was a double blind RCT that compared norepinephrine and epinephrine in critically ill adults requiring a vasopressor.[5] The trial did not find a significant difference in the primary outcome of achievement of the MAP target within 24 hours. However, rates of lactic acidosis, tachycardia, and failure to achieve the target parameters were higher in the epinephrine group. These factors led to a higher study withdrawal rate within the epinephrine group (18/139 [12.9%] vs 4/138 [2.8%]; $p = 0.002$). Given these undesirable effects of epinephrine and the lack of a primary outcome or mortality benefit versus norepinephrine, epinephrine is generally used as a second-line agent in adult septic shock.

Dopamine: Low-Dose Dopamine

At low doses (1-2 μg/kg/min), dopamine exerts significant dopaminergic D_1-mediated vasodilation of renal vasculature and raises urine output. This led to the hypothesis that it may be useful in preventing AKI.[6] However, a meta-analysis of 61 RCTs (n = 3,359) of low-dose dopamine (≤5 μg/kg/min) found an improvement in urine output, but no difference in mortality or initiation of KRT.[7]

Dopamine in Vasodilatory Shock

Dopamine, at medium doses (~3-10 μg/kg/min), primarily acts on β-1-adrenergic receptors, resulting in an inotropic effect with increased CO. It also indirectly releases norepinephrine. At higher doses (>10 μg/kg/min), the balance shifts with predominant α-1-adrenergic agonists and an increased SVR. High variation in the clearance of dopamine contributes to a significant overlap of the receptor response curves.[8] Thus, many patients receiving infusions at low "dopaminergic" doses will experience mixed effects and be susceptible to β-1-adrenoceptor-induced arrhythmias.

Dopamine was previously widely used in the treatment of vasodilatory shock. In the **SOAP II** trial (see **Visual Abstract 13.2**), 1,679 patients were randomized to either dopamine or norepinephrine as the first-line vasopressor. There was no significant difference in the primary outcome of 28-day mortality. However, an increased rate of arrhythmias (207 [24.1%] events in the dopamine group vs 102 [12.4%] events in the norepinephrine group) was observed ($p < 0.001$).[9] This contributed to the Surviving Sepsis Guidelines recommendation to restrict use of dopamine to highly selected cases of septic shock with a low arrhythmia risk.

Phenylephrine

Phenylephrine is a specific α-1 agonist that is useful for its rapid vasopressor effects. It can be given as boluses of 50 to 100 μg or as an infusion of 0.1 to 10 μg/kg/min. Phenylephrine has a half-life of 5 to 10 minutes after IV injection. Its uses include counteracting the vasodilatory effects of anesthetic agents and treating vasodilatory states. It is recommended by the Surviving Sepsis Guidelines in the setting of norepinephrine-associated arrhythmias and high CO with hypotension or refractory hypotension. Disadvantages include the risk of a reflex bradycardia and reduced CO. A small clinical trial randomized patients to either norepinephrine or phenylephrine infusion to achieve an MAP target of 65 to 75 mm Hg. It found no difference in the primary outcome of hepatosplanchnic perfusion, but higher doses of phenylephrine were required to obtain MAP targets.[10]

Vasopressin

Vasopressin (antidiuretic hormone or ADH) acts on G-protein-coupled V receptors in vascular smooth muscle. This results in an increase in intracellular calcium and induces significant vasoconstriction. Vasopressin plasma levels have been reported to be low in septic shock, perhaps reflecting an acquired deficiency, prompting interest in the therapeutic use of exogenous vasopressin in vasodilatory shock to supplement and spare dosing of catecholamine vasopressors. It is given at a dose of 0.01 to 0.1 U/min as an IV infusion. Vasopressin was removed from the 2015 ACLS cardiac arrest guidelines because of a lack of evidence of benefit over epinephrine.

The use of vasopressin in septic shock is supported by the results of two large RCTs: the Vasopressin and Septic Shock Trial (VASST) and the VAsopressin versus Noradrenaline as Initial therapy in Septic sHock (VANISH) trials.

Vasopressin and Septic Shock Trial

The VASST ($n = 778$) investigated the addition of blinded low-dose vasopressin or norepinephrine to open-label vasopressors.[11] It found no change in the primary outcomes of mortality rates between the vasopressin and norepinephrine groups, at day 28 (35.4% and 39.3%, respectively; $p = 0.26$) or day 90 (43.9% and 49.6%, respectively; $p = 0.11$). A subgroup analysis of the predefined lower severity septic shock group found a trend toward lower mortality in those treated with adjuvant vasopressin (relative risk [RR] 0.74; 95% CI, 0.55-1.01; $p = 0.05$). In addition to these interesting findings, a post hoc analysis showed an interaction effect between vasopressin and hydrocortisone.[12]

VAsopressin versus Noradrenaline as Initial therapy in Septic sHock Trial

The VANISH trial ($n = 409$) sought to determine whether vasopressin could increase kidney failure–free days (Acute Kidney Injury Network [AKIN] stage 3) during the 28-day period after randomization (see **Visual Abstract 13.3**). Patients with septic shock were randomized to vasopressin (titrated up to 0.06 U/min) and/or hydrocortisone or norepinephrine (titrated up to 12 μg/min) and/or hydrocortisone in a 2×2 factorial design. There was no significant difference in the primary outcome of kidney failure in either survivors or nonsurvivors. In the survivor analysis, 94/165 patients (57.0%) in the vasopressin group never developed kidney failure as opposed to 93/157 patients (59.2%) in the norepinephrine group (difference, −2.3%; 95% CI, −13.0% to 8.5%). In a subgroup analysis, vasopressin reduced KRT requirements, although the effect was only seen in nonsurvivors.

In summary, vasopressin has not demonstrated a benefit over norepinephrine in clinical trials. It is typically used as an adjunctive agent to supplement norepinephrine in the management of vasodilatory shock (for recommended dosing, see **Table 13.1**). Vasopressin and phenylephrine are nonchronotropic vasopressors that do not increase heart rate. They are also treatment options in the initial management of cardiogenic shock (CS) secondary to aortic/mitral stenosis and left ventricular outflow tract obstruction. In these conditions, these agents maintain perfusion pressure without inducing tachycardia.[13] Studies have shown significant hypotension on discontinuing vasopressin. It is thus recommended to slowly titrate down infusions by 0.01 U/min every 30 to 60 minutes.

Angiotensin II

Angiotensin II is produced by the renin-angiotensin-aldosterone system in response to low kidney perfusion, decreased sodium delivery to the macula densa or β1 stimulation. It exerts its main actions via AT_1 and, to a lesser extent, AT_2 receptors. Highly potent vasoconstriction, reduced reuptake of norepinephrine, and increased ADH, aldosterone, and adrenocorticotropic hormone (ACTH) secretion result. In the ATHOS-3 trial, 321 patients on high-dose vasopressors were randomized to either an infusion of angiotensin II or placebo.[14] The primary outcome was an MAP target of 75 mm Hg or an increase of 10 mm Hg from baseline. The majority (69.9%) achieved the target MAP in the angiotensin group, versus only 23.4% in the placebo group ($p < 0.001$; OR, 7.95; 95% CI, 4.76-13.3). A post hoc analysis of patients with AKI requiring KRT found improved 28-day survival in the angiotensin arm (53% [95% CI, 38%-67%] vs 30% [95% CI, 19%-41%]; $p = 0.012$).[15] Further large RCTs that compare angiotensin II with other second-line vasopressors are needed. Efficacy data using patient-centered end points are essential to determine the clinical role of angiotensin II, which is currently licensed in the United States for the treatment of vasodilatory shock. Angiotensin has been shown to be prothrombotic in animal models.[16] Furthermore, angiotensin II carries a Food and Drug Administration (FDA) warning as a higher rate of thrombotic events, particularly deep vein thrombosis (DVT), was observed in the ATHOS-3 trial (13.5% in angiotensin II vs 5% in placebo).

TABLE 13.1 Recommended Dosing, Receptor Affinities, Hemodynamic Effects and Adverse Effects of Commonly Used Vasoactive Medications

		β-Adrenergic[b]		α-Adrenergic	Dopamine		
Medication[a]	**Dosage**	**β-1**	**β-2**	**α-1**	**DA**	**Actions**	**Major Side Effects**
Vasopressors							
Norepinephrine	Initially: 0.05 to 0.15 μg/kg/minute Maintenance: 0.01-3 μg/kg/min	++	+	++++	–	↑**SVR**, ↑CO	Digital ischemia Arrhythmias Bradycardia
Epinephrine	0.01-0.7 μg/kg/min	++++	+++	++++	–	↑**SVR**, ↑**CO**	Ventricular arrhythmias Severe hypertension Cardiac ischemia Splanchnic hypoperfusion ↑ Lactate
Vasopressin	0.03-0.07 Units/min	V1 receptors ++++ V2 receptors +++				↑**SVR**	Arrhythmias Peripheral, pulmonary, splanchnic vasoconstriction Hyponatremia ↓CO at high doses Hypotension on cessation
Phenylephrine	0.1-10 μg/kg/min	–	–	+++	–	↑**SVR**, may ↓HR	Reflex bradycardia Severe peripheral vasoconstriction
Low-dose dopamine	0.5-3 μg/kg/min	+	–	–	+++	↑CO	Arrhythmias
Moderate-dose dopamine	3-10 μg/kg/min	+++	+	+	++	↑**CO**, ↑SVR	Hypotension
High-dose dopamine	10-20 μg/kg/min	++	–	+++	++	↑**SVR**, ↑CO	Myocardial ischemia Peripheral ischemia

(*continued*)

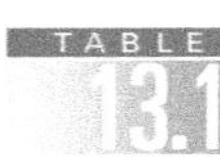

TABLE 13.1 Recommended Dosing, Receptor Affinities, Hemodynamic Effects and Adverse Effects of Commonly Used Vasoactive Medications (*continued*)

Medication[a]	Dosage	β-Adrenergic[b] β-1	β-Adrenergic[b] β-2	α-Adrenergic α-1	Dopamine DA	Actions	Major Side Effects
Angiotensin II	10-40 ng/kg/min	Angiotensin (AT_1 and AT_2) receptors				↑**SVR**	Thrombosis, DVT Thrombocytopenia Tachycardia
Inotropes	**Acute Heart Failure Dosing[c]**						
Dobutamine	2-20 μg/kg/min	++++	++	+	–	↑**CO**, ↓SVR, ↓PVR	Tachycardia Ventricular arrhythmias Cardiac ischemia
Levosimendan	Initial: 0.1 μg/kg/min Maintenance: 0.05-0.2 μg/kg/min	↑ Myocardial filament Ca^{2+} sensitivity				↑CO, ↓SVR, ↓PVR	Arrhythmias, ↑AV conduction Tachycardia Hypotension
Milrinone	0.375-0.75 μg/kg/min	PDE-3 inhibition				↑CO, ↓SVR, ↓PVR	Ventricular arrhythmias Supraventricular arrhythmias Hypotension Cardiac ischemia
Enoximone	5-20 μg/kg/min	PDE-3 inhibition				↑CO, ↓SVR, ↓PVR	Nausea Arrhythmias Headache

Vasodilators	Acute Heart Failure Dosing[c]			
Nitroglycerin (GTN)	Initial: 10-20 μg/min, increase up to 200 μg/min	Prodrug of NO, ↑cGMP GTN: Venous >> arterial vasodilation Sodium nitroprusside: Venous > arterial	↓**SVR**, ↑CO, ↓PVR	Headache Hypotension Dizziness/syncope
Sodium nitroprusside	Initial: 0.3 μg/kg/min Max: 5 μg/kg/min		↓**SVR**, ↑CO, ↓PVR	Cyanide toxicity Severe hypotension Brady-/tachycardia
Carperitide (ANP)	Initial: 0.025 μg/kg/min[d] Max: 0.2 μg/kg/min	↑cGMP, inhibits catecholamines Vasodilation: Arterial = venous	↓**SVR**, ↑CO, ↓PVR	Hypotension Acute kidney injury Headache
Inhaled NO	5-20 ppm	↑cGMP → selective pulmonary vasodilation	↓**PVR**	Hypotension Hypoxemia Methemoglobinemia
Vasodilators	**Acute Hypertensive Emergency Dosing[d]**			
Fenoldopam	Initial: 0.1-0.3 μg/kg/min; increased in increments of 0.05-0.1 μg/kg/min Max. rate 1.6 μg/kg/min	D_1-receptor selective agonist	↓**SVR**, ↑CO, ↓PVR	Hypotension Angina ↑Intraocular and intracranial pressure

ANP, atrial natriuretic peptide; AV, atrioventricular; cGMP, cyclic guanosine monophosphate; CO, cardiac output; DVT, deep vein thrombosis; GTN, glyceryl trinitrate; HR, heart rate; HTN, hypertension; NO, nitric oxide; PVR, pulmonary vascular resistance; SVR, systemic vascular resistance.

[a]Examples of recommended vasodilator, inotrope, or vasopressor dosing are provided in Table 13.1. Clinicians should individualise dosing to the indication and patient requirements. We recommend either weight-based dosing or non-weight-based dosing of vasoactive drugs where indicated.

[b]van Diepen S, Katz JN, Albert NM, et al. Contemporary management of cardiogenic shock: a scientific statement from the American Heart Association. *Circulation*. 2017;136:e232-e268.

[c]2016 ESC Guidelines for the diagnosis and treatment of acute and chronic heart failure.

[d]JCS Joint Working Group. Guidelines for treatment of acute heart failure (JCS 2011). *Circ J*. 2013;77:2157-2201.

[e]2017 ACC/AHA Guideline for the Prevention, Detection, Evaluation, and Management of High Blood Pressure in Adults.

ADMINISTRATION

Vasopressor medications should be administered via a continuous infusion through a central venous catheter (CVC). Limited evidence suggests that under highly controlled conditions, peripheral administration of norepinephrine, dopamine, and phenylephrine has a relatively low incidence of extravasation (2%).[17] However, currently, no international guideline recommends the use of peripheral vasopressor medications in critical care patients.

Extravasation Injury of Vasoactive Medications

Extravasation of vasopressors is a serious event that causes extreme vasoconstriction and may cause tissue necrosis. In the event of extravasation, the infusion should be immediately stopped, the cannula aspirated, irrigated with saline, and a warm compressor applied.[18] Phentolamine is the only FDA-approved treatment for extravasation injury, and 10 to 15 mL of 0.9% normal saline with 5 to 10 mg phentolamine should be infiltrated subcutaneously as soon as possible after detection.[18]

INOTROPES

Inotropes are a class of medications whose primary action is to increase myocardial contractility and thus CO. The primary role of inotropes is in the management of LCOS and CS.

Dobutamine

Dobutamine is a powerful inotrope with 3:1 selectivity for the β-1-adrenergic receptor over β-2. β-2-Adrenergic agonist causes peripheral vasodilation and a reduction in SVR at doses lesser than or equal to 5 μg/kg/min. There is usually little change in SVR at doses between 5 and 15 μg/kg/min. Above 15 μg/kg/min, α-1-mediated vasoconstriction predominates.[19]

It is a treatment option in cases of LCOS and CS. β-2-Adrenergic-mediated vasodilation may exacerbate hypotension in some patients. Concerns regarding increased rates of arrhythmias mean that it should not be used in routine cases of acute heart failure (AHF).

A trial of dobutamine therapy is suggested in cases of septic shock refractory to fluid therapy and vasopressors, although the underlying evidence is limited. Dobutamine should be titrated to the minimum dosage necessary and therapy reduced/discontinued if hypotension or arrhythmias occur. Continuous electrocardiogram (ECG) monitoring is necessary to detect myocardial ischemia or arrhythmias. The British National Formulary advises that low concentration (0.5-1 mg/mL) of dobutamine may be administered through a peripheral line.[20] Concentrations above this require a CVC.

Levosimendan

Levosimendan acts on cardiac myofilaments, increasing sensitivity to calcium and acting as a positive inotropic agent. It is currently not FDA approved. The SURVIVE trial, the largest trial of levosimendan in acute decompensated heart failure (ADHF), did not show any difference in clinical outcome against placebo. A recent Cochrane review (n = 1,552) compared the efficacy of vasodilatory and inotropic agents in the setting of LCOS and CS.[21] The main finding based on six studies (n = 1,776) was that levosimendan may improve short-term mortality over dobutamine (RR 0.60; 95% CI, 0.37-0.95; low-quality evidence). However, this effect should be interpreted with caution as it was driven by small, low-quality trials with a high risk of bias caused by a lack of blinding in four studies, loss to follow-up in one study, and baseline imbalance in another. Levosimendan has significant vasodilatory effects. For this reason, the European Society of Cardiology Guidelines recommend avoiding its use in patients with systolic blood pressure (SBP) less than 85 mm Hg or CS unless combined with another vasopressor/inotrope. Large, high-quality RCTs are needed to establish the optimal role of inotropes and vasopressors in the management of CS.

Phosphodiesterase Inhibitors

Phosphodiesterase-3 (PDE3) enzyme inhibition causes an accumulation in intracellular cyclic adenosine monophosphate (cAMP). This results in increased myocardial inotropy and peripheral vasodilation. The most common PDE3 inhibitors in critical care are milrinone and enoximone. As a result of their vasodilatory properties, these agents should be avoided in hypotensive patients. A meta-analysis of clinical trials of milrinone versus any comparator in critically ill adults with cardiac dysfunction found no difference in all-cause mortality (RR 0.96; 95% CI, 0.76-1.21; $p = 0.73$) among the 14 small trials ($n = 1,611$) that reported this outcome.[22] The included trials had a high risk of bias, mainly because of a lack of reporting of bias protection, and most had increased risk of random errors.

VASODILATORS

Vasodilators are agents that induce peripheral vasodilation (Table 13.1). A detailed review on the use of vasodilators is beyond the scope of this chapter. Nitrovasodilators such as nitroglycerin and sodium nitroprusside effectively reduce preload and afterload. Their core role is in the management of hypertensive emergencies (see Chapter 44). Vasodilators are also useful as a temporizing measure in the management of acute aortic and mitral regurgitation.

Recombinant Natriuretic Peptides

Nesiritide, a recombinant B-type natriuretic peptide (BNP), produces balanced arterial and venous vasodilation. It was most commonly used in the United States in the early 2000s for the treatment of ADHF. The ASCEND-HF trial ($n = 7,141$) randomized patients with AHF to either nesiritide infusion or placebo. There was a small change in dyspnea, but no difference in mortality or readmission within 30 days. Nesiritide was discontinued by Janssen in 2018.

Carperitide

Carperitide is a recombinant A-type natriuretic peptide. It has similar effects to nesiritide, producing vasodilation and natriuresis. It is widely used in Japan, with the ATTEND registry showing its use in 58.2% of AHF patients.[23] Carperitide should be avoided in cases of CS or SBP less than 90 mm Hg. RCT support is limited to small studies, and a propensity score–matched study indicated a possible increase in mortality.[24] A large RCT is needed before it should be used more widely.

Inhaled Nitric Oxide

Inhaled nitric oxide (iNO) is a potent selective pulmonary vasodilator. iNO is used to reduce pulmonary vascular resistance in conditions such as right ventricular failure, severe pulmonary hypertension, and graft failure after lung transplantation. RCT evidence of efficacy is currently lacking, although some reports have shown hemodynamic improvements, including decreased pulmonary arterial pressure, pulmonary vascular resistance, and CO.[25]

Fenoldopam

Fenoldopam is a selective D_1-receptor agonist. It is used in the management of acute hypertensive emergencies (see Chapter 44). Early trials indicated a potential role in the setting of cardiac surgery, with a 2012 meta-analysis (n = 440; six studies) showing a reduction in AKI (OR = 0.41; 95% CI, 0.23-0.74; p = 0.003).[26] However, a large Italian trial (n = 667) was stopped for futility owing to a lack of efficacy in the primary outcome of KRT and an increase in the incidence of hypotension in the fenoldopam group (85 [26%] vs 49 [15%]) compared to the placebo group (p = 0.001).[27] In summary, fenoldopam has no proven renoprotective effect in patients with shock requiring pressor support and significant potential for harm in this setting. Finally, fenoldopam is contraindicated in patients with glaucoma and in the presence of raised intracranial pressure.

References

1. Asfar P, Meziani F, Hamel J-F, et al. High versus low blood-pressure target in patients with septic shock. *N Engl J Med.* 2014;370(17):1583-1593.
2. Lamontagne F, Richards-Belle A, Thomas K, et al. Effect of reduced exposure to vasopressors on 90-day mortality in older critically ill patients with vasodilatory hypotension: a randomized clinical trial. *JAMA.* 2020;323:938-949.
3. Rhodes A, Evans LE, Alhazzani W, et al. Surviving sepsis campaign: international guidelines for management of sepsis and septic shock: 2016. *Intensive Care Med.* 2017;43(3):304-377.
4. Permpikul C, Tongyoo S, Viarasilpa T, et al. Early use of norepinephrine in septic shock resuscitation (CENSER). A randomized trial. *Am J Respir Crit Care Med.* 2019;199(9):1097-1105.
5. Myburgh JA, Higgins A, Jovanovska A, et al. A comparison of epinephrine and norepinephrine in critically ill patients. *Intensive Care Med.* 2008;34(12):2226-2234.
6. Dasta JF, Kirby MG. Pharmacology and therapeutic use of low-dose dopamine. *Pharmacotherapy.* 1986;6(6):304-310.
7. Friedrich JO, Adhikari N, Herridge MS, et al. Meta-analysis: low-dose dopamine increases urine output but does not prevent renal dysfunction or death. *Ann Intern Med.* 2005;142(7):510-524.
8. Juste RN, Moran L, Hooper J, et al. Dopamine clearance in critically ill patients. *Intensive Care Med.* 1998;24(11):1217-1220.
9. De Backer D, Biston P, Devriendt J, et al. Comparison of dopamine and norepinephrine in the treatment of shock. *N Engl J Med.* 2010;362(9):779-789.
10. Morelli A, Ertmer C, Rehberg S, et al. Phenylephrine versus norepinephrine for initial hemodynamic support of patients with septic shock: a randomized, controlled trial. *Crit Care.* 2008;12(6):R143.
11. Russell JA, Walley KR, Singer J, et al. Vasopressin versus norepinephrine infusion in patients with septic shock. *N Engl J Med.* 2008;358(9):877-887.
12. Russell JA, Walley KR, Gordon AC, et al. Interaction of vasopressin infusion, corticosteroid treatment, and mortality of septic shock. *Crit Care Med.* 2009;37(3):811-818.
13. Diepen SV, Katz JN, Albert NM, et al. Contemporary management of cardiogenic shock: a scientific statement from the American Heart Association. *Circulation.* 2017;136(16):e232-e268.
14. Khanna A, English SW, Wang XS, et al. Angiotensin II for the treatment of vasodilatory shock. *N Engl J Med.* 2017;377(5):419-430.
15. Tumlin JA, Murugan R, Deane AM, et al. Outcomes in Patients with Vasodilatory Shock and Renal Replacement Therapy Treated with Intravenous Angiotensin II. *Crit Care Med.* 2018;46(6):949–957.
16. Mogielnicki A, Chabielska E, Pawlak R, et al. Angiotensin II enhances thrombosis development in renovascular hypertensive rats. *Thromb Haemost.* 2005;93(6):1069-1076.
17. Cardenas-Garcia J, Schaub KF, Belchikov YG, et al. Safety of peripheral intravenous administration of vasoactive medication. *J Hosp Med.* 2015;10(9):581-585.
18. Plum M, Moukhachen O. Alternative pharmacological management of vasopressor extravasation in the absence of phentolamine. *P T.* 2017;42(9):581-592.
19. Overgaard CB, Džavík V. Inotropes and vasopressors. *Circulation.* 2008;118(10):1047-1056.

20. Joint Formulary Committee. British National Formulary. 2020. http://www.medicinescomplete.com/
21. Schumann J. Cochrane corner: inotropic agents and vasodilator strategies for cardiogenic shock or low cardiac output syndrome. *Heart.* 2019;105(3):178-179.
22. Koster G, Bekema HJ, Wetterslev J, et al. Milrinone for cardiac dysfunction in critically ill adult patients: a systematic review of randomised clinical trials with meta-analysis and trial sequential analysis. *Intensive Care Med.* 2016;42(9):1322-1335.
23. Sato N, Kajimoto K, Keida T, et al. Clinical features and outcome in hospitalized heart failure in Japan (from the ATTEND Registry). *Circ J.* 2013;77(4):944-951.
24. Matsue Y, Kagiyama N, Yoshida K, et al. Carperitide is associated with increased in-hospital mortality in acute heart failure: a propensity score-matched analysis. *J Card Fail.* 2015; 21(11):859-864.
25. Hill NS, Preston IR, Roberts KE. Inhaled therapies for pulmonary hypertension. *Respir Care.* 2015;60(6):794-805.
26. Zangrillo A, Biondi-Zoccai GG, Frati E, et al. Fenoldopam and acute renal failure in cardiac surgery: a meta-analysis of randomized placebo-controlled trials. *J Cardiothorac Vasc Anesth.* 2012;26(3):407-413.
27. Bove T, Zangrillo A, Guarracino F, et al. Effect of fenoldopam on use of renal replacement therapy among patients with acute kidney injury after cardiac surgery: a randomized clinical trial. *JAMA.* 2014;312(21):2244-2253.

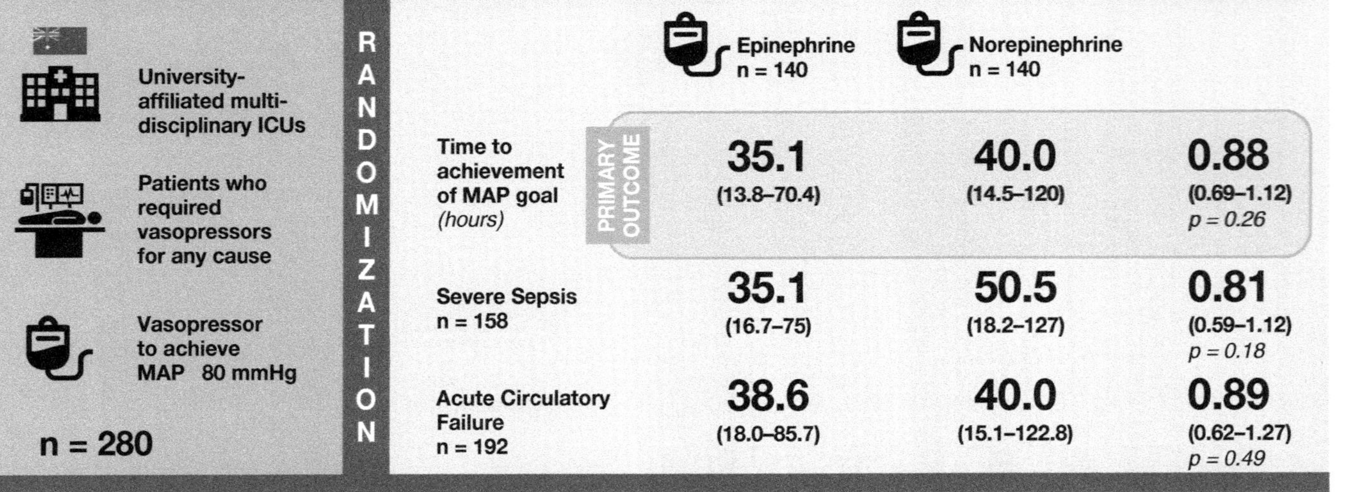

Conclusion: Despite the development of potential drug-related effects with epinephrine, there was no difference in the achievement of a MAP goal between epinephrine and norepinephrine in a heterogenous population of ICU patients.

Myburgh JA, Higgins A, Jovanovska A, Lipman J, et al. ***A comparison of epinephrine and norepinephrine in critically ill patients.*** Intensive Care Med. 2008 Dec;34(12):2226-34.

VISUAL ABSTRACT 13.1

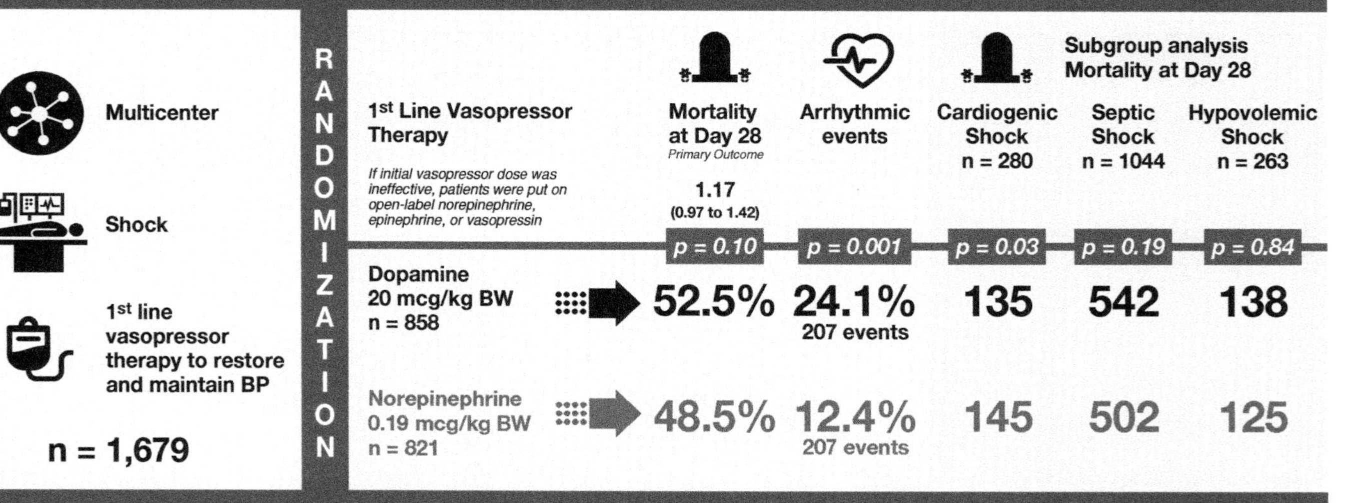

Conclusion: Although there was no significant difference in the rate of death between patients with shock who were treated with dopamine as the first-line vasopressor agent and those who were treated with norepinephrine, the use of dopamine was associated with a greater number of adverse events.

De Backer D, Biston P, Devriendt J, Mdl C, et al. ***Comparison of dopamine and norepinephrine in the treatment of shock.*** N Engl J Med 2010 Mar 4;362(9):779-89.

VISUAL ABSTRACT 13.2

Comparison of the effect of early vasopressin vs norepinephrine on kidney failure in patients with septic shock: The VANISH Randomized Clinical Trial

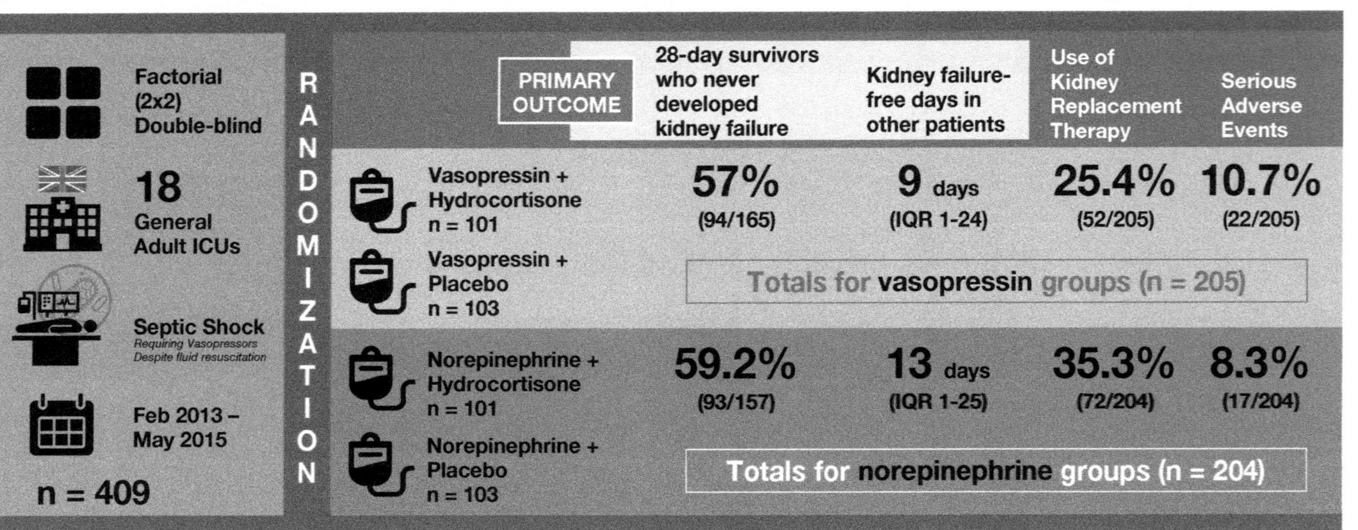

Conclusion: Among adults with septic shock, the early use of vasopressin compared with norepinephrine did not improve the number of kidney failure–free days.

Gordon AC, Mason AJ, Thirunavukkarasu N, Perkins GD, et al. VANISH investigators. ***Effect of Early Vasopressin vs Norepinephrine on Kidney Failure in Patients With Septic Shock: The VANISH Randomized Clinical Trial.*** JAMA 2016 Aug 2;316(5):509-18.

VISUAL ABSTRACT 13.3

14 Anticoagulants in the Intensive Care Unit

Paul Mark Adams and Javier A. Neyra

INTRODUCTION: ANTICOAGULATION AND KIDNEY DYSFUNCTION

Anticoagulation in the setting of kidney dysfunction presents a challenge. Low glomerular filtration rate (GFR) reduces drug clearance, making safe and effective dosing difficult. Sudden drop in GFR seen in critically ill patients with acute kidney injury (AKI) adds another level of complexity. Patients with kidney disease not only have decreased drug clearance but can also be coagulopathic, displaying both hemophilic and hypercoagulable tendencies (**Table 14.1**).[1,2] Anticoagulated patients with kidney disease have more bleeding events and higher mortality, regardless of the anticoagulant chosen.[3-5] Given these complications, management of anticoagulation in the intensive care unit (ICU) requires extra attention when kidney disease is present.

PARENTERAL AGENTS: HEPARINS

Unfractionated Heparin

Pharmacology

Unfractionated heparin (UFH) is given parenterally or subcutaneously, with the subcutaneous route yielding a longer half-life.[6] UFH binds antithrombin, accelerating inactivation of thrombin (IIa) and factor Xa. Response to UFH can be unpredictable because binding of positively charged surfaces reduces bioavailability.[5] Larger UFH molecules can also interfere with platelet-endothelial interaction, prolonging bleeding time.[6] Given UFH's variable activity and short half-life

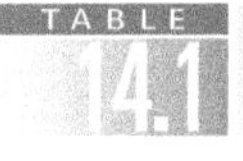

TABLE 14.1 Coagulopathy of Kidney Disease

Thrombophilic	Hemophilic
Increased fibrinogen[2]	Uremic platelet dysfunction[1]
Increased factors XIIa and VIIa	Poor von Willebrand factor adhesion[2]
Reduced antithrombin activity	Increased nitric oxide activity with poor vasoconstriction[2]
Activated, inflamed endothelium	
Anticardiolipin, antiphospholipid antibodies[1]	

(60-150 minutes), it requires careful monitoring, usually through following activated partial thromboplastin time (aPTT) or anti-Xa levels.

UFH is cleared through two main pathways: (a) a rapid but saturable endothelial cell and macrophage-mediated depolymerization process and (b) slower urinary clearance, eliminating remaining UFH.[6] Supratherapeutic anticoagulation can occur with impaired kidney function when creatinine clearance (CrCl) or estimated GFR (eGFR) is below 50 mL/min/1.73 m^2, becoming more significant at lower GFRs.[5]

Dosing and Use

For venous thromboembolism (VTE) and general systemic anticoagulation needs, a loading dose of 75 to 80 U/kg, followed by 18 U/kg/hr infusion, usually leads to therapeutic anticoagulation in patients with normal kidney function.[6,7] A reduced 60 U/kg loading dose and 12 U/kg/hr maintenance dose is recommended for patients with kidney dysfunction (CrCl <50 mL/min).[5] This reduced dose still offers therapeutic anticoagulation, but avoids supratherapeutic anticoagulation. Acute coronary syndrome (ACS) requires lower doses, given concomitant use of fibrinolytics and/or antiplatelet agents, but does not require adjustment for kidney function.[8,9]

An aPTT of 1.5 to 2.5 times the normal range is widely accepted for UFH monitoring.[6,10] Anti-Xa levels can also monitor heparin levels, with anti-Xa range of 0.3 to 0.7 U/mL usually indicating therapeutic anticoagulation. Both aPTT and anti-Xa targets vary based on local laboratory practices and may not provide a reliable reference for monitoring. Neither aPTT nor anti-Xa has been proven superior, and clinical practice should follow institutional protocols for heparin monitoring after a loading dose is given.[6,7,11,12]

Reversal and Safety

The advantages of UFH for critically ill patients with kidney failure come from its short half-life and easy reversibility with protamine. Supratherapeutic anticoagulation and minor bleeding can be managed by stopping UFH infusion. More serious bleeding associated with supratherapeutic UFH levels can be reversed with protamine; 1 mg of intravenous (IV) protamine neutralizes about 100 U of UFH. Given UFH's short half-life, only the UFH dose given within the previous 4 to 6 hours should be considered for reversal. Protamine should be given slowly (<20 mg/min) to avoid hypotension or bradycardia.[6,13] Although UFH can be used for hemodialysis (HD) and continuous kidney replacement therapy (CKRT) anticoagulation, extracorporeal clearance has a limited role in correcting supratherapeutic UFH levels and should not be utilized. UFH is not dialyzable and does not need adjustments in the setting of KRT. More information regarding anticoagulation for KRT can be found in Chapter 33.

Heparin-induced thrombocytopenia (HIT) is a rare but serious complication of UFH therapy, leading to a coagulopathic state. All heparin products, including low-molecular-weight heparin (LMWH), should be avoided during the prothrombotic HIT state, necessitating anticoagulation with nonheparin-based alternatives. In patients with severe kidney failure, argatroban is the preferred agent for acute therapy because it relies on extensive hepatic clearance rather than urinary elimination.[14] Warfarin is then used for chronic anticoagulation as other agents have not been proven for patients with kidney disease.

Low-Molecular-Weight Heparin

Pharmacology

LMWHs are shorter heparin chains with a stronger affinity for factor Xa but lower affinity for thrombin. Interaction with antithrombin III induces a conformational change, accelerating inactivation of factor Xa and factor II.[15] Interactions with platelets, macrophages, endothelium, and plasma proteins are reduced, thus making systemic anticoagulation with LMWH more predictable and less prone to adverse effects, such as HIT.[5,6] LMWHs require less monitoring as therapeutic anticoagulation is easier to achieve.

The half-life of LMWH is 2 to 4 hours after IV administration and 3 to 6 hours after more common subcutaneous injection.[6,15] LMWHs are primarily cleared by the kidneys, prolonging half-life in patients with kidney failure.[6,16] Although LMWHs have more predictable action than UFH, variation exists between formulations with different molecular weights.

Dosing and Use

Convenience and high bioavailability make subcutaneous injection the preferred route of administration.[17] The various LMWHs differ in their properties and dosing regimens, but no clear differences in outcomes exist.[6] LMWHs have not been proven superior to UFH or other anticoagulants for most acute indications, such as ACS or VTE.[8,9,18,19] Nonetheless, LMWH is the preferred anticoagulation for patients with malignancy-associated VTE.[18-20]

Because these drugs are eliminated by the kidneys, LMWHs accumulate with increasing dose and decreasing kidney function.[6,21] Patients with CrCl greater than or equal to 30 mL/min usually do not require dose adjustment, whereas LMWHs should be adjusted in patients with CrCl less than 30 mL/min.[2,4,6,22,23] Enoxaparin has the most evidence supporting safe use in kidney failure, with a general dose reduction of 50% being recommended when CrCl is less than 30 mL/min (**Table 14.2**).[5,7-9,18,24] LMWHs are not approved by the U.S. Food and Drug Administration (FDA) for dialysis patients; therefore, extra care and anti-Xa monitoring should be used when dialysis is required.[5,17,25]

Reversal and Safety

There is no proven LMWH reversal method. Protamine may normalize aPTT and anti-Xa levels but has limited clinical efficacy.[6,17] If life-threatening bleeding occurs, IV protamine sulfate may be trialed. For LMWH given within 8 hours, 1-mg protamine per 100 anti-Xa units of LMWH can be used. Enoxaparin reversal is relatively straightforward as 1-mg enoxaparin equals approximately 100

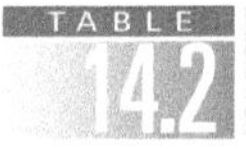
TABLE 14.2 Enoxaparin Dosing for CrCl <30 mL/min

Indication	**Dose**
VTE prophylaxis	30 mg administered SC once daily
Acute VTE treatment	1 mg/kg administered SC once daily
ACS: NSTEMI	1 mg/kg administered SC once daily
ACS: STEMI age <75 yr	30 mg single IV bolus plus a 1 mg/kg SC dose followed by 1 mg/kg administered SC once daily
ACS: STEMI age ≥75 yr	1 mg/kg administered SC once daily (no bolus)

ACS, acute coronary syndrome; CrCl, creatinine clearance; IV, intravenous; NSTEMI, non–ST-elevation myocardial infarction; SC, subcutaneously; STEMI, ST-elevation myocardial infarction; VTE, venous thromboembolism.

From FDA, CDER. Fachinformation Lovenox (enoxaparin sodium injection) for subcutaneous and intravenous use 3000 IU. Stand: 10/2013. sanofi-aventis U.S. LLC, Bridgewater. National Drug Code: 0075-0624-30. Accessed June 24, 2019. www.fda.gov/medwatch

anti-Xa units; 1 mg of protamine can be used for every 1 mg of enoxaparin.[6,17] LMWHs are not cleared by dialysis; therefore, it should not be used for correction of supratherapeutic LMWH anticoagulation.

Contraindicated or Rarely Used Agents in Kidney Failure

Fondaparinux is a synthetic antithrombin analog with the minimum chain length for factor Xa inactivation. It is used for the prevention and treatment of VTE, ACS, and HIT. It can be dose reduced for CrCl 30 to 50 mL/min but contraindicated when CrCl is less than 30 mL/min.[17,26]

PARENTERAL AGENTS: DIRECT THROMBIN INHIBITORS

Hirudin, Lepirudin, and Desirudin

Hirudin is a polypeptide isolated from medical leeches that inhibits thrombin.[6] Lepirudin and desirudin are two recombinant forms with pharmacologic properties identical to hirudin.[27,28] In the United States, lepirudin is used for HIT-associated thrombosis or VTE prophylaxis. All hirudins are cleared by the kidneys with rapid accumulation when CrCl is less than 60 mL/min and should not be used during severe kidney failure (acute or chronic).[6,27]

Bivalirudin

Bivalirudin is a shorter synthetic analog of hirudin that inactivates thrombin.[6,29] Bivalirudin is mainly used for ACS with percutaneous coronary intervention (PCI) or for anticoagulation in the setting of HIT.[6,8,9] Bivalirudin is also gaining popularity for extracorporeal membrane oxygenation (ECMO) anticoagulation, but published data are limited for this off-label use. Bivalirudin is short acting with a half-life of about 25 minutes after IV administration and relies on urinary elimination for only 20% of clearance.[30] For PCI, an IV bolus dose of 0.75 mg/kg followed by a maintenance infusion of 1.75 mg/kg/hr for the duration of the procedure is recommended.[31] For CrCl less than 30 mL/min, the bolus dose does not need to be changed, whereas maintenance dose should be reduced to a rate of 1 mg/kg/hr. Patients requiring KRT should use a reduced infusion rate of 0.25 mg/kg/hr.[30,31]

Bivalirudin use for HIT is off-label but commonly utilized. An initial dose of 0.15 to 0.2 mg/kg/hr is adjusted to accommodate an aPTT 1.5 to 2.5 times the baseline value. This strategy is used as a bridge to warfarin after about 5 days of bivalirudin therapy.[32,33] Recommended dosing during kidney failure is outlined in **Table 14.3**.[33,34]

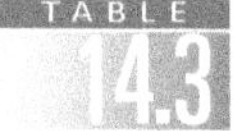

TABLE 14.3 Bivalirudin HIT Dosing in Kidney Failure

Kidney Function	Dose
CrCl >60 mL/min	0.13 mg/kg/hr
CrCl 30-60 mL/min	0.08-0.1 mg/kg/hr
CrCl <30 mL/min	0.04-0.05 mg/kg/hr
Intermittent hemodialysis	0.07 mg/kg/hr
CKRT (CVVH or CVVHDF)	0.03-0.07 mg/kg/hr

CKRT, continuous kidney replacement therapy; CrCl, creatinine clearance; CVVH, continuous venovenous hemofiltration; CVVHDF, continuous venovenous hemodiafiltration; HIT, heparin-induced thrombocytopenia.

Argatroban

Argatroban reversibly binds and inhibits thrombin. Argatroban is mainly used for anticoagulation in HIT and during PCI when heparin is contraindicated because of a recent history of HIT.[6] Argatroban is not excreted by the kidneys, with clearance dependent on hepatic metabolism. It should be avoided when hepatic failure is a concern, but can be used without adjustment when kidney failure is present.[35] Argatroban is administered with a continuous IV infusion. An initial dose of 1 to 2 mg/kg/min is adjusted to maintain aPTT in the range of 1.5 to 2.5.[32]

ORAL ANTICOAGULANTS: WARFARIN

Pharmacology

Warfarin inhibits vitamin K epoxide reductase, depleting the reduced form of vitamin K that acts as a coagulation cofactor. Several coagulation factors depend on vitamin K for action, and without vitamin K, these factors cannot adequately bind calcium to phospholipid membranes. Production of new vitamin K is required before clotting factors are again functional.[36]

Dosing and Use

Warfarin is mainly used for outpatient anticoagulation, but is often encountered in the ICU. A loading dose between 5 and 10 mg seems safe and effective. Doses as low as 5 mg daily can achieve anticoagulation within 4 to 5 days for hospitalized, elderly patients.[37,38] A higher 10 mg dose can achieve anticoagulation faster, but is associated with higher bleeding risk.[36] In general, an initial dose of 7.5 mg daily is recommended, then titrated to an international normalized ratio (INR) of 2.0 to 3.0 for most indications. A slower, lower dose approach may be more desirable in patients with kidney dysfunction.[5,36] INR should be checked daily until a stable level and dose are achieved.

Multiple factors can influence individual patient response to warfarin, including other medications, diet, hepatic function, and genetics. Warfarin's significant drug-drug interactions are especially important, given the polypharmacy common in critically ill patients and patients with kidney disease.

Safety and Reversal

Despite the FDA black box warning for increased bleeding risk with warfarin use in patients with kidney dysfunction, warfarin is still widely used and is often the recommended anticoagulant for chronic kidney disease (CKD) patients.[39] Safety is unclear, as patients with kidney failure using warfarin have an increased risk of bleeding, stroke, and other hemorrhagic complications.[40,41] One such complication is anticoagulant-related nephropathy (ARN), an increasingly recognized condition associated with chronic oral anticoagulant use, leading to glomerular hemorrhage and inflammation. Most cases are associated with warfarin and present as an unexplained AKI, or rarely as unusually progressive CKD. Unexplained AKI in patients experiencing supratherapeutic anticoagulation should prompt investigation with a high degree of suspicion for ARN.[42]

A stepwise approach is taken for patients on warfarin with supratherapeutic anticoagulation. A minimally supratherapeutic INR of 3 to 4 can be monitored without significant changes in dose.[36,43] Risk of unprovoked hemorrhage even with an INR up to 10 is low. An INR of 4 to 10 without overt bleeding is managed by reducing warfarin dose or skipping a dose.[43] Because hemorrhagic effects can be prolonged in patients with AKI or CKD, close monitoring is recommended.[44]

If mild bleeding or other need for reversal is present, vitamin K can be administered at a dose that will quickly lower the INR but avoid excessive resistance once warfarin is restarted, as detailed further in Chapter 27.[45,46] To prevent anaphylaxis, low doses of vitamin K and slow infusion rates are recommended.[47,48] A vitamin K dose of 1.0 to 2.5 mg is recommended when the INR is 5.0 to 9.0, but larger doses (2.5-5 mg) may be required for INRs greater than 9.0. Oral dosing may minimize anaphylaxis, but IV infusion allows more rapid delivery.[36]

For active, life-threatening bleeding, immediate correction of warfarin anticoagulation with fresh-frozen plasma (FFP) or more potent factor concentrates is indicated. FFP is given at an initial dose of 15 to 30 mL/kg.[49,50] Although FFP has traditionally anchored warfarin-associated bleeding management, concentrated or recombinant factor formulations require less overall volume and act faster than traditional FFP.[51-55] Factor 3 or 4 prothrombin complex concentrate (PCC) or recombinant factor 7 should be considered when available for life-threatening warfarin-associated bleeding.[36]

DIRECT ORAL ANTICOAGULANTS

Direct oral anticoagulants (DOACs) inhibiting thrombin (dabigatran) or factor Xa (rivaroxaban, apixaban, and edoxaban) are becoming widely used. Although mainly outpatient anticoagulants, their growing utilization ensures considerations for critically ill patients. As all DOACs depend on urinary clearance, patients with kidney failure are often vulnerable to their supratherapeutic effects.[5]

Dabigatran—Direct Thrombin Inhibitor

Dabigatran was approved in 2010 for stroke prevention in patients with atrial fibrillation. However, patients with an eGFR less than 30 mL/min were excluded from the trial.[56] Dabigatran is mainly excreted by the kidneys, with urinary elimination making up to 80% of clearance.[57] This urinary clearance makes dabigatran a poor choice for anticoagulation in the setting of kidney failure. Studies show a direct relationship between kidney failure and bleeding risk, with dabigatran causing more bleeding than warfarin.[58,59]

Dabigatran reversal is often necessary in patients with kidney failure. The efficacy of FFP or PCC is questionable for supratherapeutic dabigatran anticoagulation.[60] Fortunately, dabigatran can be eliminated through KRT, with 49% to 68% cleared though HD. Although HD provides more efficient initial clearance compared to CKRT, significant dabigatran rebound has been reported with HD alone, whereas CKRT provides slower but more steady clearance.[61-63] KRT should be considered for therapeutic clearance of dabigatran when life-threatening bleeding is present. The monoclonal antibody idarucizumab has also been approved for dabigatran neutralization, with a dose of 5 g IV used, regardless of kidney function.[64]

Direct Xa Inhibitors

General Safety and Reversal

Life-threatening bleeding related to direct Xa inhibitors does not generally respond to traditional FFP. Instead, unactivated four-factor PCC is recommended. The novel agent andexanet alfa has also been approved for rivaroxaban and apixaban reversal and has some data supporting the use for edoxaban.[65]

Rivaroxaban—Factor Xa Inhibitor

Rivaroxaban is a factor Xa inhibitor approved for stroke prevention in atrial fibrillation as well as for the prevention and treatment of deep venous thrombosis (DVT) and pulmonary embolism (PE). However, rivaroxaban is not recommended for uses other than atrial fibrillation when CrCl is less than 30 mL/min and is contraindicated for patients with CrCl less than 15 mL/min. Rivaroxaban accumulates in patients with reduced kidney function and is poorly cleared by HD or CKRT.[41]

Apixaban—Factor Xa Inhibitor

Apixaban is approved for stroke prevention in patients with atrial fibrillation and for DVT/PE prophylaxis and treatment. Apixaban can be used in patients with kidney failure with some caution. If serum creatinine is greater than 1.5 mg/dL, age above 80 years, or body weight less than 60 kg, a reduced dose of 2.5 mg twice daily is recommended (standard dose of 5 mg twice daily).[66] Although data are limited, KRT-dependent patients may safely tolerate a reduced dose of 2.5 mg of apixaban twice daily.[67]

Edoxaban—Factor Xa Inhibitor

Edoxaban is approved for stroke prevention in patients with atrial fibrillation and for the treatment of DVT/PE, but only after initial 5- to 10-day treatment with parenteral anticoagulation. For patients with CrCl of 50 to 95 mL/min, 60 mg once daily is recommended, whereas 30 mg daily can be used for patients with CrCl of 15 to 50 mL/min.[66] Although edoxaban is a small molecule, its large volume of distribution and protein binding limit clearance with KRT.[68]

References

1. Molino D, De Lucia D, De Santo NG. Coagulation disorders in uremia. *Semin Nephrol.* 2006;26(1):46-51. doi:10.1016/j.semnephrol.2005.06.011
2. Lutz J, Menke J, Sollinger D, et al. Haemostasis in chronic kidney disease. *Nephrol Dial Transplant.* 2014;29(1):29-40. doi:10.1093/ndt/gft209
3. Thorevska N, Amoateng-Adjepong Y, Sabahi R, et al. Anticoagulation in hospitalized patients with renal insufficiency: a comparison of bleeding rates with unfractionated heparin vs enoxaparin. *Chest.* 2004;125(3):856-863. doi:10.1378/chest.125.3.856
4. Spinler SA, Inverso SM, Cohen M, et al. Safety and efficacy of unfractionated heparin versus enoxaparin in patients who are obese and patients with severe renal impairment: analysis from the ESSENCE and TIMI 11b studies. *Am Heart J.* 2003;146(1):33-41. doi:10.1016/S0002-8703(03)00121-2
5. Hughes S, Szeki I, Nash MJ, et al. Anticoagulation in chronic kidney disease patients—the practical aspects. *Clin Kidney J.* 2014;7(5):442-449. doi:10.1093/ckj/sfu080
6. DeLoughery TG. Other parenteral anticoagulants. In: DeLoughery TG, ed. *Hemostasis and Thrombosis.* 3rd ed. Springer; 2015:117-119. doi:10.1007/978-3-319-09312-3_23
7. Raschke RA, Reilly BM, Guidry JR, et al. The weight-based heparin dosing nomogram compared with a standard care nomogram. *Ann Intern Med.* 1993;119(9):874. doi:10.7326/0003-4819-119-9-199311010-00002
8. O'Gara PT, Kushner FG, Ascheim DD, et al. 2013 ACCF/AHA guideline for the management of ST-elevation myocardial infarction: executive summary. *Circulation.* 2012;127(4):529-555. doi:10.1161/cir.0b013e3182742c84
9. Amsterdam EA, Wenger NK, Brindis RG, et al. 2014 AHA/ACC guideline for the management of patients with non–ST-elevation acute coronary syndromes: executive summary. *Circulation.* 2014;130(25):2354-2394. doi:10.1161/CIR.0000000000000133
10. Basu D, Gallus A, Hirsh J, et al. A prospective study of the value of monitoring heparin treatment with the activated partial thromboplastin time. *N Engl J Med.* 2010;287(7):324-327. doi:10.1056/nejm197208172870703
11. Raschke R, Hirsh J, Guidry JR. Suboptimal monitoring and dosing of unfractionated heparin in comparative studies with low-molecular-weight heparin. *Ann Intern Med.* 2003;138(9):720. doi:10.7326/0003-4819-138-9-200305060-00008

12. Zehnder J, Price E, Jin J. Controversies in heparin monitoring. *Am J Hematol.* 2012;87(S1):S137-S140. doi:10.1002/ajh.23210
13. Heparin and LMW heparin: dosing and adverse effects—UpToDate. Accessed June 22, 2019. https://www.uptodate.com/contents/heparin-and-lmw-heparin-dosing-and-adverse-effects?search=protamine§ionRank=1&usage_type=default&anchor=H81746&source=machineLearning&selectedTitle=2~99&display_rank=2#H81746
14. Reddy BV, Grossman EJ, Trevino SA, et al. Argatroban anticoagulation in patients with heparin-induced thrombocytopenia requiring renal replacement therapy. *Ann Pharmacother.* 2005;39(10):1601-1605. doi:10.1345/aph.1G033
15. Effrey J, Eitz IW. Drug therapy low-molecular-weight heparins. Accessed June 23, 2019. https://www.nejm.org/doi/pdf/10.1056/NEJM199709043371007?articleTools=true
16. Handeland GF, Abildgaard U, Holm HA, et al. Dose adjusted heparin treatment of deep venous thrombosis: a comparison of unfractionated and low molecular weight heparin. *Eur J Clin Pharmacol.* 1990;39(2):107-112. Accessed June 23, 2019. http://www.ncbi.nlm.nih.gov/pubmed/2174783
17. Hirsh J, Bauer KA, Donati MB, et al. Parenteral anticoagulants: American College of Chest Physicians evidence-based clinical practice guidelines (8th edition). *Chest.* 2008;133(6 suppl 6):141S-159S. doi:10.1378/chest.08-0689
18. Kearon C, Akl EA, Ornelas J, et al. Antithrombotic therapy for VTE disease. *Chest.* 2016;149(2):315-352. doi:10.1016/j.chest.2015.11.026
19. Holbrook A, Schulman S, Witt DM, et al. Evidence-based management of anticoagulant therapy: antithrombotic therapy and prevention of thrombosis, 9th ed: American College of Chest Physicians evidence-based clinical practice guidelines. *Chest.* 2012;141(2 suppl):e152S-e184S. doi:10.1378/chest.11-2295
20. Kahale LA, Hakoum MB, Tsolakian IG, et al. Anticoagulation for the long-term treatment of venous thromboembolism in people with cancer. *Cochrane Database Syst Rev.* 2018;2018(6):CD006650. doi:10.1002/14651858.CD006650.pub5
21. Chow SL, Zammit K, West K, et al. Correlation of antifactor Xa concentrations with renal function in patients on enoxaparin. *J Clin Pharmacol.* 2003;43(6):586-590. Accessed June 23, 2019. http://www.ncbi.nlm.nih.gov/pubmed/12817521
22. Gerlach AT, Pickworth KK, Seth SK, et al. Enoxaparin and bleeding complications: a review in patients with and without renal insufficiency. *Pharmacotherapy.* 2000;20(7):771-775. Accessed June 23, 2019. http://www.ncbi.nlm.nih.gov/pubmed/10907967
23. Cestac P, Bagheri H, Lapeyre-Mestre M, et al. Utilisation and safety of low molecular weight heparins. *Drug Saf.* 2003;26(3):197-207. doi:10.2165/00002018-200326030-00005
24. Lachish T, Rudensky B, Slotki I, et al. Enoxaparin dosage adjustment in patients with severe renal failure: antifactor Xa concentrations and safety. *Pharmacotherapy.* 2007;27(10):1347-1352. doi:10.1592/phco.27.10.1347
25. FDA, CDER. Fachinformation Lovenox (enoxaparin sodium injection) for subcutaneous and intravenous use 3000 IU. Stand: 10/2013. sanofi-aventis U.S. LLC, Bridgewater. National Drug Code: 0075-0624-30. Accessed June 24, 2019. www.fda.gov/medwatch
26. Nijkeuter M, Huisman MV. Pentasaccharides in the prophylaxis and treatment of venous thromboembolism: a systematic review. *Curr Opin Pulm Med.* 2004;10(5):338-344. doi:10.1097/01.mcp.0000136901.80029.37
27. Wallis RB. Hirudins: from leeches to man. *Semin Thromb Hemost.* 1996;22(2):185-196. doi:10.1055/s-2007-999007
28. Toschi V, Lettino M, Gallo R, et al. Biochemistry and biology of hirudin. *Coron Artery Dis.* 1996;7(6):420-428. Accessed June 25, 2019. http://www.ncbi.nlm.nih.gov/pubmed/8889357
29. Maraganore JM, Bourdon P, Jablonski J, et al. Design and characterization of hirulogs: a novel class of bivalent peptide inhibitors of thrombin. *Biochemistry.* 1990;29(30):7095-7101. doi:10.1021/bi00482a021
30. Robson R. The use of bivalirudin in patients with renal impairment. *J Invasive Cardiol.* 2000;12 suppl F:33F-6. Accessed June 26, 2019. http://www.ncbi.nlm.nih.gov/pubmed/11156732
31. FDA. Highlights of prescribing information-bivalirudin®. *FDA.* 1997:1-33. doi:10.1017/CBO9781107415324.004
32. Linkins L-A, Dans AL, Moores LK, et al. Treatment and prevention of heparin-induced thrombocytopenia. *Chest.* 2012;141(2):e495S-e530S. doi:10.1378/chest.11-2303
33. Kiser TH, Burch JC, Klem PM, et al. Safety, efficacy, and dosing requirements of bivalirudin in patients with heparin-induced thrombocytopenia. *Pharmacotherapy.* 2008;28(9):1115-1124. doi:10.1592/phco.28.9.1115
34. Tsu LV, Dager WE. Bivalirudin dosing adjustments for reduced renal function with or without hemodialysis in the management of heparin-induced thrombocytopenia. *Ann Pharmacother.* 2011;45(10):1185-1192. doi:10.1345/aph.1Q177

35. Swan SK, Hursting MJ. The pharmacokinetics and pharmacodynamics of argatroban: effects of age, gender, and hepatic or renal dysfunction. *Pharmacotherapy.* 2000;20(3):318-329. doi:10.1592/phco.20.4.318.34881
36. Ansell J, Hirsh J, Hylek E, et al. Pharmacology and management of the vitamin K antagonists: American College of Chest Physicians Evidence-Based Clinical Practice Guidelines (8th edition). *Chest.* 2008;133(6 suppl 6):160S-198S. doi:10.1378/chest.08-0670
37. Harrison L, Johnston M, Massicotte MP, et al. Comparison of 5-mg and 10-mg loading doses in initiation of Warfarin therapy. *Ann Intern Med.* 1997;126(2):133. doi:10.7326/0003-4819-126-2-199701150-00006
38. Crowther MA, Ginsberg JB, Kearon C, et al. A randomized trial comparing 5-mg and 10-mg warfarin loading doses. *Arch Intern Med.* 1999;159(1):46-48. Accessed June 28, 2019. http://www.ncbi.nlm.nih.gov/pubmed/9892329
39. January CT, Wann LS, Alpert JS, et al. 2014 AHA/ACC/HRS Guideline for the management of patients with atrial fibrillation: executive summary. *Circulation.* 2014;130(23):2071-2104. doi:10.1161/CIR.0000000000000040
40. Chan KE, Lazarus JM, Thadhani R, et al. Warfarin use associates with increased risk for stroke in hemodialysis patients with atrial fibrillation. *J Am Soc Nephrol.* 2009;20(10):2223-2233. doi:10.1681/ASN.2009030319
41. Jain N, Reilly RF. Clinical pharmacology of oral anticoagulants in patients with kidney disease. *Clin J Am Soc Nephrol.* 2018;14(2):278-287. doi:10.2215/cjn.02170218
42. Brodsky S, Eikelboom J, Hebert LA. Anticoagulant-related nephropathy. *J Am Soc Nephrol.* 2018;29(12):2787-2793. doi:10.1681/ASN.2018070741
43. Md Arif K, Rahman MA. A review of warfarin dosing and monitoring. *Faridpur Med Coll J.* 2018;13(1):40-43. doi:10.3329/fmcj.v13i1.38018
44. Limdi NA, Nolin TD, Booth SL, et al. Influence of kidney function on risk of supratherapeutic international normalized ratio-related hemorrhage in warfarin users: a prospective cohort study. *Am J Kidney Dis.* 2015;65(5):701-709. doi:10.1053/j.ajkd.2014.11.004
45. Fan J, Armitstead JA, Adams AG, et al. A retrospective evaluation of vitamin K1 therapy to reverse the anticoagulant effect of warfarin. *Pharmacotherapy.* 2003;23(10):1245-1250. Accessed June 28, 2019. http://www.ncbi.nlm.nih.gov/pubmed/14594342
46. Shetty HG, Backhouse G, Bentley DP, et al. Effective reversal of warfarin-induced excessive anticoagulation with low dose vitamin K1. *Thromb Haemost.* 1992;67(1):13-15. Accessed June 28, 2019. http://www.ncbi.nlm.nih.gov/pubmed/1615468
47. Britt RB, Brown JN. Characterizing the severe reactions of parenteral vitamin K1. *Clin Appl Thromb.* 2018;24(1):5-12. doi:10.1177/1076029616674825
48. Fiore LD, Scola MA, Cantillon CE, et al. Anaphylactoid reactions to vitamin K. *J Thromb Thrombolysis.* 2001;11(2):175-183. Accessed June 28, 2019. http://www.ncbi.nlm.nih.gov/pubmed/11406734
49. Duguid J, O'Shaughnessy DF, Atterbury C, et al. Guidelines for the use of fresh-frozen plasma, cryoprecipitate and cryosupernatant. *Br J Haematol.* 2004;126(1):11-28. doi:10.1111/j.1365-2141.2004.04972.x
50. Rashidi A, Tahhan HR. Fresh frozen plasma dosing for warfarin reversal: a practical formula. *Mayo Clin Proc.* 2013;88:244-250. doi:10.1016/j.mayocp.2012.12.011
51. Mayer SA, Brun NC, Begtrup K, et al. Recombinant activated factor VII for acute intracerebral hemorrhage. *N Engl J Med.* 2005;352(8):777-785. doi:10.1056/NEJMoa042991
52. Dager WE, King JH, Regalia RC, et al. Reversal of elevated international normalized ratios and bleeding with low-dose recombinant activated factor VII in patients receiving warfarin. *Pharmacotherapy.* 2006;26(8):1091-1098. doi:10.1592/phco.26.8.1091
53. Wozniak M, Kruit A, Padmore R, et al. Prothrombin complex concentrate for the urgent reversal of warfarin. Assessment of a standard dosing protocol. *Transfus Apher Sci.* 2012;46(3):309-314. doi:10.1016/j.transci.2012.03.021
54. Yasaka M, Sakata T, Naritomi H, et al. Optimal dose of prothrombin complex concentrate for acute reversal of oral anticoagulation. *Thromb Res.* 2005;115(6):455-459. doi:10.1016/j.thromres.2004.09.002
55. Aguilar MI, Hart RG, Kase CS, et al. Treatment of warfarin-associated intracerebral hemorrhage: literature review and expert opinion. *Mayo Clin Proc.* 2007;82(1):82-92. doi:10.4065/82.1.82
56. Connolly SJ, Ezekowitz MD, Yusuf S, et al. Dabigatran versus warfarin in patients with atrial fibrillation. *N Engl J Med.* 2009;361(12):1139-1151. doi:10.1056/NEJMoa0905561
57. Changes M. PRADAXA® (dabigatran etexilate mesylate) capsules [package insert on internet]. *Ridgef Boehringer Ingelheim Pharm Inc.* 2015. https://www.accessdata.fda.gov/drugsatfda_docs/label/2015/022512s028lbl.pdf
58. Chan KE, Edelman ER, Wenger JB, et al. Dabigatran and rivaroxaban use in atrial fibrillation patients on hemodialysis. *Circulation.* 2015;131(11):972-979. doi:10.1161/CIRCULATIONAHA.114.014113

59. Hijazi Z, Hohnloser SH, Oldgren J, et al. Efficacy and safety of dabigatran compared with warfarin in relation to baseline renal function in patients with atrial fibrillation: a RE-LY (Randomized evaluation of long-term anticoagulation therapy) trial analysis. *Circulation.* 2014;129(9):961-970. doi:10.1161/CIRCULATIONAHA.113.003628
60. Eerenberg ES, Kamphuisen PW, Sijpkens MK, et al. Reversal of rivaroxaban and dabigatran by prothrombin complex concentrate. *Circulation.* 2011;124(14):1573-1579. doi:10.1161/CIRCULATIONAHA.111.029017
61. Bouchard J, Ghannoum M, Bernier-Jean A, et al. Comparison of intermittent and continuous extracorporeal treatments for the enhanced elimination of dabigatran. *Clin Toxicol.* 2015;53(3):156-163. doi:10.3109/15563650.2015.1004580
62. Khadzhynov D, Wagner F, Formella S, et al. Effective elimination of dabigatran by haemodialysis. A phase I single-centre study in patients with end-stage renal disease. *Thromb Haemost.* 2013;109(4):596-605. doi:10.1160/TH12-08-0573
63. Stangier J, Rathgen K, Stähle H, et al. Influence of renal impairment on the pharmacokinetics and pharmacodynamics of oral dabigatran etexilate. *Clin Pharmacokinet.* 2010;49(4):259-268. doi:10.2165/11318170-000000000-00000
64. Pollack CV, Reilly PA, van Ryn J, et al. Idarucizumab for dabigatran reversal—full cohort analysis. *N Engl J Med.* 2017;377(5):431-441. doi:10.1056/NEJMoa1707278
65. Cuker A, Burnett A, Triller D, et al. Reversal of direct oral anticoagulants: guidance from the anticoagulation forum. *Am J Hematol.* 2019;94(6):697-709. doi:10.1002/ajh.25475
66. FDA, CDER. FDA label. 2012:1-46. Accessed July 10, 2019. www.fda.gov/medwatch
67. Mavrakanas TA, Samer CF, Nessim SJ, et al. Apixaban pharmacokinetics at steady state in hemodialysis patients. *J Am Soc Nephrol.* 2017;28(7):2241-2248. doi:10.1681/asn.2016090980
68. Parasrampuria DA, Marbury T, Matsushima N, et al. Pharmacokinetics, safety, and tolerability of edoxaban in end-stage renal disease subjects undergoing haemodialysis. *Thromb Haemost.* 2015;113(4):719-727. doi:10.1160/TH14-06-0547

15 The Metabolic Management and Nutrition of Acute Kidney Injury

Wilfred Druml and Kamyar Kalantar-Zadeh

Acute kidney injury (AKI) is a heterogeneous syndrome with a broad pattern of etiologies and clinical presentations, which is defined by three distinct stages. This necessitates an individualized approach regarding the metabolic and nutritional management, which must be meticulously adapted for each patient at each time point of therapy. Nutrition is more than maintaining a good nutritional state; it should be viewed as part of the metabolic management of a patient and must also integrate volume therapy, acid-base and electrolyte balance, and hemodynamic/respiratory care.[1,2]

In this chapter, we propose a stage-specific approach in the metabolic management—including infusion therapy and both enteral and parenteral nutrition support—in the therapy of patients with acute kidney dysfunction and its prevention.

Many or even most of the statements are not based on randomized controlled trials (RCTs) and are expert opinions only.

PREVENTION AND THERAPY OF STAGE 1 ACUTE KIDNEY INJURY

There is no effective pharmacologic therapy available for AKI. Therefore, the general management of the AKI patient consists of: optimization of hemodynamic and volume status, the avoidance of nephrotoxic drugs; maintaining metabolic balance and nutrition support (**Table 15.1**).[3]

Volume Management

Within the context of prevention of AKI, volume management plays a central role. However, the association of volume status and risk of AKI follows a U-shaped curve, so both hypovolemia and hypervolemia play an important role in the deterioration and outcome of kidney function. As discussed elsewhere, the type (e.g., balanced vs saline) and volume of fluid can impact renal outcomes (Chapter 10).

Electrolyte Homeostasis and Acid-Base Balance

In experimental models, deficiencies of magnesium, potassium, and phosphate can augment kidney injury.[4] Thus, electrolyte derangements should be prevented and/or corrected in all ICU patients.

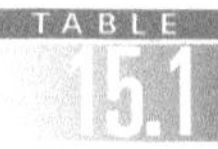

TABLE 15.1 Infusion Therapy and Metabolic Management in the Prevention of AKI and Therapy of Stage 1 AKI (Risk Stage)

- Volume therapy
  - Infusion solutions: balanced, no artificial colloids
  - Avoidance of both hypovolemia and hypervolemia
- Prevention/correction of electrolyte imbalances
  - Potassium, phosphate, magnesium
- Prevention/correction deficiency states
  - Thiamine, vitamin D, vitamin C
- Prevention/correction of metabolic acidosis
- Prevention/correction of hyperglycemia
- Early start of (whenever possible) enteral nutrition
- Avoidance of hypercaloric nutrition in the early phase
- Higher protein/amino acid intake in the early phase

AKI, acute kidney injury.

In animal models, acidosis aggravates kidney injury after ischemia reperfusion injury. In a large prospective randomized trial, correction of severe metabolic acidosis (pH ≤ 7.2) using bicarbonate infusions in ICU patients reduced the risk of AKI and improved prognosis in kidney replacement therapy (KRT).[5-8] It is unclear whether these improved outcomes are from the bicarbonate-related avoidance of hyperkalemia or systemic alkalinization.

Hyperglycemia

Hyperglycemia interferes with endothelial structure and function, promotes inflammation, and may aggravate kidney injury.[6,7] Thus, in any critically ill patient, blood glucose concentration should be lower than 180 mg/dL.[8] Because blood glucose concentrations have diurnal variation, some institutions aim for 150 mg/dL to keep the level reliably below 180 mg/dL. These higher-than-euglycemia targets stem, in part, from the Normoglycemia in Intensive Care Evaluation—Survival Using Glucose Algorithm Regulation (NICE-SUGAR) trial. This multicenter trial randomized patients to conventional (<180 mg/dL) versus intensive (81–108 mg/dL) glucose control and demonstrated increased risk of hypoglycemic events and death with tighter control.

Nutrition in the Prevention of Acute Kidney Injury and as Therapy for Stage 1 Acute Kidney Injury

Nutrition therapy (oral/enteral/parenteral) in this early stage of AKI is not fundamentally different from that in other patient groups. Nevertheless, in respect to preservation of kidney function, some points should be considered:

Initiation and route of nutrition support: Whenever possible, enteral nutrition should be used. In animal models, enteral feeds are associated with improved kidney perfusion and kidney function.[9,10] Although older randomized multicenter data demonstrate that later initiation of parental nutrition is associated with faster recovery and fewer complications compared to early initiation,[11] we believe that in ICU patients, nutrition support should be started early, but at a low rate (trophic nutrition), and infusion rate should be increased slowly according to the individual metabolic and gastrointestinal tolerance.[12]

Early high-energy intake may increase the risk of developing AKI.[13] Preexisting deficiency states (electrolytes and micronutrients such as thiamine) should be corrected to avoid untoward side effects of nutrition and the development of refeeding syndrome.[14]

Amino acid/protein intake: Currently, there is a lot of interest in determining the optimal protein/amino acid intake in patients at risk of developing AKI and those with Stage 1 AKI. A high amino acid infusion/protein intake dilates afferent arterioles and increases kidney perfusion and glomerular filtration—a phenomenon designated renal reserve capacity (i.e., the percentage increase in kidney function in a postabsorptive patient after a defined protein load).[15]

It was hypothesized that this mechanism could support kidney function and help to prevent the evolution of AKI. An earlier small pilot study had suggested that a higher amino acid intake (about 2 g/kg/d) lowers serum creatinine, increases diuresis, and lowers the need for diuretics.[16] A large randomized controlled study using an intravenous amino acid infusion of 1 g/kg/d in addition to the protein intake of (about 1 g/kg/d) improved kidney function during the first 4 days but had no effects on the need for KRT, length of hospital stay, or survival.[17]

In a post hoc analysis of this study, the increased amino acid intake protected against the development of AKI and improved survival in those patients who did not show kidney injury at the start of therapy.[18] In a more recent study, cardiac surgery patients received an amino acid infusion immediately after the induction of anesthesia.[19] The duration of AKI was shortened, estimated glomerular filtration rate (eGFR) and urine output were significantly improved after surgery, but again, no additional clinical end-points were affected.

More evidence derived from RCTs is needed, and for the time being, no definite recommendations can be given concerning an increased protein/amino acid infusion in ICU patients for the prevention of AKI or as therapy for Stage 1 AKI (see below for discussion around more severe stages of AKI).

Nutrition solutions: In ICU patients with Stage 1 AKI, no specific nutrition preparations should be used for enteral or parenteral nutrition.

INFUSION THERAPY AND NUTRITION SUPPORT IN STAGE 2 AND 3 ACUTE KIDNEY INJURY WITHOUT THE NEED FOR KIDNEY REPLACEMENT THERAPY

Although Stage 2 and 3 AKI without the need for KRT is common, there are limited systematic data on the optimal metabolic management and nutritional therapy in this cohort. Careful, fastidious ICU management guides the care in patients with Stage 2 and 3 AKI (Table 15.1). Most measures are not fundamentally different from those used in the management of other unstable critically ill patients.[20]

These patients often exhibit volume intolerance, that is, both too little and too much fluids will have immediate consequences for hemodynamics/microcirculation and also for the kidney.[21] It is pivotal to prevent volume overload, which compromises microcirculation and kidney function. In a European cohort, patients with AKI had better survival if they were not fluid overloaded at the time of initiation of KRT.[22]

Maintaining a balanced metabolic environment (electrolytes, glucose, triglycerides, and acid-base balance) is an essential goal of therapy. Use of sodium bicarbonate in patients with sepsis and severe AKI and severe metabolic acidosis (pH < 7.2) may improve outcomes.[5]

Metabolic Alterations Specifically Induced by Acute kidney Dysfunction

AKI occurs in various clinical situations, and metabolism in these patients is affected not only by AKI but also by the underlying disease process, associated comorbidities, and further complications/organ dysfunctions such as infections. The main metabolic alterations associated with AKI are summarized in **Table 15.2**. Basically, severe AKI is a systemic syndrome in which all physiologic functions and endocrine and metabolic pathways are affected. AKI presents a proinflammatory, pro-oxidative, and hypercatabolic state, which exerts a profound impact on the course of disease.

Energy metabolism is not grossly affected by AKI, even in those patients requiring KRT. Energy metabolism is largely determined by the underlying disease process and associated complications.[23,24] Protein catabolism is stimulated, especially in those patients with additional catabolic factors such as acidosis or infections. Thus, protein catabolic rate can vary considerably in patients with AKI; on average it is estimated to be around 1.5 g/kg/d.[25] Moreover, severe AKI induces a state of insulin resistance, which is associated with decreased survival.[26]

A fundamental difference in the metabolic characteristics of other acutely ill patients is the fact that in AKI, lipolysis is impaired, potentially resulting in hypertriglyceridemia.[27] Lipid oxidation, however, is maintained in these patients and lipids can be used both in enteral and parenteral nutrition at currently recommended infusion rates.[27,28] Nevertheless, when additional factors are present, such as sedation therapy using propofol or a high-energy intake, hypertriglyceridemia may evolve.

Because of the heterogeneity of AKI and the multifaceted clinical presentation, both nutrient disposal and nutritional requirements can vary fundamentally between individual patients. Furthermore, AKI is a dynamic process and the metabolic situation can change within the same patient during the course of disease. Thus, metabolic management/nutrition must be individualized and continually assessed in patients with Stage 2 and 3 AKI.

The previously held opinion that KRT should be started early in order to enable sufficient nutrition therapy cannot be maintained any unnecessary KRT should be avoided.[29]

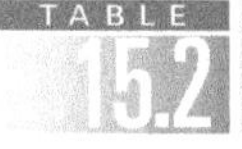

Main Metabolic Alterations in Patients With Acute Kidney Injury

- Induction/augmentation of an inflammatory state
- Activation of protein catabolism
- Peripheral insulin resistance/increased gluconeogenesis
- Impairment of lipolysis and intestinal lipid absorption
- Depletion of antioxidative systems
- Metabolic acidosis
- Endocrine alterations: hyperparathyroidism, reduced vitamin D (calcitriol) synthesis, erythropoietin resistance, growth hormone resistance

Nutrition Support in Stage 2 and 3 Acute Kidney Injury Without the Need for Kidney Replacement Therapy

Again, whenever possible, enteral nutrition should be used in these patients. However, kidney dysfunction is associated with impairment of gastrointestinal motility that often can limit full enteral nutrition.[30,31] Prokinetic drugs should be given early (potentially even prophylactically) to facilitate successful enteral nutrition. In many patients, a supplemental or total parenteral nutrition will be necessary.[32]

Energy intake: In Stage 2 and 3 AKI without the need for KRT, a full "normocaloric" nutrition should not be pursued or forced. In analogy with other critically ill patients, rather a mild "permissive" hypoalimentation should be the target with a prescription for 60% to 80% of calculated or measured energy expenditure.[33] An exaggerated energy intake can induce a further deterioration of kidney function in these stages.[13]

Protein intake: As demonstrated in animal models and confirmed by recent clinical trials, a high protein/amino acid intake during an active AKI can aggravate kidney damage and uremic toxicity ("amino acid paradox").[18,34] Moreover, a high protein intake in this phase may enhance the necessity of KRT by increasing urea generation.[35] Intake of protein/amino acids must be monitored regularly by measuring plasma urea concentrations and be adapted accordingly. Protein intake should not be higher than 0.8 to 1.2 g/kg/d.[25] Neither intravenous nor enteral glutamine should be provided in patients with Stage 2 and 3 AKI.[36]

Nutrition solutions: International societies do not recommend the use of specific "nephro" diets but rather standard solutions for both enteral and parenteral nutrition in patients with severe AKI. Amino acid solutions adapted to uremic metabolism and with a high content of anabolic essential and conditionally essential amino acids are available in some countries.[36,37] Theoretical advantages are a normalization of plasma amino acid pattern, a reduction of urea formation, and improved protein synthesis, but these specific solutions have not been proven to exert an impact on patient outcome.

METABOLIC MANAGEMENT AND NUTRITION SUPPORT IN PATIENTS WITH ACUTE KIDNEY INJURY-3 (AND CHRONIC KIDNEY DISEASE-5) REQUIRING KIDNEY REPLACEMENT THERAPY

Management of the fluid, electrolyte, and acid-base status is regulated in patients on KRT by the extracorporeal device. However, aside from the metabolic alterations induced by AKI, all extracorporeal treatment modalities exert a profound impact on metabolism, nutrient balances, and resulting nutrient requirements (**Table 15.3**).

Electrolytes: Obviously, in any patient with kidney dysfunction, electrolyte balance has to be monitored closely and intake has to be adapted accordingly. Plasma levels of phosphate, magnesium, and potassium should be monitored regularly.

There is increased risk of hypophosphatemia with continuous KRT (CKRT) and also with intermittent hemodialysis (HD).[38,39] Hypophosphatemia is associated with an increased risk of complications, a retardation of the weaning from artificial ventilation, and decreased survival (see Chapter 23). Because of the high prevalence of this derangement, either a systematic phosphate supplementation or phosphate-containing substitution fluids for CKRT or dialysates should be used.[40]

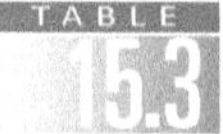

TABLE 15.3 Impact of Kidney Replacement Therapy on Metabolism and Nutrient Balances

Intermittent Hemodialysis

- Loss of water-soluble substances:
  - Amino acids, water-soluble vitamins, L-carnitine, etc.
- Activation of protein catabolism:
  - Loss of amino acids, proteins, blood
  - Release of cytokines (tumor necrosis factor-α)
  - Impairment of protein synthesis
- Depletion of antioxidative potential
  - Loss of antioxidants
  - Stimulation of reactive oxygen species (ROS) production

Continuous Kidney Replacement Therapy

- Heat loss
- Increased intake of substrates
  - Glucose, citrate, lactate
- Loss of nutrients
  - Amino acids, vitamins, selenium, etc.
- Loss of albumin
- Elimination of peptides:
  - Hormones, cytokines
- Loss of electrolytes (phosphate, magnesium)

Metabolic Consequences of Bioincompatibility

- Induction of a "low-grade" inflammation, activation of protein catabolism, formation of ROS

Nutrition Therapy

In designing a nutritional regimen for patients on KRT, nutrient losses associated with KRT must be considered. Guiding values for nutrient requirements are summarized in **Table 15.4**. Again, the nutrition support must be adapted to individual needs and tolerance. Whenever possible, enteral nutrition should be preferred in AKI patients on KRT, but because of the gastrointestinal intolerance, in many patients a supplement of total parenteral nutrition may be required.

Protein intake: Nutritional protein intake for patients on KRT must consider the therapy-associated losses of amino acids/protein. Depending on the type and intensity of KRT, loss of amino acids is highly variable. A loss of about 2 g of amino acids per hour during intermittent HD and about 0.2 g/L effluent during CKRT or sustained low-efficiency dialysis (SLED) should be accounted for.[41-43] Depending on the type of membranes used and the transmembrane pressure, additional protein losses may account for up to 20 g/d. To compensate these losses, an increase in protein intake of 0.2 g/kg/d is generally recommended.[25]

For optimal protein intake, considerable variations exist between recommendations from international societies. The American Society of Parenteral and Enteral Nutrition (ASPEN) recommends a protein/amino acid intake of 2.0 to 2.5 g/kg/d (or even higher) in AKI patients on KRT.[8] This statement is more or less based on a single study.[12] It is not clear why the protein intake should be so much higher than that in other critically ill patients. An exaggerated protein intake can induce serious complications such as hyperammonemia and associated coma.

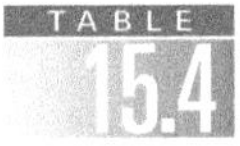

Nutritional Requirements in Patients With Stage 2 and 3 AKI (Without/With KRT)

Energy intake	20-25[a] max. 30 kcal/kg/d	
Glucose	2-3 g/kg/d	
Lipids[b]	0.8-1.2 g/kg/d	
Protein/amino acids		
Without KRT	0.8–1.2 g/kg/d	
+ KRT	1.2-1.5 g/kg/d	
+ Hypercatabolism max. 1.7 g/kg/d		
Vitamins combination products according to RDA		
Water-soluble vitamins		2 × RDA/d
Lipid-soluble vitamins		1-2 × RDA/d
Higher for vitamins D, E		
Trace elements combination products according to RDA		
1 × RDA/d		
Selenium 200-600 µg/d		
Electrolytes intake must be individualized		

These can be guiding values only, nutrition must be individualized; requirements can vary between patients and in the same patient often during the dynamic course of disease.
AKI, acute kidney injury; KRT, kidney replacement therapy; RDA, recommended dietary allowance.
[a]Consider energy intake during citrate anticoagulation.
[b]When using propofol, consider therapy-associated lipid intake.

In contrast, European nutrition societies recommend an intake of 1.2 to 1.5 g/kg/d or a maximum of 1.7 g/kg/d in hypercatabolic patients with a high severity of disease, a dosage which includes 0.2 g/kg/d for compensation of KRT-associated losses[25] (Table 15.4).

Energy intake: Energy expenditure in patients with AKI on KRT is not fundamentally different from other disease states. As in other intensive care patients, the goal of energy intake should be 25 kcal/kg/d (20 kcal/kg/d in patients >60 years).[8,33] Indirect calorimetry, which is often recommended to measure energy expenditure, is rarely available in the clinical setting. Currently available formulas for calculations of energy expenditure in critically ill patients tend to overestimate the energy needs.

Concerning the calculation of energy supply in patients on KRT, it should be noted that during anticoagulation with citrate—which is increasingly used as a standard for CKRT—energy is provided by citrate infusion.[44] This extra energy intake can be very variable depending on the type and dose of therapy and may account for roughly 200 kcal/d.

Despite the presence of an impairment of lipolysis in AKI, lipids can be given by enteral or parenteral nutrition. However, plasma levels have to be monitored during nutrition therapy. If a patient develops severe hypertriglyceridemia (>800 mg/dL), this can interfere with KRT and cause the filter to clot.[45]

Micronutrients: There is a profound depletion of the antioxidative potential in patients on KRT.[46] KRT contributes to this deficiency by removing water-soluble vitamins, trace elements, and other nutrients, with this being exacerbated in those with CKRT.[47,48]

In the absence of systematic investigation, recommendations for intake are based on expert opinion only. Standard multivitamin and multitrace element preparations should be used. For water-soluble vitamins, an intake of double the standard daily allowances is proposed.[25] During the early phase of nutrition, even higher amounts of thiamine may be required.[14] The optimal dose of vitamin C in AKI patients remains undefined.

As in chronic kidney disease (CKD), vitamin D activation is also impaired in patients with AKI.[49] Vitamin D deficiency aggravates tubular injury, and supplementation may exert a protective potential.[50] In patients with decreased plasma concentrations of 25-OH-vitamin D_3, supplementation is recommended. The optimal formulation and dose remain unknown. Other fat-soluble vitamins should be provided according to standard recommended dietary allowances.

Concerning trace elements, some replacement fluids and dialysates may contain various elements, such as zinc, nickel, copper, or manganese. Selenium is eliminated during CKRT and potentially should be provided in higher amounts (i.e., 600 μg/d).[48]

Nutrition solutions: Because energy intake should be increased gradually and the presence of non-nutritional energy intake (i.e., citrate, propofol, and glucose) should be counted, using protein-rich diets may be advantageous during the first days of nutrition to ensure an adequate protein and amino acid intake.[51] In selected patients, enteral protein supplement or a separate infusion of amino acids may be required to achieve this goal.[32]

International societies recommend the use of standard solutions for enteral and parenteral nutrition. Nevertheless, specific enteral diets designed as oral nutritional supplements (ONS) for enteral nutrition of chronic HD patients can be used especially in a noninflammatory stable patient with AKI on KRT. These ONS are energy-rich (2 kcal/mL), protein-rich, and electrolyte-reduced sources of nutrition and can facilitate nutrition in stable patients with prolonged AKI.

As stated earlier, there are specific "nephro" amino acid solutions available in some countries, which are adapted to the uremic metabolism and have a high concentration in essential anabolic amino acids and a low content of "cheap" glucoplastic amino acids and may exert several metabolic advantages. However, these kidney-specific formulations have not been proven to have an impact on outcomes.[37]

MONITORING OF NUTRITION SUPPORT

Because of the multiple metabolic alterations, disturbances in electrolyte and acid base balance, volume intolerance and the gastrointestinal side effects of kidney dysfunction the metabolic management and nutrition support in patients with AKI requires especially tight clinical and metabolic monitoring.

Because AKI is associated with insulin resistance, patients often develop hyperglycemia, and insulin infusions become necessary. The impairment of lipolysis in patients with AKI increases plasma concentrations of triglycerides—especially if additional factors such as infections, pancreatitis, hyperglycemia, a high-energy intake, or supplemental lipid infusions (e.g., propofol) are present.

Many of the side effects and complications associated with nutrition can be prevented by starting nutrition support at a low rate and by gradually increasing the infusion rate according to the individual metabolic and gastrointestinal tolerance. By this approach, an adaptation of nutritional intake for individual needs and clinical monitoring is facilitated.

References

1. Druml W, Joannidis M, John S, et al. Metabolic management and nutrition in critically ill patients with renal dysfunction: recommendations from the renal section of the DGIIN, OGIAIN, and DIVI. *Med Klin Intensivmed Notfmed.* 2018;113(5):393-400.
2. Ostermann M, Macedo E, Oudemans-van Straaten H. How to feed a patient with acute kidney injury. *Intensive Care Med.* 2019;45(7):1006-1008.
3. Kidney Disease: Improving Global Outcomes (KDIGO) Acute Kidney Injury Work Group. KDIGO clinical practice guideline for acute kidney injury. *Kidney Int Suppl (2011).* 2012;2(1):1-138.
4. Seguro AC, de Araujo M, Seguro FS, Rienzo M, Magaldi AJ, Campos SB. Effects of hypokalemia and hypomagnesemia on zidovudine (AZT) and didanosine (ddI) nephrotoxicity in rats. *Clin Nephrol.* 2003;59(4):267-272.
5. Jaber S, Paugam C, Futier E, et al. Sodium bicarbonate therapy for patients with severe metabolic acidaemia in the intensive care unit (BICAR-ICU): a multicentre, open-label, randomised controlled, phase 3 trial. *Lancet.* 2018;392(10141):31-40.
6. Vanhorebeek I, Gunst J, Ellger B, et al. Hyperglycemic kidney damage in an animal model of prolonged critical illness. *Kidney Int.* 2009;76(5):512-520.
7. Schetz M, Vanhorebeek I, Wouters PJ, Wilmer A, Van den Berghe G. Tight blood glucose control is renoprotective in critically ill patients. *J Am Soc Nephrol.* 2008;19(3):571-578.
8. Taylor BE, McClave SA, Martindale RG, et al. Guidelines for the provision and assessment of nutrition support therapy in the adult critically ill patient: Society of Critical Care Medicine (SCCM) and American Society for Parenteral and Enteral Nutrition (A.S.P.E.N.). *Crit Care Med.* 2016;44(2):390-438.
9. Mouser JF, Hak EB, Kuhl DA, Dickerson RN, Gaber LW, Hak LJ. Recovery from ischemic acute renal failure is improved with enteral compared with parenteral nutrition. *Crit Care Med.* 1997;25(10):1748-1754.
10. Roberts PR, Black KW, Zaloga GP. Enteral feeding improves outcome and protects against glycerol-induced acute renal failure in the rat. *Am J Respir Crit Care Med.* 1997;156(4 Pt 1):1265-1269.
11. Casaer MP, Mesotten D, Hermans G, et al. Early versus late parenteral nutrition in critically ill adults. *N Engl J Med.* 2011;365(6):506-517.
12. Reintam Blaser A, Starkopf J, Alhazzani W, et al. Early enteral nutrition in critically ill patients: ESICM clinical practice guidelines. *Intensive Care Med.* 2017;43(3):380-398.
13. Al-Dorzi HM, Albarrak A, Ferwana M, Murad MH, Arabi YM. Lower versus higher dose of enteral caloric intake in adult critically ill patients: a systematic review and meta-analysis. *Crit Care.* 2016;20(1):358.
14. Moskowitz A, Andersen LW, Cocchi MN, Karlsson M, Patel PV, Donnino MW. Thiamine as a renal protective agent in septic shock. A secondary analysis of a randomized, double-blind, placebo-controlled trial. *Ann Am Thorac Soc.* 2017;14(5):737-741.
15. Sharma A, Mucino MJ, Ronco C. Renal functional reserve and renal recovery after acute kidney injury. *Nephron Clin Pract.* 2014;127(1-4):94-100.
16. Singer P. High-dose amino acid infusion preserves diuresis and improves nitrogen balance in non-oliguric acute renal failure. *Wien Klin Wochenschr.* 2007;119(7-8):218-222.
17. Doig GS, Simpson F, Bellomo R, et al. Intravenous amino acid therapy for kidney function in critically ill patients: a randomized controlled trial. *Intensive Care Med.* 2015;41(7):1197-1208.
18. Zhu R, Allingstrup MJ, Perner A, Doig GS; Nephro-Protective Trial Investigators Group. The effect of IV amino acid supplementation on mortality in ICU patients may be dependent on kidney function: post hoc subgroup analyses of a multicenter randomized trial. *Crit Care Med.* 2018;46(8):1293-1301.
19. Pu H, Doig GS, Heighes PT, et al. Intravenous amino acid therapy for kidney protection in cardiac surgery patients: a pilot randomized controlled trial. *J Thorac Cardiovasc Surg.* 2019;157(6):2356-2366.
20. Joannidis M, Druml W, Forni LG, et al. Prevention of acute kidney injury and protection of renal function in the intensive care unit: update 2017: Expert opinion of the Working Group on Prevention, AKI section, European Society of Intensive Care Medicine. *Intensive Care Med.* 2017;43(6):730-749.
21. Prowle JR, Kirwan CJ, Bellomo R. Fluid management for the prevention and attenuation of acute kidney injury. *Nat Rev Nephrol.* 2014;10(1):37-47.
22. Vaara ST, Korhonen AM, Kaukonen KM, et al. Fluid overload is associated with an increased risk for 90-day mortality in critically ill patients with renal replacement therapy: data from the prospective FINNAKI study. *Crit Care.* 2012;16(5):R197.

23. Schneeweiss B, Graninger W, Stockenhuber F, et al. Energy metabolism in acute and chronic renal failure. *Am J Clin Nutr.* 1990;52(4):596-601.
24. Sabatino A, Theilla M, Hellerman M, et al. Energy and protein in critically ill patients with AKI: a prospective, multicenter observational study using indirect calorimetry and protein catabolic rate. *Nutrients.* 2017;9(8):802.
25. Cano NJ, Aparicio M, Brunori G, et al. ESPEN guidelines on parenteral nutrition: adult renal failure. *Clin Nutr.* 2009;28(4):401-414.
26. Basi S, Pupim LB, Simmons EM, et al. Insulin resistance in critically ill patients with acute renal failure. *Am J Physiol Renal Physiol.* 2005;289(2):F259-F264.
27. Druml W, Fischer M, Sertl S, et al. Fat elimination in acute renal failure: long-chain vs medium-chain triglycerides. *Am J Clin Nutr.* 1992;55(2):468-472.
28. Hellerman M, Sabatino A, Theilla M, Kagan I, Fiaccadori E, Singer P. Carbohydrate and lipid prescription, administration, and oxidation in critically ill patients with acute kidney injury: a post hoc analysis. *J Ren Nutr.* 2019;29(4):289-294.
29. Gaudry S, Quenot JP, Hertig A, et al. Timing of renal replacement therapy for severe acute kidney injury in critically ill patients. *Am J Respir Crit Care Med.* 2019;199(9):1066-1075.
30. Nagib EM, El-Sayed MH, Ahmed MA, Youssef MH. Intestinal motility in acute uremia and effects of erythropoietin. *Saudi Med J.* 2012;33(5):500-507.
31. Silva AP, Freire CC, Gondim FA, et al. Bilateral nephrectomy delays gastric emptying of a liquid meal in awake rats. *Ren Fail.* 2002;24(3):275-284.
32. Wong Vega M, Juarez Calderon M, Tufan Pekkucuksen N, Srivaths P, Akcan Arikan A. Feeding modality is a barrier to adequate protein provision in children receiving continuous renal replacement therapy (CRRT). *Pediatr Nephrol.* 2019;34(6):1147-1150.
33. Singer P, Blaser AR, Berger MM, et al. ESPEN guideline on clinical nutrition in the intensive care unit. *Clin Nutr.* 2019;38(1):48-79.
34. Zager RA, Venkatachalam MA. Potentiation of ischemic renal injury by amino acid infusion. *Kidney Int.* 1983;24(5):620-625.
35. Gunst J, Vanhorebeek I, Casaer MP, et al. Impact of early parenteral nutrition on metabolism and kidney injury. *J Am Soc Nephrol.* 2013;24(6):995-1005.
36. Heyland DK, Elke G, Cook D, et al. Glutamine and antioxidants in the critically ill patient: a post hoc analysis of a large-scale randomized trial. *JPEN J Parenter Enteral Nutr.* 2014;39:401-409.
37. Smolle KH, Kaufmann P, Fleck S, et al. Influence of a novel amino acid solution (enriched with the dipeptide glycyl-tyrosine) on plasma amino acid concentration of patients with acute renal failure. *Clin Nutr.* 1997;16(5):239-246.
38. Schiffl H, Lang SM. Severe acute hypophosphatemia during renal replacement therapy adversely affects outcome of critically ill patients with acute kidney injury. *Int Urol Nephrol.* 2013;45(1):191-197.
39. Demirjian S, Teo BW, Guzman JA, et al. Hypophosphatemia during continuous hemodialysis is associated with prolonged respiratory failure in patients with acute kidney injury. *Nephrol Dial Transplant.* 2011;26(11):3508-3514.
40. Pistolesi V, Zeppilli L, Polistena F, et al. Preventing continuous renal replacement therapy-induced hypophosphatemia: an extended clinical experience with a phosphate-containing solution in the setting of regional citrate anticoagulation. *Blood Purif.* 2017;44(1):8-15.
41. Frankenfield DC, Badellino MM, Reynolds HN, Wiles CE 3rd, Siegel JH, Goodarzi S. Amino acid loss and plasma concentration during continuous hemodiafiltration. *JPEN J Parenter Enteral Nutr.* 1993;17(6):551-561.
42. Oh WC, Mafrici B, Rigby M, et al. Micronutrient and amino acid losses during renal replacement therapy for acute kidney injury. *Kidney Int Rep.* 2019;4(8):1094-1108.
43. Stapel SN, de Boer RJ, Thoral PJ, Vervloet MG, Girbes ARJ, Oudemans-van Straaten HM. Amino acid loss during continuous venovenous hemofiltration in critically ill patients. *Blood Purif.* 2019:1-9.
44. New AM, Nystrom EM, Frazee E, Dillon JJ, Kashani KB, Miles JM. Continuous renal replacement therapy: a potential source of calories in the critically ill. *Am J Clin Nutr.* 2017;105(6):1559-1563.
45. Bassi E, Ferreira CB, Macedo E, Malbouisson LM. Recurrent clotting of dialysis filter associated with hypertriglyceridemia induced by propofol. *Am J Kidney Dis.* 2014;63(5):860-861.
46. Metnitz GH, Fischer M, Bartens C, Steltzer H, Lang T, Druml W. Impact of acute renal failure on antioxidant status in multiple organ failure. *Acta Anaesthesiol Scand.* 2000;44(3):236-240.
47. Morena M, Cristol JP, Bosc JY, et al. Convective and diffusive losses of vitamin C during haemodiafiltration session: a contributive factor to oxidative stress in haemodialysis patients. *Nephrol Dial Transplant.* 2002;17(3):422-427.

48. Berger MM, Shenkin A, Revelly JP, et al. Copper, selenium, zinc, and thiamine balances during continuous venovenous hemodiafiltration in critically ill patients. *Am J Clin Nutr.* 2004;80(2):410-416.
49. Druml W, Schwarzenhofer M, Apsner R, Horl WH. Fat-soluble vitamins in patients with acute renal failure. *Miner Electrolyte Metab.* 1998;24(4):220-226.
50. Reis NG, Francescato HDC, de Almeida LF, Silva C, Costa RS, Coimbra TM. Protective effect of calcitriol on rhabdomyolysis-induced acute kidney injury in rats. *Sci Rep.* 2019;9(1):7090.
51. Looijaard W, Denneman N, Broens B, Girbes ARJ, Weijs PJM, Oudemans-van Straaten HM. Achieving protein targets without energy overfeeding in critically ill patients: a prospective feasibility study. *Clin Nutr.* 2019;38(6):2623-2631.

SECTION IV

Special Labs

16

Biomarkers of Acute Kidney Injury

Ravi Kodali and Dennis G. Moledina

INTRODUCTION

Acute kidney injury (AKI) encompasses various triggers, insults, and types of kidney injuries that result in an acute reduction in glomerular filtration rate (GFR). AKI affects one in five hospitalized patients and half of the patients admitted to intensive care unit (ICU) and is associated with increased morbidity, mortality, and health care cost.[1,2] The current standard of care to detect and monitor AKI is by measuring serum creatinine (SCr) and/or urine output (UO), which has remained unchanged for nearly a century.[3] Defining AKI using changes in SCr has several limitations, including the entities termed "hemodynamic" or "prerenal" AKI, where a rise in SCr is not associated with tubular injury, and "subclinical" AKI, where tubular injury occurs without SCr rise[4] (**Figure 16.1**).

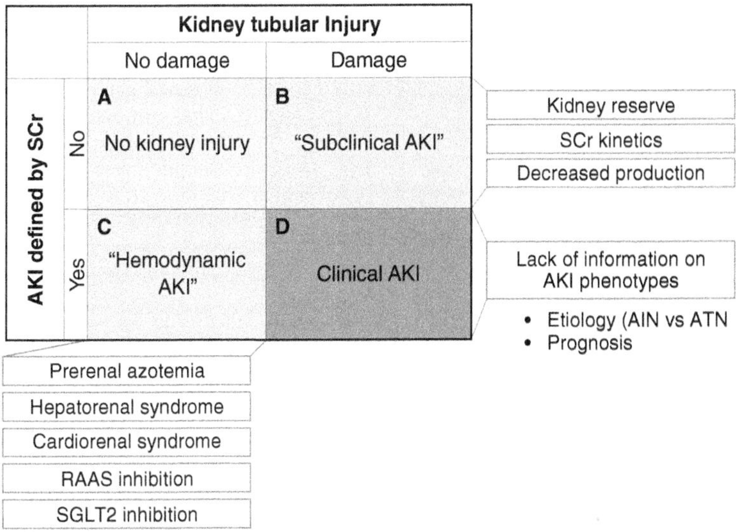

		Kidney tubular Injury	
		No damage	Damage
AKI defined by SCr	No	A No kidney injury	B "Subclinical AKI"
	Yes	C "Hemodynamic AKI"	D Clinical AKI

Kidney reserve
SCr kinetics
Decreased production

Lack of information on AKI phenotypes
- Etiology (AIN vs ATN
- Prognosis

Prerenal azotemia
Hepatorenal syndrome
Cardiorenal syndrome
RAAS inhibition
SGLT2 inhibition

FIGURE 16.1: Limitations of serum creatinine (SCr)–based acute kidney injury (AKI) definition. **A.** No AKI. **B.** Patients with subclinical AKI wherein SCr does not rise despite tubular injury. **C.** "Hemodynamic AKI" wherein rise in SCr is not associated with tubular injury. **D.** Clinical AKI wherein there is true tubular injury and rise in SCr. AIN, acute interstitial nephritis; ATN, acute tubular necrosis; RAAS, renin-angiotensin-aldosterone system; SGLT2, sodium-glucose cotransporter 2.

Adapted from Moledina DG, Parikh CR. Phenotyping of acute kidney injury: beyond serum creatinine. *Semin Nephrol.* 2018;38(1):3-11.

NOVEL BIOMARKERS FOR ACUTE KIDNEY INJURY

Given the limitations of SCr-based AKI definition, kidney disease researchers have focused on discovering and validating novel biomarkers of AKI. These biomarkers can be classified based on their primary role in AKI into markers of reduced glomerular or tubular function, markers of tubular injury, or markers of inflammation.

a) Markers of reduced glomerular filtration: An ideal marker of GFR should be either endogenously produced at a constant rate or injected exogenously, freely filtered by the glomeruli, and neither absorbed nor secreted by the renal tubules. In addition to SCr, serum cystatin C is a marker of GFR that has been extensively evaluated as it is produced by most nucleated cells in the body and is unaffected by muscle mass, freely filtered across glomeruli, and is completely reabsorbed by tubular cells and catabolized.[5] A meta-analysis showed that serum cystatin C showed good discrimination for AKI diagnosis, with an area under the curve (AUC) of 0.89.[6] However, cystatin C is limited in clinical availability, not standardized across laboratories (unlike SCr), and expensive. Where available, the most accurate estimate of GFR is obtained by averaging the GFR estimates obtained using SCr and cystatin C.[7] Several newer methods of "real-time" GFR assessment are currently being tested. Inulin clearance is considered the gold standard for measuring GFR; however, it is only used in research given the need for continuous injection of exogenous substance. Recently, visible fluorescent injectate (VFI) has also shown reliable results in measuring GFR when given as single-dose intravenous injection.[8]

b) Markers of tubular function: Injured tubules lose their normal capacity to reabsorb various electrolytes, including sodium, whereas intact tubules can reabsorb sodium, particularly in states of volume depletion. This forms the basis of fractional excretion of sodium (FENa) to distinguish prerenal azotemia (PRA) AKI from acute tubular necrosis (ATN). However, FENa has only been validated in oliguric AKI patients and may lose accuracy in the setting of diuretic use. A newer test of tubular function and integrity is the furosemide stress test, which evaluates UO 2 hours after administration of high-dose loop diuretic furosemide (1-1.5 mg/kg) in patients with stage 1 or 2 AKI. Low UO (defined in this study as ≤100 mL/hr for 2 hours) was associated with progression to stage 3 AKI and need for kidney replacement therapy and outperformed most other biomarkers of AKI (**Visual Abstract 16.1**).[9]

c) Markers of tubular injury and inflammation: Several proteins are upregulated in response to kidney injury and have been evaluated as biomarkers of tubular injury, including neutrophil gelatinase–associated lipocalin (NGAL), kidney injury molecule 1 (KIM-1), tissue inhibitor of metalloproteinases (TIMP-2), and insulin-like growth factor binding protein 7 (IGFBP-7). Interleukin-18 (IL-18) and YKL-40 are inflammatory markers that are also upregulated in patients with AKI.

APPLICATION OF BIOMARKERS TO SPECIFIC CLINICAL QUESTIONS IN ACUTE KIDNEY INJURY

Can Biomarkers Identify Acute Kidney Injury Earlier Than Serum Creatinine?

SCr tends to rise slowly after kidney injury, and SCr-based AKI is detected on average 2 to 3 days after initial kidney insult. This could lead to administration of potential nephrotoxins before AKI is diagnosed by SCr. Moreover, if a specific therapy for AKI were to be tested in clinical trials, this delay would prevent enrollment of patients immediately after the injury before irreversible damage occurs. As such, many AKI biomarker studies have focused on diagnosing this disease before SCr. Translational Research Investigating Biomarker Endpoints in AKI (TRIBE-AKI) consortium is one of the largest prospective cohort populations used to study various utilities of biomarkers in AKI. In the TRIBE-AKI study, biomarkers such as NGAL, KIM-1, and IL-18 detected AKI within 6 hours of the kidney insult (i.e., cardiac surgery).[10] Nephrocheck (Astute Medical/BioMerieux), the product of urine TIMP-2 and IGFBP-7, is a Food and Drug Administration (FDA)–approved biomarker to detect risk of AKI in patients at the time of admission to the ICU.[11] The positive predictive value of the test for occurrence of AKI at a cutoff of 0.3 is 0.25, which increases to 0.50 at cutoff of 2.0 (**Visual Abstract 16.2**).

Can Biomarkers Distinguish Hemodynamic Acute Kidney Injury From Acute Tubular Necrosis?

The two forms of AKI commonly encountered in clinical practice are PRA and ATN. Molecular pathways activated in these two conditions have minimal overlap, indicating that therapeutic targets may be different in these two common forms of AKI.[12] Studies have found IL-18 and NGAL to be elevated in clinician-adjudicated and histologic ATN as compared to PRA.[12-14]

Can Biomarkers Differentiate Various Causes of Acute Kidney Injury in Cirrhosis?

Differentiating between various causes of AKI in cirrhosis is a common clinical challenge. In a study by Belcher et al,[15] urinary biomarkers including NGAL, KIM-1, IL-18, and L-FABP were able to distinguish ATN from PRA and hepatorenal syndrome (HRS) in patients with cirrhosis (**Visual Abstract 16.3**). The levels of all these biomarkers were significantly higher in ATN patients as compared with those without ATN. In addition, very low FENa (≤0.1%) also distinguished HRS from PRA and ATN, whereas a high urine albumin distinguished ATN from PRA/HRS (**Table 16.1**).

Can Biomarkers Detect "Subclinical" Acute Kidney Injury?

"Subclinical" AKI refers to the phenomenon in which structural kidney injury occurs in the absence of detectable SCr rise/UO decrease. Patients with elevated urine NGAL levels but with normal SCr were found to have higher rates of kidney replacement therapy and mortality.[16-19] In a study of 581 deceased donor kidneys who were biopsied at the time of organ procurement,[14] about half of the donors with biopsy-proven acute tubular injury (ATI) did not have SCr-based AKI, whereas urinary NGAL levels were higher with increasing severity of histologic ATI.

TABLE 16.1 Distinguishing Between PRA, HRS, and ATN Using Traditional and Novel Biomarkers

	Urine NGAL	Urine IL-18	FENa	Urine Albumin
PRA	↓↓	↓↓	↓	↓↓
HRS	–	–	↓↓	↓↓
ATN	↑↑	↑↑	↓↓	↑↑

ATN, acute tubular necrosis; FENa, fractional excretion of sodium; HRS, hepatorenal syndrome; IL, interleukin; NGAL, neutrophil gelatinase–associated lipocalin; PRA, prerenal azotemia.

Can Biomarkers Provide Prognostic Information?

Biomarkers also provide information regarding short- and long-term prognosis in terms of kidney replacement therapy, mortality, and duration of AKI.

a) Short-term prognosis: In TRIBE-AKI study, plasma NGAL had an AUC of 0.80 for AKI progression and highest tertile of plasma NGAL had an odds ratio of 7.7 (95% confidence interval [CI] 2.6-22.5) for AKI progression.[20] Perazella et al[21] noted that patients with granular casts and renal tubular epithelial cells on urine sediment microscopy had a 7.3-fold higher risk of AKI progression. The test "Nephrocheck" discussed above predicted development of stage 2 or 3 AKI in the next 12 hours, when the test is performed at admission to ICU.
b) Long-term prognosis: Biomarkers can also augment clinician judgment in determining chronic kidney disease (CKD) development and long-term mortality. Higher levels of plasma NGAL, urine NGAL, IL-18, and KIM-1 at the time of AKI were associated with higher 3-year mortality.[18,22]

Can Biomarkers Distinguish Acute Interstitial Nephritis From Acute Tubular Necrosis?

Distinguishing acute interstitial nephritis (AIN) from other causes of AKI is challenging; however, it is important to clinicians as management strategies are quite different. Moledina et al[23] analyzed cytokines in the T helper cell pathway in patients with AKI who underwent a kidney biopsy, of whom 15% had AIN upon adjudication by pathologists. Higher urine IL-9 and tumor necrosis factor α (TNF-α) levels were independently associated with AIN and improved diagnosis of AIN over currently available clinical tests as well as clinician's prebiopsy diagnosis with an AUC of 0.84. In a subsequent analysis comparing AIN to ATN, urine IL-9 value less than 0.41 reduced post-test probability of AIN to 0.07 if pretest probability was 0.25 ruling out AIN, whereas a value above 2.53 would increase post-test probability to 0.84 and avoid the need for a kidney biopsy.[24]

PHENOTYPING ACUTE KIDNEY INJURY IN THE SETTING OF THERAPEUTIC INTERVENTIONS

Biomarkers also helped demonstrate that AKI that occurs in the setting of therapeutic interventions, such as diuresis in acute decompensated heart failure (ADHF) and intensive blood pressure control, may not be associated with structural kidney damage. First, biomarkers NGAL and KIM-1 were not elevated in patients who developed AKI in response to diuresis in ADHF as compared to those who did not develop AKI, indicating that AKI in response to diuresis lacked tubular injury and may not be of concern.[25] Second, biomarkers were used to demonstrate that the higher incidence of AKI and CKD that occurred in patients randomized to intensive blood pressure control arm in the SPRINT trial was because of hemodynamic increases in SCr rather than tubular injury. For example, YKL-40 and KIM-1 levels were lower in those who developed CKD in intensive blood pressure control group than in those in the standard group. This likely explains the apparent discrepancy in the SPRINT trial where patients randomized to intensive blood pressure control arm had lower cardiovascular events and mortality despite higher CKD and AKI.[26]

FUTURE DIRECTIONS

Future studies should attempt to better phenotype AKI into its subtypes using biomarkers. Studies should test the accuracy of biomarkers against histology or patient-focused outcomes rather than the flawed "gold standard" of SCr.[27] Finally, studies need to demonstrate improved patient outcomes with biomarker use. This approach may bring us closer to finding AKI biomarkers with meaningful application to clinical care.

Acknowledgment

This study is supported by the National Institutes of Health (NIH) award K23DK117065 (DGM).

References

1. Hoste EA, Bagshaw SM, Bellomo R, et al. Epidemiology of acute kidney injury in critically ill patients: the multinational AKI-EPI study. *Intensive Care Med.* 2015;41(8):1411-1423.
2. Nisula S, Kaukonen K-M, Vaara ST, et al. Incidence, risk factors and 90-day mortality of patients with acute kidney injury in Finnish intensive care units: the FINNAKI study. *Intensive Care Med.* 2013;39(3):420-428.
3. Winkler AW, Parra J. The measurement of glomerular filtration: the creatinine, sucrose and urea clearances in subjects with renal disease. *J Clin Invest.* 1937;16(6):869-877.
4. Moledina DG, Parikh CR. Phenotyping of acute kidney injury: beyond serum creatinine. *Semin Nephrol.* 2018;38(1):3-11.
5. Koyner JL, Bennet MR, Worcester EM, et al. Urinary cystatin C as an early biomarker of acute kidney injury following adult cardiothoracic surgery. *Kidney Int.* 2008;74(8):1059-1069.
6. Yong Z, Pei X, Zhu B, et al. Predictive value of serum cystatin C for acute kidney injury in adults: a meta-analysis of prospective cohort trials. *Sci Rep.* 2017;7:41012.
7. Fan L, Levey AS, Gudnason V, et al. Comparing GFR estimating equations using cystatin c and creatinine in elderly individuals. *J Am Soc Nephrol.* 2015;26(8):1982-1989.
8. Rizk DV, Meier D, Sandoval RM, et al. A novel method for rapid bedside measurement of GFR. *J Am Soc Nephrol.* 2018;29(6):1609-1613.
9. Koyner JL, Davison DL, Brasha-Mitchell E, et al. Furosemide stress test and biomarkers for the prediction of AKI severity. *J Am Soc Nephrol.* 2015;26(8):2023-2031.
10. Parikh CR, Coca SG, Thiessen-Philbrook H, et al. Postoperative biomarkers predict acute kidney injury and poor outcomes after adult cardiac surgery. *J Am Soc Nephrol.* 2011;22(9): 1748-1757.
11. Kashani K, Al-Khafaji A, Ardiles T, et al. Discovery and validation of cell cycle arrest biomarkers in human acute kidney injury. *Crit Care.* 2013;17(1):R25.
12. Xu K, Rosenstiel P, Paragas N, et al. Unique transcriptional programs identify subtypes of AKI. *J Am Soc Nephrol.* 2017;28(6):1729-1740.
13. Parikh CR, Jani A, Melnikov VY, et al. Urinary interleukin-18 is a marker of human acute tubular necrosis. *Am J Kidney Dis.* 2004;43(3):405-414.
14. Moledina DG, Hall IE, Thiessen-Philbrook H, et al. Performance of serum creatinine and kidney injury biomarkers for diagnosing histologic acute tubular injury. *Am J Kidney Dis.* 2017;70(6):807-816.
15. Belcher JM, Sanyal AJ, Peixoto AJ, et al. Kidney biomarkers and differential diagnosis of patients with cirrhosis and acute kidney injury. *Hepatology.* 2014;60(2):622-632.
16. Haase M, Kellum JA, Ronco C. Subclinical AKI—an emerging syndrome with important consequences. *Nat Rev Nephrol.* 2012;8(12):735-739.
17. Nickolas TL, Schmidt-Ott KM, Canetta P, et al. Diagnostic and prognostic stratification in the emergency department using urinary biomarkers of nephron damage: a multicenter prospective cohort study. *J Am Coll Cardiol.* 2012;59(3):246-255.
18. Coca SG, Garg AX, Thiessen-Philbrook H, et al. Urinary biomarkers of AKI and mortality 3 years after cardiac surgery. *J Am Soc Nephrol.* 2014;25(5):1063-1071.
19. Haase M, Devarajan P, Haase-Fielitz A, et al. The outcome of neutrophil gelatinase-associated lipocalin-positive subclinical acute kidney injury: a multicenter pooled analysis of prospective studies. *J Am Coll Cardiol.* 2011;57(17):1752-1761.

20. Koyner JL, Garg AX, Coca SG, et al. Biomarkers predict progression of acute kidney injury after cardiac surgery. *J Am Soc Nephrol.* 2012;23(5):905-914.
21. Perazella MA, Coca SG, Hall IE, et al. Urine microscopy is associated with severity and worsening of acute kidney injury in hospitalized patients. *Clin J Am Soc Nephrol.* 2010;5(3): 402-408.
22. Moledina DG, Parikh CR, Garg AX, et al. Association of perioperative plasma neutrophil gelatinase-associated lipocalin levels with 3-year mortality after cardiac surgery: a prospective observational cohort study. *PLoS One.* 2015;10(6):e0129619.
23. Moledina DG, Wilson FP, Pober JS, et al. Urine TNF-alpha and IL-9 for clinical diagnosis of acute interstitial nephritis. *JCI Insight.* 2019;4(10):e127456.
24. Moledina DG, Parikh CR. Differentiating acute interstitial nephritis from acute tubular injury: a challenge for clinicians. *Nephron.* 2019:1-6.
25. Ahmad T, Jackson K, Rao VS, et al. Worsening renal function in patients with acute heart failure undergoing aggressive diuresis is not associated with tubular injury. *Circulation.* 2018;137(19):2016-2028.
26. SPRINT Research Group, Wright JT Jr, Williamson JD, et al. A randomized trial of intensive versus standard blood-pressure control. *N Engl J Med.* 2015;373(22):2103-2116.
27. Waikar SS, Betensky RA, Emerson SC, et al. Imperfect gold standards for kidney injury biomarker evaluation. *J Am Soc Nephrol.* 2012;23(1):13-21.

Can the Furosemide Stress Test help predict which patients will progress to more severe stages of AKI ?

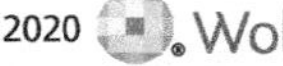

Cohort 1
Retrospective cohort who received a FST in the setting of AKI in critically ill patients as part of Southern AKI Network

Cohort 2
Prospective multicenter group of critically ill patients who received their FST in the setting of early AKI.

Furosemide Stress Test (FST)
1.0 or 1.5 mg/kg

n = 77

AUC ± SEM*	AUCs for prediction of progression to AKI stage 3	AUCs for prediction of receipt of inpatient KRT	AUCs for prediction of AKI stage 3 and death
FST Urine Output	0.87 ± 0.09 $p < 0.001$	0.86 ± 0.08 $p = 0.0001$	0.81 ± 0.06 $p < 0.0001$
FST Urine Output + ↑ TIMP-2x IGFBP-7	0.90 ± 0.06 $p < 0.001$	0.91 ± 0.08 $p = 0.009$	0.81 ± 0.10 $p = 0.003$
FST Urine Output + ↑ NGAL	0.86 ± 0.06 $p < 0.001$	0.91 ± 0.06 $p < 0.001$	0.89 ± 0.06 $p < 0.001$

Conclusion: Overall, in the setting of early AKI, FST urine output outperformed biochemical biomarkers for prediction of progressive AKI, need for KRT, and inpatient mortality. Using a FST in patients with increased biomarker levels improves risk stratification, although further research is needed.

Koyner JL, Davison DL, Brasha-Mitchell E, et al. ***Furosemide Stress Test and Biomarkers for the Prediction of AKI Severity.*** J Am Soc Nephrol. 2015 Aug;26(8):2023-31.

VISUAL ABSTRACT 16.1

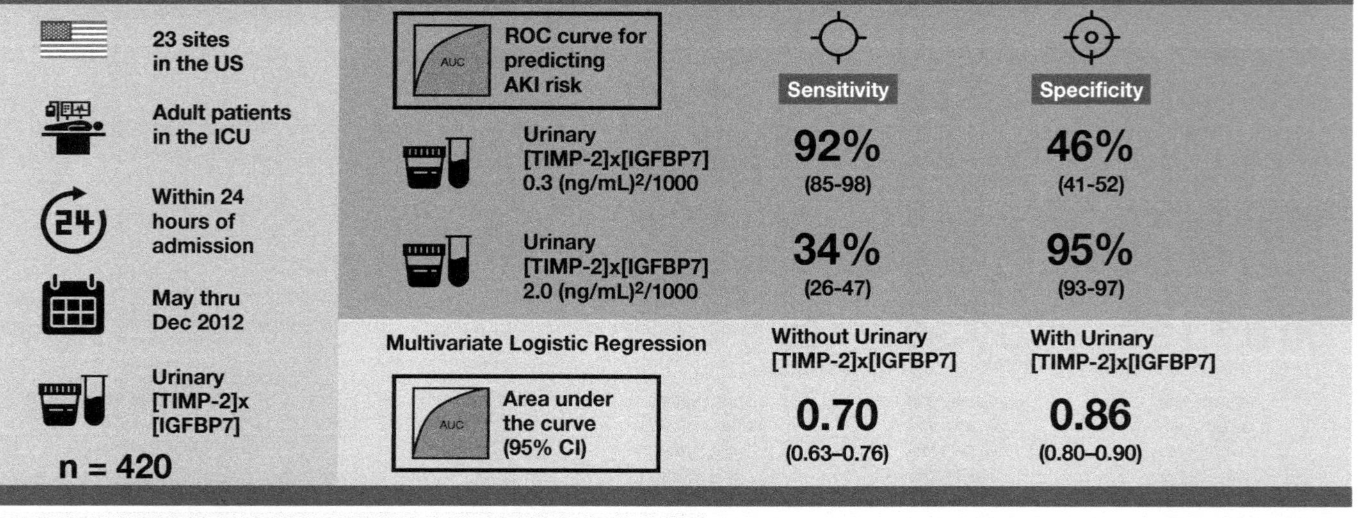

VISUAL ABSTRACT 16.2

Do Kidney Biomarkers aid in the Differential Diagnosis of Patients With Cirrhosis and Acute Kidney Injury ?

PROSPECTIVE

- Multicenter
- Cirrhosis and AKI
- Multiple biomarkers of clinically adjudicated AKI

n = 188

BIOMARKER	TUBULAR INJURY				TUBULAR FUNCTION	GLOMERULAR FUNCTION
	NGAL *ng/mL*	IL-1 *pg/mL*	KIM-1 *ng/mL*	L-FABP *ng/mL*	FE Na %	Albumin *(mgs/dL)*
Prerenal n = 55	54 *(17–180)*	15 *(15–49)*	4.4 *(1.8–11.7)*	9 *(4–18)*	0.27 *(0.13–0.58)*	21 *(4–70)*
Hepatorenal n = 16	115 *(51–373)*	37 *(15–90)*	7.6 *(4.5–10.1)*	14 *(6–20)*	0.10 *(0.02–0.23)*	24 *(13–129)*
ATN n = 39	565 *(76–1000)*	124 *(15–325)*	8.4 *(4.1–18.3)*	27 *(8–103)*	0.31 *(0.12–0.65)*	92 *(44–253)*
	$p < 0.001$	$p < 0.001$	$p = 0.03$	$p = 0.002$	$p = 0.01$	$p < 0.001$

Conclusion: Urinary biomarkers of kidney injury are elevated in patients with cirrhosis and AKI due to ATN. Incorporating biomarkers into clinical decision making has the potential to more accurately guide treatment by establishing which patients have structural injury underlying their AKI.

Belcher JM, Sanyal AJ, Peixoto AJ. ***Kidney Biomarkers and Differential Diagnosis of Patients With Cirrhosis and Acute Kidney Injury.*** Hepatology 2014 Aug;60(2):622-32.

VISUAL ABSTRACT 16.3

17 Biomarkers of Critical Illness

Rajit K. Basu

INTRODUCTION

Optimal management of critically ill patients is dependent on accurate and timely diagnostics. Despite tremendous research efforts dedicated to the identification and validation of newer diagnostic tests, integration into real practice has been slow.[1] A number of biomarkers capable of providing a diagnostic and prognostic advance for earlier recognition of critical illness have been studied. The varied ability of these novel biomarkers to demonstrate high levels of reproducibility across the heterogeneity of illness for some of the major syndromes affecting intensive care unit (ICU) patients (e.g., sepsis, acute respiratory distress syndrome [ARDS], acute kidney injury [AKI]) has precluded widespread acceptance and incorporation into care pathways.[2-7] In addition, problematically, although most of the novel biomarkers demonstrate robust sensitivity for injury, few consistently are highly specific. Finally, although a majority of the reported literature has focused on the change in *outcome* of care for patients via inclusion of biomarkers (for prediction, diagnostics, or management), less effort has been expended to report on how biomarkers can result in improvements in the *process* of care. In this chapter, the existing inertia opposing incorporation of biomarkers into practice is explained. The potential value of biomarker integration into the process of managing critically ill patients (ICU) is also highlighted. Finally, this chapter illustrates the next step of precision medicine, facilitated by biomarker-directed prognostic and predictive population enrichment.

THE HETEROGENEITY CONUNDRUM

Critically ill patients demonstrate marked heterogeneity. Patients admitted to the medical ICU are by nature complex and diverse. Unlike the general hospital wards where patients are often admitted for single-organ injury, or in focused surgical ICUs–medical ICU, patients vary considerably by age, demographics, background conditions, comorbid conditions, and ongoing concurrent diagnosis. Many critical illnesses are actually syndromes—residing under umbrella catch-all diagnoses, such as sepsis, ARDS, traumatic brain injury (TBI), AKI, or delirium. For a myriad of reasons, each critically ill patient is unique. Patient age and size can significantly influence the host response to complex illness. For instance, data indicate patients at the extremes of age (i.e., very young or very old) and the extremes of size (i.e., low body mass index or high body mass index) differ considerably from each other and also from the middle in terms of critical illness demographics (mainly outcome) and also response to illness.[4,8,9] Background conditions can modulate critical illness. In adult and geriatric populations, chronic immunosuppression and cardiopulmonary, kidney, or hepatic dysfunction are not uncommon and can potentiate acute sickness. Although the abovementioned conditions are less common, children have unique comorbidities related to oncologic and immunodysregulatory conditions, birth and developmental issues, and, most importantly, less physiologic reserve to counter acute decompensation. Problematically, a majority of diagnostic markers currently used in management (e.g., pH, lactate, C-reactive protein [CRP], partial pressure of oxygen [Pao2], erythrocyte sedimentation rate [ESR], white blood cell count, platelet count) do not adjudicate for comorbid conditions (**Table 17.1**). For instance, the importance in a change in CRP in an adult patient with sepsis may be different if the patient is otherwise healthy or has rheumatoid arthritis as a baseline condition. As mentioned previously, physiologic reserve and the ability to compensate for loss of homeostasis vary across age, yet existing diagnostics are relatively crude in sophistication with regard to patient age. Finally, the relationship between time and illness progression and/or severity changes dramatically in the first few days of ICU course, regardless of patient demographic. For most ICU patients, the predictability of how illness will change is unclear—particularly in those patients with complex medical background.[10,11] Unfortunately, diagnostics as they are currently used offer very little data specificity in relation to patient, background, and time as they are markers oriented toward overall patient homeostasis (best example is pH). Thus, in addition to the heterogeneity of comorbidity and patient age, time adds a very real "third dimension" to critical illness, complicating the adjudication of injury in the current diagnostic landscape. The next generation

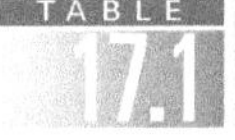
TABLE 17.1 Current and Novel Biomarkers for Intensive Care Unit Syndromes

Time Frame	Sepsis	ARDS	TBI
Current	pH Lactate CRP ESR PCT	P/F ratio CXR Chest CT Spo_2 Pao_2	
Novel	PCT IL-18 HMGB1 sTREM IL-6, IL-8 Caspase-3	ICAM VEGF IGFBP3 S100 SP-A SP-B Ang-2 e-Selectin p-Selectin HMGB1 Ang-1, Ang-2	S100β GFAP GBDP

AKI, acute kidney injury; ARDS, acute respiratory distress syndrome; CRP, C-reactive protein; CT, computed tomography; CXR, chest x-ray; ESR, erythrocyte sedimentation rate; GFAP-GBDP, glial fibrillary acidic protein-breakdown products; HMGB1, high mobility group box 1; ICAM, intercellular adhesion molecule; IGFBP3, insulin-like growth factor binding protein 3; IL, interleukin; PCT, patient care technician; P/F, Pao_2/Fio_2; SP-A, surfactant protein A; SP-B, surfactant protein B; sTREM, soluble triggering receptor on myeloid cells; TBI, traumatic brain injury; VEGF, vascular endothelial growth factor.

of diagnostic tests, novel biomarkers, is generally initially identified, derived, and validated in isolation of the patient—using in vitro or ex vivo modeling—and then tested in specific patient populations at very fixed time intervals. The complexities of patient age, myriad comorbid conditions, and time of illness are not initially examined in the clinical adjudication of these biomarkers. For the major ICU disease processes, a number of biomarkers have been identified and studied at least in limited populations (Table 17.1).

Critical illness itself is heterogeneous. Appreciation of the diversity and spectrum of illnesses has led to injury complexes now being classified as "syndromes." For instance, sepsis, AKI, and ARDS are not manifest similarly in patients, even when present in patients with relatively same demographic and comorbid background. The pathophysiologic drivers of each syndrome can be quite diverse—molecular underpinnings are wide ranging, clinical manifestations of these perturbations varied, and relationship of injury process to the patient inconsistent.[12] For instance, although sepsis recognition has advanced considerably, the criteria have traditionally been fixed and do not account for patient-level variability. The manifestation of sepsis between patients can be wide ranging—evidenced by the constellation of symptoms that vary by time of ascertainment, evolution of injury, and interventions performed. In addition, the syndromes do not consistently affect one organ system versus multiple other systems. Many ICU syndromes—ARDS and AKI, for example, in which injury processes are theoretically confined to a "single-organ system"—are often present in the context of other critical illnesses and, on a molecular level, demonstrate endocrine effects on distal organ systems. Unfortunately, current diagnostic tests do not adjudicate systematic illness from single-organ injury.

Critical illness varies by time. As opposed to complex surgery or trauma, when the onset of an insult is known, many critically ill patients have poorly defined "onset" times and, as a result, present to medical attention and, ultimately, the ICU at various points in their course. Both biologic models of critical illness and the clinical course of patients demonstrate evolution of disease over time.[12,13] The progression of disease can lead to significant variability in the values obtained in the marker(s) used for diagnosis. For instance, in matching patients with urosepsis and shock, the value of a serum lactate level can be dramatically different based on the time of presentation, the onset of the infection, and the time of the measurement.

Taken together, critical illness is highly complex—heterogeneous by patient background, disease, time, and evolution. By comparison, the existing paradigm for diagnostic testing is overly simplistic. Testing is focused primarily on diagnosis by comparing a singular point in time using fixed cutoff values, without the context of other organ dysfunction, for the prediction of a singular end point (most commonly, mortality). The biomarkers that are actually used currently are sensitive for critical illness, but not specific for the injury syndrome. For instance, lactate, utilized to connote the balance between anaerobic and aerobic metabolism, is a biomarker for sepsis, ARDS, cardiac dysfunction, and TBI—almost all ICU syndromes. Similarly, the other markers for sepsis and ARDS generally provide a reference for host homeostasis and are not necessarily reflective of the injuries themselves (i.e., how the syndrome is evolving or being controlled). The lack of reliable, consistently successful therapeutics in nearly all ICU syndromes is likely in part driven by these unsophisticated and imprecise diagnostics. It is possible that the use of biomarkers with greater specificity for the unique illness itself may help manage the heterogeneity synonymous with ICU disease (**Figure 17.1**).

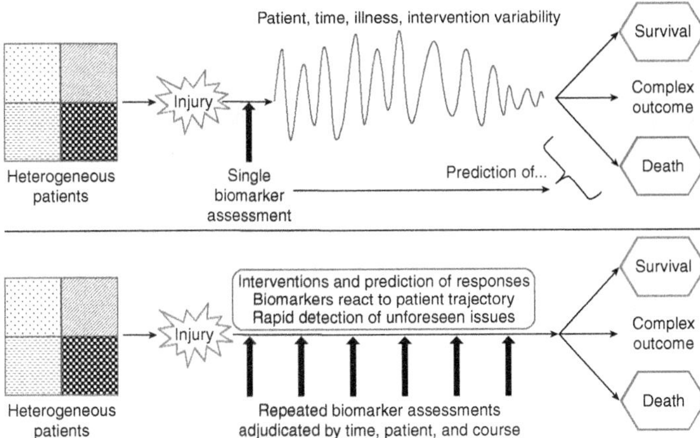

FIGURE 17.1: Comparison of biomarker strategies. Top: Demonstration of how current biomarkers are utilized—single value, single time point, single cutoff, for a remote singular end point. Bottom: Depiction of how incorporation of biomarkers can serve to guide management more directly—multiple markers, multiple time points, for more proximal end points.

INTENSIVE CARE UNIT SYNDROMES AND NOVEL BIOMARKERS

The desire to improve the care of critically ill patients based on earlier detection, improve the specificity of diagnosis, and target efficacious therapies has driven the push to identify new biomarkers (Table 17.1). Although current diagnostic tests are used to drive supportive management, the benefit of novel biomarkers is theoretically to identify injury in its early stages, allowing providers to expedite mitigative therapies.

For the major ICU syndromes, advances in diagnostics could change how patients are managed. Sepsis is an apt example for how diagnostic change could improve patient care and outcome. Early recognition in sepsis is now the cornerstone of care. Early recognition relies on a combination of provider education, awareness of sepsis risk, and clinical markers of illness (qSOFA or quick Sequential Organ Function Assessment)—a combination of which leads a provider to initiate antimicrobial therapy and supportive care measures.[14] Existing markers such as lactate, in the right patient context, can help adjudicate the decision to initiate antibiotics. Unfortunately, markers such as lactate do not generally offer significant insight into the disease process itself. For instance, in a patient with septic shock, the level of elevation of a lactate has never been proven to be associated with the severity or mechanism of the sepsis. Newer biomarkers in the field of sepsis, such as soluble triggering receptor on myeloid cells-1 (sTREM-1) derived from both molecular (genetic microarray and proteomic study) and animal models, have demonstrated high degrees of specificity for sepsis disease progression; the degree of elevation in sTREM-1 has been found to be correlated with the severity of the sepsis.[15] Microarray and genomics have identified groups of markers that can also separate populations of patients by sepsis severity. In these studies, the balance of inflammatory and anti-inflammatory markers can be adjudicated, the expression of steroid receptors elucidated, and the progression of cellular apoptosis (vs necrosis) detailed.[8,16,17] All of these have obvious downstream ramifications to guide therapy. Compared to sepsis, unfortunately, other ICU syndromes have far fewer existing clinical markers and novel biomarkers. ARDS diagnosis and prognosis has relied extensively on clinical indices of patient stability, specific to respiratory disease. Identification of TBI markers has lagged behind, but markers are now emerging, describing direct injury to glial cells (S100β and glial fibrillary acidic protein [GFAP]).[18] Novel biomarkers for AKI, discussed elsewhere in this text, may elucidate the location, mechanism, and progression of injury within the kidney.

The inertia preventing incorporation of novel biomarkers into practice results from a combination of factors. Across the ICU literature, a plethora of literature discusses risk versus benefit or pro versus con assessment of biomarkers into practice, if these markers are ready for use and integration into practice. Despite the available evidence, few, if any, have made it in "prime time."[1] How these tests are studied is problematic. The current practice is to assess efficacy by testing a biomarker at a single time point against a single cutoff value. This standard does not match how ICU patients change over time. A dynamic approach, similar to how blood gas measurements track respiratory variation, would match the dynamic nature of patients more appropriately (**Figure 17.2**). The second is the reliance on evaluating performance of a biomarker via analyzing the prediction of outcomes heavily confounded by factors both related and unrelated to the patient (e.g., 28-day mortality, length of stay). Biomarkers are rarely studied using methods akin to quality improvement methodology, determining the effect on process metrics rather than on outcome metrics. Critical care management is a real-time process, adjudicated multiple times daily, making identification of consistently functional and beneficial short-term interventions or tests possible. Instead of attempting to pair a point-of-care biomarker at the time of admission to the outcome of death at 28 days, matching the biomarker to the evolution of the disease or effect of therapies may be more practical. Third, randomized clinical trial (RCT) remains the gold-standard level of evidence to drive practice change. Unfortunately, very few RCTs in critical care have ever demonstrated compelling, practice-changing evidence in the management of most ICU syndromes. In addition, most RCTs have historically failed to account for disease heterogeneity and, therefore, have been designed in an imprecise manner. The goal of demonstrating

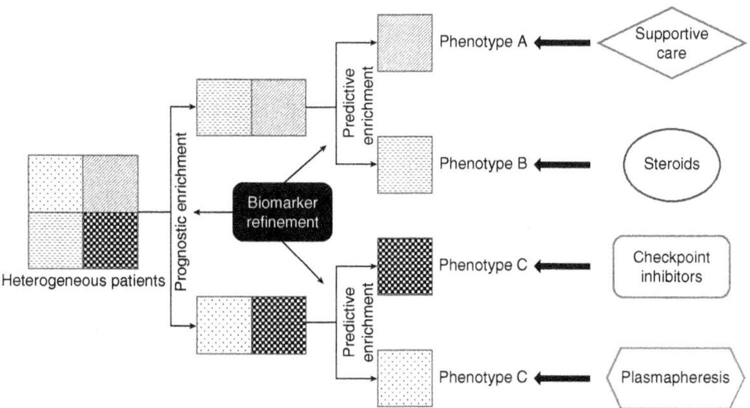

FIGURE 17.2: Practical implementation of current and novel biomarkers. Use of novel diagnostics may refine a population through prognostic and predictive enrichment. Targeted therapies can be focused on defined, refined populations and biomarkers functional for assessing patient homeostasis and injury progression used to help guide the process of management. The example depicted is for septic shock.

outcome improvement in a complex patient via incorporation of a single diagnostic test for a heavily confounded final metric (mortality) is likely unrealistic. Finally, the financial aspect of incorporating a new diagnostic into management cannot be understated. Value-based care, to optimize quality and minimize curtailable costs, has become the focus, particularly in the United States. Absent data demonstrating a financial benefit to patient care, an additional cost incursion of a new diagnostic test is a fiscal liability for many institutions.

INTEGRATION THROUGH ENRICHMENT

The integration of biomarkers in critical care management will require a contemporary and pragmatic application. The purpose of novel biomarkers should be specific to the nature of the test itself and the context of the patient. If prognosis, diagnosis, and theragnosis are distinct characteristics of a given biomarker test, it is unlikely that a single test could be used for all three purposes, especially if that given test is measured once and compared to a specific cutoff value. Although troponin-I is often used as a gold-standard reference for biomarker research, troponin isoenzyme measurement is not used for all aspects of tracking care of the patient with acute coronary syndrome. In addition, troponin testing in the patient without risk factors for heart disease or other clinical symptoms of disease demonstrates a high false-positive rate and poor utilization practice. Patient context drives biomarker testing. In sepsis recognition, the utilization of patient care technician for the purpose of diagnosis can be improved when tested in the patient with higher pretest probability for sepsis complications.[3,19] The parallel has been demonstrated for AKI biomarkers and the renal angina prodrome of AKI risk.[20] In TBI, for example, S100β and GFAP levels are indicative of unique aspects of glial injury.[18] Prognostic and predictive enrichment using novel biomarkers is possible in sepsis, AKI, and ARDS.[2,8,21] If biomarkers are used in this way, populations could be refined from a diverse, heterogeneous mix of patients via multiple sequential categorical classifications to a more precise illness severity, targeting for potential therapies and, in general, populations of interest (in whom therapeutic intervention would be of the most "significant" consequence) (Figure 17.2).

The novel biomarkers for ICU syndromes can be used to guide management. For instance, in the management of sepsis and multiorgan failure, the markers of platelet count and ADAMTS-13 (a disintegrin and metalloproteinase with a thrombospondin type 1 motif, member 13) can be used to drive the use of plasmapheresis—a practice that has resulted in improvement in recovery from sepsis and reduction in duration and severity of organ failure.[22] Management of fluid balance in the context of AKI is possible using a sequential assessment of novel AKI biomarkers.[23] The focus of critical care diagnostic markers could, therefore, be on process. The commonsense plausibility of a clinical index or biomarker measured at the time of ICU admission or early in ICU course carrying a one-to-one association with ICU outcome is low, regardless of statistical association. A combination of the existing diagnostics that render an adjudication of host stability and changes in homeostasis with the incorporation of novel biomarkers specific for injury may be practical, pragmatic, and lead to advances in management (Figure 17.2).

CONCLUSION

In this brief narrative, the heterogeneity of critical illness has been described amid the context of recent advances in biomarker development. The field of intensive care medicine will require coordinated and forward-thinking movement to improve patient care—inclusion of novel diagnostics is central to this work. Only through a reframed vision for how these diagnostics can be studied will the integration into practice be made possible.

References

1. Honore PM, Jacobs R, Hendrickx I, et al. Biomarkers in critical illness: have we made progress? *Int J Nephrol Renovasc Dis.* 2016;9:253-256.
2. Sarma A, Calfee CS, Ware LB. Biomarkers and precision medicine: state of the art. *Crit Care Clin.* 2020;36(1):155-165.
3. Lam SW, Bauer SR, Fowler R, et al. Systematic review and meta-analysis of procalcitonin-guidance versus usual care for antimicrobial management in critically ill patients: focus on subgroups based on antibiotic initiation, cessation, or mixed strategies. *Crit Care Med.* 2018;46(5):684-690.
4. Sims CR, Nguyen TC, Mayeux PR. Could biomarkers direct therapy for the septic patient? *J Pharmacol Exp Ther.* 2016;357(2):228-239.
5. Sinha P, Calfee CS. Phenotypes in acute respiratory distress syndrome: moving towards precision medicine. *Curr Opin Crit Care.* 2019;25(1):12-20.
6. Metwaly S, Cote A, Donnelly SJ, et al. Evolution of ARDS biomarkers: will metabolomics be the answer? *Am J Physiol Lung Cell Mol Physiol.* 2018;315(4):L526-L534.
7. Honore PM, Joannes-Boyau O, Boer W, et al. Acute kidney injury in the ICU: time has come for an early biomarker kit! *Acta Clin Belg.* 2007;62(suppl 2):318-321.
8. Wong HR, Caldwell JT, Cvijanovich NZ, et al. Prospective clinical testing and experimental validation of the Pediatric Sepsis Biomarker Risk Model. *Sci Transl Med.* 2019;11(518). doi:10.1126/scitranslmed.aax9000
9. Meyer NJ, Calfee CS. Novel translational approaches to the search for precision therapies for acute respiratory distress syndrome. *Lancet Respir Med.* 2017;5(6):512-523.
10. Yende S, Kellum JA, Talisa VB, et al. Long-term host immune response trajectories among hospitalized patients with sepsis. *JAMA Netw Open.* 2019;2(8):e198686.
11. Sakr Y, Reinhart K, Bloos F, et al. Time course and relationship between plasma selenium concentrations, systemic inflammatory response, sepsis, and multiorgan failure. *Br J Anaesth.* 2007;98(6):775-784.
12. Leligdowicz A, Matthay MA. Heterogeneity in sepsis: new biological evidence with clinical applications. *Crit Care.* 2019;23(1):80.
13. Donahoe M. Acute respiratory distress syndrome: a clinical review. *Pulm Circ.* 2011;1(2):192-211.
14. Seymour CW, Liu VX, Iwashyna TJ, et al. Assessment of clinical criteria for sepsis: for the Third International Consensus Definitions for Sepsis and Septic Shock (Sepsis-3). *JAMA.* 2016;315(8):762-774.
15. Su L, Liu D, Chai W, et al. Role of sTREM-1 in predicting mortality of infection: a systematic review and meta-analysis. *BMJ Open.* 2016;6(5):e010314.
16. Vassiliou AG, Floros G, Jahaj E, et al. Decreased glucocorticoid receptor expression during critical illness. *Eur J Clin Invest.* 2019;49(4):e13073.
17. Alder MN, Opoka AM, Wong HR. The glucocorticoid receptor and cortisol levels in pediatric septic shock. *Crit Care.* 2018;22(1):244.
18. Mondello S, Sorinola A, Czeiter E, et al. Blood-based protein biomarkers for the management of traumatic brain injuries in adults presenting to emergency departments with mild brain injury: a living systematic review and meta-analysis. *J Neurotrauma.* 2018. doi:10.1089/neu.2017.5182
19. Liu D, Su L, Han G, et al. Prognostic value of procalcitonin in adult patients with sepsis: a systematic review and meta-analysis. *PLoS One.* 2015;10(6):e0129450.
20. Basu RK, Wang Y, Wong HR, et al. Incorporation of biomarkers with the renal angina index for prediction of severe AKI in critically ill children. *Clin J Am Soc Nephrol.* 2014;9(4):654-662.
21. Shankar-Hari M, Rubenfeld GD. Population enrichment for critical care trials: phenotypes and differential outcomes. *Curr Opin Crit Care.* 2019;25(5):489-497.
22. Nguyen TC, Han YY, Kiss JE, et al. Intensive plasma exchange increases a disintegrin and metalloprotease with thrombospondin motifs-13 activity and reverses organ dysfunction in children with thrombocytopenia-associated multiple organ failure. *Crit Care Med.* 2008;36(10):2878-2887.
23. Varnell CD, Goldstein SL, Devarajan P, et al. Impact of near real-time urine neutrophil gelatinase-associated lipocalin assessment on clinical practice. *Kidney Int Rep.* 2017;2(6):1243-1249.

SECTION V

Imaging in the Intensive Care Unit

18 Ultrasound Imaging in the Intensive Care Unit

Sharad Patel, Gurkeerat Singh, and Nathaniel C. Reisinger

INTRODUCTION

Point-of-care ultrasound (POCUS) is an important tool for the intensivist. The proverbial "fifth pillar" of the physical exam, POCUS is used by the treating physician at the bedside to augment diagnosis, particularly in the rapid assessment of shock and hypoxemia.[1] In contradistinction to traditional referral radiology, POCUS is limited in scope to focused questions with binary, yes-or-no answers intended to drive immediate decision-making in time-sensitive situations.[2] The emergence of ultraportable devices at reduced cost has made POCUS ubiquitous.[3] The noninvasive nature of ultrasound with no ionizing radiation makes it benign and repeatable.[4] This draws the physician back to the bedside, decreasing fragmentation of care and enhancing the patient experience.[2,3] The majority of medical schools have implemented POCUS curricula.[5] Indeed, the American College of Chest Physicians has recognized POCUS as a core competency since 2009.[6] We aim to describe selected uses of POCUS in critical care and how they may be adapted to add value to the nephrologist practicing in this setting.

PHYSICS

Knowledge of the principles underpinning image generation is important to interpret ultrasound imaging. Ultrasound is a form of tomography, imaging by sections using a penetrating wave.[7] Ultrasound devices use crystals termed "piezoelectrics" that emit a vibration when a current is applied and vice versa.[8] Piezoelectrics, chiefly lead zirconate titanate, are arrayed across the ultrasound transducer generating ultrasound waves in response to pulses of alternating current.[9] Ultrasound waves have frequencies of 1 to 20 MHz.[8] These waves propagate through media such as tissues and about 1% are reflected to return to the transducer and stimulate the piezoelectric, generating an image.[9] The velocity of ultrasound waves is determined by the physical properties of the media they are examining. In human tissues, it averages 1,540 m/s.[8] The strength of the returning signal corresponds to the brightness of the pixel on the screen, termed "echogenicity."[9] Objects that appear bright are hyperechoic, objects that appear dark are "hypoechoic" or anechoic if they are black.[7]

Understanding the inverse relationship between frequency and wavelength is important for understanding the limitations of ultrasound imaging. Higher frequency ultrasound waves (6-20 MHz) have shorter wavelengths giving poorer penetration, but better spatial resolution, ideal for superficial structures and vascular imaging.[7] Lower frequency ultrasound waves (1-6 MHz) have longer wavelengths achieving better penetration depth at the cost of decreased spatial resolution, permitting visualization of deeper structures, ideal for abdominal imaging and echocardiography.[7] Ultrasound transducers are customized in terms of both frequency and the actual footprint of the transducer.[7] Linear transducers are typically of higher frequency, whereas abdominal and cardiac transducers are of lower frequency, the latter having a foreshortened footprint to fit between ribs.[7]

The most commonly used modes are B-mode, M-mode, and Doppler ultrasonography.[9] B-mode (brightness mode) generates a two-dimensional cross section with brightness determined by the intensity of the returning signal and depth determined based on time to return of the signal.[9] M-mode (motion mode) generates images from a single transducer tracked over time charting the motion over time.[9] Doppler mode is used to detect and evaluate movement.[9] Echoes returning from a moving structure have a different frequency as compared to the original frequency of the echo signal.[9] This difference is called the Doppler shift, which can be used to calculate flow velocities that are useful for cardiac and vascular applications.[9] Interaction of sound waves with anatomic structures gives rise to a variety of ultrasound artifacts, which are seen in daily practice. Some give clues to the underlying pathology, whereas others can lead to mismanagement if not correctly interpreted. Clinically relevant artifacts are discussed in the lung section.

KIDNEYS AND BLADDER

Focused ultrasound of the kidneys and bladder is useful in the workup of acute kidney injury (AKI) to identify structural abnormalities and exclude ureteral or bladder outlet obstruction.[10] The kidney is scanned with an abdominal probe just subcostally in the coronal plane (oriented superoinferiorly) with the patient supine taking care to fan through the entire organ in two planes using the liver as an acoustic window (permitting ready transmission of sound waves) on the right and the spleen on the left.[11] Hydronephrosis is visualized as confluent, arborizing anechoic spaces within the medullary sinus fat and can be graded as mild, moderate, or severe.[10,12] False positives include parapelvic cysts that appear as discrete anechoic structures with posterior acoustic enhancement and prominent kidney vasculature, which can be identified with Doppler.[11,13] Mild hydronephrosis can be observed under states of high urinary flow such as with diuresis or diabetes insipidus, in pregnancy, or in the transplanted kidney because of denervation.[10] False negatives can arise in early obstruction, malignancy, or with retroperitoneal fibrosis[10] (**Figures 18.1** and **18.2**) (**Visual Abstract 18.1**).

The bladder is best visualized with an abdominal transducer just above the pubic symphysis appearing as a rounded anechoic structure.[11] Ultrasound can be used to estimate the bladder volume scanning in two planes (**Visual Abstract 18.2**).[12] Size can be ascertained approximating as an ellipse using the following formula: volume $= 0.52 \times$ length $\times$ width $\times$ height.[12] Inappropriate distention can suggest obstruction because of prostatic hypertrophy, medications, or a malfunctioning urethral catheter.[14] Presence of bilateral ureteral jets on Doppler ultrasonography argues against but does not exclude ureteral obstruction.[14]

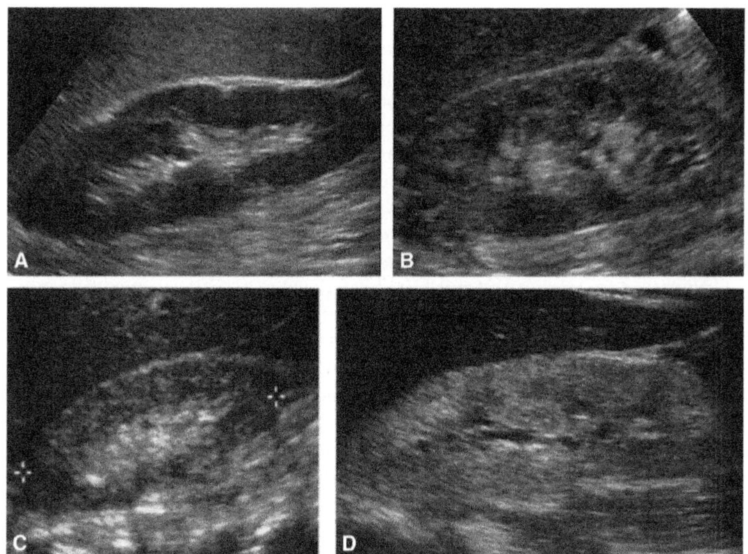

FIGURE 18.1: **A:** Normal kidney with parenchyma hypoechoic to the liver. **B:** Normal kidney with parenchyma isoechoic to the liver. **C:** Diseased kidney with parenchyma hyperechoic to the liver. **D:** Diseased kidney with parenchyma markedly hyperechoic to the liver.

From Khati NJ, Hill MC, Kimmel PL. The role of ultrasound in kidney insufficiency: the essentials. *Ultrasound Q.* 2005;21(4):227-244. Figure 2.

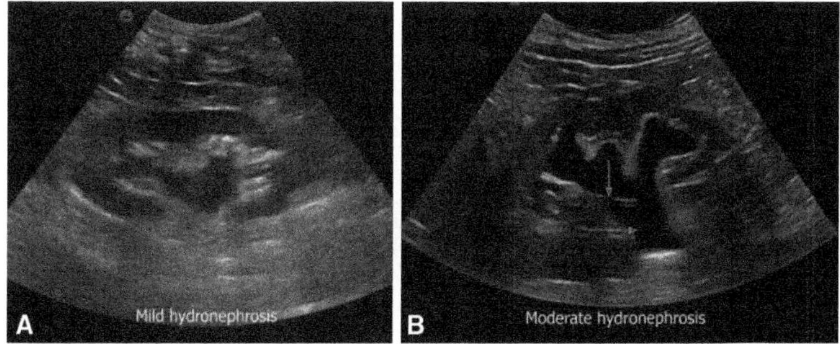

FIGURE 18.2: **A:** Mild hydronephrosis, note dilatation of minor calyces appearing as an anechoic space within the hyperechoic kidney sinus fat. Reproduced with permission. **B:** Moderate hydronephrosis, note dilatation of major and minor calyces appearing as anechoic space displacing hyperechoic kidney sinus fat. White arrow indicates ureteral stent. Yellow arrow indicates dilated proximal ureter. From Koratala A, Bhattacharya D, Kazory A. Point of care renal ultrasonography for the busy nephrologist: a pictorial review. *World J Nephrol.* 2019;8(3):44-58.

LUNG

Originally thought to be valueless because of the presence of ultrasound artifacts, in the past 30 years lung ultrasound has become integral to the practice of critical care medicine. Lung ultrasound can detect and diagnose pneumothorax, pleural effusion, consolidation, acute cardiogenic pulmonary edema (ACPE), and acute respiratory distress syndrome (ARDS).[15-18]

Normal lung can be scanned using most ultrasound transducers, with cardiac transducers fitting between two rib spaces and linear transducers giving higher resolution of the pleural line.[19] Deep to the skin, the visceral and parietal pleura are visible as a single hyperechoic line with to-and-fro motion visible with respiration termed "lung sliding."[18] Deep to the pleural line, no anatomic detail is visible under normal circumstances because of reverberation artifacts arising from the high-impedance mismatch between the pleural surface and air in the alveoli.[18] These reverberation artifacts are visualized as hyperechoic horizontal lines at integer multiples of the pleural depth and termed A-lines.[18] A-lines represent a well-aerated lung but can be present in patients with dyspnea because of pneumothorax or airways disease.[18,20]

Numerous scanning patterns have been developed with varying utility based on indication. The bedside lung ultrasound in emergency (BLUE) protocol scans three points in each hemithorax and has been demonstrated to be a useful algorithm for rapidly differentiating causes of acute dyspnea.[17] In addition to A-lines, the BLUE protocol relies on observation of other lung ultrasound artifacts to parse the differential diagnosis.[17] The presence of lung sliding rules out pneumothorax at that point.[20] The absence of lung sliding is suggestive of pneumothorax and when paired with a "lung point" (the junction between lung sliding and absent sliding) is 100% specific for pneumothorax, outperforming CXR[20-22] (**Figure 18.3**).

B-lines are hyperechoic vertically oriented reverberation artifacts arising from impedance mismatch at the pleural surface and radiating to the edge of the ultrasound field, abolishing A-lines.[17] One B-line per field is normal, whereas more than two are pathologic, with number of B-lines rising quantitatively with increased fluid in the lung.[23-25] When present focally, B-lines are suggestive of

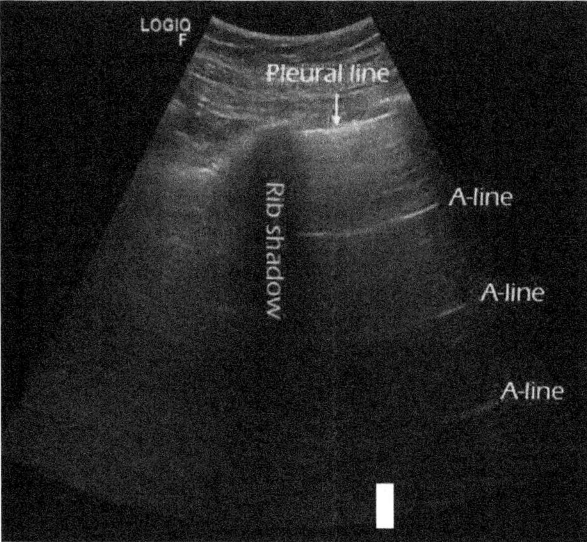

FIGURE 18.3: Normal lung ultrasound appearance. Note the hyperechoic pleural line with A-lines arising as horizontal lines at integer intervals of the pleural depth. This is a normal, well-aerated lung, though this pattern can arise in airways disease such as chronic obstructive pulmonary disease and asthma. Reproduced with permission from nephropocus.com. Accessed November 5, 2020.

pneumonia or atelectasis and when present diffusely suggest ACPE when homogeneous or ARDS when nonhomogeneous and are associated with thickened pleural lines and subpleural consolidations.[26-28] One potential confounder is the presence of diffuse interstitial lung disease, which presents as a diffuse homogeneous B-line pattern associated with thickened pleural line.[29]

B-lines are correlated with the extent of extravascular lung water. In hemodialysis patients, B-lines outperform the physical exam in the detection of fluid overload, decrease dynamically with ultrafiltration, and correlate in a dose-dependent fashion with adverse cardiovascular outcomes.[30-32] More broadly, lung ultrasound outperforms CXR for the identification of acute heart failure, and in combination with lower extremity venous compression study, the BLUE protocol correctly diagnosed 90.5% of intensive care unit (ICU) patients with acute dyspnea.[16,17,33]

A pleural effusion is visualized as an anechoic space displacing the lung artifact pattern described earlier.[23] A pleural effusions transmit sound waves well and often the vertebral spine can be visualized posteriorly though it is not normally obscured, termed “spine sign.”[34] Lung ultrasound can easily detect even small pleural effusions and outperforms physical exam and chest x-ray.[29] Ultrasound often distinguishes transudative from exudative pleural effusions, the latter more likely to have echogenic material and contain loculations and septations.[23] Finally, ultrasound is useful to quantify pleural effusions and guide thoracentesis with lowered rate of complications.[35]

Most lung consolidations reach the pleura and are visible on lung ultrasound. Depending on position and size, they can appear as small pleural-based densities to tissue-like consolidations.[36] Consolidations appear with an irregular border with normal well-aerated lung termed the “shred sign” or C-profile often associated with B-lines deep to the consolidation.[36] Again, lung ultrasound outperforms CXR, with meta-analyses studying lung ultrasound for pneumonia consistently demonstrating sensitivities and specificities in the 80% to 90% range[37-41] (**Figure 18.4**) (**Visual Abstract 18.3**).

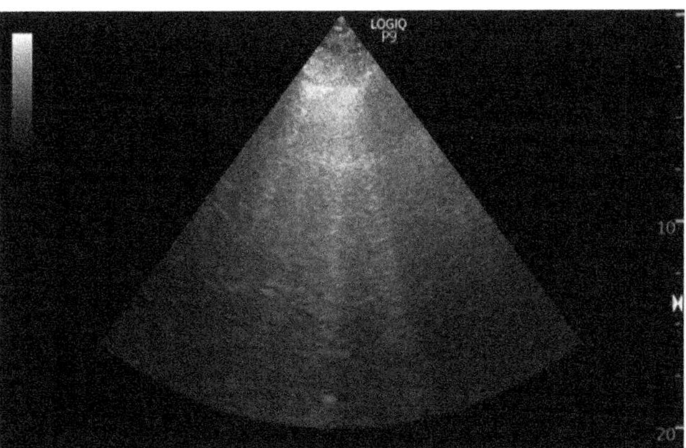

FIGURE 18.4: Lung ultrasound with B-lines. This image is taken from a patient with cardiogenic pulmonary edema. Note the hyperechoic B-lines running vertically and emanating from the pleural line. Reproduced with permission from nephropocus.com. Accessed November 5, 2020.

CARDIAC

Distinct from traditional referral transthoracic echocardiography (TTE), focused cardiac ultrasound (FOCUS) is limited cardiac ultrasound performed at the bedside by the treating intensivist as the case unfolds, guiding therapy in real time especially for patients with undifferentiated shock. FOCUS is not meant to replace referral TTE for comprehensive valvular assessment, assessment for wall motion abnormalities, or other primary cardiac indications. The four basic FOCUS views are the parasternal long axis (PSLA), parasternal short axis (PSSA), apical 4-chamber (A4C), and subcostal (SC) views. Each view is obtained systematically with a dedicated cardiac transducer.[42-44]

The first view is the PSLA view obtained with the transducer in the second to fourth intercostal space precordially on the patient's left with indicator to the right shoulder. This view includes images of the mitral valve (MV) and aortic valve (AV) as well as permitting the assessment of left ventricle (LV) size and function. LV ejection fraction (EF) is estimated visually based on fractional shortening of the LV and excursion of the MV toward the ventricular septum termed E-point septal separation (EPSS). The right ventricle (RV), left ventricular outflow tract (LVOT), and left atrium (LA) are also visible to the right, allowing for gross comparisons of chamber sizes. Pericardial effusion can be seen as anechoic fluid anterior or posterior to the heart, though fluid posterior to the descending aorta is a left-sided pleural effusion (**Figure 18.5**).

From the PSLA, the transducer is rotated so that the indicator is facing the patient's left shoulder to obtain the PSSA view. In the PSSA, the LV appears as a circle with the RV up and to the left. Here EF is visually estimated at the level of the papillary muscles. Bowing of the interventricular wall in the LV can give an indication of severely elevated right-sided pressures (D-sign). Additional information can be obtained by angling the transducer up toward the AV or down to the cardiac apex[44,45] (**Figure 18.6**).

Next is the A4C obtained with transducer lateral to the midclavicular line at the fourth and fifth intercostal space ideally at the patient's point of maximal impulse, indicator toward the patient's left axilla. Left lateral decubitus positioning is preferred. Here the atria and ventricles are seen side by side, allowing for chamber size comparisons across the interventricular septum. A normal RV to

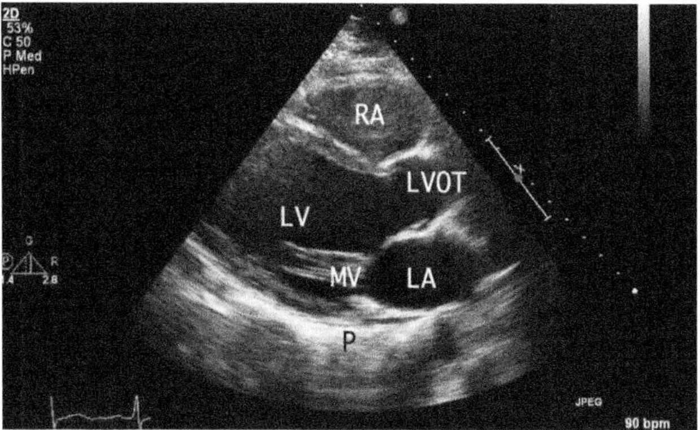

FIGURE 18.5: Parasternal long-axis view. LA, left atrium; LV, left ventricle; LVOT, left ventricular outflow tract; MV, mitral valve; P, pericardium; RA, right atrium. Original by SP. Altered by NR.

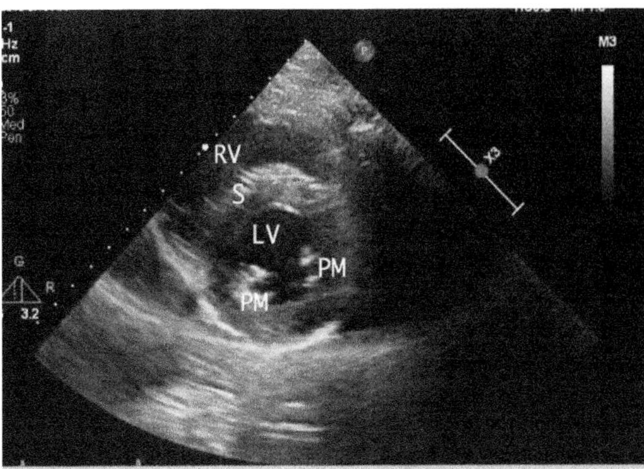

FIGURE 18.6: Parasternal short-axis view at the level of the papillary muscles. LV, left ventricle; RV, right ventricle. S, septum; PM, papillary muscle. Original by SP. Altered by NR.

LV ratio is 0.6 to 1. The MV and tricuspid valve (TV) are seen separating the atria and ventricles. Tricuspid annular plane systolic excursion (TAPSE) is the extent of up-and-down motion of the TV between systole and diastole and can be used to estimate RV systolic function, most often using M-mode. By angling the transducer toward the bed, the LVOT can be visualized permitting measurements of cardiac output using the velocity-time integral (VTI)[44,45] (**Figure 18.7**).

The final FOCUS view is the SC view with transducer just inferior to the xiphoid process with horizontal orientation, indicator toward the patient's left using the liver as an acoustic window. With all four chambers again visualized, the SC view can be a good view for overall cardiac function and may be the only feasible view in patients with hyperinflated lungs because of airways disease or positive pressure ventilation as well as patients undergoing cardiopulmonary resuscitation (**Figure 18.8**). From here the transducer is rotated to view the inferior vena cava (IVC) in long axis. To confirm the IVC, continuity

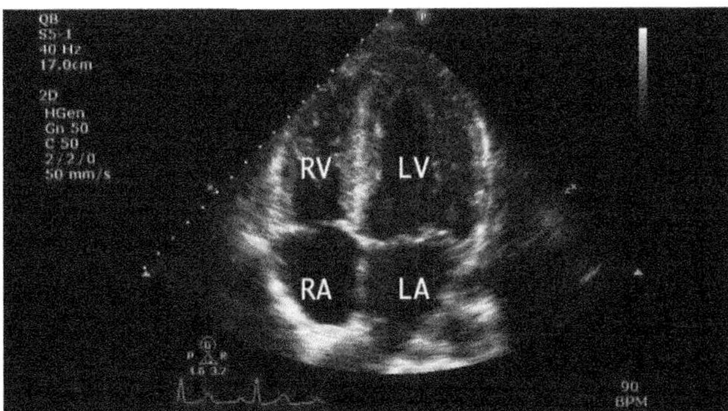

FIGURE 18.7: Apical four-chamber view. LA, left atrium; LV, left ventricle; RA, right atrium; RV, right ventricle. Original by SP. Altered by NR.

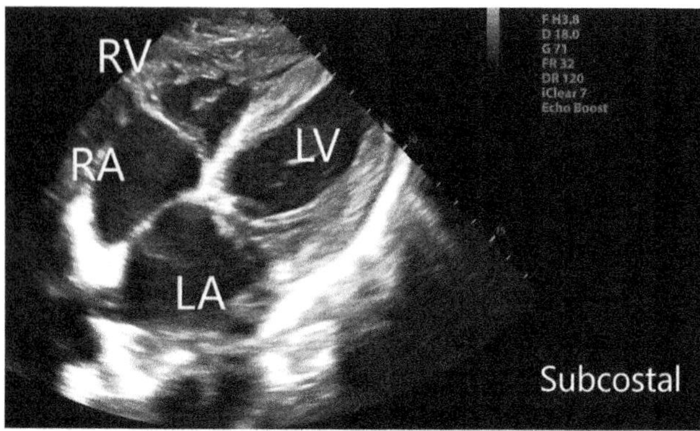

FIGURE 18.8: Subcostal view. LA, left atrium; LV, left ventricle; RA, right atrium; RV, right ventricle. Original by SP.

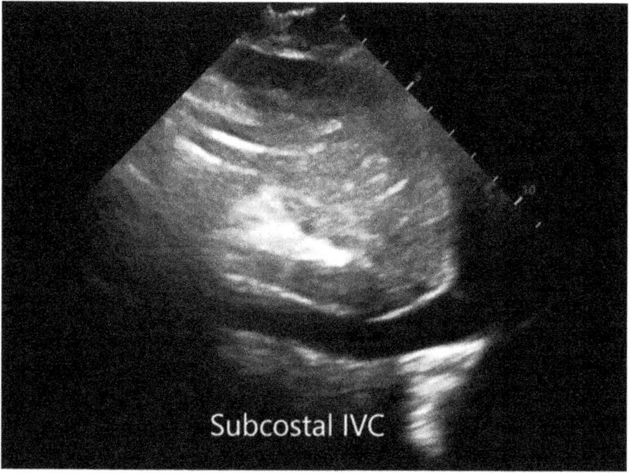

FIGURE 18.9: Inferior vena cava (IVC) in long axis. Original by SP.

with hepatic veins is noted, and the aorta is visualized immediately to the patient's left. The IVC is gauged 2 cm below the diaphragm. Though IVC assessment is confounded by multiple factors, a flat and collapsible IVC can suggest a volume responsive state, whereas a distended and noncollapsing IVC can be seen with intravascular volume expansion, cardiac tamponade, or pulmonary embolism[44,45] (**Figure 18.9**).

INTEGRATIVE ULTRASOUND

In the ICU, FOCUS can be combined with lung ultrasound, abdominal ultrasound for free fluid, and vascular assessment in the Rapid Ultrasound in Shock (RUSH) protocol. Systematic multiorgan assessments such as the RUSH protocol are complementary to the history and physical exam in patients with shock. As the physician gathers information, patterns emerge.

For instance, a large pericardial effusion with dilated IVC and B-line pattern on lung ultrasound suggests obstructive shock because of cardiac tamponade. In another scenario, a dilated and hypocontractile RV is seen on FOCUS with dilated IVC and A-line pattern, which together push the observer toward considering pulmonary embolism. Finally, consider a patient with a hyperdynamic LV with a flat and collapsing IVC and lung consolidation with subjacent pleural effusion, which speaks toward septic shock because of pneumonia. Although these cases are illustrative, outcomes data are limited to date. However, available data demonstrate that such protocols add or confirm clinical information and guide decision-making in patients with shock.[43,46-48]

CONCLUSION

POCUS is a crucial skill to master in the critical care setting. Significant information can be obtained on cardiac function and volume status, allowing for rapid narrowing of differential diagnosis in hypoxemia, shock states, and AKI. The falling cost of high-quality ultraportable ultrasound devices will mean that they are regularly available. Medical students and residents are integrating POCUS into their daily practice and medical decision-making. Critical care nephrologists must develop the skill set needed for both image acquisition and interpretation just to keep up with evolving practice patterns. The current pace of innovation and adoption makes outcomes research in POCUS of crucial importance. The time is now to establish the evidence base for future applications.

References

1. Narula J, Chandrashekhar Y, Braunwald E. Time to add a fifth pillar to bedside physical examination. *JAMA Cardiol.* 2018;3(4):346-350. doi:10.1001/jamacardio.2018.0001
2. Moore CL, Copel JA. Current concepts: point-of-care ultrasonography. *N Engl J Med.* 2011;364(8):749-757. doi:10.1056/NEJMra0909487
3. Solomon SD, Saldana F. Point-of-care ultrasound in medical education—stop listening and look. *N Engl J Med.* 2014;370(12):1083-1085. doi:10.1056/NEJMp1311944
4. Phillips RA, Stratmeyer ME, Harris GR. Safety and U.S. regulatory considerations in the nonclinical use of medical ultrasound devices. *Ultrasound Med Biol.* 2010;36(8):1224-1228. doi:10.1016/j.ultrasmedbio.2010.03.020
5. Bahner DP, Goldman E, Way D, Royall NA, Liu YT. The state of ultrasound education in U.S. medical schools: results of a national survey. *Acad Med.* 2014;89(12):1681-1686. doi:10.1097/ACM.0000000000000414
6. Mayo PH, Beaulieu Y, Doelken P, et al. American College of Chest Physicians/la societédé réanimation de langue française statement on competence in critical care ultrasonography. *Chest.* 2009;135(4):1050-1060. doi:10.1378/chest.08-2305
7. Sargsyan AE, Blaivas M, Lumb P, Karakitsos D. *Concepts and Capability.* 1st ed. Elsevier Inc; 2020. doi:10.1155/2018/2764907
8. Aldrich JE. Basic physics of ultrasound imaging. *Crit Care Med.* 2007;35(5 suppl):131-137. doi:10.1097/01.CCM.0000260624.99430.22
9. Mayette M, Mohabir PK. *Ultrasound Physics.* In: Soni NJ, Arntfield R, & Kory P, eds. *Point-of-Care Ultrasound.* 2nd ed. Philadelphia: Elsevier, 2020:7-20.
10. Faubel S, Patel NU, Lockhart ME, Cadnapaphornchai MA. Renal relevant radiology: use of ultrasonography in patients with AKI. *Clin J Am Soc Nephrol.* 2014;9(2):382-394. doi:10.2215/CJN.04840513
11. Hassani B. Kidneys. In: Soni NJ, Arntfield R, & Kory P, eds. *Point-of-Care Ultrasound.* 2nd ed. Philadelphia: Elsevier, 2020:229-238.
12. O'Neill WC. Renal relevant radiology: use of ultrasound in kidney disease and nephrology procedures. *Clin J Am Soc Nephrol.* 2014;9(2):373-381. doi:10.2215/CJN.03170313
13. Koratala A, Alquadan KF. Parapelvic cysts mimicking hydronephrosis. *Clin Case Rep.* 2018;6(4):760-761. doi:10.1002/ccr3.1431

14. Hassani B. Bladder. In: Soni NJ, Arntfield R, & Kory P, ed. *Point-of-Care Ultrasound.* 2nd ed. Philadelphia: Elsevier, 2020:239-245.
15. Baston C, Eoin West T. Lung ultrasound in acute respiratory distress syndrome and beyond. *J Thorac Dis.* 2016;8(12):E1763-E1766. doi:10.21037/jtd.2016.12.74
16. Maw AM, Hassanin A, Ho PM, et al. Diagnostic accuracy of point-of-care lung ultrasonography and chest radiography in adults with symptoms suggestive of acute decompensated heart failure: a systematic review and meta-analysis. *JAMA Netw Open.* 2019;2(3):e190703. doi:10.1001/jamanetworkopen.2019.0703
17. Lichtenstein D. Lung ultrasound in the critically ill. *Curr Opin Crit Care.* 2014;20(3):315-322. doi:10.1097/MCC.0000000000000096
18. Lichtenstein DA. Ultrasound in the management of thoracic disease. *Crit Care Med.* 2007; 35(5 suppl). doi:10.1097/01.CCM.0000260674.60761.85
19. Ketelaars R, Gülpinar E, Roes T, Kuut M, van Geffen GJ. Which ultrasound transducer type is best for diagnosing pneumothorax? *Crit Ultrasound J.* 2018;10(1):1-9. doi:10.1186/s13089-018-0109-0
20. Lichtenstein DA, Mezière G, Lascols N, et al. Ultrasound diagnosis of occult pneumothorax. *Crit Care Med.* 2005;33(6):1231-1238. doi:10.1097/01.CCM.0000164542.86954.B4
21. Lichtenstein D, Mezière G, Biderman P, Gepner A. The "lung point": an ultrasound sign specific to pneumothorax. *Intensive Care Med.* 2000;26(10):1434-1440. doi:10.1007/s001340000627
22. Ding W, Shen Y, Yang J, He X, Zhang M. Diagnosis of pneumothorax by radiography and ultrasonography: a meta-analysis. *Chest.* 2011;140(4):859-866. doi:10.1378/chest.10-2946
23. Volpicelli G, Elbarbary M, Blaivas M, et al. International evidence-based recommendations for point-of-care lung ultrasound. *Intensive Care Med.* 2012;38(4):577-591. doi:10.1007/s00134-012-2513-4
24. Picano E, Pellikka PA. Ultrasound of extravascular lung water: a new standard for pulmonary congestion. *Eur Heart J.* 2016;37(27):2097-2104. doi:10.1093/eurheartj/ehw164
25. Covic A, Siriopol D, Voroneanu L. Use of lung ultrasound for the assessment of volume status in CKD. *Am J Kidney Dis.* 2018;71(3):412-422. doi:10.1053/j.ajkd.2017.10.009
26. Copetti R, Soldati G, Copetti P. Chest sonography: a useful tool to differentiate acute cardiogenic pulmonary edema from acute respiratory distress syndrome. *Cardiovasc Ultrasound.* 2008;6:1-10. doi:10.1186/1476-7120-6-16
27. Lichtenstein DA, Mezière GA. Relevance of lung ultrasound in the diagnosis of acute respiratory failure the BLUE protocol. *Chest.* 2008;134(1):117-125. doi:10.1378/chest.07-2800
28. Lichtenstein D, Goldstein I, Mourgeon E, Cluzel P, Grenier P, Rouby JJ. Comparative diagnostic performances of auscultation, chest radiography, and lung ultrasonography in acute respiratory distress syndrome. *Anesthesiology.* 2004;100(1):9-15. doi:10.1097/00000542-200401000-00006
29. Hasan AA, Makhlouf HA. B-lines: transthoracic chest ultrasound signs useful in assessment of interstitial lung diseases. *Ann Thorac Med.* 2014;9(2):99-103. doi:10.4103/1817-1737.128856
30. Torino C, Gargani L, Sicari R, et al. The agreement between auscultation and lung ultrasound in hemodialysis patients: the LUST study. *Clin J Am Soc Nephrol.* 2016;11(11):2005-2011. doi:10.2215/CJN.03890416
31. Noble VE, Murray AF, Capp R, Sylvia-Reardon MH, Steele DJR, Liteplo A. Ultrasound assessment for extravascular lung water in patients undergoing hemodialysis: time course for resolution. *Chest.* 2009;135(6):1433-1439. doi:10.1378/chest.08-1811
32. Zoccali C, Torino C, Tripepi R, et al. Pulmonary congestion predicts cardiac events and mortality in ESRD. *J Am Soc Nephrol.* 2013;24(4):639-646. doi:10.1681/ASN.2012100990
33. Al Deeb M, Barbic S, Featherstone R, Dankoff J, Barbic D. Point-of-care ultrasonography for the diagnosis of acute cardiogenic pulmonary edema in patients presenting with acute dyspnea: a systematic review and meta-analysis. *Acad Emerg Med.* 2014;21(8):843-852. doi:10.1111/acem.12435
34. Dickman E, Terentiev V, Likourezos A, Derman A, Haines L. Extension of the thoracic spine sign: a new sonographic marker of pleural effusion. *J Ultrasound Med.* 2015;34(9):1555-1561. doi:10.7863/ultra.15.14.06013
35. Vignon P, Chastagner C, Berkane V, et al. Quantitative assessment of pleural effusion in critically ill patients by means of ultrasonography. *Crit Care Med.* 2005;33(8):1757-1763. doi:10.1097/01.CCM.0000171532.02639.08
36. Lichtenstein DA, Lascols N, Mezière G, Gepner A. Ultrasound diagnosis of alveolar consolidation in the critically ill. *Intensive Care Med.* 2004;30(2):276-281. doi:10.1007/s00134-003-2075-6
37. Long L, Zhao HT, Zhang ZY, Wang GY, Zhao HL. Lung ultrasound for the diagnosis of pneumonia in adults: a meta-analysis. *Med (United States).* 2017;96(3):e5713. doi:10.1097/MD.0000000000005713

38. Staub LJ, Mazzali Biscaro RR, Kaszubowski E, Maurici R. Lung ultrasound for the emergency diagnosis of pneumonia, acute heart failure, and exacerbations of chronic obstructive pulmonary disease/asthma in adults: a systematic review and meta-analysis. *J Emerg Med.* 2019;56(1):53-69. doi:10.1016/j.jemermed.2018.09.009
39. Llamas-Álvarez AM, Tenza-Lozano EM, Latour-Pérez J. Accuracy of lung ultrasonography in the diagnosis of pneumonia in adults: systematic review and meta-analysis. *Chest.* 2017;151(2):374-382. doi:10.1016/j.chest.2016.10.039
40. Winkler MH, Touw HR, van de Ven PM, Twisk J, Tuinman PR. Diagnostic accuracy of chest radiograph, and when concomitantly studied lung ultrasound, in critically ill patients with respiratory symptoms: a systematic review and meta-analysis. *Crit Care Med.* 2018;46(7):e707-e714. doi:10.1097/CCM.0000000000003129
41. Xia Y, Ying Y, Wang S, Li W, Shen H. Effectiveness of lung ultrasonography for diagnosis of pneumonia in adults: a systematic review and meta-analysis. *J Thorac Dis.* 2016;8(10):2822-2831. doi:10.21037/jtd.2016.09.38
42. Arntfield RT, Millington SJ. Point of care cardiac ultrasound applications in the emergency department and intensive care unit—a review. *Curr Cardiol Rev.* 2012;8(2):98-108. doi:10.2174/157340312801784952
43. Cardenas-Garcia J, Mayo PH. Bedside ultrasonography for the intensivist. *Crit Care Clin.* 2015;31(1):43-66. doi:10.1016/j.ccc.2014.08.003
44. Baston C, Moore C, Krebs EA, et al. *Pocket Guide to POCUS: Point-of-Care Tips for Point-of-Care Ultrasound (eBook).* McGraw Hill Professional; 2019.
45. Millington S. *Cardiac Ultrasound Technique.* In: Soni NJ, Arntfield R, & Kory P, ed. *Point-of-Care Ultrasound.* 2nd eds. Philadelphia: Elsevier, 2020: 111-125.
46. Shokoohi H, Boniface KS, Pourmand A, et al. Bedside ultrasound reduces diagnostic uncertainty and guides resuscitation in patients with undifferentiated hypotension. *Crit Care Med.* 2015;43(12):2562-2569. doi:10.1097/CCM.0000000000001285
47. Gidwani H, Gómez H. The crashing patient: hemodynamic collapse. *Curr Opin Crit Care.* 2017;23(6):533-540. doi:10.1097/MCC.0000000000000451
48. Narasimhan M, Koenig SJ, Mayo PH. A whole-body approach to point of care ultrasound. *Chest.* 2016;150(4):772-776. doi:10.1016/j.chest.2016.07.040

Ultrasonography versus Computed Tomography for Suspected Nephrolithiasis

 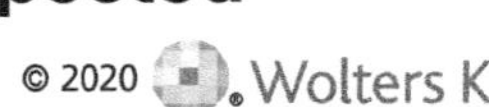

		PRIMARY OUTCOMES		SECONDARY OUTCOMES	
Multicenter (ER visits)	Randomization	High-risk diagnosis with complication *(First 30 days)*	Cumulative radiation exposure (m5v) *(6-months)*	Serious Adverse Events	Average Pain Score *(7 days)*
Comparative Effectiveness Trial	Point-of-Care Ultrasonography *(ER Physicians)* n = 908	6 (0.7%)	10.1 ± 14.1	113 (12.4%)	2.0 ± 2.9
	Radiology Ultrasonography *(Radiologists)* n = 853	3 (0.3%)	9.3 ± 13.4	96 (10.8%)	2.0 ± 2.8
Suspected Nephrolithiasis	Abdominal CT n = 958	2 (0.2%)	17.2 ± 13.4	107 (11.2%)	2.0 ± 2.8
n = 2759		*p = 0.30*	*p < 0.001*	*p = 0.50*	

Conclusion: Initial ultrasonography was associated with lower cumulative radiation exposure than initial CT, without significant differences in high-risk diagnoses with complications, serious adverse events, pain scores, return emergency department visits, or hospitalizations.

Smith-Bindman R, Aubin C, Bailitz J, et al. ***Ultrasonography Versus Computed Tomography for Suspected Nephrolithiasis.*** N Engl J Med 2014 Sep 18;371(12):1100-10.

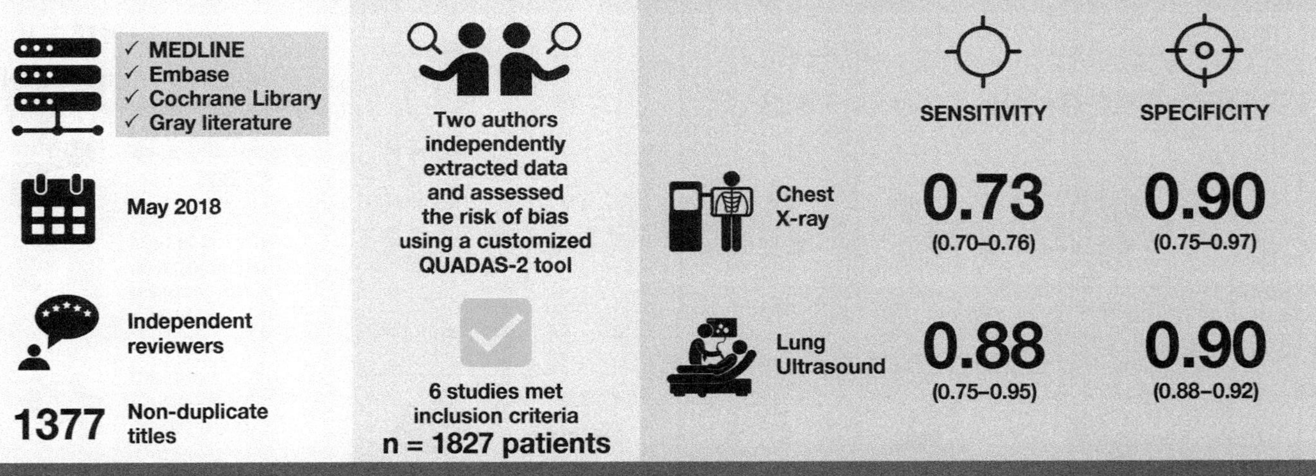

Conclusion: The findings suggest that LUS is more sensitive than CXR in detecting pulmonary edema in ADHF; LUS should be considered as an adjunct imaging modality in the evaluation of patients with dyspnea at risk of ADHF.

Maw AM, Hassanin A, Ho PM, et al. ***Diagnostic Accuracy of Point-of-Care Lung Ultrasonography and Chest Radiography in Adults With Symptoms Suggestive of Acute Decompensated Heart Failure: A Systematic Review and Meta-analysis*** JAMA Netw Open 2019 Mar 1;2(3):e190703.

VISUAL ABSTRACT 18.2

Effect of dry-weight reduction with a lung-ultrasound-guided strategy on ambulatory BP in patients with hypertension who are on hemodialysis

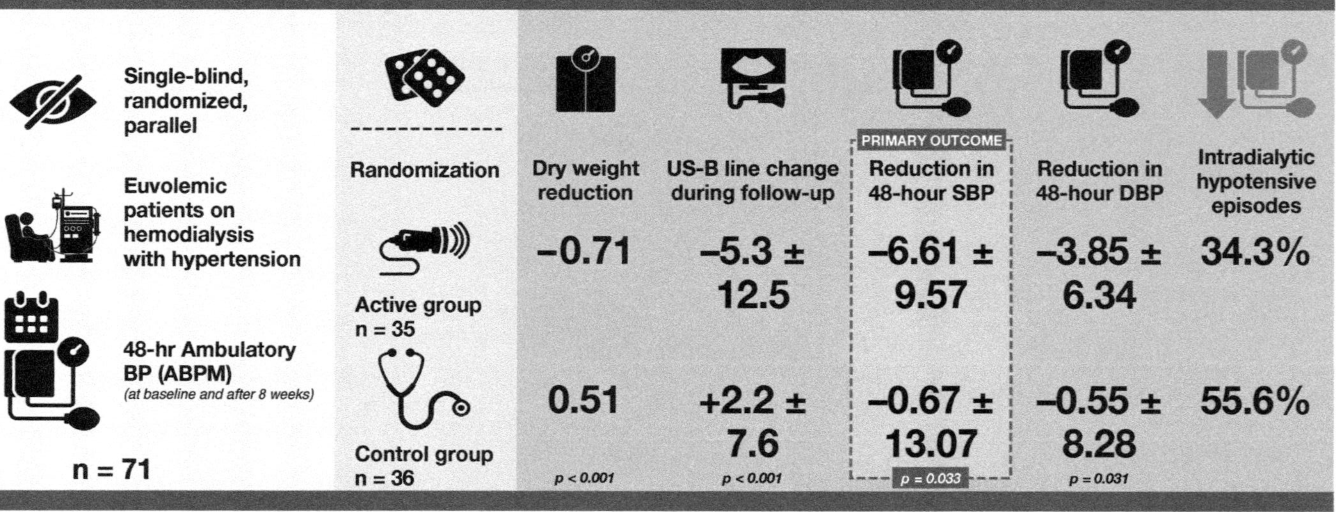

Conclusion: A lung-ultrasound-guided strategy for dry-weight reduction can effectively and safely reduce ambulatory BP levels in patients on hemodialysis.

Loutradis C, Sarafidis PA, Ekart R, et al. ***The Effect of Dry-Weight Reduction Guided by Lung Ultrasound on Ambulatory Blood Pressure in Hemodialysis Patients: A Randomized Controlled Trial.*** Kidney Int. 2019 Jun;95(6):1505-1513.

VISUAL ABSTRACT 18.3

SECTION VI

Electrolytes and Acid-Base Disorders

19

Sodium Homeostasis and Hyponatremia in the Intensive Care Unit

Mohammad Y. Alsawah, Awais Zaka, and Joel M. Topf

SODIUM PHYSIOLOGY

Dysnatremia refers to abnormal sodium concentration. Edelman defined the determinants of serum sodium concentration in 1958 in a landmark study[1] (see **Equation 19.1**).

$$[Na] = [1.03\,(Na_e + K_e)/TBW] - 23.8 \qquad \text{(Eq 19.1)}$$

where Na_e is the exchangeable sodium, K_e is the exchangeable potassium (essentially the sodium and potassium that are in solution rather than locked in bones), and TBW is total body water. Simplified, Edelman showed that the sodium concentration is proportional to the total exchangeable sodium plus exchangeable potassium divided by total body water. Total body water normally represents 60% of body mass in a lean male, less in women, more in children and infants. Total body water also is decreased in the elderly and the obese. In response to changes in tonicity, the homeostatic mechanisms adjust total body water. Increases in tonicity stimulate the release of both antidiuretic hormone (ADH) and thirst. In response to decreases in tonicity, ADH is suppressed, increasing renal water excretion. Sodium concentration is regulated by changing the denominator (total body water), not by changing the numerator (total body exchangeable sodium and potassium).

Not all solutes are osmotically active. Urea, ethanol, and glucose (in the presence of adequate insulin) are all ineffective osmoles and can accumulate without influencing the movement of water across body compartments. Effective osmoles are particles that are functionally impermeable to the membrane and can osmotically move water.

- **Osmolality** is the *concentration of all particles* in solution regardless of whether or not they can osmotically move water. The important osmoles in plasma are sodium, chloride, albumin, urea, and glucose.
- **Tonicity** is the concentration of *osmotically active particles* in solution. The principal tonic particles in plasma are sodium and chloride.

Changes in sodium concentration cause symptoms by causing a change in tissue size. Increases in plasma sodium cause water to flow out of the intracellular compartment into the extracellular compartment. Decreases in the extracellular sodium concentration cause water to move into the relatively hypertonic intracellular compartment, increasing tissue size. This has particular relevance in the brain where the calvaria limits brain swelling, resulting in increased intracellular pressure and causing the most prominent and dangerous symptoms of hyponatremia. The symptoms of dysnatremia are largely due to the consequences of redistributing total body water between the intracellular and extracellular compartments.

Electrolyte Free Water Clearance

Evaluating dysnatremia requires sophisticated assessment of water balance. Urinary excretion of hypotonic urine raises the serum sodium as total body water falls, whereas excretion of hypertonic urine actually represents the generation of free water and can lower plasma sodium. However, in addition to effective osmoles, urine can contain significant urea, an ineffective osmole, so urine osmolality may not be a good clue as to how urine production affects serum sodium. For example, in heart failure, the kidneys produce concentrated urine with only modest amounts of sodium and potassium, but this urine will raise the serum sodium despite being concentrated. The opposite situation occurs with syndrome of inappropriate antidiuretic hormone secretion (SIADH) where the concentrated urine is composed of a high concentration of urine sodium, so the production of this urine lowers serum sodium (see **Figure 19.1**).

What is important is tracking the tonicity of the urine (urine Na + urine K) that will affect serum tonicity. The best way to differentiate these cases is the use of *electrolyte free water clearance* (see **Equation 19.2**). The idea is to divide the urine output into an electrolyte component and an electrolyte free water component. The electrolyte component contains all of the urinary cations at the same concentration as the plasma sodium concentration. Loss of this isotonic component does not change serum tonicity and, in regard to its effect on serum sodium, it can be ignored. The balance of the urine output is the electrolyte free water component and this does affect serum sodium and is the key number when looking at regulating serum sodium.

$$\text{Electrolyte free water clearance} = \text{urine output} \times [1 - ([\text{urine Na} + \text{urine K}]/\text{serum Na})] \qquad \text{(Eq 19.2)}$$

When the urine sodium plus urine potassium is greater than the serum sodium, the electrolyte free water clearance will be negative, meaning that despite making urine the patient is *generating* electrolyte free water (not clearing it) and producing this urine will dilute the serum sodium further. This effect is usually only seen in SIADH, where the elevated urine sodium pushes the electrolyte free water clearance negative; in both heart failure and volume depletion, the urine sodium is low enough that the electrolyte free water clearance does not become negative. This is clinically relevant because patients with a negative free water clearance will not correct their sodium with fluid restriction alone.

HYPONATREMIA

Hyponatremia is the most common electrolyte abnormality, affecting roughly 15% to 20% of emergency hospital admissions.[2] Hyponatremia is associated with increased length of stay, as well as increased hospital morbidity and worse outcomes in heart failure and cirrhosis.[3] So hyponatremia is both common and dangerous. What makes hyponatremia particularly frightening is that inadequate therapy in acute hyponatremia can be dangerous and life threatening but being too aggressive in chronic hyponatremia can be just as dangerous and devastating.[4]

Heart Failure	SIADH
▪ Urine osmolality: 800	▪ Urine osmolality: 800
▪ Serum osmolality: 270	▪ Serum osmolality: 270
▪ Urine volume: 800	▪ Urine volume: 800
▪ Serum Na: 125	▪ Seum Na: 125
▪ Urine Na: 5	▪ Urine Na: 125
▪ Urine K: 40	▪ Urine K: 40

$$Cl_{efw} = U_{vol} \times \left(1 - \frac{Na_{urine} + K_{urine}}{Na_{serum}}\right)$$

Heart Failure:

$$Cl_{efw} = 0.8 \times \left(1 - \frac{5 + 40}{125}\right)$$

$$Cl_{efw} = 0.5\ \text{L}$$

SIADH:

$$Cl_{efw} = 0.8 \times \left(1 - \frac{125 + 40}{125}\right)$$

$$Cl_{efw} = -0.25\ \text{L}$$

FIGURE 19.1: Comparison of the electrolyte free water clearance in a typical case of heart failure–induced hyponatremia and a case of syndrome of inappropriate antidiuretic hormone secretion (SIADH). In heart failure, the kidney is appropriately getting rid of electrolyte free water, but the patient develops hyponatremia because there is insufficient production of this appropriate urine. In SIADH, the kidney is producing urine with a negative electrolyte free water clearance, so at least in this example, for every 800 mL of urine the patient makes, they are actually adding 250 mL of water to the body, further diluting the sodium.

Clinical Signs and Symptoms

In hyponatremia, the drop in serum sodium causes water to move into the intracellular compartment. This is most problematic in the brain where hyponatremia results in increased intracranial pressure, driving most of the symptoms of the hyponatremia. In addition to increases in intracranial pressure, other findings include gait disturbances, increased fall risk, cognitive deficits, osteoporosis, and increased risk for fractures.[5,6]

Management of Symptomatic Hyponatremia

Management of hyponatremia depends on the severity of symptoms. Therefore, it is crucial to understand the symptoms of hyponatremia and be able to classify them as severe or moderate (**Table 19.1**). Also, because many of the symptoms of hyponatremia are nonspecific, it is important to try to establish causality between hyponatremia and symptoms. For example, if hyponatremia is mild and symptoms are severe, there may be an additional underlying etiology. Likewise, if the symptoms persist despite an increase in the serum sodium, an alternative etiology should be sought.[2]

Management of Hyponatremia With Severe Symptoms

Severe symptomatic hyponatremia can lead to permanent brain damage and death. Severe symptoms result from cerebral edema because of an acute drop in effective osmolality.[7] Observational studies and clinical experience indicate that a 5 mmol/L increase in serum sodium concentration is sufficient to improve symptoms and can reduce intracranial pressure by 50% within an hour.[8,9] This can be achieved by using small infusions of 3% saline. For example, the European Clinical Practice Guidelines on Hyponatremia recommend repeatedly giving 150 mL of 3% NaCl for severe symptomatic hyponatremia every 20 minutes until the sodium has gone up by 5 mmol/L or the symptoms improve.[2]

If the symptoms improve, then further correction of hyponatremia depends on determining the specific etiology of the hyponatremia and treating appropriately with care not to increase sodium more than 8 mmol/L over any 24-hour period to minimize the risk of osmotic demyelination syndrome (ODS).

If the symptoms do not improve after the sodium has gone up by 5 mmol/L, the sodium should be increased at 1 mmol/L/hr until the sodium has gone up by

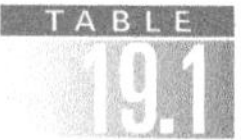

TABLE 19.1 Classification of Symptoms of Hyponatremia

Moderately Severe Hyponatremia	Severe
Nausea without vomiting	Vomiting
Confusion	Cardiorespiratory distress
Headache	Abnormal and deep somnolence
	Seizures
	Coma (Glasgow coma scale $\leq$8)

Because many of these symptoms are nonspecific, clinicians must adjudicate whether any symptom is due to the hyponatremia. Attention should be spent on the temporal relationship between the symptoms and the hyponatremia to ensure that symptoms attributed to hyponatremia do not precede the hyponatremia.

From Spasovski G, Vanholder R, Allolio B, et al. Clinical practice guideline on diagnosis and treatment of hyponatraemia. *Eur J Endocrinol.* 2014;170(3):G1-G47.

a total of 10 mmol/L. If the symptoms still have not improved, it is unlikely that the symptoms are due to the hyponatremia and alternative explanations should be sought. Adrogué and Madias' change in sodium formula (**Equation 19.3**) can be used to estimate the amount the serum sodium would rise with an infusion of 1 L of 3% saline.[10] From this information, a rate can be estimated. In typical adults, this should be around 1 mmol/L increase for every 100 mL of 3% saline. In multiple retrospective reviews, this widely used equation was shown to profoundly *underestimate* the change in sodium; thus, frequent reassessment of the serum sodium and adjustment of the infusion rate are necessary to prevent inadvertent overcorrection of hyponatremia.[11,12]

$$\text{Change in serum sodium} = [(\text{infusate Na} + \text{infusate K}) - \text{serum Na}/\text{total body water}] \qquad \text{(Eq 19.3)}$$

This calculates how much the sodium will rise following an infusion of 1 L.

Management of Hyponatremia With Moderately Severe Symptoms

In patients with less severe, non–life-threatening symptoms, the focus should be on determining the specific etiology followed by cause-specific therapy. The European Guidelines point out that any further drop could worsen the symptoms and recommend an initial bolus of 150 mL of 3% saline over 20 minutes. Care should be taken to prevent the sodium from going up by more than 8 mmol/L in 24 hours to prevent ODS.[2] In patients at high risk of ODS (see **Table 19.2**), consideration should be given to correcting the sodium even slower.[13] Cases of ODS despite guideline-based correction speeds have been reported.[2,14]

If a patient is at risk of ODS and the sodium has increased too fast, consideration should be given to relowering the sodium. This reduces mortality from ODS in rats and has been done successfully in humans.[15-17] Steroids, specifically dexamethasone, have been suggested as an alternate or additional therapy for rapid increases in sodium, though human and animal data are thin.[13]

Management of Asymptomatic Hyponatremia

Chronic hyponatremia is common and is associated with an increased risk of death, both in and out of the hospital.[3] It remains unclear, however, whether it is the hyponatremia itself or the underlying disease that is the cause of the poor outcomes. There are no data pointing to improved patient outcomes following

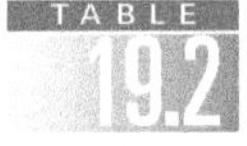

TABLE 19.2 Risk Factors for Osmotic Demyelination Syndrome

Risk Factors for Osmotic Demyelination Syndrome
Serum sodium <120 mmol/L
Rapid correction of hyponatremia (>8 mmol/L/d)
Hypokalemia
Alcohol abuse
Malnutrition
Liver disease (and especially liver transplant)

the treatment of hyponatremia, whereas mistreatment is associated with devastating patient outcomes.

The absence of hyponatremic symptoms in the face of significant hyponatremia indicates that the patient has adapted to the decreased serum tonicity by ejecting osmotically active solutes from the intracellular compartment, allowing the cells to return to its normal size. However, this puts these cells at risk of becoming relatively hypotonic if the serum sodium is rapidly corrected. Water then leaves the cells, causing them to shrink, resulting in a neurologic syndrome called ODS (see **Figure 19.2**). Preventing this complication becomes the overriding concern in the management of asymptomatic hyponatremia. Instead of intervening to raise the serum sodium, the focus is on determining the etiology and reversing it while preventing the sodium from rising too quickly. It is often difficult to be certain if the hyponatremia is acute or chronic, but in asymptomatic patients, the conservative approach is to assume it is chronic and to limit the increase in sodium to no more than 8 mmol/L/d.

The speed of correction of chronic hyponatremia is not the only risk factor for ODS. Malnutrition, hypokalemia, and liver disease all increase the risk of ODS (see Table 19.2).

In some situations, specific treatments of hyponatremia are so effective that patients will autocorrect their hyponatremia faster than 8 mmol/L/d. Diagnosis where this is common include: psychogenic polydipsia, tea and toast syndrome, volume depletion, thiazide-induced hyponatremia, and adrenal insufficiency. In these situations, preventing rapid increases in serum sodium is the primary concern. The traditional method of handling this is to monitor urine output and serum sodium and to add D5W and desmopressin (DDAVP) if the sodium starts to rise too fast or the urine output starts to increase.[18] DDAVP is a synthetic form of ADH that is a

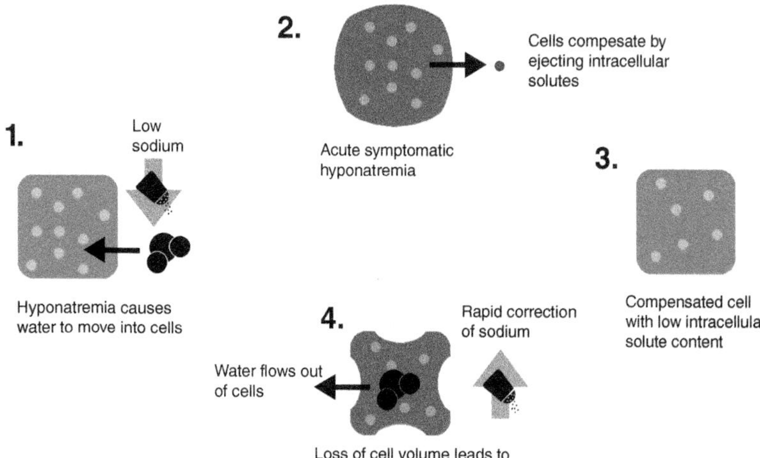

FIGURE 19.2: In acute hyponatremia, cells are hypotonic to plasma so water flows into them, causing cerebral edema. Cells compensate by ejecting intracellular solutes, resulting in restoration of cell volume at a lower intracellular tonicity. If the sodium is rapidly corrected, the cells are now relatively hypotonic to the extracellular compartment and water leaves the cell, causing the cell to shrink leading to osmotic demyelination syndrome (ODS).

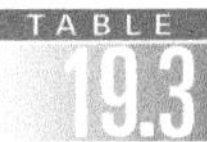

TABLE 19.3 DDAVP Clamp Protocol

Stop any maintenance fluids.
Start DDAVP 2 μg IV q8h.
Start 3% NaCl (1-1.5 mL/kg over 6 hr).
Fluid restrict patient to 1.2 L/d.
Monitor sodium q2h initially. Once the sodium is rising predictably, decrease frequency to q4-6h.
Adjust 3% NaCl infusion rate to achieve correction of <8 mmol/L/d. Try to avoid adjusting the rate more than q6h. Look at the sodium trend rather than the latest value.
Continue 3% and DDAVP until the sodium is 125-130.

DDAVP, desmopressin; IV, intravenous.
Not to be used in patients with volume overload or symptomatic hyponatremia.

selective V2 agonist. DDAVP increases collecting duct water permeability, resulting in a small volume of concentrated urine but does not trigger the V1-induced vasoconstriction. A more proactive approach is to start DDAVP at the outset of the treatment of hyponatremia; this is called a DDAVP clamp (**Table 19.3**).[19] In addition to the DDAVP, the patients require a 3% saline infusion to correct the hyponatremia.

Cause-Specific Treatment

General Management

After the immediate treatment of symptomatic hyponatremia, physicians should determine the cause of the hyponatremia and provide specific therapies directed at the etiology.

The cause of hyponatremia can be quickly sketched out in flowcharts (see **Figure 19.3**), but none of the tests have sufficient sensitivity or specificity to make an accurate diagnosis straightforward. A thorough history, a careful assessment of the patient, and judicious use of the laboratory can allow cagey physicians to come up with a preliminary diagnosis.

After finding low serum sodium, a serum osmolality should be checked. A normal or elevated osmolality is unexpected and has a narrow differential that should be explored.[21] One explanation is systematic lab error that occurs with elevated lipids or proteins in the blood sample. This is a case of pseudohyponatremia and should be addressed by looking at serum glucose, lipids, and total protein. The increased glucose will osmotically draw water from the intracellular compartment and dilute the serum sodium. This is reversible and the sodium will go back up when the glucose is corrected. What the sodium will be with a normal glucose can be calculated from the current sodium and the serum glucose (see **Equation 19.4**).

$$\text{Adjusted sodium} = \text{Na} + 1.6 \times (\text{glucose}/100) \qquad \text{(Eq 19.4)}$$

After low serum osmolality is confirmed, urine osmolality should be assessed. A urine osmolality less than 100 indicates suppressed ADH, leaving a limited differential for hyponatremia including insufficient solute intake (beer

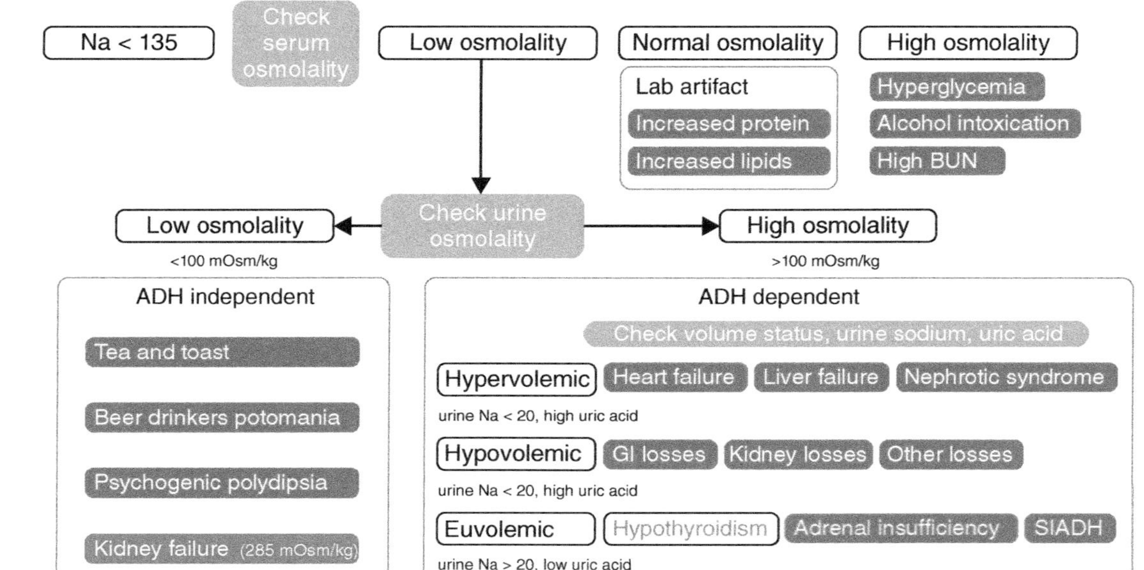

FIGURE 19.3: Hyponatremia diagnostic algorithm. Hypothyroidism is grayed out because though it has traditionally been included as a cause of euvolemic hyponatremia, lately this has been questioned and best evidence suggests this is rarely a cause of clinically significant hyponatremia and when it does cause hyponatremia it is through associated heart failure so these patients will be hypervolemic, not euvolemic.[20] Kidney failure is in orange to point out that though it is ADH independent, these patients will not have the dilute urine seen in the other causes of ADH-independent hyponatremia. The urine in kidney failure is close to isosmotic with plasma. ADH, antidiuretic hormone; BUN, blood urea nitrogen; GI, gastrointestinal; SIADH, syndrome of inappropriate antidiuretic hormone secretion.

drinker's potomania, tea and toast syndrome) or primary polydipsia. Kidney failure is on this list, as these patients develop hyponatremia from oliguria because of decreased glomerular filtration rate (GFR), rather than increased ADH.

A urine osmolality greater than 100 indicates increased ADH as the driving factor in hyponatremia. There are a number of diagnoses here and they are best categorized by volume status. However, caution is urged before overindexing on perceived volume status as even experienced clinicians make mistakes with this assessment.[22] Hypervolemic and hypovolemic causes of hyponatremia will typically have low urine sodium and elevated serum uric acid. Euvolemic hyponatremia will be associated with high urine sodium and low serum uric acid.

Expanded Extracellular Fluid Volume

Patients with expanded extracellular fluid volume have a primary condition that causes intense renal sodium conservation. Giving these patients 3% saline risks worsening the fluid overload. Interventions should focus on restoring normal volume status and correcting the primary condition.

Heart Failure

In hyponatremia associated with acute decompensated heart failure, the primary therapy is fluid restriction along with loop diuretics, in addition to other treatments to improve the underlying heart failure (i.e., vasodilators, inotropes). If serum sodium does not improve, consideration should be given to tolerating mild to moderate asymptomatic hyponatremia without further intervention. Hyponatremia in heart failure is a poor prognostic sign, but no data show improved outcomes with correcting hyponatremia. ADH receptor antagonists, either intravenous (IV) conivaptan or oral tolvaptan, would be appropriate agents to increase serum sodium although they have not been shown to improve heart failure outcomes.[23]

Cirrhosis

Fluid restriction is the primary therapy for hyponatremia in cirrhosis. Hypertonic saline should be used with caution in cirrhosis as it will increase ascites. The use of vaptans in cirrhosis should be done only with caution because of the risk of hepatotoxicity. Additionally, conivaptan, a combined V1a/V2 receptor antagonist, can increase portal blood flow by blocking V1 in the splanchnic circulation, which may precipitate variceal bleeding.

Contracted Extracellular Volume

Significant hypovolemia stimulates the release of ADH that reduces the electrolyte free water clearance, which is the source of the hyponatremia. Correcting the volume depletion suppresses ADH releases, resulting in a water diuresis and rapid correction of hyponatremia. In hemodynamically unstable patients, the direct risk of decreased organ perfusion outweighs the potential risk of rapid increases in the serum sodium level so volume resuscitation with isotonic crystalloids should continue until blood pressure is restored and the patient has clinical euvolemia. This is an ideal clinical scenario to consider a DDAVP clamp, to prevent resuscitation fluids from rapidly raising the serum sodium.

In patients with an equivocal volume estimate, it is not always easy to differentiate between volume depletion and euvolemic causes of hyponatremia like SIADH. A fluid challenge in these situations can be both diagnostic and therapeutic. With volume depletion, administering isotonic saline leads to an increase in both the serum sodium and urine sodium. In SIADH, administering saline also results in an increase in urine sodium; however, serum sodium may fall as the administered sodium is excreted in a small volume of concentrated urine and the water is retained. In cases where there is a possibility that the primary diagnosis is SIADH and the plan is to give a fluid challenge as a diagnostic maneuver, consideration should be given to using 3% saline in cases where the sodium is already critically low (<120 mmol/L) to avoid dropping the sodium even further.

Gastrointestinal and Diuretic-Induced Hyponatremia

After urgent fluid resuscitation to stabilize blood pressure, tailor the repletion fluid to correct additional electrolyte abnormalities. Because potassium has the same effect on serum sodium as sodium does (see the Edelman formula, Eq 19.1), correcting hypokalemia puts patients at risk for inadvertent, rapid correction of hyponatremia. This may contribute to hypokalemia being an independent risk factor for ODS.

Patients with thiazide-induced hyponatremia are at high risk for recurrence of sodium abnormality and should not be rechallenged with a thiazide agent.[24]

Cerebral Salt-Wasting Syndrome

Patients who develop hemodynamic instability and frank volume depletion in response to fluid restriction have cerebral salt wasting (CSW), and patients whose urine volume decreases and sodium improves with fluid restriction have SIADH. The overwhelming majority of patients in the neurosurgical setting with hyponatremia after subarachnoid hemorrhage, trauma, or surgery have SIADH, not CSW. A high urine output and urinary sodium content during sodium infusion are insufficient evidence to differentiate between CSW and SIADH because patients with SIADH will excrete any administered sodium and fluid to maintain balance. Similarly, reduced uric acid and blood urea nitrogen (BUN) in serum occur in both CSW and SIADH, offering no help in diagnosis. Diagnosis of CSW requires demonstration of a period of inappropriate renal sodium and fluid loss preceding the development of volume depletion and hyponatremia.

Mineralocorticoid Deficiency

Mineralocorticoid deficiency is typically a chronic hyponatremia. Volume repletion with isotonic saline is the mainstay of therapy. A spontaneous aquaresis with rapid correction of hyponatremia may occur once the volume deficit is replete; frequent monitoring of serum sodium is essential. Acquired mineralocorticoid deficiency severe enough to lead to volume depletion and hyponatremia occurs only with bilateral adrenal failure from adrenal destruction or adrenalectomy. As such, patients presenting with mineralocorticoid deficiency should be suspected to have glucocorticoid deficiency as well. Presumptive glucocorticoid deficiency should be treated with stress-dose hydrocortisone (e.g., 50-100 mg of hydrocortisone given parenterally every 8 hours). Once the diagnosis is confirmed, treatment can be started with fludrocortisone.

Management of Euvolemic Hyponatremia

Syndrome of Inappropriate Antidiuretic Hormone Secretion

In SIADH, patients have unregulated release of ADH, which results in continuous renal water retention. These patients are roughly in sodium balance, so that sodium intake is equivalent to sodium excretion; however, the sodium is excreted in a small volume of urine because of excess, unregulated ADH. The sodium excretion in a small volume of concentrated urine creates the high urine sodium,

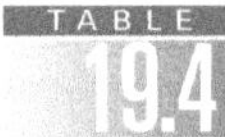

Causes of SIADH

Malignancy	Pulmonary Disease	CNS Disease	Medications
Lung cancer	Pneumonia	Infection	**ADH agonists**
Head and neck cancer	Asthma	Vascular bleeds	DDAVP
GI tract	Cystic fibrosis	Mass lesions	Oxytocin
GU tract	Positive pressure ventilation	Trauma	Terlipressin
Lymphoma		GBS	Vasopressin
Sarcoma			**CNS**
Neuroblastoma			SSRI
			Tricyclics
			MAOI
			Venlafaxine
			Carbamazepine
			Valproic acid
			MDMA
			Opiates
			Cancer
			Platinum compounds
			Ifosfamide
			Cyclophosphamide
			Melphalan
			Methotrexate
			Diabetes
			Chlorpropamide
			Tolbutamide

ADH, antidiuretic hormone; CNS, central nervous system; DDAVP, desmopressin; GBS, Guillain-Barré syndrome; GI, gastrointestinal; GU, gastrourinary; MAOI, monoamine oxidase inhibitor; MDMA, 3,4-methylene-dioxy-methamphetamine; SIADH, syndrome of inappropriate antidiuretic hormone secretion; SSRI, selective serotonin reuptake inhibitor.

Adapted from Liamis G, Milionis H, Elisaf M. A review of drug-induced hyponatremia. *Am J Kidney Dis.* 2008;52(1):144-153.

differentiating it from the hypo- and hypervolemic etiologies of hyponatremia. SIADH occurs in a variety of circumstances including malignancy, central nervous system (CNS) disease, pulmonary disease, and as medication induced (see **Table 19.4**).[25]

Restricting water intake below urine volume should get patient's sodium to rise. However, this often means highly restrictive and uncomfortable fluid restrictions. Because urine osmolality is fixed in SIADH, the only way to increase urine volume is by increasing the solute load. This can be done with salt tablets, high-protein diet, or urea tablets. Alternatelively, one could look to vaptans to block ADH and allow patients to lower urine osmolality.

Urea has been used to treat hyponatremia for a variety of conditions. Urea is freely filtered by the glomerulus and quickly cleared in patients with normal kidney function. The molecular weight of urea is 60 g/mol so a 15 g dose has 250 mOsm of solute. If the patient has a urine osmolarity of 500, this will increase urine output by half a liter.[26] To get a similar osmolar load from sodium chloride tablets would require seven 1-g tablets (there are 17 mmol of NaCl per 1 g NaCl, which dissociates to 17 mmol of sodium and 17 mmol of chloride). In a retrospective study of urea used for hyponatremia among inpatients, Rondon-Berrios et al showed it to be safe and effective for a variety of diagnoses including SIADH, heart failure, and cirrhosis.[27]

Antidiuretic Hormone–Independent Hyponatremia

In most cases of hyponatremia, the kidneys cannot clear excess water because of the activity of excess ADH, either physiologic (hypovolemic and heart failure) or nonphysiologic (SIADH). There are a few causes of ADH-independent hyponatremia. In these cases, ADH is fully suppressed, the urine is dilute but the patient is unable to make enough urine to compensate for water intake. There are two clinical scenarios where this is seen, compulsive water drinkers and low-solute hyponatremia.

Primary Polydipsia

A healthy adult kidney is able to make 18 L of urine a day. Some patients drink more than this, exceeding the maximum water clearance. This is often seen in schizophrenia. Treatment can be accomplished with simple water restriction. As soon as water intake is curtailed, the body will rapidly clear the excess water and the sodium will rise.

Low-solute hyponatremia results from low-solute intake such that urine output is limited by the lack of solute. The lowest urine osmolality in most patients is between 50 and 100 mOsm/L. In a patient where this number is 50, a low-osmolar diet with only 100 mOsm/d, the patient would only be able to make 2 L of urine, far short of the 14 L possible with a normal osmolar load of 700 mOsm/d. Diets low in osmoles include those based on carbohydrate as seen in alcoholics, or in patients with minimal intake. Because the insufficient urine output is due to decreased solute, increasing the solute load will result in an immediate and brisk diuresis. In patients with a urine osmolality of 50 mOsm/kg H_2O, a liter of normal saline will result in 6 L of urine production. This will rapidly (often too rapidly) raise the serum sodium.

References

1. Edelman IS, Leibman J, O'Meara MP, Birkenfeld LW. Interrelations between serum sodium concentration, serum osmolarity and total exchangeable sodium, total exchangeable potassium and total body water. *J Clin Invest.* 1958;37(9):1236-1256. doi:10.1172/jci103712
2. Spasovski G, Vanholder R, Allolio B, et al. Clinical practice guideline on diagnosis and treatment of hyponatraemia. *Eur J Endocrinol.* 2014;170(3):G1-G47.
3. Liamis G, Rodenburg EM, Hofman A, Zietse R, Stricker BH, Hoorn EJ. Electrolyte disorders in community subjects: prevalence and risk factors. *Am J Med.* 2013;126(3):256-263.
4. Berl T. Treating hyponatremia: damned if we do and damned if we don't. *Kidney Int.* 1990;37(3):1006-1018.
5. Renneboog B, Musch W, Vandemergel X, Manto MU, Decaux G. Mild chronic hyponatremia is associated with falls, unsteadiness, and attention deficits. *Am J Med.* 2006;119(1):71.E1-71.E8.
6. Hoorn EJ, Rivadeneira F, van Meurs JBJ, et al. Mild hyponatremia as a risk factor for fractures: the Rotterdam Study. *J Bone Miner Res.* 2011;26(8):1822-1828.
7. Arieff AI. Hyponatremia, convulsions, respiratory arrest, and permanent brain damage after elective surgery in healthy women. *N Engl J Med.* 1986;314(24):1529-1535.
8. Sterns RH, Nigwekar SU, Hix JK. The treatment of hyponatremia. *Semin Nephrol.* 2009;29(3):282-299.
9. Koenig MA, Bryan M, Lewin JL 3rd, Mirski MA, Geocadin RG, Stevens RD. Reversal of transtentorial herniation with hypertonic saline. *Neurology.* 2008;70(13):1023-1029.
10. Adrogué HJ, Madias NE. Hyponatremia. *N Engl J Med.* 2000;342(21):1581-1589.
11. Hanna RM, Yang W-T, Lopez EA, Riad JN, Wilson J. The utility and accuracy of four equations in predicting sodium levels in dysnatremic patients. *Clin Kidney J.* 2016;9(4):530-539.

12. Mohmand HK, Issa D, Ahmad Z, Cappuccio JD, Kouides RW, Sterns RH. Hypertonic saline for hyponatremia: risk of inadvertent overcorrection. *Clin J Am Soc Nephrol.* 2007;2(6):1110-1117.
13. King JD, Rosner MH. Osmotic demyelination syndrome. *Am J Med Sci.* 2010;339(6):561-567.
14. Reijnders TDY, Janssen WMT, Niamut SML, Kramer AB. Role of risk factors in developing osmotic demyelination syndrome during correction of hyponatremia: a case study. *Cureus.* 2020;12(1):e6547.
15. Gankam Kengne F, Soupart A, Pochet R, Brion J-P, Decaux G. Re-induction of hyponatremia after rapid overcorrection of hyponatremia reduces mortality in rats. *Kidney Int.* 2009;76(6):614-621.
16. Oya S, Tsutsumi K, Ueki K, Kirino T. Reinduction of hyponatremia to treat central pontine myelinolysis. *Neurology.* 2001;57(10):1931-1932.
17. Soupart A, Ngassa M, Decaux G. Therapeutic relowering of the serum sodium in a patient after excessive correction of hyponatremia. *Clin Nephrol.* 1999;51(6):383-386.
18. Perianayagam A, Sterns RH, Silver SM, et al. DDAVP is effective in preventing and reversing inadvertent overcorrection of hyponatremia. *Clin J Am Soc Nephrol.* 2008;3(2):331-336.
19. Sood L, Sterns RH, Hix JK, Silver SM, Chen L. Hypertonic saline and desmopressin: a simple strategy for safe correction of severe hyponatremia. *Am J Kidney Dis.* 2013;61(4):571-578.
20. Pantalone KM, Hatipoglu BA. Hyponatremia and the thyroid: causality or association? *J Clin Med Res.* 2014;4(1):32-36.
21. Rohrscheib M, Rondon-Berrios H, Argyropoulos C, Glew RH, Murata GH, Tzamaloukas AH. Indices of serum tonicity in clinical practice. *Am J Med Sci.* 2015;349(6):537-544.
22. Chung HM, Kluge R, Schrier RW, Anderson RJ. Clinical assessment of extracellular fluid volume in hyponatremia. *Am J Med.* 1987;83(5):905-908.
23. Konstam MA, Gheorghiade M, Burnett JC Jr, et al. Effects of oral tolvaptan in patients hospitalized for worsening heart failure: the EVEREST Outcome Trial. *JAMA.* 2007;297(12):1319-1331.
24. Friedman E, Shadel M, Halkin H, Farfel Z. Thiazide-induced hyponatremia. Reproducibility by single dose rechallenge and an analysis of pathogenesis. *Ann Intern Med.* 1989;110(1):24-30.
25. Liamis G, Milionis H, Elisaf M. A review of drug-induced hyponatremia. *Am J Kidney Dis.* 2008;52(1):144-153.
26. Sterns RH, Silver SM, Hix JK. Urea for hyponatremia? *Kidney Int.* 2015;87(2):268-270.
27. Rondon-Berrios H, Tandukar S, Mor MK, et al. Urea for the treatment of hyponatremia. *Clin J Am Soc Nephrol.* 2018;13(11):1627-1632.

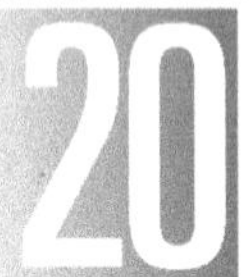

Hypernatremia in the Intensive Care Unit

Joel M. Topf

Compared to hyponatremia, hypernatremia is easy. There is minimal concern about acute versus chronic hypernatremia, mistreatment is not associated with devastating clinical outcomes, and the diagnosis is usually pretty straightforward.

The body protects itself from increases in tonicity by increasing water intake by stimulating thirst and decreasing renal excretion of water mediated through the action of antidiuretic hormone (ADH) binding to V2 receptors primarily in the medullary collecting duct. Thirst and water drinking are so effective that even with a total absence of ADH activity, as in complete diabetes insipidus (DI), people are able to maintain normal tonicity through increased water intake. However, in the intensive care unit (ICU), patients are often unable to respond to normal thirst because of altered mentation, sedation, or intubation, so that primary defense is lost. Although hypernatremia is incredibly uncommon in general laboratory findings, it is seen in 6% to 25% of ICU patients, making this a common electrolyte abnormality in the ICU.[1-3]

CLINICAL SIGNS AND SYMPTOMS

Increases in extracellular swelling cause water to move out of the cells, causing cells to shrink, altering their function. The primary symptoms are neurologic, including lethargy, weakness, irritability, seizures, and coma.[4] It also decreases insulin sensitivity.[5] It can cause cramps, rhabdomyolysis, and has been associated with decreased left ventricular function.[6] The most prominent symptom is thirst. Most worrisome finding is that really acute rises in serum sodium can result in osmotic demyelination syndrome, as seen with mismanagement of chronic hyponatremia.[7]

One of the most worrisome manifestations of hypernatremia is increased morbidity and mortality. In study after study, hypernatremia comes up as a risk factor for death.[3,8,9] Although most believe this is a marker of underlying severity of illness, this association persists despite being controlled for all known confounders. Some have advocated using hypernatremia as a marker of poor quality of care in the ICU.[10]

MANAGEMENT

The treatment for hypernatremia, like the treatment for most electrolytes, is not grounded in solid randomized controlled trials or interventional trials. Recommendations come from retrospective observational trials, combined with basic physiology and expert opinion. The standard therapy for hypernatremia is to provide enough electrolyte-free water to bring the sodium concentration down to normal. In addition to providing water to correct the deficit, water also needs to be provided to cover ongoing water losses from renal or extrarenal sources. In cases of DI, this may be substantial.

Calculating the Fluid Deficit

The calculation of the fluid deficit gives the percentage the sodium has risen over normal (140 mmol/L) and then multiplies that percentage by the estimated total body water. Total body water is estimated from the weight, gender, and age of the patient. Gender and age are used to help estimate percent body fat as adipose is largely anhydrous, so as percent body fat goes up, the percent total body water goes down. Elderly and women tend to have a higher percentage of body fat, though individuals vary. The standard formula is shown in **Equation 20.1.**

$$\text{Water deficit} = \text{Wt (kg)} \times (0.6 \text{ in children and men, } 0.5 \text{ in women and elderly men, } 0.45 \text{ for elderly women}) \times (\text{Serum Na}/140 - 1) \qquad \text{(Eq 20.1)}$$

When treating obese patients, use lower constants than listed in **Equation 20.2.**

Calculating Ongoing Losses

If patients have modest urine output, it is not so important to consider the correction of hypernatremia, but as the urine output rises, it becomes more and more important to include it in the treatment plan. A quick method to estimate how to correct for ongoing losses is to ignore the first liter of urine output. For urine output from 1 to 3 L, replace half the volume with electrolyte-free water and then replace all the urine output greater than 3 L. For example, for a patient making 6 L of urine a day,

- 0-1 L: ignore
- 1-3 L: replace half: 1 L
- 3-6 L: replace 3 L
- Total replacement: 4 L of free water

A more precise calculation for replacing ongoing losses is to use the electrolyte-free water clearance, see Equation 20.2.

$$\text{Electrolyte-free water clearance} = \text{urine output} \times [1 - ([\text{urine Na} + \text{urine K}]/\text{serum Na})] \qquad \text{(Eq 20.2)}$$

Administer the Fluid

The ideal fluid is enteral water. Often patients in the ICU have various contraindications to enteral intake and in that case D5W can be used. However, care should be used. Hypernatremia can increase insulin resistance resulting in hyperglycemia, which can raise the osmolality and stimulate osmotic diuresis, further increasing the serum sodium.[11] Expert consensus is to correct hypernatremia no faster than 0.5 mmol/L/hr or 12 mmol/d.[12] However, a 2019 publication did not find any excess mortality or morbidity in patients who were corrected faster than 0.5 mmol/L/hr.[13] There are some data showing increased risk of seizure with rapid correction in infants, but there are no case series or even anecdotal data to suggest worse outcomes with rapid correction in adults.[14] There are, however, some data showing worse outcomes with slow correction.[15] Another difference between the treatment of hypernatremia and hyponatremia is that hyponatremia often spontaneously resolves during treatment and the kidneys regain the ability to clear excess free water, so overcorrection is common. This spontaneous resolution is rare in hypernatremia and undertreatment is far more common than overtreatment.

Look for and Correct Causes of Increased Water Losses

Although a failure to drink water and respond to the normal thirst response is the ultimate cause of hypernatremia, in most cases there is an additional factor, that is, increasing water loss, either essentially electrolyte-free water as with DI (central or nephrogenic) or hypotonic fluid as with diuretics or osmotic diuresis. Steps should be taken to identify and correct this ongoing water loss.

- Correct osmotic diuresis (treat hyperglycemia, stop sodium-glucose cotransporter 2 inhibitors [SGLT2i], stop mannitol)
- Correct hypokalemia and hypercalcemia
- Stop loop diuretics
- Stop lithium

If the patient has nephrogenic diabetes insipidus (NDI), decrease urine output with:

- Thiazide diuretics and a low sodium diet
- Nonsteroidal anti-inflammatory drugs (NSAIDs)
- Acetazolamide. This newer therapy is particularly effective in lithium-induced NDI.[16]

DIAGNOSIS

The cause of hypernatremia is always a failure to drink and the etiology is then typically obvious from the clinical scenario: altered mental status, unconsciousness, intubated on a ventilator, increased insensible losses from burns, surgical wounds, or other losses. But often there is an additional factor that drives the hypernatremia. It fits in one of three categories:

1. Extrarenal water loss because of diarrhea, sweating, large open (usually abdominal) wounds, fever, burns.
2. Renal water losses because of an inability to adequately concentrate urine, resulting in loss of hypotonic fluid. This happens with loop diuretics, osmotic diuresis, and the polyuric phase of recovery from acute tubular necrosis (ATN). This also occurs with DI discussed more later.
3. Excess sodium intake. A number of intravenous (IV) infusions can increase the sodium load predisposing to hypernatremia. A 50 mL ampule of sodium bicarbonate has a sodium concentration of 1,000 mmol/L. Resuscitation efforts that use multiple doses of sodium bicarbonate can leave a patient with hypernatremia. Sodium ingestions, intension or accidental, can also cause hypernatremia.[17,18] Some drugs also contain a significant sodium load—ticarcillin has 5 mmol/g, resulting in almost 70 mmol of sodium a day at 3.375 g q6h. Ciprofloxacin has 78 mmol of sodium per gram.

DIABETES INSIPIDUS

DI is an inability of the kidney to conserve water. These patients make large amounts of dilute urine, up to a liter an hour. If patients are able to drink, they will keep their sodium in the normal range at the expense of profound polyuria and polydipsia. If these patients are made NPO (nil per os), lose consciousness, or for some other reason cease to have access to water, they will rapidly dehydrate as they produce high volumes of hypotonic urine and become hypernatremic. The diagnosis can be made by finding hypotonic urine in the presence of hypernatremia. To differentiate central from NDI, a dose of desmopressin (dDAVP) can be given and patients will have one of two responses: either the urine volume will fall and the urine concentration will rise (look for the urine osmolality to rise 200 mOsm/kg H_2O or above 600 mOsm/kg H_2O), indicating central DI (CDI), or nothing will happen to the urine concentration or flow rate, indicating NDI. (See **Table 20.1**).[19]

Central Diabetes Insipidus

CDI is due to damage or alteration in function of either the posterior pituitary or hypothalamus. Causes include: mass lesions, trauma, infiltrative disease, infections, ischemic diseases, and postsurgical damage.[20] Postsurgical CDI may follow a triphasic response:

1. Initially patients have diabetes insipidus with high urine output and a rising sodium because of the acute insult to the pituitary, preventing any release of ADH.

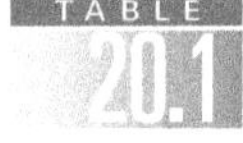

TABLE 20.1 dDAVP Challenge in Hypernatremia

Condition	Urine Osmolality Before dDAVP	Response to dDAVP
Normal	1,200 mOsm/kg H_2O, but may be lower in patients with CKD	No increase in urine osmolality or volume as patients are already at maximal ADH activity
Complete central diabetes insipidus	Below 290 mOsm/kg H_2O	Urine osmolality rises by 200 mOsm/kg H_2O and usually above 500 mOsm/kg H_2O
Complete nephrogenic diabetes insipidus		No change in urine osmolality
Partial central diabetes insipidus	400-500 mOsm/kg H_2O	Urine osmolality rises by 200 mOsm/kg H_2O
Partial nephrogenic diabetes insipidus		No change in urine osmolality

ADH, antidiuretic hormone; CKD, chronic kidney disease; dDAVP, desmopressin.

2. Following this, the pituitary breaks down, releasing stored ADH causing the second phase resembling syndrome of inappropriate antidiuretic hormone secretion (SIADH) with decreased urine output and falling serum sodium.
3. After that comes the final stage of permanent CDI when the patient can no longer produce or release ADH.

Patients with CDI following neurosurgery should get careful follow-up as many times this is only temporary and water balance improves in the perioperative period.

CDI is managed by pharmaceutical vasopressin 2 agonist, dDAVP. (See **Table 20.2**).

Nephrogenic Diabetes Insipidus

NDI is end-organ resistance to ADH. There are some rare congenital causes of NDI because of mutations in the V2 receptor or the aquaporin-2 channel. Additionally, the congenital salt wasting nephropathy, Bartter syndrome, will cause NDI. More common in the ICU will be acquired forms of DI. These can be drug induced, electrolyte induced, or during the recovery from acute kidney injury.

Drug-Induced Nephrogenic Diabetes Insipidus

The prototypical cause of NDI is lithium. Lithium causes NDI in 55% of long-term users.[19] Initially this NDI is reversible but eventually it becomes permanent. Loop diuretics prevent the generation of a concentrated medullary interstitium, essential for making urine hypertonic to plasma. Tolvaptan, an ADH antagonist used to slow the progression of polycystic kidney disease, causes NDI. Demeclocycline, foscarnet, and amphotericin B are also reported to cause NDI. See the systematic review by Garofeanu et al for a more thorough list of drugs that cause NDI.[21] Drug-induced NDI is generally reversible with stopping the offending agent.

Electrolyte-Induced Nephrogenic Diabetes Insipidus

Hypercalcemia and hypokalemia both cause NDI. Additionally, osmotic diuresis can resemble NDI, so correcting hyperglycemia and stopping mannitol can help. Additionally, SGLT2i cause glucosuria and have caused hypernatremia in at least one case.[22]

TABLE 20.2 Use of dDAVP

Oral dDAVP	IV	Nasal Spray
Start with 100 µg HS, titrate up to 200 µg to prevent nocturia Patients may need to increase the frequency to BID or TID to control polyuria	1-2 µg IV bid	10 µg per spray 1-4 sprays divided over three doses

dDAVP, desmopressin; IV, intravenous.

Recovery from AKI can cause NDI

As patients recover from AKI, they often go through a polyuric phase, during which time they are unable to concentrate their urine and are predisposed to hypernatremia, as well as hypokalemia and other electrolyte losses. This is especially common with postobstructive diuresis.[23]

References

1. Palevsky PM, Bhagrath R, Greenberg A. Hypernatremia in hospitalized patients. *Ann Intern Med.* 1996;124(2):197-203.
2. Funk G-C, Lindner G, Druml W, et al. Incidence and prognosis of dysnatremias present on ICU admission. *Intensive Care Med.* 2010;36(2):304-311.
3. Lindner G, Funk G-C, Schwarz C, et al. Hypernatremia in the critically ill is an independent risk factor for mortality. *Am J Kidney Dis.* 2007;50(6):952-957.
4. Liamis G, Filippatos TD, Elisaf MS. Evaluation and treatment of hypernatremia: a practical guide for physicians. *Postgrad Med.* 2016;128(3):299-306.
5. Hoorn EJ, De Vogel S, Zietse R. Insulin resistance in an 18-year-old patient with Down syndrome presenting with hyperglycaemic coma, hypernatraemia and rhabdomyolysis. *J Intern Med.* 2005;258(3):285-288.
6. Kozeny GA, Murdock DK, Euler DE, et al. In vivo effects of acute changes in osmolality and sodium concentration on myocardial contractility. *Am Heart J.* 1985;109(2):290-296.
7. Shah MK, Mandayam S, Adrogué HJ. Osmotic demyelination unrelated to hyponatremia. *Am J Kidney* Dis. 2018;71(3):436-440.
8. Darmon M, Timsit J-F, Francais A, et al. Association between hypernatraemia acquired in the ICU and mortality: a cohort study. *Nephrol Dial Transplant.* 2010;25(8):2510-2515.
9. O'Donoghue SD, Dulhunty JM, Bandeshe HK, Senthuran S, Gowardman JR. Acquired hypernatraemia is an independent predictor of mortality in critically ill patients. *Anaesthesia.* 2009;64(5):514-520.
10. Polderman KH, Schreuder WO, Strack van Schijndel RJ, Thijs LG. Hypernatremia in the intensive care unit: an indicator of quality of care? *Crit Care Med.* 1999;27(6):1105-1108.
11. Bratusch-Marrain PR, DeFronzo RA. Impairment of insulin-mediated glucose metabolism by hyperosmolality in man. *Diabetes.* 1983;32(11):1028-1034.
12. Adrogué HJ, Madias NE. Hypernatremia. *N Engl J Med.* 2000;342(20):1493-1499.
13. Chauhan K, Pattharanitima P, Patel N, et al. Rate of correction of hypernatremia and health outcomes in critically ill patients. *Clin J Am Soc Nephrol.* 2019;14(5):656-663.
14. Sterns RH. Evidence for managing hypernatremia. *Clin J Am Soc Nephrol.* 2019;14(5):645-647.
15. Bataille S, Baralla C, Torro D, et al. Undercorrection of hypernatremia is frequent and associated with mortality. *BMC Nephrol.* 2014;15:37.
16. Gordon CE, Vantzelfde S, Francis JM. Acetazolamide in lithium-induced nephrogenic diabetes insipidus. *N Engl J Med.* 2016;375(20):2008-2009.
17. Carlberg DJ, Borek HA, Syverud SA, Holstege CP. Survival of acute hypernatremia due to massive soy sauce ingestion. *J Emerg Med.* 2013;45(2):228-231.
18. Baugh JR, Krug EF, Weir MR. Punishment by salt poisoning. *South Med J.* 1983;76(4):540-541.
19. Sands JM, Bichet DG; American College of Physicians, American Physiological Society. Nephrogenic diabetes insipidus. *Ann Intern Med.* 2006;144(3):186-194.
20. Garrahy A, Moran C, Thompson CJ. Diagnosis and management of central diabetes insipidus in adults. *Clin Endocrinol.* 2019;90(1):23-30.
21. Garofeanu CG, Weir M, Rosas-Arellano MP, Henson G, Garg AX, Clark WF. Causes of reversible nephrogenic diabetes insipidus: a systematic review. *Am J Kidney Dis.* 2005;45(4):626-637.
22. Kaur A, Winters SJ. Severe hypercalcemia and hypernatremia in a patient treated with canagliflozin. *Endocrinol Diabetes Metab Case Rep.* 2015;2015:150042.
23. Moeller HB, Rittig S, Fenton RA. Nephrogenic diabetes insipidus: essential insights into the molecular background and potential therapies for treatment. *Endocr Rev.* 2013;34(2):278-301.

21 Dyskalemias in the Intensive Care Unit

Benjamin Ko

Hypokalemia and hyperkalemia are among the most common electrolyte disorders encountered in the intensive care unit (ICU). Nearly 50% of ICU patients have hyperkalemia alone and hypokalemia, hyperkalemia, and potassium variability are independently associated with increased mortality.[1,2] Furthermore, potassium concentrations are a strong predictor of all-cause mortality 30 days following admission to the ICU.[3] Although potassium is the most abundant cation in the human body, only a small fraction resides within the serum. The remaining 98% is intracellular; this difference (60 mEq intracellularly vs 3,000 mEq extracellularly) is the primary determinant of cellular resting membrane potential. As such, serum potassium must be tightly regulated, and both hypokalemia and hyperkalemia require immediate attention in the ICU.

NORMAL POTASSIUM HOMEOSTASIS

The vast difference between intracellular and extracellular potassium concentrations is maintained by the action of Na^+/K^+-ATPase, the activity of which is regulated by insulin, catecholamines, osmolality, and acid-base status. Insulin and β-adrenergic stimulation promote K^+ influx in cells, whereas α-adrenergic stimulation and increased tonicity stimulate K^+ efflux.[4-6] The relationship between acid-base and K^+ is more complex, with a mineral acidosis (nongap acidosis) causing K^+ efflux to a far greater extent than an organic acidosis (lactic acidosis) or a respiratory acidosis.

In the kidney, potassium is freely filtered and reabsorbed in the proximal tubule and thick ascending limb.[7,8] Under conditions of hypokalemia, further potassium reabsorption can occur in the intercalated cells of the collecting duct.[7,8] Potassium is secreted in the collecting duct via the renal outer medulla potassium (ROMK) channel in principal cells and big potassium (BK) channels in the principal and intercalated cells, stimulated by aldosterone and high tubular flow rates.[7,8] These generally opposing stimuli for potassium secretion allow for adequate potassium secretion, independent of volume status.[8]

HYPOKALEMIA

Clinical Sequelae

Hypokalemia is defined as a serum K^+ concentration less than 3.5 mEq/L. The clinical manifestations of hypokalemia correlate well with the severity of hypokalemia. Muscle weakness and rhabdomyolysis typically occur with serum K levels of 2.5 mEq/L, whereas the feared ICU complication of respiratory muscle weakness is rare until serum K reaches 2.0 mEq/L or less.[9,10] Impaired renal electrolyte handling and glucose intolerance are also the known complications of hypokalemia, but these effects are more chronic in nature.

By contrast, cardiac conduction abnormalities do not correlate with the degree of hypokalemia.[11] Thus, premature atrial and ventricular beats, sinus bradycardia, junctional rhythms, atrioventricular (AV) block, and ventricular tachycardia occur variably with hypokalemia.[12] The presence of digoxin, magnesium depletion, or cardiac ischemia has been shown to potentiate hypokalemic arrhythmias.[13] Electrocardiogram (ECG) findings are classic: ST-segment depression, decreased T-wave amplitude, and increased U-wave amplitude (**Figure 21.1**).[12,14]

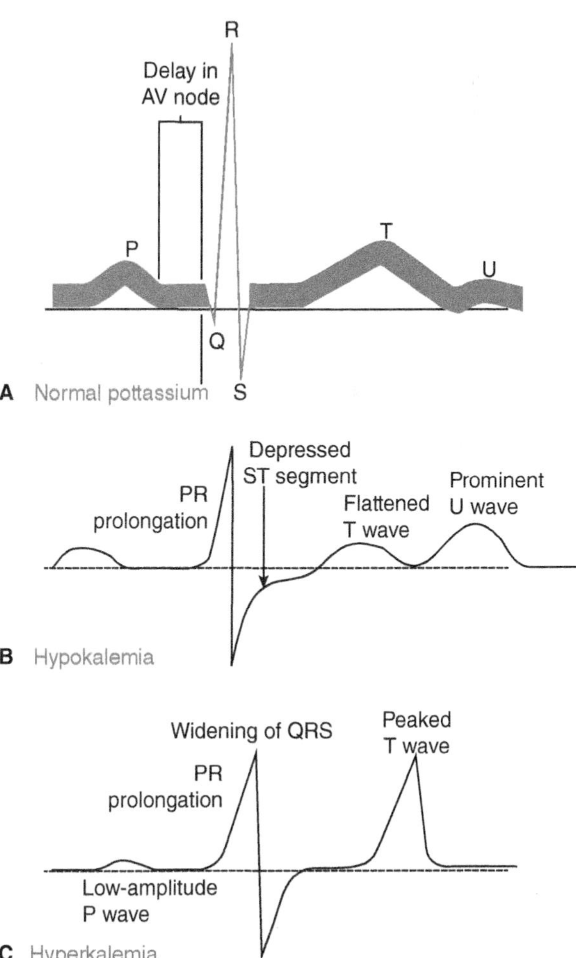

FIGURE 21.1: Electrocardiogram changes in hypokalemia/hyperkalemia. AV, atrioventricular.

Etiologies/Diagnosis

Hypokalemia is typically caused by a disruption in normal potassium handling at any or all sites, decreased intake, increased excretion, or increased intracellular shift. The most common etiologies are listed in **Table 21.1**.

The diagnosis of the cause of hypokalemia is based on history, physical examination, and laboratory evaluation. An assessment of renal response is useful in determining the etiology of hypokalemia. A 24-hour urinary potassium measurement of less than 25 mEq/d is a normal renal response to hypokalemia, but spot determinations of renal potassium handling are more useful in an ICU setting. These, however, are limited by urinary concentration and so they need to be indexed.

A spot K^+-to-creatinine (Cr) ratio can be used. A urinary K^+/Cr less than 13 mEq/mg Cr (2.5 mEq/mmol Cr) is an appropriate renal response to hypokalemia.[15] Values greater than this suggest renal potassium wasting.[15]

Alternatively, the transtubular K^+ gradient (TTKG) of less than 3 in the setting of hypokalemia is a normal response to hypokalemia.[16] The TTKG, however, requires that the urine osmolality be greater than the serum osmolality and the urinary sodium be greater than 25 mEq/L. In addition, the TTKG assumes that there is no appreciable solute reabsorption in the medullary collecting duct so that any increase in osmolality is due purely to water reabsorption. Because there is urea reabsorption in this segment, the validity of the TTKG has been called into question.[17]

$$\text{TTKG} = ((\text{urine } [K^+]/\text{serum } [K^+]) / (\text{urine osmolality}/\text{serum osmolality}))$$[18]

Treatment

Not surprisingly, except in the cases of hypokalemia caused by cellular shift (Table 21.1), treatment of hypokalemia consists primarily of potassium repletion. Of the various available formulations, potassium chloride is the preferred agent. Oral KCl administration is preferred and gives a peak increase of 1 to 1.5 mEq/L with a 40 to 60 mEq dose.[19] Intravenous KCl can also be used but should be given with

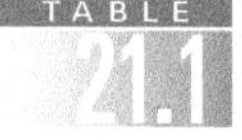

Common Causes of Hypokalemia in the Intensive Care Unit

Decreased Intake	Increased Renal Excretion	Increased Extrarenal Excretion	Cellular Shift
Malnutrition	Diuretic use	Diarrhea	Alkalosis
Malabsorption	Metabolic alkalosis	Fistulas	β-agonist
Alcoholism	Urinary ketones	Bowel resection/ostomy	Insulin
	Hypomagnesemia	Excessive perspiration	Periodic paralysis
	Mineralocorticoid excess		Thyrotoxicosis
			Theophylline/caffeine

saline rather than dextrose because the dextrose will stimulate insulin secretion and increased intracellular shift of potassium. Rates of infusion can be as high as 20 to 40 mEq/hr, although great caution needs to be used during administration at these rates.[20]

In addition to potassium repletion, attention should be given to the serum magnesium level. Magnesium normally acts to inhibit potassium secretion, and so in hypomagnesemia, there is obligate renal potassium wasting.[21]

Although rare, hypokalemia because of intracellular redistribution of potassium as in the case of thyrotoxic periodic paralysis or hypokalemic periodic paralysis can often result in severe rebound hyperkalemia; therefore, all hypokalemic patients need careful monitoring of serum potassium levels following treatment.

HYPERKALEMIA

Clinical Sequelae

Hyperkalemia is defined as a serum K^+ concentration greater than 5.3 mEq/L. Elevated serum potassium can cause muscle weakness and metabolic acidosis, but most concerningly, hyperkalemia is associated with conduction abnormalities and arrhythmias, most notably sinus bradycardia, sinus arrest, slow idioventricular rhythms, ventricular tachycardia, ventricular fibrillation, and asystole.

A number of ECG abnormalities are seen with hyperkalemia (peaked T waves, shortened QT interval, lengthened PR and QRS), but interestingly, ECG changes do not correlate well with the degree of hyperkalemia (Figure 21.1).[14,22] The chronicity of the hyperkalemia seems to provide a protective effect of hyperkalemia, but how this occurs is not well understood. The unpredictability and severity of hyperkalemia's effects on the heart make hyperkalemia a true medical emergency.

Etiologies and Diagnosis

Hyperkalemia is typically caused by a decreased potassium excretion or increased intracellular shift of potassium. The most common causes are listed in **Table 21.2**. Unlike with hypokalemia, dietary intake rarely causes hyperkalemia alone in the absence of advanced chronic kidney disease (CKD) or end-stage kidney disease (ESKD).

Prior to the diagnosis of the etiology of hyperkalemia, pseudohyperkalemia must be ruled out. This is commonly due to cellular hemolysis during the blood draw, but also occurs with thrombocytosis or marked leukocytosis.[23]

As in the case of hyperkalemia, the renal contribution to hyperkalemia can be assessed using the TTKG (with its associated caveats). Here, a TTKG less than 6 is consistent with impaired renal secretion and, ultimately, excretion of potassium.[16,24] It is, however, important to note that potassium balance is the net effect of intake, cellular distribution, and renal secretion, and so except in cases of extreme reductions of renal potassium secretion (e.g., anuric acute kidney injury [AKI] and ESRD), hyperkalemia is generally multifactorial in nature. In mild-to-moderate CKD, there is K^+ adaptation that enhances renal tubular K^+ secretion such that hyperkalemia is unusual by itself until glomerular filtration rate (GFR) falls below 10 mL/min.[25] As such, in most cases of hyperkalemia, examination of the TTKG (and more specifically the urine potassium) should not be relied on for clinical decision making.

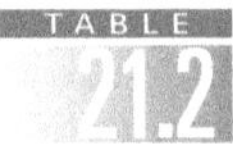

Common Causes of Hyperkalemia in the Intensive Care Unit

Increased Intake	Decreased Renal Excretion	Cellular Shift
Diet	AKI	Inorganic acidemia
Potassium supplementation	Advanced CKD	Cell ischemia/necrosis
Tube feeds	Volume depletion	Rhabdomyolysis
TPN	Effective decreased circulating volume	Tumor lysis
Blood transfusions	ACE inhibitors/ARBs	Hemolysis
	Hypoaldosteronism	Insulin deficiency
	Heparin	Digoxin
	Triamterene	Succinylcholine
	Spironolactone	
	Calcineurin inhibitors	
	Amiloride	

ACE, angiotensin-converting enzyme; AKI, acute kidney injury; ARBs, angiotensin receptor blockers; CKD, chronic kidney disease; TPN, total parenteral nutrition.

Treatment

Hyperkalemia is a true medical emergency, and prompt attention is required. Acutely, the treatment is the same, regardless of the etiology, and so treatment should be initiated as soon as it is recognized (**Figure 21.2; Table 21.3**).

Calcium acts to stabilize the cardiac membrane and acts as a buffer against the cardiac conduction abnormalities seen with hyperkalemia and normalize the ECG. Theoretically, calcium chloride is more effective than gluconate because of a higher availability of free calcium, but calcium gluconate is the agent of choice because of a higher rate of vein sclerosis with calcium chloride. Calcium should be re-dosed if ECG changes persist and every hour thereafter until hyperkalemia is resolved.

Insulin, albuterol, and sodium bicarbonate all act by inducing a transcellular shift of potassium. Insulin acts within 15 minutes, with a peak effect by 1 hour.[26] It should be administered with dextrose to prevent hypoglycemia, typically 10 units of insulin along with 25 g of dextrose. Albuterol acts by stimulating β2 receptors.[27] Its use is often limited by its major side effect of tachycardia. Bicarbonate is classically thought of as inducing a transcellular shift of potassium, but at the doses commonly given (50 to 100 mEq), this has not been shown to be effective.[26,28] These agents can work together, but owing to their similar mechanisms of action, the effects are additive and not synergistic.[29]

Oral agents such as sodium polystyrene (SPS), patiromer, and zirconium cyclosilicate bind intestinal potassium and can be helpful in removing potassium from the body.[30-32] Although commonly used in clinical practice, there remains

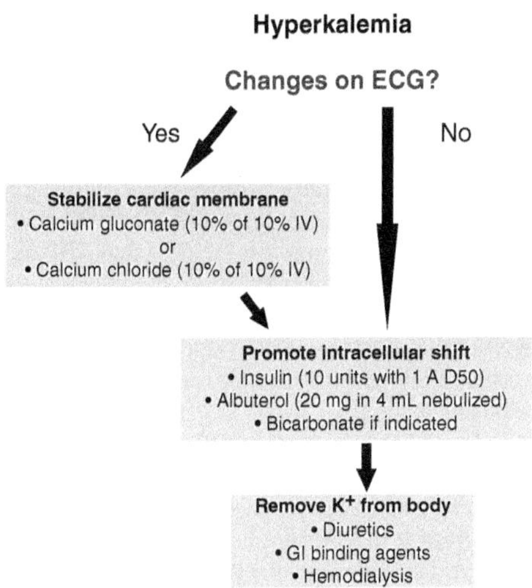

FIGURE 21.2: Approach to the treatment of hyperkalemia. ECG, electrocardiogram; GI, gastrointestinal; IV, intravenous.

controversy in their onset of action and best use. SPS has been shown in historic studies to be effective in lowering serum K chronically, whereas more recent studies have shown little impact of SPS on serum K.[33,34] Patiromer may have a role in the acute treatment of hyperkalemia, but the data have yet to establish this. Zirconium cyclosilicate is effective in both CKD and ESKD and has been shown to lower potassium as early as 1 hour in studies, but this has not been established in a hyperkalemic ICU population.[31,35] While published data around their use in the setting of AKI or ICU is lacking, anectdotally they are tolerated in hospitalized patients and we anticipate future studies evaluating their efficacy in this patient population.

As potassium secretion is dependent on both aldosterone and distal sodium delivery, agents that cause a mismatch of high aldosterone and high distal

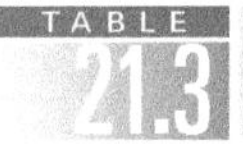

TABLE 21.3 Agents for Acute Treatment of Hyperkalemia

Treatment	Dose	Peak Onset	Duration
Calcium	1 g as Ca gluconate or chloride	Immediate	60 min
Insulin/dextrose	10 units insulin/25 g dextrose	1 hr	6 hr
Albuterol	10 mg in 5 mL nebulized treatment	1-2 hr	3-6 hr
Sodium bicarbonate	400 mEq	3 hr	6+ hr
Sodium polystyrene sulfate	15-30 g (orally or rectally)	2 hr	4-6 hr
Zirconium cyclosilicate	10 g	1 hr	6+ hr

sodium delivery, such as loop diuretics, are an attractive therapy for hyperkalemic patients without severe kidney impairment. Despite this, no published data show clear acute increase in kaliuresis with diuretic therapy.

In the case of continued life-threatening hyperkalemia, despite the above-mentioned treatments or in the case of severe kidney impairment, dialysis should be utilized to lower serum potassium. Studies have shown that dialysis is the quickest method to remove potassium, lowering K by 1.34 mEq/L at 1 hour and 60 to 140 mEq total over a 4-hour session.[26,36] The use of a 1K dialysate bath is controversial owing to concerns of precipitating arrhythmias. However, the association between sudden cardiac death and 1K dialysate was not seen in the ICU population but seen in the chronic ESRD population.[37,38] Furthermore, a randomized crossover study showed that premature ventricular contractions (PVCs) decreased during dialysis using a 1K bath.[37,39,40] For patients who cannot tolerate intermittent hemodialysis (IHD), continuous kidney replacement therapy (CKRT) has been shown to be an effective treatment.[41]

With dialysis and, to some degree, gastrointestinal (GI)-binding agents and diuretics, serum potassium levels rebound some 6 hours after treatment because of a lowered serum K and a favorable electrochemical gradient for extracellular shifts of potassium.[42] This effect is often magnified by agents that cause intracellular shifts of potassium, such as insulin and albuterol, resulting in clinically significant rebound hyperkalemia. In the case of ongoing hemolysis, cell death, or rhabdomyolysis, these effects may require frequent repeated IHD or perhaps transition to CKRT to maintain normokalemia.

Once hyperkalemia has been treated acutely, chronic management of hyperkalemia is largely aimed at identifying underlying causes and removing exacerbating conditions whenever possible. In addition, oral potassium-binding agents, as previously discussed, under acute treatment can indeed be used chronically. SPS sulfate is still commonly used for this purpose, often given 1 to 2 times/day, although there are recent concerns regarding its safety.[43,44] Zirconium cyclosilicate (Lokelma) performs well in the chronic setting.[31] Patiromer (Veltassa), which has limited use acutely, also represents a well-tolerated chronic option.[30,32]

SUMMARY

- Disorders of potassium handling are common in the ICU and associated with significant mortality.
- Dyskalemias are due to disturbances in potassium intake, cellular shifts, and renal potassium handling.
- Spot urinary potassium-to-Cr ratios or TTKG can be used to determine the contribution of renal handling to the dyskalemia.
- Prompt treatment of hypokalemia and hyperkalemia is essential.

References

1. Hessels L, Hoekstra M, Mijzen LJ, et al. The relationship between serum potassium, potassium variability and in-hospital mortality in critically ill patients and a before-after analysis on the impact of computer-assisted potassium control. *Crit Care.* 2015;19:4.
2. Tongyoo S, Viarasilpa T, Permpikul C. Serum potassium levels and outcomes in critically ill patients in the medical intensive care unit. *J Int Med Res.* 2018;46:1254-1262.
3. McMahon GM, Mendu ML, Gibbons FK, et al. Association between hyperkalemia at critical care initiation and mortality. *Intensive Care Med.* 2012;38:1834-1842.
4. Palmer BF, Clegg DJ. Electrolyte and acid-base disturbances in patients with diabetes mellitus. *N Engl J Med.* 2015;373:548-559.

5. Williams ME, Gervino EV, Rosa RM, et al. Catecholamine modulation of rapid potassium shifts during exercise. *N Engl J Med.* 1985;312:823-827.
6. Zierler KL, Rabinowitz D. Effect of very small concentrations of insulin on forearm metabolism. Persistence of its action on potassium and free fatty acids without its effect on glucose. *J Clin Invest.* 1964;43:950-962.
7. Giebisch G, Wang W. Potassium transport: from clearance to channels and pumps. *Kidney Int.* 1996;49:1624-1631.
8. Palmer BF. Regulation of potassium homeostasis. *Clin J Am Soc Nephrol.* 2015;10:1050-1060.
9. Comi G, Testa D, Cornelio F, et al. Potassium depletion myopathy: a clinical and morphological study of six cases. *Muscle Nerve.* 1985;8:17-21.
10. Shintani S, Shiigai T, Tsukagoshi H. Marked hypokalemic rhabdomyolysis with myoglobinuria due to diuretic treatment. *Eur Neurol.* 1991;31:396-398.
11. Siegel D, Hulley SB, Black DM, et al. Diuretics, serum and intracellular electrolyte levels, and ventricular arrhythmias in hypertensive men. *JAMA.* 1992;267:1083-1089.
12. Helfant RH. Hypokalemia and arrhythmias. *Am J Med.* 1986;80:13-22.
13. Shapiro W. Correlative studies of serum digitalis levels and the arrhythmias of digitalis intoxication. *Am J Cardiol.* 1978;41:852-859.
14. Porth CM. *Essentials of Pathophysiology.* 3rd ed. Wolters Kluwer/Lippincott Williams and Wilkins; 2011.
15. Lin SH, Lin YF, Chen DT, et al. Laboratory tests to determine the cause of hypokalemia and paralysis. *Arch Intern Med.* 2004;164:1561-1566.
16. Ethier JH, Kamel KS, Magner PO, et al. The transtubular potassium concentration in patients with hypokalemia and hyperkalemia. *Am J Kidney Dis.* 1990;15:309-315.
17. Kamel KS, Halperin ML. Intrarenal urea recycling leads to a higher rate of renal excretion of potassium: an hypothesis with clinical implications. *Curr Opin Nephrol Hypertens.* 2011;20:547-554.
18. West ML, Marsden PA, Richardson RM, et al. New clinical approach to evaluate disorders of potassium excretion. *Miner Electrolyte Metab.* 1986;12:234-238.
19. Keith NM, Osterberg AE, Burchell HB. Some effects of potassium salts in man. *Ann Intern Med.* 1942;16:879-892.
20. Hamill RJ, Robinson LM, Wexler HR, et al. Efficacy and safety of potassium infusion therapy in hypokalemic critically ill patients. *Crit Care Med.* 1991;19:694-699.
21. Huang CL, Kuo E. Mechanism of hypokalemia in magnesium deficiency. *J Am Soc Nephrol.* 2007;18:2649-2652.
22. Montague BT, Ouellette JR, Buller GK. Retrospective review of the frequency of ECG changes in hyperkalemia. *Clin J Am Soc Nephrol.* 2008;3:324-330.
23. Palmer BF, Clegg DJ. Hyperkalemia. *JAMA.* 2015;314:2405-2406.
24. Palmer BF, Clegg DJ. The use of selected urine chemistries in the diagnosis of kidney disorders. *Clin J Am Soc Nephrol.* 2019;14(2):306-316.
25. Stanton BA. Renal potassium transport: morphological and functional adaptations. *Am J Physiol.* 1989;257:R989-R997.
26. Blumberg A, Weidmann P, Shaw S, et al. Effect of various therapeutic approaches on plasma potassium and major regulating factors in terminal renal failure. *Am J Med.* 1988;85:507-512.
27. Allon M, Dunlay R, Copkney C. Nebulized albuterol for acute hyperkalemia in patients on hemodialysis. *Ann Intern Med.* 1989;110:426-429.
28. Allon M, Shanklin N. Effect of bicarbonate administration on plasma potassium in dialysis patients: interactions with insulin and albuterol. *Am J Kidney Dis.* 1996;28:508-514.
29. Allon M, Copkney C. Albuterol and insulin for treatment of hyperkalemia in hemodialysis patients. *Kidney Int.* 1990;38:869-872.
30. Bakris GL, Pitt B, Weir MR, et al. Effect of Patiromer on serum potassium level in patients with hyperkalemia and diabetic kidney disease: the AMETHYST-DN Randomized Clinical Trial. *JAMA.* 2015;314:151-161.
31. Kosiborod M, Rasmussen HS, Lavin P, et al. Effect of sodium zirconium cyclosilicate on potassium lowering for 28 days among outpatients with hyperkalemia: the HARMONIZE randomized clinical trial. *JAMA.* 2014;312:2223-2233.
32. Weir MR, Bakris GL, Bushinsky DA, et al. Patiromer in patients with kidney disease and hyperkalemia receiving RAAS inhibitors. *N Engl J Med.* 2015;372:211-221.
33. Batterink J, Lin J, Au-Yeung SHM, et al. Effectiveness of sodium polystyrene sulfonate for short-term treatment of hyperkalemia. *Can J Hosp Pharm.* 2015;68:296-303.
34. Scherr L, Ogden DA, Mead AW, et al. Management of hyperkalemia with a cation-exchange resin. *N Engl J Med.* 1961;264:115-119.
35. Fishbane S, Ford M, Fukagawa M, et al. A phase 3b, randomized, double-blind, placebo-controlled study of sodium zirconium cyclosilicate for reducing the incidence of predialysis hyperkalemia. *J Am Soc Nephrol.* 2019;30:1723-1733.

36. Ahmed J, Weisberg LS. Hyperkalemia in dialysis patients. *Semin Dial.* 2001;14:348-356.
37. Karnik JA, Young BS, Lew NL, et al. Cardiac arrest and sudden death in dialysis units. *Kidney Int.* 2001;60:50-357.
38. Pun PH, Lehrich RW, Honeycutt EF, et al. Modifiable risk factors associated with sudden cardiac arrest within hemodialysis clinics. *Kidney Int.* 2011;79:218-227.
39. Hou S, McElroy PA, Nootens J, et al. Safety and efficacy of low-potassium dialysate. *Am J Kidney Dis.* 1989;13:137-143.
40. Redaelli B, Locatelli F, Limido D, et al. Effect of a new model of hemodialysis potassium removal on the control of ventricular arrhythmias. *Kidney Int.* 1996;50:609-617.
41. John AK, Raghavan M, Mitra KN. *Indications, Timing, and Patient Selection Continuous Renal Replacement Therapy.* Oxford: Oxford University Press.
42. Blumberg A, Roser HW, Zehnder C, et al. Plasma potassium in patients with terminal renal failure during and after haemodialysis; relationship with dialytic potassium removal and total body potassium. *Nephrol Dial Transplant.* 1997;12:1629-1634.
43. Abraham SC, Bhagavan BS, Lee LA, et al. Upper gastrointestinal tract injury in patients receiving kayexalate (sodium polystyrene sulfonate) in sorbitol: clinical, endoscopic, and histopathologic findings. *Am J Surg Pathol.* 2001;25:637-644.
44. Harel Z, Harel S, Shah PS, et al. Gastrointestinal adverse events with sodium polystyrene sulfonate (Kayexalate) use: a systematic review. *Am J Med.* 2013;126:264.e29-264.e24.

22

Calcium Management in the Intensive Care Unit

Anna L. Zisman

Calcium is a divalent cation critical for homeostasis. In addition to being a core component of the bony skeleton, calcium modulates the activation threshold of Na^+ channels, including those responsible for cardiac action potentials, neurologic activity, muscle function, and bowel motility. In its role as a second messenger, it regulates countless intracellular proteins, while also playing a central role in cell injury and death.[1] Serum calcium levels are tightly regulated by parathyroid hormone (PTH), vitamin D (calcitriol), and, to a lesser degree, calcitonin. These endocrine factors modify calcium movement across the gastrointestinal (GI) mucosa, kidney tubules, and bone.[2]

More than 99% of the body's calcium stores are in the skeleton, whereas less than 1% is found intracellularly. Only 0.1% of total calcium is found in the extracellular fluid (ECF), which is the compartment accessed via laboratory testing. Within the ECF, approximately 50% of calcium is in the form of ionized calcium, the biologically active form. Approximately 45% of calcium is protein bound, with the remainder complexed to anions, such as citrate, phosphate, sulfate, and bicarbonate.[2] The ionized calcium fraction is thus dependent on the serum pH and protein concentrations, with hypoalbuminemia and acidosis increasing the ionized calcium.[3,4] In the setting of a low serum albumin, adjusted serum calcium can be estimated[4]:

$$\text{Corrected calcium} = \text{Serum calcium} + 0.8 \times (4.0 - \text{serum albumin [g/dL]})$$

However, poor correlation between estimated calcium and measured ionized calcium values is not uncommon in the critical care setting. Disturbances in acid-base status or changes in total serum protein, common in the critically ill, will not lead to changes in the total serum calcium concentration, so potentially significant changes in the biologically active ionized calcium concentration may be missed with routine serum testing in the intensive care unit (ICU).[5] Owing to these concerns, critical care teams often rely on measurement of ionized calcium.[6]

EPIDEMIOLOGY AND SIGNIFICANCE OF ABNORMALITIES IN SERUM CALCIUM IN CRITICAL CARE

Perturbations in ionized calcium levels are common in the critical care setting and are present in more than 50% of patients at some juncture during their ICU stay.[7-9] Most often, however, these abnormalities are not due to significant underlying disorders of calcium homeostasis, but rather reflect the critically ill state.[8,10,11] Mostly, the abnormality is hypocalcemia, which has been repeatedly identified as a risk factor for ICU mortality.[7,8,11,12] More recent studies have noted an attenuated mortality effect once adjusted for the significant correlation of ionized hypocalcemia with illness severity scores.[7,8]

HYPOCALCEMIA IN THE INTENSIVE CARE UNIT

Clinical Manifestations

The clinical symptoms of hypocalcemia are dependent on the severity and chronicity of the abnormality. The classic complication of tetany reflects neuromuscular irritability.[7] Early symptoms include perioral numbness, paresthesias of the distal extremities, and muscle cramps. More severe symptoms can include focal or generalized seizures, bronchospasm, and arrhythmia resulting from prolongation of the QT interval.[13] Patients who have had a chronic course with gradual decline in serum values may note fatigue, irritability, anxiety, and depression or may be asymptomatic.

Differential Diagnosis

The differential diagnosis of hypocalcemia is broad (**Table 22.1**), though, as noted earlier, the vast majority of patients who are critically ill do not have an underlying abnormality of calcium homeostasis. Although the etiology of hypocalcemia is sometimes obvious, such as in the patient post parathyroidectomy or a radical neck dissection, the general approach to evaluation of hypocalcemia is to ascertain whether the PTH values are low or high (Table 22.1). Further evaluation can proceed as appropriate based on the results and clinical picture.

In critically ill patients with hypocalcemia, the etiology of hypocalcemia may remain indeterminate in more than 50%.[11] Sepsis has been strongly associated with the presence of hypocalcemia,[14-16] with vitamin D deficiency and resistance,[16,17] acquired hypoparathyroidism,[18,19] and 1-alpha-hydroxylase deficiency all implicated as potential mechanisms in the inflammatory state.[16]

Treatment

The approach to therapy of hypocalcemia in the ICU is contingent on the degree of hypocalcemia, severity of symptoms, and etiology.

For patients with severe hypocalcemia who are acutely symptomatic with tetany, arrhythmia, or seizure, administration of 100 to 200 mg of elemental calcium over 10 to 20 minutes is warranted, followed by a calcium infusion of 0.5 to 1.5 mg elemental calcium/kg/hr to prevent rebound hypocalcemia.[11,20] The two commonly used calcium solutions are 10% calcium chloride (272 mg elemental calcium per 10 mL vial) and 10% calcium gluconate (90 mg elemental calcium per 10 mL vial).[11,20] Both solutions are hyperosmolar and should be administered via a central vein, if possible. If injecting peripherally, calcium gluconate is the preferred agent.[11,20] Patients receiving intravenous calcium administration need to be closely monitored because infusions of calcium may precipitate bradycardia and cardiac arrhythmias.[11,20] As magnesium depletion contributes to hypocalcemia and is common in the critical care setting, it must be corrected concurrently.[11,21] Serum levels of 25-hydroxyvitamin D should also be checked and repleted, and treatment with activated vitamin D (calcitriol) can be considered to increase intestinal absorption of calcium to facilitate earlier liberation from continuous calcium infusion.[11,20]

Treatment of critically ill hypocalcemic patients who are asymptomatic is controversial. Hypocalcemia has been associated with cardiac dysfunction and hypotension,[16,22] and calcium administration has been noted to improve blood

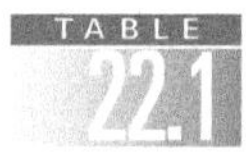

TABLE 22.1 Differential Diagnosis of Hypocalcemia in Adults

Associated with low PTH
- Loss of active parathyroid tissue
  - Postsurgical (thyroid, parathyroid, neck dissection)
  - Autoimmune
  - Infiltrative
  - Genetic disorders
    - X-linked or autosomal recessive hypoparathyroidism
    - DiGeorge syndrome
- Abnormal PTH regulation
  - Hypomagnesemia
  - X-linked or autosomal recessive hypoparathyroidism
  - Mutations in calcium-sensing receptor (CaSR)

Associated with high PTH
- Chronic kidney disease
- Vitamin D deficiency
- PTH resistance (pseudohypoparathyroidism)
- Critical illness or sepsis
- Extravascular deposition
  - Acute pancreatitis
  - Rhabdomyolysis
  - Hyperphosphatemia
  - Metastatic osteoblastic disease

Medications or therapies
- Parenteral phosphate supplementation
- Bisphosphonates
- Denosumab
- Calcimimetics
- Foscarnet
- Pentamidine
- Cisplatin
- Doxorubicin
- Aminoglycosides
- Citrate (massive blood transfusion, pheresis, dialysis)

PTH, parathyroid hormone.

pressure and ventricular function in ICU patients with ionized calcium less than 1.05 mmol/L.[23] However, a 2008 Cochrane review that included five randomized controlled trials with 159 subjects found no clear evidence that calcium supplementation impacted outcomes in critically ill patients,[24] as none of the studies evaluated mortality, organ dysfunction, or length of hospital stay. Furthermore, data suggest that the hypocalcemia of the critically ill is not amenable to treatment.[25] In one study, during a single month at one hospital, there were approximately 4,700 ionized calcium tests performed, of which about half were abnormal. During the same time frame, approximately 20,000 of 10-mL vials of calcium gluconate were dispensed. The authors noted only a minimal effect of the intravenous administration of calcium on the subsequent ionized calcium levels.[25,26] Some data indicate that repletion of calcium may, in fact, be harmful, because several animal models of sepsis have demonstrated increased mortality with calcium supplementation.[27-29] Mortality was also significantly higher with calcium supplementation in a retrospective cohort study of critically ill patients in Pittsburgh with ionized hypocalcemia.[27] Of the 526 patients with sepsis and an ionized calcium measurement, 377 (72%) were hypocalcemic. Ninety-three patients received intravenous calcium supplementation during their ICU stay. After adjusting for severity of illness and other comorbidities, those who had received calcium supplementation had an increased risk of death, an increased risk of kidney dysfunction, and a significant decrease in ventilator-free days.[27]

Special circumstances of hypocalcemia that may warrant a targeted treatment approach where supplementation is reasonable include hypocalcemia secondary to hemodialysis or due to chelation with citrate during a massive transfusion protocol (MTP).[25] In secondary analysis of a large trial of patients with acute kidney injury (AKI) requiring kidney replacement therapy, severe hypocalcemia predicted mortality even with adjustment for disease severity, though it is unknown whether calcium repletion would modify this relationship.[30] In the setting of trauma-associated MTP, lower ionized calcium values are also associated with higher mortality (and higher transfusion volumes).[31] The optimal calcium replacement strategy during MTP remains uncertain; however, it is likely that at least 2 g of calcium chloride (~6 g of calcium gluconate) is needed for every 2 to 4 units of blood products transfused, especially if a transfusion requirement of greater than 15 units is anticipated. This is particularly relevant if hepatic function is impaired, further compromising citrate metabolism, though it is unknown whether repletion impacts morbidity and mortality.[31]

HYPERCALCEMIA

Clinical Manifestations

Clinical manifestations of hypercalcemia are diverse and involve multiple organ systems, with higher serum concentrations increasing the likelihood of symptoms. Generally, patients are asymptomatic below serum calcium levels of 11.5 mg/dL, with levels above that necessitating more urgent correction owing to the risks of complications. With higher levels, altered mental status with somnolence, confusion, and psychosis may be present from the neurologic perspective, whereas the cardiovascular signs may include hypertension and arrhythmias with shortening of the QT interval, heart block, and cardiac arrest. Notably, hypercalcemia may increase the risk of digitalis toxicity (see Chapter 27). The GI symptoms may include constipation, nausea and vomiting, loss of appetite, abdominal pain, pancreatitis, and peptic ulcer disease. Acute and chronic kidney disease may be present, along with kidney stones and nephrocalcinosis. Polyuria and polydipsia may be noted because of an inability to maximally concentrate the urine. This stems from a calcium-mediated downregulation of aquaporin-2 channels[32] and inhibition of the $Na^+K^+:2Cl^-$ cotransporter,[33] leading to perturbation of the countercurrent concentrating mechanism. Bone pain, fractures, and loss of bone mineralization leading to osteoporosis may complicate the clinical course.

Differential Diagnosis

Although there is a broad differential of hypercalcemia (**Table 22.2**), by far, the most common etiologies in a hospitalized patient are primary hyperparathyroidism and malignancy-associated hypercalcemia. In the ICU setting, prolonged

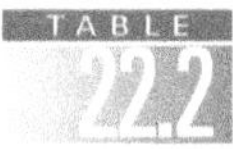

Differential Diagnosis of Hypercalcemia

PTH-Dependent Hypercalcemia
- Primary hyperparathyroidism
  - Sporadic
    - Adenoma or hyperplasia
  - Familial
    - Isolated primary hyperparathyroidism
    - Associated with multiple endocrine neoplasia I or II
- Tertiary hyperparathyroidism
- Lithium
- Familial hypocalciuric hypercalcemia

PTH-Independent Hypercalcemia
- Malignancy
  - Endocrine hypercalcemia
    - PTH-related protein
    - 1,25-hydroxyvitamin D excess
  - Malignant osteolysis
    - Diffuse marrow infiltration
    - Bony metastases with cytokine release
- Prolonged immobilization
- Parenteral nutrition
- Granulomatous disease
  - Sarcoidosis
  - Tuberculosis
  - Coccidioidomycosis
- Endocrine disorders
  - Hyperthyroidism
  - Adrenal insufficiency
  - Acromegaly
  - Pheochromocytoma
- Medications
  - Vitamin D and vitamin D analogs
  - Calcium (milk-alkali syndrome)
  - Vitamin A
  - Thiazide diuretics

PTH, parathyroid hormone.

immobility and parenteral nutrition may also contribute. Diagnostically, it is important to determine whether the disease process is PTH dependent versus independent, with additional testing proceeding depending on the results.

Management

General

Treatment of hypercalcemia in the ICU is dependent on the etiology and severity of hypercalcemia, degree of symptoms, and underlying comorbidities, including hypoalbuminemia and congestive heart failure. Initial management should generally include removal of any offending agents, such as calcium supplements, and volume resuscitation that will ultimately result in a saline (and calcium) diuresis, as long as no signs of volume overload are present. Although patients in the ICU with mild hypercalcemia (albumin-adjusted serum calcium <12 mg/dL [3 mmol/L]) may be asymptomatic and do not require urgent therapy, clinicians should be cognizant of the values when choosing fluid strategies or addition of potential offending agents. Those with moderate hypercalcemia (albumin-adjusted serum calcium <14 mg/dL [3.5 mmol/L]) and severe hypercalcemia (albumin-adjusted serum calcium >14 mg/dL [3.5 mmol/L]) typically require fluids and additional medical therapy. Consideration of likely underlying diagnosis and overall clinical course should guide clinical judgment on treatment selection.

Intravenous Fluids and Diuretics

Targets of 4 to 6 L of intravenous isotonic fluid administration during the first 24 hours have historically been advised, though limited data support these recommendations.[34-37] More recently, recommendations target infusion rates of 200 to 300 mL/hr initially until volume replete, then decreasing to rates targeting urine outputs of 100 to 150 mL/hr.[38,39] In those with hypoalbuminemia, particularly those with advanced malignancy, it may be prudent to limit the rate of infusion to 75 to 150 mL/hr to limit further complications.[40] Traditionally, concomitant use of high-dose loop diuretics[41] has been advised to promote further calciuresis once volume replete, but little evidence-based data exist on the efficacy of this approach with lower doses, which has generally been adopted.[42]

Medications

Calcitonin: Calcitonin has a rapid onset of action and can decrease serum calcium by 1 to 2 mg/dL beginning within 6 hours by blocking osteoclastic resorption of bone and increasing calcium excretion by the kidneys.[43,44] Typical calcitonin dosing is 4 IU/kg either intramuscularly or subcutaneously every 12 hours, but can be increased to 8 IU/kg every 6 to 12 hours if insufficient effect is noted after 24 hours.[38] The use of calcitonin is limited to 24 to 48 hours because of rapid tachyphylaxis.[44]

Bisphosphonates: Bisphosphonates lower serum calcium by blocking various osteoclastic functions, including bone resorption,[45] and have become the standard therapy for severe hypercalcemia. Onset of action is approximately 48 to 72 hours, so alternate agents may be required in the hyperacute setting. Various bisphosphonates have been studied for hypercalcemia of malignancy,[46,47] with all showing greater efficacy in calcium lowering than intravenous hydration or calcitonin. In addition, bisphosphonates have been used successfully in the treatment of a variety of other etiologies of hypercalcemia, including vitamin D intoxication,[48,49] vitamin A intoxication,[50,51] immobility,[52,53] hyperparathyroidism,[54,55] and granulomatous disease.[56,57] In patients with kidney dysfunction, bisphosphonates must be used cautiously owing to the risk of AKI and potentially prolonged duration of action.[58]

Glucocorticoids: Glucocorticoids lower serum calcium by decreasing synthesis of 1,25-hydroxyvitamin D, ultimately limiting intestinal calcium absorption. Given the efficacy of bisphosphonates in lowering serum calcium, these agents have been less utilized, but remain a key therapeutic tool for hypercalcemia related to granulomatous disease or vitamin D intoxication.[59]

Denosumab: Denosumab, a human monoclonal antibody against the receptor activator of nuclear factor-κB (RANK) ligand (a stimulator of osteoclast activity), has been shown to reduce serum calcium levels acutely in multiple case reports.[60,61] It is not cleared by the kidney and thus can be used in patients with kidney impairment.

Calcimimetics: Cinacalcet and etelcalcetide mimic the role of calcium by activating the calcium-sensing receptor and suppressing PTH. Although typically not utilized in the acute setting, there have been reports of successful use in severe hypercalcemia in parathyroid carcinoma[62] and in primary hyperparathyroidism.[63]

Kidney Replacement Therapy

If the abovementioned measures are unsuccessful or if severe hypercalcemia with coma is present, dialysis against a low or zero calcium dialysate is efficacious to acutely lower serum calcium.[64-66] Identification and treatment of the underlying etiology of hypercalcemia will be critical because dialysis will serve only as a temporizing measure.

SUMMARY AND CONCLUSIONS

Perturbations in serum calcium levels are common in the critical care setting. The majority of patients with hypocalcemia in the ICU do not have an underlying disorder of calcium regulation, and correction of asymptomatic hypocalcemia is not warranted in the acute care setting. For patients with hypercalcemia in the ICU, evaluation hinges on whether PTH is appropriately suppressed. Treatment may include judicious volume replacement, calcitonin, and bisphosphonates.

References

1. Marban E, Koretsune Y, Corretti M, Chacko VP, Kusuoka H. Calcium and its role in myocardial cell injury during ischemia and reperfusion. *Circulation.* 1989;80(6 Suppl):IV17-IV22.
2. Favus MJ, Goltzman D. Regulation of calcium and magnesium. In Rosen CJ, ed. *Primer on the Metabolic Bone Diseases and Disorders of Mineral Metabolism.* Hoboken, NJ: American Society for Bone and Mineral Research; 2008:104-108.
3. Moore EW. Ionized calcium in normal serum, ultrafiltrates, and whole blood determined by ion-exchange electrodes. *J Clin Invest.* 1970;49(2):318-334.
4. Payne RB, Little AJ, Williams RB, Milner JR. Interpretation of serum calcium in patients with abnormal serum proteins. *Br Med J.* 1973;4(5893):643-646.
5. Slomp J, van der Voort PH, Gerritsen RT, Berk JA, Bakker AJ. Albumin-adjusted calcium is not suitable for diagnosis of hyper-and hypocalcemia in the critically ill. *Crit Care Med.* 2003;31(5):1389-1393.
6. Zaloga GP, Chernow B, Cook D, Snyder R, Clapper M, O'Brian JT. Assessment of calcium homeostasis in the critically ill surgical patient. The diagnostic pitfalls of the McLean-Hastings nomogram. *Ann Surg.* 1985;202(5):587-594.
7. Zivin JR, Gooley T, Zager RA, Ryan MJ. Hypocalcemia: a pervasive metabolic abnormality in the critically ill. *Am J Kidney Dis.* 2001;37(4):689-698.
8. Egi M, Kim I, Nichol A, et al. Ionized calcium concentration and outcome in critical illness. *Crit Care Med.* 2011;39(2):314-321.
9. Ferreira-Junior M, Lichtenstein A, Sales MM, et al. Rational use of blood calcium determinations. *Sao Paulo Med J.* 2014;132(4):243-248.
10. Kelly A, Levine MA. Hypocalcemia in the critically ill patient. *J Intensive Care Med.* 2013;28(3):166-177.
11. Desai TK, Carlson RW, Geheb MA. Prevalence and clinical implications of hypocalcemia in acutely ill patients in a medical intensive care setting. *Am J Med.* 1988;84(2):209-214.
12. Burchard KW, Gann DS, Colliton J, Forster J. Ionized calcium, parathormone, and mortality in critically ill surgical patients. *Ann Surg.* 1990;212(4):543-549.
13. Tohme JF, Bilezikian JP. Hypocalcemic emergencies. *Endocrinol Metab Clin North Am.* 1993;22(2):363-375.
14. Zaloga GP. Ionized hypocalcemia during sepsis. *Crit Care Med.* 2000;28(1):266-268.
15. Taylor B, Sibbald WJ, Edmonds MW, Holliday RL, Williams C. Ionized hypocalcemia in critically ill patients with sepsis. *Can J Surg.* 1978;21(5):429-433.
16. Zaloga GP, Chernow B. The multifactorial basis for hypocalcemia during sepsis. Studies of the parathyroid hormone-vitamin D axis. *Ann Intern Med.*1987;107(1):36-41.

17. Desai TK, Carlson RW, Geheb MA. Parathyroid-vitamin D axis in critically ill patients with unexplained hypocalcemia. *Kidney Int Suppl.* 1987;22:S225-S228.
18. Canaff L, Hendy GN. Calcium-sensing receptor gene transcription is up-regulated by the proinflammatory cytokine, interleukin-1beta. Role of the NF-kappaB PATHWAY and kappaB elements. *J Biol Chem.* 2005;280(14):14177-14188.
19. Canaff L, Zhou X, Hendy GN. The proinflammatory cytokine, interleukin-6, up-regulates calcium-sensing receptor gene transcription via Stat1/3 and Sp1/3. *J Biol Chem.* 2008;283(20): 13586-13600.
20. Topf J, Worcester EM. Disorders of calcium, phosphorus, and magnesium. In Murray PT, Brady HR, Hall JB, eds. *Intensive Care in Nephrology*. London: Taylor & Francis; 2006:383-389.
21. Hermans C, Lefebvre C, Devogelaer JP, Lambert M. Hypocalcaemia and chronic alcohol intoxication: transient hypoparathyroidism secondary to magnesium deficiency. *Clin Rheumatol.* 1996;15(2):193-196.
22. Desai TK, Carlson RW, Thill-Baharozian M, Geheb MA. A direct relationship between ionized calcium and arterial pressure among patients in an intensive care unit. *Crit Care Med.* 1988;16(6):578-582.
23. Jankowski S, Vincent JL. Calcium administration for cardiovascular support in critically ill patients: when is it indicated? *J Intensive Care Med.* 1995;10(2):91-100.
24. Forsythe RM, Wessel CB, Billiar TR, Angus DC, Rosengart MR. Parenteral calcium for intensive care unit patients. *Cochrane Database Syst Rev.* 2008;(4):CD006163.
25. Aberegg SK. Ionized calcium in the ICU: should it be measured and corrected? *Chest.* 2016;149(3):846-855.
26. Baird GS, Rainey PM, Wener M, Chandler W. Reducing routine ionized calcium measurement. *Clin Chem.* 2009;55(3):533-540.
27. Collage RD, Howell GM, Zhang X, et al. Calcium supplementation during sepsis exacerbates organ failure and mortality via calcium/calmodulin-dependent protein kinase signaling. *Crit Care Med.* 2013;41(11):e352-e360.
28. Zaloga GP, Sager A, Black KW, Prielipp R. Low dose calcium administration increases mortality during septic peritonitis in rats. *Circ Shock.* 1992;37(3):226-229.
29. Malcolm DS, Zaloga GP, Holaday JW. Calcium administration increases the mortality of endotoxic shock in rats. *Crit Care Med.* 1989;17(9):900-903.
30. Afshinnia F, Belanger K, Palevsky PM, Young EW. Effect of ionized serum calcium on outcomes in acute kidney injury needing renal replacement therapy: secondary analysis of the acute renal failure trial network study. *Ren Fail.* 2013;35(10):1310-1318.
31. Giancarelli A, Birrer KL, Alban RF, Hobbs BP, Liu-DeRyke X. Hypocalcemia in trauma patients receiving massive transfusion. *J Surg Res.* 2016;202(1):182-187.
32. Rosen S, Greenfeld Z, Bernheim J, Rathaus M, Podjarny E, Brezis M. Hypercalcemic nephropathy: chronic disease with predominant medullary inner stripe injury. *Kidney Int.* 1990;37(4):1067-1075.
33. Hebert SC. Extracellular calcium-sensing receptor: implications for calcium and magnesium handling in the kidney. *Kidney Int.* 1996;50(6):2129-2139.
34. Hosking DJ, Cowley A, Bucknall CA. Rehydration in the treatment of severe hypercalcaemia. *Q J Med.* 1981;50(200):473-481.
35. Andersen M. Rehydration as a diagnostic and therapeutic measure in hypercalcemia including an assessment of the calcium-lowering effect of porcine calcitonin. *Acta Med Scand.* 1972;192(4):347-351.
36. Sleeboom HP, Bijvoet OL, van Oosterom AT, Gleed JH, O'Riordan JL. Comparison of intravenous (3-amino-1-hydroxypropylidene)-1, 1-bisphosphonate and volume repletion in tumour-induced hypercalcaemia. *Lancet.* 1983;2(8344):239-243.
37. Maier JD, Levine SN. Hypercalcemia in the intensive care unit: a review of pathophysiology, diagnosis, and modern therapy. *J Intensive Care Med.* 2015;30(5):235-252.
38. Bilezikian JP. Clinical review 51: management of hypercalcemia. *J Clin Endocrinol Metab.* 1993;77(6):1445-1449.
39. Bilezikian JP. Management of acute hypercalcemia. *N Engl J Med.* 1992;326(18):1196-1203.
40. Legrand SB. Modern management of malignant hypercalcemia. *Am J Hosp Palliat Care.* 2011;28(7):515-517.
41. Suki WN, Yium JJ, Von MM, Saller-Hebert C, Eknoyan G, Martinez-Maldonado M. Acute treatment of hypercalcemia with furosemide. *N Engl J Med.* 1970;283(16):836-840.
42. Legrand SB, Leskuski D, Zama I. Narrative review: furosemide for hypercalcemia: an unproven yet common practice. *Ann Intern Med.* 2008;149(4):259-263.
43. Kammerman S, Canfield RE. Effect of porcine calcitonin on hypercalcemia in man. *J Clin Endocrinol Metab.* 1970;31(1):70-75.
44. Austin LA, Heath H III. Calcitonin: physiology and pathophysiology. *N Engl J Med.* 1981;304(5):269-278.

45. Fleisch H. Bisphosphonates: mechanisms of action. *Endocr Rev.* 1998;19(1):80-100.
46. Saunders Y, Ross JR, Broadley KE, Edmonds PM, Patel S. Systematic review of bisphosphonates for hypercalcaemia of malignancy. *Palliat Med.* 2004;18(5):418-431.
47. Major P, Lortholary A, Hon J, et al. Zoledronic acid is superior to pamidronate in the treatment of hypercalcemia of malignancy: a pooled analysis of two randomized, controlled clinical trials. *J Clin Oncol.* 2001;19(2):558-567.
48. Selby PL, Davies M, Marks JS, Mawer EB. Vitamin D intoxication causes hypercalcaemia by increased bone resorption which responds to pamidronate. *Clin Endocrinol.* 1995;43(5):531-536.
49. Rizzoli R, Stoermann C, Ammann P, Bonjour JP. Hypercalcemia and hyperosteolysis in vitamin D intoxication: effects of clodronate therapy. *Bone.* 1994;15(2):193-198.
50. Bhalla K, Ennis DM, Ennis ED. Hypercalcemia caused by iatrogenic hypervitaminosis A. *J Am Diet Assoc.* 2005;105(1):119-121.
51. Cordoba R, Ramirez E, Lei SH, et al. Hypercalcemia due to an interaction of all-trans retinoic acid (ATRA) and itraconazole therapy for acute promyelocytic leukemia successfully treated with zoledronic acid. *Eur J Clin Pharmacol.* 2008;64(10):1031-1032.
52. Alborzi F, Leibowitz AB. Immobilization hypercalcemia in critical illness following bariatric surgery. *Obes Surg.* 2002;12(6):871-873.
53. Meythaler JM, Tuel SM, Cross LL. Successful treatment of immobilization hypercalcemia using calcitonin and etidronate. *Arch Phys Med Rehabil.* 1993;74(3):316-319.
54. Witteveen JE, Haak HR, Kievit J, Morreau H, Romijn JA, Hamdy NA. Challenges and pitfalls in the management of parathyroid carcinoma: 17-year follow-up of a case and review of the literature. *Horm Cancer.* 2010;1(4):205-214.
55. Fitzpatrick LA, Bilezikian JP. Acute primary hyperparathyroidism. *Am J Med.* 1987;82(2):275-282.
56. Gibbs CJ, Peacock M. Hypercalcaemia due to sarcoidosis corrects with bisphosphonate treatment. *Postgrad Med J.* 1986;62(732):937-938.
57. Zhang JT, Chan C, Kwun SY, Benson KA. A case of severe 1,25-dihydroxyvitamin D-mediated hypercalcemia due to a granulomatous disorder. *J Clin Endocrinol Metab.* 2012;97(8):2579-2583.
58. Perazella MA, Markowitz GS. Bisphosphonate nephrotoxicity. *Kidney Int.* 2008;74(11):1385-1393.
59. Vucinic V, Skodric-Trifunovic V, Ignjatovic S. How to diagnose and manage difficult problems of calcium metabolism in sarcoidosis: an evidence-based review. *Curr Opin Pulm Med.* 2011;17(5):297-302.
60. Bech A, de Boer H. Denosumab for tumor-induced hypercalcemia complicated by renal failure. *Ann Intern Med.* 2012;156(12):906-907.
61. Boikos SA, Hammers HJ. Denosumab for the treatment of bisphosphonate-refractory hypercalcemia. *J Clin Oncol.* 2012;30(29):e299.
62. Silverberg SJ, Rubin MR, Faiman C, et al. Cinacalcet hydrochloride reduces the serum calcium concentration in inoperable parathyroid carcinoma. *J Clin Endocrinol Metab.* 2007;92(10):3803-3808.
63. Marcocci C, Bollerslev J, Khan AA, Shoback DM. Medical management of primary hyperparathyroidism: proceedings of the fourth International Workshop on the Management of Asymptomatic Primary Hyperparathyroidism. *J Clin Endocrinol Metab.* 2014;99(10):3607-3618.
64. Camus C, Charasse C, Jouannic-Montier I, et al. Calcium free hemodialysis: experience in the treatment of 33 patients with severe hypercalcemia. *Intensive Care Med.* 1996;22(2):116-121.
65. Koo WS, Jeon DS, Ahn SJ, Kim YS, Yoon YS, Bang BK. Calcium-free hemodialysis for the management of hypercalcemia. *Nephron.* 1996;72(3):424-428.
66. Wang CC, Chen YC, Shiang JC, Lin SH, Chu P, Wu CC. Hypercalcemic crisis successfully treated with prompt calcium-free hemodialysis. *Am J Emerg Med.* 2009;27(9):1174.e1-1174.e3.

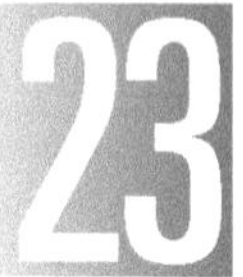

Phosphorus Management in the Intensive Care Unit

Mina El Kateb and Joel M. Topf

INTRODUCTION

Phosphorus is an essential element required for almost every reaction in the human body. In the form of adenosine triphosphate (ATP), it is the body's major form of energy transfer. Phosphate is also important for the structural integrity of the cell and its genetic content, in the form of phospholipid bilayer and ribonucleic and deoxyribonucleic acid (RNA and DNA), respectively. Most of the body's phosphorus is stored in bones and teeth, with only about 0.1% of it free in the extracellular space reflecting, under normal circumstance, a serum level of 2.5 to 4.5 mg/dL (0.8-1.45 mmol/L or 1.45-2.61 mEq/L).

Clinically, phosphorus levels are an indicator of nutritional status, with hypophosphatemia seen in the critically ill.[1] Low levels in the intensive care unit (ICU) are associated with poor cardiac function, difficult extubation, and rhabdomyolysis.[2-4] Replacing phosphorus has caveats and limitations, with the major complication being hyperphosphatemia. Hyperphosphatemia has an equally negative impact on patient outcomes in the ICU.[5] It is closely linked to kidney dysfunction and dialysis, which at times, may be the only cure for severe, symptomatic hyperphosphatemia.[6,7] This chapter reviews hypo- and hyperphosphatemia, its impact, treatment, causes, workup, and signs and symptoms, while placing emphasis on prompt ICU management.

HYPOPHOSPHATEMIA

Low phosphorus levels (<2.5 mg/dL, 0.32 mmol/L or 1.45 mEq/L) can be seen in 20% of ICU patients, with certain populations having more pronounced and more frequent hypophosphatemia including patients with diabetic ketoacidosis, cardiac surgery, sepsis, continuous kidney replacement therapy, refeeding syndrome, and an especially high rate in patients with major hepatic surgery.[1,8-10] Even though it may be a general marker of illness, replacement has improved clinical outcomes, including cardiac morbidity and mortality.[3]

Refeeding Syndrome

Commonly encountered in the ICU, refeeding has been specifically addressed by the guidelines put forth by the National institute for Health and Care Excellence (NICE).[11] In these guidelines, NICE identifies the risk factors shown in **Table 23.1** for the development of refeeding syndrome. For these patients, the recommendation is to reduce their maximum nutritional support to 10 kcal/kg/d

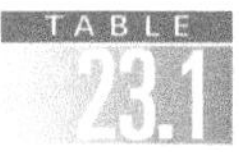

Risk Factors for Refeeding Syndrome

Any patient with at least one of the following:

- Body mass index (BMI) < 16 kg/m^2
- Unintentional weight loss >15% over the last 3-6 mo
- Little intake >10 d
- Low K, P, or Mg prior to feeding

Any patient with at least two of the following:

- BMI < 18.5 kg/m^2
- Unintentional weight loss >10% over the last 3-6 mo
- Little intake >5 d
- History of alcohol abuse or drugs such as insulin, chemotherapy, antacids, or diuretics

while slowly increasing that goal over 1 week, so as to minimize the potential for hypophosphatemia. They also recommend empirically adding 0.3 to 0.6 mmol/kg/d of phosphorus in patients whose phosphorus is not elevated.

Kidney Replacement Therapy

Patients receiving continuous kidney replacement theray (CKRT) are at increased risk of developing hypophosphatemia, as phosphorus is directly removed with dialysis. This risk can exceed 50% and can be as high as 65% in those receiving dialysis with a high effluent rate.[12] The hypophosphatemia of CKRT is associated with nearly twice the rates of prolonged respiratory failure (defined by the requirement of tracheostomy).[13] Although standard dialysate does not contain phosphorus, clinicians should consider using dialysate with a phosphorus concentration of 1 mmol/L in patients without hyperphosphatemia.

Factitious Hypophosphatemia

High doses of mannitol, used in the treatment of increased intracranial or intraocular pressure, can lead to a false drop in the serum phosphorus level, and so hypophosphatemia should be interpreted cautiously in this setting.[14]

Causes

The causes of hypophosphatemia can be categorized into three broad categories: decreased intestinal absorption, urinary wasting, and cellular shift (see **Tables 23.2** and **23.3**).

Decreased Intestinal Absorption

Phosphorus is found in a wide variety of foods and so dietary deficiency is rare; additionally, in these circumstances, tunbular reabsorption is upregulated and urinary phosphate loss approaches zero.[15] More commonly, gastrointestinal loss or lack of intestinal absorption can result in hypophosphatemia. Malabsorption syndromes also result in hypovitaminosis D and a secondary hyperparathyroidism; parathyroid hormone (PTH) is phosphaturic, leading to tubular phosphate wasting. Thus, in chronic diarrhea or steatorrhea, intestinal loss is

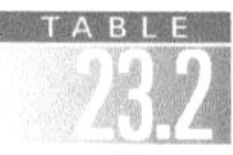

TABLE 23.2 Common Causes of Hypophosphatemia in the Intensive Care Unit

Sepsis	Respiratory alkalosis
Aggressive intravenous fluids (IVF)	Metabolic acidosis
Trauma	Glucose/insulin therapy
Refeeding	Catecholamines
Postoperative	Diuretics
Kidney replacement therapy	

combined with urinary wasting, leading to significant hypophosphatemia.[16] Calcium, magnesium, and aluminum-based antacids also act as phosphate binders, leading to hypophosphatemia through decreased intestinal absorption.

Cellular Shift

Internal redistribution of phosphorus occurs in several situations such as refeeding syndrome, treatment of diabetic ketoacidosis, respiratory alkalosis, and hungry bone syndrome. Insulin shifts phosphorus intracellularly. Refeeding syndrome is often encountered in malnourished, anorexic, and alcoholic patients whose phosphorus stores are low. With the reintroduction of carbohydrates after a period of starvation, the endogenous insulin release shifts phosphorus intracellularly, resulting in significant hypophosphatemia.[17] Similarly, in diabetic ketoacidosis, the insulin infusion shifts phosphorus intracellularly, which can induce hypophosphatemia. In hungry bone syndrome, calcium and phosphorus redeposit back into bone once the PTH falls following a parathyroidectomy. The administration of denosumab, a monoclonal antibody that antagonizes the activity of receptor activator nuclear factor kappa B ligand (RANKL), prevents maturation of osteoclasts.[18] This prevents bone breakdown in states of bony metastases and allows reconstitution of bone, resulting in hypocalcemia and hypophosphatemia, similar to hungry bone syndrome.[19]

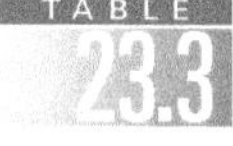

TABLE 23.3 Causes of Hypophosphatemia

Intestinal Absorption	Internal Redistribution	Urinary Wasting
Malabsorption syndromes	Refeeding	Hyperparathyroidism
Steatorrhea	Glucose/insulin therapy	Volume expansion
Vitamin D deficiency	Hungry bone syndrome	Vitamin D deficiency
Antacids	Respiratory alkalosis	Metabolic acidosis
Malnutrition		Diuretics
Gastric suction		Fanconi syndrome

Urinary Phosphate Wasting

Urinary phosphate reabsorption occurs predominantly in the proximal tubule via sodium phosphate cotransporters.[15,20] Hypophosphatemia results in increased activity and number of these transporters. On the other hand, PTH and phosphatonins (such as fibroblast growth factor 23, FGF23) result in decreased activity of these same Na/P cotransporters.[21,22] Hence, hyperparathyroidism, primary or secondary, leads to urinary phosphate wasting. Tumor-induced (oncogenic) osteomalacia is a rare paraneoplastic syndrome wherein the mesenchymal tumor releases FGF23, leading to urinary phosphate wasting.[23] Dialysis patients with long-standing secondary hyperparathyroidism often continue to have hyperparathyroidism even after transplantation. Referred to as tertiary hyperparathyroidism, autonomous hyperactive parathyroid glands continue secreting PTH after transplantation, leading to marked hypophosphatemia. Low vitamin D leads to increased PTH release (secondary hyperparathyroidism) but additionally decreases the intestinal absorption of phosphorus, leading to both increased urinary wasting and decreased intestinal absorption.

There are several primary urinary phosphate wasting syndromes. They are rare and tend to have normal calcium balance. For a detailed discussion, refer to the review article by Tenenhouse and Murer.[24] A more common form of urinary phosphate wasting occurs in Fanconi syndrome, which is a generalized proximal tubular dysfunction leading to normoglycemic glucosuria, amino aciduria, renal tubular acidosis, and hypokalemia.[25] Fanconi syndrome can be seen in multiple myeloma, heavy metal exposure, and certain drugs, such as tenofovir.

Workup

Oftentimes, the history and presentation reveal the cause. However, if the source of the hypophosphatemia is not readily apparent, one can determine the degree of urinary wasting with a 24-hour urine phosphate collection or the fractional excretion of phosphorus ($FePO_4$). In the setting of hypophosphatemia, the 24-hour urine phosphate should be less than 100 mg, and the $FePO_4$ should be less than 5%; values greater than these suggest a kidney origin of phosphorus deficiency.[26]

Signs and Symptoms

Hypophosphatemia can lead to a wide variety of symptoms, most of them subtle and difficult to isolate entirely. In the ICU, poor diaphragmatic contractility, ventilator dependence, and failure to wean have been associated with hypophosphatemia.[27,28] One study, looking at intubated patients with acute exacerbation of chronic obstructive pulmonary disease, found a significantly higher rate of failure-to-extubate of the mechanical ventilator in patients with hypophosphatemia versus those with normal serum phosphorus levels (34% vs 10%, $p < 0.05$).[2] Furthermore, the investigator linked this failure-to-extubate to weakness of the respiratory muscles, evidenced by a decreased tidal volume of spontaneous respiration, reduced static lung compliance, and impaired pulmonary function. Other muscles affected by hypophosphatemia include the heart. One study conducted in the ICU showed improved cardiac index (by an average of 18%) after normalizing serum phosphorus.[3] Peripheral muscles can be so disturbed by hypophosphatemia that they break down, leading to rhabdomyolysis, typically within 72 hours of the onset of hypophosphatemia. Red blood cells can also lyse in the setting of hypophosphatemia, leading to hemolysis. Central nervous system manifestations are uncommon but have included confusion, lethargy, encephalopathy, seizures, as well as central pontine myelinolysis.[4]

Treatment

Prospective studies, conducted in the ICU setting, suggest that weight-based intravenous (IV) replacement with a single infusion over a 6-hour period is a safe (with fewer cases of hyperphosphatemia) and effective (with >75% efficacy) way to correct severe hypophosphatemia[29] (see **Table 23.4**). If quicker correction is required, for example, in the setting of active hemolysis or rhabdomyolysis, a one-time 15 mmol infusion over a 2-hour period is a safe method of correcting hypophosphatemia. Quicker rates of correction can result in periodic hyperphosphatemia that can lead to hypocalcemia, ECG changes, and acute kidney injury.

HYPERPHOSPHATEMIA

Hyperphosphatemia is defined by a serum phosphate level greater than 4.5 mg/dL (1.45 mmol/L). The incidence of hyperphosphatemia is quite variable based on the setting, but correlates closely with kidney function. In a study of 2,390 hospitalized patients, 9% had hyperphosphatemia.[30] Those with hyperphosphatemia had a significantly lower estimated glomerular filtration rate (eGFR), averaging 22 mL/min/1.73 m^2, as compared to the normophosphatemic patients whose average eGFR was 93 mL/min/1.73 m^2. Those with hyperphosphatemia also had a significantly higher mortality rate (11% vs 2%). In a study of patients with underlying coronary artery disease, with normal kidney function, the incidence of hyperphosphatemia was 0.9% and was associated with a graded risk of death and cardiovascular events.[5] Among dialysis patients, hyperphosphatemia is much more common, with incidence rates as high as 47%.[6] In these patients, chronic exposure to high phosphorus level results in a variety of complications ranging from hypocalcemia, hyperparathyroidism, bone demineralization as well as bone deposits (calcification) in blood vessels and soft tissue, leading to premature heart disease and death.

Lab Errors

Hyperglobulinemia has been associated with falsely elevated phosphorus levels.[31] Cases of Waldenström macroglobulinemia and multiple myeloma cause pseudohyperphosphatemia as high as 32 mg/dL.[32,33] Spurious hyperphosphatemia can also be seen with high-dose liposomal amphotericin B.[34] Hyperlipidemia also causes spurious elevations in serum phosphorus.[35] Treating hyperphosphatemia in these settings without evidence of hyperphosphatemia (concomitant hypocalcemia or acute kidney injury) is discouraged.[36]

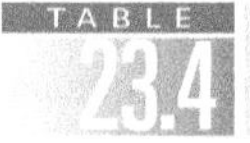
TABLE 23.4 Suggested Replacement Rates for Phosphorus

Phosphorus Level		Weight-Based Replacement		
mg/dL	mmol/L	40-60 kg	61-80 kg	81-120 kg
1.0	<0.32	30 mmol P	40 mmol P	50 mmol P
1.0-1.7	0.32-0.54	20 mmol P	30 mmol P	40 mmol P
1.7-2.2	0.55-0.70	10 mmol P	15 mmol P	20 mmol P

Causes

Similar to hypophosphatemia, the causes of hyperphosphatemia can be traced to the gastrointestinal tract, the kidneys, and transcellular shifts or redistribution.

Increased Intestinal Intake

Sodium phosphate–based cathartics, such as fleet enema, contain high amounts of phosphorus, with a standard dose of 250 mL having as much as 32 g of phosphorus.[37] Despite its magnitude, this load is generally well tolerated and the hyperphosphatemia is only transient with most of the phosphorus not being absorbed, acting only as an osmotic cathartic, and any absorbed phosphorus is promptly cleared by the kidneys. However, in patients with impaired kidney function, the elderly, and those with impaired gut motility, the consequences of using sodium phosphate bowel preps can be catastrophic, with hypocalcemia, shock, and even death.[38,39] In one case series of 11 elderly patients who received fleet enema for constipation, serum phosphorus levels rose as high as 45 mg/dL and calcium fell as low as 2 mg/dL. Of the 11 patients, 5 died as a direct consequence of the hyperphosphatemia.[40]

In patients with advanced kidney failure and those on dialysis, the kidney's ability to excrete phosphorus dwindles and the daily phosphorus load starts to accumulate. The recommended dietary intake should be reduced to 800 mg in dialysis patients (the typical American diet contains 1,300-1,700 mg phosphorus daily).[41] Intravenous fosphenytoin, an antiepileptic, is metabolized into phenytoin and phosphorus and, in the setting of kidney impairment, can lead to significant hyperphosphatemia.[42]

Cellular Shift

Three commonly encountered causes of hyperphosphatemia in the ICU are a result of cell lysis and the release of intracellular phosphorus: tumor lysis syndrome, hemolytic anemia, and rhabdomyolysis. These also can cause kidney failure because of the nephrotoxic nature of uric acid, hemoglobin, and myoglobin, respectively. Treatment often requires dialysis, especially in the setting of concomitant hyperkalemia and oliguria. Other causes of hyperphosphatemic shift include lactic and diabetic acidosis.[43,44] This is in part explained by organ ischemia seen in lactic acidosis, resulting in reduced glycolysis and cell death, leading to intracellular phosphorus release.[44] In diabetic ketoacidosis, the relative insulin deficiency prevents the entry of phosphorus into the cell from the extracellular space.

Kidney Retention

Kidney failure, acute or chronic, is ubiquitous in the development of hyperphosphatemia. In the setting of preserved kidney function, hypoparathyroidism is a leading cause of hyperphosphatemia. The PTH induces urinary phosphate wasting, and so deficiency or resistance to PTH (as seen in pseudohypoparathyroidism) leads to increased tubular reabsorption of phosphorus. Hypoparathyroidism can be congenital, as in the setting of DiGeorge syndrome, manifesting in infancy and childhood.[45] Hypoparathyroidism can also be the result of autoimmune disease (very rare) or acquired, postsurgically (more common), following partial parathyroidectomy, thyroidectomy, or other neck surgery.[45,46] Likewise, hypervitaminosis D directly inhibits the production of PTH while increasing intestinal and tubular absorption of phosphorus. Acromegaly, by way of excess of growth hormone and insulin-like growth factor production, results in increased tubular reabsorption of phosphorus.[47] Hyperphosphatemic familial tumoral calcinosis is a disease characterized by hyperphosphatemia, normal calcium level,

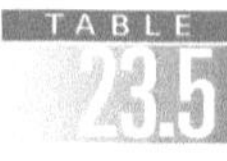

Causes of Hyperphosphatemia

Intestinal Intake	Internal Redistribution	Kidney Retention
Sodium phosphate cathartics	Rhabdomyolysis	Acute or chronic kidney failure
>800 mg in dialysis patients	Tumor lysis syndrome	Hypoparathyroidism
Vitamin D toxicity	Hemolysis	Pseudohyperparathyroidism
	Lactic acidosis	Vitamin D toxicity
	Diabetic ketoacidosis	Acromegaly
		Tumoral calcinosis

and multiple calcified, painful nodules. Several mutations have been characterized, ultimately leading to decreased number or effect of FGF23 and its phosphaturic effects[48] (see **Table 23.5**).

Workup

In the setting of normal kidney function, it is important to rule out intracellular release by checking uric acid (for tumor lysis syndrome); creatinine kinase (for rhabdomyolysis); and lactate dehydrogenase, haptoglobin levels (for hemolysis), and, when appropriate, a serum lactate. Additional testing should include PTH, vitamin D, and insulin-like growth factor levels (a normal level, rules out acromegaly).

Signs and Symptoms

Acute hyperphosphatemia has little to no symptoms, and the symptoms that may manifest are largely due to hypocalcemia. The central nervous system signs and symptoms of hypocalcemia include: irritability, numbness, tingling, laryngospasms, seizures, and coma. Cardiovascular signs include: prolonged QTc, bradycardia, decreased contractility, hypotension, and shock.

Severe hyperphosphatemia has also been linked to development of acute and chronic kidney disease, with pathology showing tubular calcium phosphate deposits on a background of diffuse chronic tubulointerstitial injury.[49]

Chronic hyperphosphatemia occurring in advanced chronic kidney disease and those undergoing dialysis is a much more intricate disease, resulting in bone demineralization, ectopic calcification, chronic inflammation, cardiovascular disease, and premature death. Renal osteodystrophy manifests as weaker bones, which are more susceptible to fracture as well as to bone pain and generalized fatigue. Calciphylaxis, formally known as calcific uremic arteriolopathy, is a complex disease where smooth muscles are replaced by bone-forming cells, resulting in painful deep tissue nodules and necrotic tissue. The tissue necrosis can be extensive, affecting areas as large as the entire abdomen and often becoming infected. It frequently is fatal.

Treatment

Prevention is key and maintaining kidney function is fundamental. Aggressive intravenous fluid is often used to preserve kidney function and augment urinary clearance of phosphorus. However, in cases with severe, symptomatic

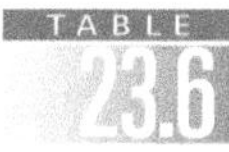

Treatment of Severe Hyperphosphatemia

Modality	When to Use It
Intravenous (IV) fluid hydration	Whenever possible
Kidney replacement therapy (continuous > intermittent)	With significant kidney failure
Insulin + dextrose	Only as an adjunct

hyperphosphatemia, when kidney function is compromised, dialysis is used to remove phosphorus. Continuous kidney replacement has better efficacy than conventional or intermittent hemodialysis with fewer instances of rebound hyperphosphatemia.[7] Because insulin therapy can temporarily shift phosphorus intracellularly, it has been used in conjunction with dextrose to mitigate hyperphosphatemia[50] (see **Table 23.6**).

References

1. Suzuki S, Egi M, Schneider AG, Bellomo R, Hart GK, Hegarty C. Hypophosphatemia in critically ill patients. *J Crit Care.* 2013;28(4):536.e9-536.e19.
2. Zhao Y, Li Z, Shi Y, et al. Effect of hypophosphatemia on the withdrawal of mechanical ventilation in patients with acute exacerbations of chronic obstructive pulmonary disease. *Biomed Rep.* 2016;4(4):413-416.
3. Zazzo JF, Troché G, Ruel P, Maintenant J. High incidence of hypophosphatemia in surgical intensive care patients: efficacy of phosphorus therapy on myocardial function. *Intensive Care Med.* 1995;21(10):826-831.
4. Michell AW. Central pontine myelinolysis temporally related to hypophosphataemia. *J Neurol Neurosurg Psychiatry.* 2003;74(6):820. doi:10.1136/jnnp.74.6.820
5. Tonelli M, Sacks F, Pfeffer M, Gao Z, Curhan G. Relation between serum phosphate level and cardiovascular event rate in people with coronary disease. *Circulation.* 2005;112(17): 2627-2633. doi:10.1161/circulationaha.105.553198
6. Port FK, Pisoni RL, Bommer J, et al. Improving outcomes for dialysis patients in the international Dialysis Outcomes and Practice Patterns Study. *Clin J Am Soc Nephrol.* 2006;1(2):246-255.
7. Tan HK, Bellomo R, M'Pis DA, Ronco C. Phosphatemic control during acute renal failure: intermittent hemodialysis versus continuous hemodiafiltration. *Int J Artif Organs.* 2001;24(4):186-191.
8. Cohen J, Kogan A, Sahar G, Lev S, Vidne B, Singer P. Hypophosphatemia following open heart surgery: incidence and consequences. *Eur J Cardiothorac Surg.* 2004;26(2):306-310.
9. Yang Y, Zhang P, Cui Y, et al. Hypophosphatemia during continuous veno-venous hemofiltration is associated with mortality in critically ill patients with acute kidney injury. *Crit Care.* 2013;17(5):R205.
10. Salem RR, Tray K. Hepatic resection-related hypophosphatemia is of renal origin as manifested by isolated hyperphosphaturia. *Ann Surg.* 2005;241(2):343-348. doi:10.1097/01.sla.0000152093.43468.c0
11. National Institute for Health and Care Excellence. Nutrition support for adults: oral nutrition support, enteral tube feeding and parenteral nutrition. Published February 22, 2006. Last updated August 4, 2017. Accessed February 6, 2020. https://www.nice.org.uk/guidance/cg32
12. RENAL Replacement Therapy Study Investigators; Bellomo R, Cass A, Cole L, et al. Intensity of continuous renal-replacement therapy in critically ill patients. *N Engl J Med.* 2009;361(17):1627-1638.
13. Demirjian S, Teo BW, Guzman JA, et al. Hypophosphatemia during continuous hemodialysis is associated with prolonged respiratory failure in patients with acute kidney injury. *Nephrol Dial Transplant.* 2011;26(11):3508-3514. doi:10.1093/ndt/gfr075
14. Donhowe JM, Freier EF, Wong ET, Steffes MW. Factitious hypophosphatemia related to mannitol therapy. *Clin Chem.* 1981;27(10):1765-1769.
15. Murer H. Homer Smith Award. Cellular mechanisms in proximal tubular Pi reabsorption: some answers and more questions. *J Am Soc Nephrol.* 1992;2(12):1649-1665.

16. Geerse DA, Bindels AJ, Kuiper MA, Roos AN, Spronk PE, Schultz MJ. Treatment of hypophosphatemia in the intensive care unit: a review. *Crit Care.* 2010;14(4):R147.
17. Marinella MA. Refeeding syndrome and hypophosphatemia. *J Intensive Care Med.* 2005;20(3):155-159.
18. Hsu H, Lacey DL, Dunstan CR, et al. Tumor necrosis factor receptor family member RANK mediates osteoclast differentiation and activation induced by osteoprotegerin ligand. *Proc Natl Acad Sci.* 1999;96(7):3540-3545. doi:10.1073/pnas.96.7.3540
19. Aude T, Thierry R, Bernard C, Aglaia K. Severe hypocalcemia after a single denosumab injection and tumor-induced persistent hypophosphatemia in a patient with metastatic prostate cancer. *Endocrine Abstracts.* 2019;64:39. doi:10.1530/endoabs.64.039
20. Murer H, Lötscher M, Kaissling B, Levi M, Kempson SA, Biber J. Renal brush border membrane Na/Pi-cotransport: molecular aspects in PTH-dependent and dietary regulation. *Kidney Int.* 1996;49(6):1769-1773.
21. Antoniucci DM, Yamashita T, Portale AA. Dietary phosphorus regulates serum fibroblast growth factor-23 concentrations in healthy men. *J Clin Endocrinol Metab.* 2006;91(8): 3144-3149.
22. Habra M, Jimenez C, Huang S-C, et al. Expression analysis of fibroblast growth factor-23, matrix extracellular phosphoglycoprotein, secreted frizzled-related protein-4, and fibroblast growth factor-7: identification of fibroblast growth factor-23 and matrix extracellular phosphoglycoprotein as major factors involved in tumor-induced osteomalacia. *Endocrine Practice.* 2008;14(9):1108-1114. doi:10.4158/ep.14.9.1108
23. Jonsson KB, Zahradnik R, Larsson T, et al. Fibroblast growth factor 23 in oncogenic osteomalacia and X-linked hypophosphatemia. *N Engl J Med.* 2003;348(17):1656-1663. doi:10.1056/nejmoa020881
24. Tenenhouse HS, Murer H. Disorders of renal tubular phosphate transport. *J Am Soc Nephrol.* 2003;14(1):240-248.
25. Clarke BL, Wynne AG, Wilson DM, Fitzpatrick LA. Osteomalacia associated with adult Fanconi's syndrome: clinical and diagnostic features. *Clin Endocrinol.* 1995;43(4):479-490. doi:10.1111/j.1365-2265.1995.tb02621.x
26. Walton RJ, Bijvoet OLM. Nomogram for derivation of renal threshold phosphate concentration. *Lancet.* 1975;306(7929):309-310. doi:10.1016/s0140-6736(75)92736-1
27. Aubier M, Murciano D, Lecocguic Y, et al. Effect of hypophosphatemia on diaphragmatic contractility in patients with acute respiratory failure. *N Engl J Med.* 1985;313(7):420-424. doi:10.1056/nejm198508153130705
28. Agusti AG, Torres A, Estopa R, Agustividal A. Hypophosphatemia as a cause of failed weaning: the importance of metabolic factors. *Crit Care Med.* 1984;12(2):142-143.
29. Taylor BE, Huey WY, Buchman TG, Boyle WA, Coopersmith CM. Treatment of hypophosphatemia using a protocol based on patient weight and serum phosphorus level in a surgical intensive care unit. *J Am Coll Surg.* 2004;198(2):198-204.
30. Haider DG, Lindner G, Wolzt M, et al. Hyperphosphatemia is an independent risk factor for mortality in critically ill patients: results from a cross-sectional study. *PLoS One.* 2015;10(8):e0133426.
31. Adler SG, Laidlaw SA, Lubran MM, Kopple JD. Hyperglobulinemia may spuriously elevate measured serum inorganic phosphate levels. *Am J Kidney Dis.* 1988;11(3):260-263.
32. Jamil MG, Abdel-Raheem MM, Potti A, Levitt R. Pseudohyperphosphatemia associated with Waldenström's macroglobulinemia. *Am J Hematol.* 2000;65(4):329.
33. Izzedine H, Camous L, Bourry E, Azar N, Leblond V, Deray G. The case | The case presentation. *Kidney Int.* 2007;72(8):1035-1036. doi:10.1038/sj.ki.5002485
34. Lane JW, Rehak NN, Hortin GL, Zaoutis T, Krause PR, Walsh TJ. Pseudohyperphosphatemia associated with high-dose liposomal amphotericin B therapy. *Clin Chim Acta.* 2008;387(1-2):145-149.
35. Leehey DJ. Spurious hyperphosphatemia due to hyperlipidemia. *Arch Intern Med.* 1985;145(4): 743-744. doi:10.1001/archinte.145.4.743
36. Larner AJ. Pseudohyperphosphatemia. *Clin Biochem.* 1995;28(4):391-393. doi:10.1016/0009-9120(95)00013-y
37. Gumurdulu Y, Serin E, Ozer B, Gokcel A, Boyacioglu S. Age as a predictor of hyperphosphatemia after oral phosphosoda administration for colon preparation. *J Gastroenterol Hepatol.* 2004;19(1):68-72. doi:10.1111/j.1440-1746.2004.03253.x
38. Mendoza J, Legido J, Rubio S, Gisbert JP. Systematic review: the adverse effects of sodium phosphate enema. *Aliment Pharmacol Ther.* 2007;26(1):9-20.
39. Beloosesky Y, Grinblat J, Weiss A, Grosman B, Gafter U, Chagnac A. Electrolyte disorders following oral sodium phosphate administration for bowel cleansing in elderly patients. *Arch Intern Med.* 2003;163(7):803-808.

40. Ori Y, Rozen-Zvi B, Chagnac A, et al. Fatalities and severe metabolic disorders associated with the use of sodium phosphate enemas: a single center's experience. *Arch Intern Med.* 2012;172(3):263-265.
41. González-Parra E, Gracia-Iguacel C, Egido J, Ortiz A. Phosphorus and nutrition in chronic kidney disease. *Int J Nephrol.* 2012;2012:597605.
42. McBryde KD, Wilcox J, Kher KK. Hyperphosphatemia due to fosphenytoin in a pediatric ESRD patient. *Pediatr Nephrol.* 2005;20(8):1182-1185. doi:10.1007/s00467-005-1947-0
43. O'Connor LR, Klein KL, Bethune JE. Hyperphosphatemia in lactic acidosis. *N Engl J Med.* 1977;297(13):707-709. doi:10.1056/nejm197709292971307
44. Kebler R, McDonald FD, Cadnapaphornchai P. Dynamic changes in serum phosphorus levels in diabetic ketoacidosis. *Am J Med.* 1985;79(5):571-576. doi:10.1016/0002-9343(85)90053-1
45. Shoback D. Hypoparathyroidism. *N Engl J Med.* 2008;359(4):391-403. doi:10.1056/nejmcp0803050
46. Hundahl SA, Cady B, Cunningham MP, et al. Initial results from a prospective cohort study of 5583 cases of thyroid carcinoma treated in the United States during 1996. *Cancer.* 2000; 89(1):202-217. doi:10.1002/1097-0142(20000701)89:1<202::aid-cncr27>3.0.co;2-a
47. Feld S, Hirschberg R. Growth hormone, the insulin-like growth factor system, and the kidney. *Endocr Rev.* 1996;17(5):423-480.
48. Sprecher E. Familial tumoral calcinosis: from characterization of a rare phenotype to the pathogenesis of ectopic calcification. *J Invest Dermatol.* 2010;130(3):652-660. doi:10.1038/jid.2009.337
49. Khurana A. The effect of oral sodium phosphate drug products on renal function in adults undergoing bowel endoscopy. *Arch Intern Med.* 2008;168(6):593. doi:10.1001/archinte.168.6.593
50. Helikson MA, Parham WA, Tobias JD. Hypocalcemia and hyperphosphatemia after phosphate enema use in a child. *J Pediatr Surg.* 1997;32(8):1244-1246.

24

Magnesium Management in the Intensive Care Unit

Mina El Kateb and Joel M. Topf

INTRODUCTION

Magnesium is the fourth most abundant cation in the human body and, behind potassium, is the second most abundant intracellular cation. In multiple studies, magnesium levels (either high[1] or low[2]) have been associated with hospital mortality. Despite these variable associations with outcomes, there are little consistent data showing improvement in outcomes with supplementing magnesium in deficient states, suggesting that altered magnesium is merely an epiphenomenon of critically ill people rather than the causative factor.

This chapter reviews the treatment of hypo- and hypermagnesemia and reviews the pathology underlying these conditions.

Normal Magnesium Levels

The average human body contains 25 g of magnesium, which is roughly equivalent to 2,000 mEq or 1 mole of magnesium. Nearly 99% of this magnesium is intracellular, with just over half trapped in bone. Only 1% is extracellular, a third of which (approximately 2.6 mmol) is present in plasma. Like calcium, only the ionized fraction of magnesium is metabolically active. Ionized magnesium ranges from 55% to 70% of serum magnesium. Although normal levels vary from laboratory to laboratory, typical lab values for various units are given in **Table 24.1**.

TABLE 24.1 Normal Magnesium Levels in Various Units

Units	Normal Magnesium Concentration
mmol/L	0.7-0.85
mEq/L	1.4-1.7
mg/dL	1.7-2.1
mg/L	17-21

HYPOMAGNESEMIA

Hypomagnesemia is defined as serum magnesium level less than 1.7 mg/dL (0.7 mmol/L). Hypomagnesemia can be found in up to two-thirds of intensive care unit (ICU) patients[3] and 11% of the general inpatient population.[4] Serum magnesium levels that represent only 0.3% of total body magnesium may not correspond with total body magnesium and therefore magnesium deficiency can be present despite a normal serum magnesium. Some experts suggest giving magnesium despite normal magnesium levels if the patient has symptoms of hypomagnesemia (e.g., hypocalcemia, hypokalemia, tachyarrhythmia). This should especially be considered in patients with risk factors for hypomagnesemia (e.g., alcoholism, diabetes, diarrhea).[5]

Causes of Hypomagnesemia

Hypomagnesemia can be due to decreased magnesium absorption or increased renal loss of magnesium (**Table 24.2**).

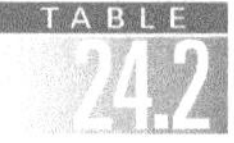

TABLE 24.2 Etiologies of Hypomagnesemia

Extrarenal Causes	Renal Causes
1. **Gastrointestinal** • Diarrhea • Steatorrhea • Congenital malabsorption • Protein calorie malnutrition • Alcoholism • Enteral nutrition • Inflammatory bowel disease • Gastric suction • Vomiting • Short bowel syndrome • Sprue • Intestinal bypass for obesity • Chronic pancreatitis 2. **Skin** • Burns • Toxic epidermal necrolysis 3. **Bone** • Hungry bone syndrome 4. **Pancreatitis**	1. **Drugs** • Proton pump inhibitors • Aminoglycoside toxicity • Pentamidine toxicity • Amphotericin B toxicity • Thiazide diuretics • Calcineurin inhibitors • Foscarnet • Cisplatin 2. **Loop of Henle** • Loop diuretics • Hypercalcemia 3. **Increased tubular flow** • Osmotic diuretics • Diabetes Type I and II • Hyperaldosteronism • Volume expansion • Diabetic ketoacidosis 4. **Tubular dysfunction** • Recovery from acute tubular necrosis • Recovery from obstruction • Recovery from transplantation 5. **Congenital renal magnesium wasting** • Bartter syndrome • Gitelman syndrome

Extrarenal Etiologies of Hypomagnesemia

Decreased oral intake, by itself, is a rare cause of hypomagnesemia. Although, in experimental settings, prolonged ingestion of a magnesium-depleted diet resulted in symptomatic hypomagnesemia, in clinical practice, this is rarely seen. However, because both upper and lower gastrointestinal (GI) secretions contain magnesium, GI losses contribute to magnesium depletion. Any malabsorption syndrome, diarrhea, enteric fistulas, surgical drainage tubes as well as steatorrhea all contribute substantially to hypomagnesemia. Similarly, small bowel resection and inflammatory bowel disease have both been associated with hypomagnesemia.[6]

In 2006 hypomagnesemia causing carpopedal spasm was found. The purported cause was a proton pump inhibitor (PPI). Two patients had been treated for a year or more prior to developing the hypomagnesemia. Switching from omeprazole to ranitidine resulted in rapid improvement in serum magnesium.[7] A systematic review and meta-analysis of 110,000 patients found the use of PPI resulted in a 43% increased risk of hypomagnesemia, though a more recent meta-analysis was unable to reproduce those findings because of the heterogeneity in the data.[8,9] The mechanism of PPI-induced hypomagnesemia has not been elucidated, but it is thought to be due to malabsorption as a result of loss of pH-dependent magnesium resorption via transient receptor potential melastatin-type magnesium channels (TRPM6) in the small bowel.[10]

Between GI losses and renal losses is only one disease, hungry bone syndrome. Following parathyroidectomy, the sudden drop in parathyroid hormone (PTH) may result in rapid reconstitution of demineralized osteoid. This can reduce serum calcium, phosphorus, and magnesium.[11]

Renal Losses

Unlike most electrolytes, where 60% to 70% of the filtered load is reabsorbed in the proximal tubule, only 10% to 20% of filtered magnesium is reabsorbed in the proximal tubule. The bulk of the filtered magnesium (70%) is reabsorbed along with calcium via a paracellular route in the thick ascending limb of the loop of Henle. The remaining 5% to 10% is reabsorbed in the distal convoluted tubule.[12]

Resorption of magnesium is inversely proportional to tubular flow, so increases in tubular flow decrease renal magnesium retention. Diuretics, hyperglycemia, nonoliguric acute tubular necrosis (ATN), volume expansion with intravenous (IV) fluids, hyperaldosteronism, and syndrome of inappropriate antidiuretic hormone (SIADH) all increase renal magnesium wasting. Given the importance of the loop of Henle in magnesium resorption, it should not be surprising to find loop diuretics as a principal cause of hypomagnesemia. Thiazide-like diuretics similarly increase renal magnesium wasting and predispose to hypomagnesemia.

Drugs and diseases that damage tubules decrease renal reabsorption of magnesium. This is seen with aminoglycosides, chronic alcohol abuse, foscarnet, cisplatin, and ATN. Genetic causes of renal wasting include Bartter and, more commonly and more severely, Gitelman syndrome.

Epithelial growth factor (EGF) increases magnesium transport through TRPM6 in the distal convoluted tubule. Anti-EGF drugs like cetuximab and panitumumab cause renal magnesium wasting and hypomagnesemia.[13]

Hypomagnesemia in alcoholics is common. De Marchi et al studied 61 patients with chronic alcoholism. A third had hypomagnesemia and urine magnesium was inappropriately elevated. The renal magnesium "leak" resolved within 4 weeks of abstinence.[14] Patients with alcohol abuse disorder also frequently experience vomiting, diarrhea, and pancreatitis, which may contribute to the high rate of hypomagnesemia.

Manifestations of Hypomagnesemia

Hypokalemia and Hypocalcemia

Hypomagnesemia causes both biochemical and clinical manifestations. The two most prominent biochemical symptoms are hypokalemia and hypocalcemia. Decreased intracellular magnesium increases renal potassium wasting. It is difficult to correct hypokalemia until the magnesium deficiency is corrected.[15] Hypocalcemia is due to decreased release of PTH and end-organ resistance to PTH in the presence of hypomagnesemia.[16]

Neuromuscular Symptoms

Neuromuscular hyperexcitability is often the earliest clinical symptoms of hypomagnesemia. Low magnesium and concomitant hypocalcemia lower the threshold for excitability. Symptoms can range from twitching, to cramps, to, in extreme cases, tetany. Chvostek and Trousseau signs may be present even in the absence of hypocalcemia.[17]

Cardiovascular Signs and Symptoms

Hypomagnesemia increases excitability of the heart and alters the electrocardiogram (ECG). Moderate hypomagnesemia causes widened QRS and peaked T waves. With more severe hypomagnesemia patients develop prolongation of the PR interval, further widening of the QRS complex, and diminution of the T wave. Low magnesium is correlated with atrial fibrillation. Ventricular arrhythmia may also be more common with hypomagnesemia.

Atrial fibrillation after coronary artery bypass is a common complication. Hypomagnesemia is also common after bypass. In a meta-analysis of seven double-blind, placebo-controlled trials, Gu et al were able to show that IV magnesium reduced postoperative atrial fibrillation by 36%.[18]

Magnesium has been a staple for the treatment of torsades de pointes; however, the 2018 focused update on Advanced Cardiovascular Life Support (ACLS) cited scant evidence to support this and stated, "The routine use of magnesium for cardiac arrest is not recommended in adult patients (Class III: No Benefit; Level of Evidence C-LD). Magnesium may be considered for torsades de pointes (i.e., polymorphic Ventricular Tachycardia associated with long-QT interval) (Class IIb; Level of Evidence C-LD)." Class IIb is weak evidence, with the likely benefit to be greater than or equal to risk.[19]

Diagnosis

Serum magnesium represents only 0.3% of total body magnesium, so it shouldn't be a surprise that serum magnesium levels do not reliably represent total magnesium stores. In some cases, patients may have clinically significant magnesium deficiency despite a normal serum magnesium. Use of ionized magnesium or erythrocyte magnesium is unable to improve the assessment of total body stores.[20,21] A 24-hour urine for magnesium can be helpful. If patients are hypomagnesemic, magnesium excretion of more than 1 mmol (24 mg) per day is suggestive of renal magnesium wasting.[22] The other commonly discussed test is the magnesium tolerance test. Here patients have their 24-hour urine magnesium checked, then get a loading dose of magnesium followed by a second 24-hour urine to see what fraction of the loading dose (0.2 mEq/kg [2.4 mg/kg]) is retained by the subject. Healthy individuals with normal magnesium status retained 14%, whereas hypomagnesemic individuals retained 85%. Patients with medical conditions predisposing them to magnesium depletion retained 51%.[23] There are little data to show if the magnesium tolerance test works in patients with renal magnesium wasting or chronic kidney disease. Given the fact that there are little data showing the advantage of using magnesium tolerance for treatment decisions and the fact that it takes at least 48 hours to complete, use of the magnesium tolerance test remains limited to research applications.

Treatment

Patients with symptomatic hypomagnesemia should be treated with IV magnesium. No trials have been done to determine the optimal regimen for magnesium replacement, but experts recommend treatment based on the level and presence of symptoms, severity of deficiency/illness.[24-26] Some recommendations for specific magnesium prescriptions are listed in **Table 24.3**. IV magnesium can be

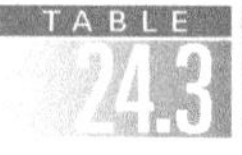

TABLE 24.3 Recommendations for Magnesium Replacement Based on Severity of Illness

Condition	**Magnesium Replacement**
Torsade de pointes	Intravenous (IV) magnesium sulfate 2 g (16 mEq) over 15 min followed by 1 g (8 mEq) hourly[26]
Cardiac arrest	No longer recommended, Class III, risk > benefit[19]
Severe, symptomatic hypomagnesemia—mg levels <1 mEq/L with neuromuscular, neurologic, or cardiac arrhythmias	2 g (16 mEq) of magnesium sulfate over 5-10 min. Alternatively, this can be given over an hour if the symptoms are not life-threatening. This initial treatment should be followed by 4-6 g (32-48 mEq) a day for 3-5 d. Use caution in patients with decreased kidney function.[24,25]
Mild to moderate hypomagnesemia—mg levels 1-1.5 mg/dL	Magnesium oxide 400 mg 2-3 times a day IV replacement is recommended if the patient develops diarrhea or has gastrointestinal disturbance.
General recommendations	Continue therapy for magnesium replacement after correction of the serum level to replace presumed intracellular magnesium depletion. Use of amiloride can minimize renal magnesium losses. Correct hypomagnesemia before correcting hypokalemia and hypocalcemia.

associated with muscle weakness, areflexia, hypotension, and decreased inotropy. One gram of IV calcium gluconate can be used as an antidote to acute toxicity of magnesium infusions.[27] Oral magnesium replacement is limited by diarrhea. As oral magnesium doses climb, the risk of diarrhea goes up. Because diarrhea is a cause of hypomagnesemia, oral magnesium can become a snake swallowing its own tail.

HYPERMAGNESEMIA

Hypermagnesemia is defined as serum magnesium over 2.4 mg/dL (1.98 mEq/L or 0.99 mmol/L). In 1,033 consecutive electrolyte determinations (not all of them with an order for a magnesium level), only 59 were more than 0.99 mmol/L.[28] Hypermagnesemia is rare because the kidney is able to increase the fractional excretion of magnesium to nearly 100% (normal 2%-4%) in response to increased levels. Hypermagnesemia is largely asymptomatic, with clinical symptoms being rare below a magnesium of 4.8 mg/dL (2 mmol/L).

Etiology of Hypermagnesemia

Hypermagnesemia can result from either increased exogenous intake or impaired excretion (see **Table 24.4**).

Increased Intake of Magnesium

Magnesium is found in laxatives and antacids. Epsom salt is magnesium sulfate and is often used as a folk remedy for abdominal pain, constipation, arthritis, and influenza. One tablespoon of Epsom salt contains approximately 35 g of magnesium sulfate.

Clark and Brown reported on eight cases of severe hypomagnesemia because of oral intake of magnesium-containing cathartics or antacids. Intake was not excessive but concurrent bowel disease allowed excess absorption. Though seven

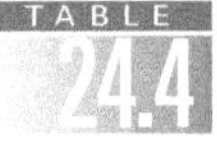

TABLE 24.4 Clinical Settings of Hypermagnesemia

Common	Acute kidney failure Chronic kidney disease with exogenous magnesium intake Preeclampsia and eclampsia therapy
Less common	Chronic kidney disease without exogenous magnesium intake Rectal administration of magnesium-containing solutions
Rare	Parasitosis with exogenous magnesium intake Lithium therapy Hypothyroidism Certain neoplasms with skeletal involvement Viral hepatitis Hyperparathyroidism with kidney disease Pituitary dwarfism Milk-alkali syndrome Perforated viscus with exogenous magnesium intake Acute diabetic ketoacidosis Addison disease

of the eight did not have preexisting diagnosis of kidney dysfunction, glomerular filtration rate (GFR) was likely compromised because of the advanced age of the patients (70 ± 6 years).[29]

Another typical setting for hypermagnesemia is the treatment of preterm labor or preeclampsia/eclampsia. Patients are routinely loaded with IV magnesium without assessing the levels. Typical infusion protocols (4-6 g load followed by 1-2 g/hr) result in serum magnesium levels of 4 to 8 mg/dL. Thankfully, patients typically have good outcomes even in cases where accidents result in very high magnesium levels.[30]

Decreased Magnesium Excretion

In most cases, decreased clearance of magnesium at least plays a role in the development of hypermagnesemia. Normally, patients with progressive kidney dysfunction insufficiency are able to maintain magnesium balance with normal magnesium intake until the GFR falls to 30 mL/min. After that, patients should be warned to avoid increased oral magnesium.[21]

Familial hypocalciuric hypercalcemia (FHH) is an autosomal dominant tubular disorder with a loss-of-function mutation of the calcium-sensing receptor (CaSR) so that serum calcium is unable to modulate calcium (and magnesium) resorption in the thick ascending limb of the loop of Henle. This unregulated calcium and magnesium result in modest hypercalcemia and hypermagnesemia, respectively.

Manifestations of Hypermagnesemia

Hypermagnesemia prevents the release of presynaptic acetylcholine-suppressing neuromuscular transmission (see **Table 24.5**). Clinically, the first place this shows up is in loss of the deep tendon reflex (usually at levels above 4.8 mg/dL). This can be followed by somnolence and ultimately muscle paralysis, including the muscles of respiration at a magnesium level around 12 mg/dL. Cardiovascular effects usually begin to be seen around 4 to 5 mg/dL and begin with hypotension. As the magnesium level rises above 7, prolonged PR intervals, increased QRS duration, and prolonged QT intervals are seen. This is followed by bradycardia. Finally, hypermagnesemia can cause complete heart block and cardiac arrest.

Magnesium is tightly linked to calcium metabolism. Hypermagnesemia inhibits PTH release, leading to mild hypocalcemia, which can worsen QT prolongation and compound cardiac arrhythmia.

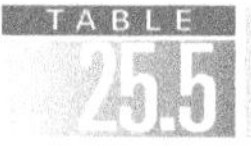

Effects of Hypermagnesemia

Serum Magnesium Level	Clinical Manifestations
1.7-2.4	Normal levels
5-8	Nausea, vomiting, headache, flushing, loss of deep tendon reflexes, somnolence, hypotension
12-15	Atrioventricular block, bradycardia, QRS widening, muscle weakness, and paralysis
>15	Cardiac arrest, respiratory arrest

Prevention and Treatment

The first rule of hypermagnesemia is preventing hypermagnesemia. Patients with compromised GFR should avoid magnesium loads. Magnesium is often delivered in antacids and cathartics.[29]

If hypermagnesemia develops in a patient with intact kidney function, stopping the magnesium should allow quick recovery. Some advocate adding a forced saline diuresis and loop diuretics with or without thiazides to increase magnesium clearance. Hypermagnesemia can cause hypotension and acute kidney injury, compromising the ability to clear magnesium via the kidney. Calcium blocks the toxic effects of magnesium so patients with severe intoxication should be given 1 g of IV calcium gluconate as a temporary antidote.[21]

If kidney function is compromised or the patient has severe symptomatic disease, dialysis should be provided. Intermittent hemodialysis lowers magnesium faster than continuous therapies.[31] Continuous Kidney replacement therapy (CKRT) has been used successfully and can prevent rebound hypermagnesemia after a session of intermittent hemodialysis; this is especially important in patients following large ingestions of magnesium citrate where retention of the magnesium-based laxative in the gut can serve as a reservoir for continuous magnesium absorption.[32] Peritoneal dialysis has also been used to successfully treat hypermagnesemia.[33]

References

1. Haider DG, Lindner G, Ahmad SS, et al. Hypermagnesemia is a strong independent risk factor for mortality in critically ill patients: results from a cross-sectional study. *Eur J Intern Med.* 2015;26(7):504-507.
2. Fairley J, Glassford NJ, Zhang L, Bellomo R. Magnesium status and magnesium therapy in critically ill patients: a systematic review. *J Crit Care.* 2015;30(6):1349-1358.
3. Ryzen E, Wagers PW, Singer FR, Rude RK. Magnesium deficiency in a medical ICU population. *Crit Care Med.* 1985;13:312-313.
4. Wong ET, Rude RK, Singer FR, Shaw ST Jr. A high prevalence of hypomagnesemia and hypermagnesemia in hospitalized patients. *Am J Clin Pathol.* 1983;79(3):348-352.
5. Agus ZS. Hypomagnesemia. *J Am Soc Nephrol.* 1999;10(7):1616-1622.
6. Kelly AP, Robb BJ, Gearry RB. Hypocalcaemia and hypomagnesaemia: a complication of Crohn's disease. *N Z Med J.* 2008;121(1287):77-79.
7. Epstein M, McGrath S, Law F. Proton-pump inhibitors and hypomagnesemic hypoparathyroidism. *N Engl J Med.* 2006;355(17):1834-1836.
8. Cheungpasitporn W, Thongprayoon C, Kittanamongkolchai W, et al. Proton pump inhibitors linked to hypomagnesemia: a systematic review and meta-analysis of observational studies. *Ren Fail.* 2015;37(7):1237-1241.
9. Liao S, Gan L, Mei Z. Does the use of proton pump inhibitors increase the risk of hypomagnesemia. *Medicine.* 2019;98(13):e15011. doi:10.1097/md.0000000000015011
10. William JH, Danziger J. Proton-pump inhibitor-induced hypomagnesemia: current research and proposed mechanisms. *World J Nephrol.* 2016;5(2):152-157.
11. Jain N, Reilly RF. Hungry bone syndrome. *Curr Opin Nephrol Hypertens.* 2017;26(4):250-255.
12. Blaine J, Chonchol M, Levi M. Renal control of calcium, phosphate, and magnesium homeostasis. *Clin J Am Soc Nephrol.* 2015;10(7):1257-1272.
13. Petrelli F, Borgonovo K, Cabiddu M, Ghilardi M, Barni S. Risk of anti-EGFR monoclonal antibody-related hypomagnesemia: systematic review and pooled analysis of randomized studies. *Expert Opin Drug Saf.* 2012;11(Suppl 1):S9-S19.
14. De Marchi S, Cecchin E, Basile A, Bertotti A, Nardini R, Bartoli E. Renal tubular dysfunction in chronic alcohol abuse—effects of abstinence. *N Engl J Med.* 1993;329(26):1927-1934.
15. Huang C-L, Kuo E. Mechanism of hypokalemia in magnesium deficiency. *J Am Soc Nephrol.* 2007;18(10):2649-2652.
16. Griffin TP, Murphy M, Coulter J, Murphy MS. Symptomatic hypocalcaemia secondary to PTH resistance associated with hypomagnesaemia after elective embolisation of uterine fibroid. *BMJ Case Rep.* 2013;2013. doi:10.1136/bcr-2013-008708
17. Hansen B-A, Bruserud Ø. Hypomagnesemia in critically ill patients. *J Intensive Care Med.* 2018;6:21.

18. Gu W-J, Wu Z-J, Wang P-F, Aung LHH, Yin R-X. Intravenous magnesium prevents atrial fibrillation after coronary artery bypass grafting: a meta-analysis of 7 double-blind, placebo-controlled, randomized clinical trials. *Trials.* 2012;13:41.
19. Panchal AR, Berg KM, Kudenchuk PJ, et al. 2018 American Heart Association focused update on advanced cardiovascular life support use of antiarrhythmic drugs during and immediately after cardiac arrest: an update to the American Heart Association Guidelines for Cardiopulmonary Resuscitation and Emergency Cardiovascular Care. *Circulation.* 2018;138(23):e740-e749.
20. Elin RJ, Hosseini JM, Gill JR Jr. Erythrocyte and mononuclear blood cell magnesium concentrations are normal in hypomagnesemic patients with chronic renal magnesium wasting. *J Am Coll Nutr.* 1994;13(5):463-466.
21. Swaminathan R. Magnesium metabolism and its disorders. *Clin Biochem Rev.* 2003;24(2):47-66.
22. Fawcett WJ, Haxby EJ, Male DA. Magnesium: physiology and pharmacology. *Br J Anaesth.* 1999;83(2):302-320.
23. Goto K, Yasue H, Okumura K, et al. Magnesium deficiency detected by intravenous loading test in variant angina pectoris. *Am J Cardiol.* 1990;65(11):709-712. doi:10.1016/0002-9149(90)91375-g
24. Ayuk J, Gittoes NJL. Treatment of hypomagnesemia. *Am J Kidney Dis.* 2014;63(4):691-695.
25. Martin KJ, González EA, Slatopolsky E. Clinical consequences and management of hypomagnesemia. *J Am Soc Nephrol.* 2009;20(11):2291-2295.
26. Tzivoni D, Banai S, Schuger C, et al. Treatment of torsade de pointes with magnesium sulfate. *Circulation.* 1988;77(2):392-397.
27. Idama TO, Lindow SW. Magnesium sulphate: a review of clinical pharmacology applied to obstetrics. *Br J Obstet Gynaecol.* 1998;105(3):260-268.
28. Whang R. Frequency of hypomagnesemia and hypermagnesemia. Requested vs routine. *JAMA.* 1990;263(22):3063-3064. doi:10.1001/jama.263.22.3063
29. Clark BA, Brown RS. Unsuspected morbid hypermagnesemia in elderly patients. *Am J Nephrol.* 1992;12(5):336-343.
30. Morisaki H, Yamamoto S, Morita Y, Kotake Y, Ochiai R, Takeda J. Hypermagnesemia-induced cardiopulmonary arrest before induction of anesthesia for emergency cesarean section. *J Clin Anesth.* 2000;12(3):224-226.
31. Schelling JR. Fatal hypermagnesemia. *Clin Nephrol.* 2000;53(1):61-65.
32. Bokhari SR, Siriki R, Teran FJ, Batuman V. Fatal hypermagnesemia due to laxative use. *Am J Med Sci.* 2018;355(4):390-395.
33. Brown AT, Campbell WA. Hazards of hypertonic magnesium enema therapy. *Arch Dis Child.* 1978;53(11):920.

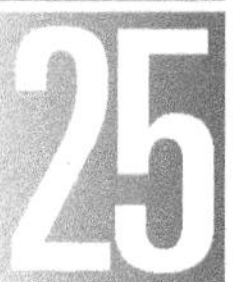

Acid-Base Management in the Intensive Care Unit

Roger A. Rodby

INTRODUCTION

Acid-base disorders are loved by nephrologists and often loathed by others, but there is no more important a place to diagnose and treat these abnormalities than in an intensive care unit (ICU) setting. Patients in an ICU frequently have derangements in $[HCO_3]$ or $[PCO_2]$ (or both) that lead to markedly abnormal pH values. It is important to recognize, however, that a normal pH does not exclude an acid-base disorder, which can be hidden and clinically significant. The clinician managing these patients needs to dissect the entire blood gas pH, $[HCO_3]$, and $[PCO_2]$ in conjunction with anion gap (AG) to best determine all components of an acid-base disorder to make the correct diagnosis. This is critical in any decision making that may be indicated based on these values. This chapter reviews the basics of determining these disorders as well as treatment approaches.

HENDERSON-HASSELBALCH SIMPLIFIED

The body regulates the pH within the narrow range of 7.38 to 7.42 through changes in the $[HCO_3]$ (kidneys) and the $[PCO_2]$ (lungs). The relationship of the pH to these values is most easily understood with a simplified version of the Henderson-Hasselbalch (H/H) equation, where

$$[H^+] = 24\,([PCO_2]/[HCO_3])$$

with the $[PCO_2]$ in mm Hg and the $[HCO_3]$ in mmol/L. Using *normal* $[HCO_3]$ and $[PCO_2]$ values of 24 and 40, respectively, this gives a *normal* $[H^+]$ of 40. The units of $[H^+]$ are in nanomoles/liter or 40×10^{-9} (Na and K values are in 10^{-3}, which speaks to just how low a concentration of $[H^+]$ exists in the blood). As pH is the negative log of the $[H^+]$, translating these nanomole $[H^+]$ values to a pH can be a bit daunting even with a calculator. However, because there are a finite number of plasma $[H^+]$ values consistent with life, these can be presented in an easy-to-use table (**Table 25.1**). Using this, you can see that a $[H^+]$ of 40×10^{-9} translates to a *normal* pH of 7.40. The relationship of $[H^+]$ to pH is logarithmic and not linear, but it is useful to know that a $[H^+]$ of 50×10^{-9} corresponds to a pH of 7.30 and 30×10^{-9} to a pH of 7.50.

Three points are worth mentioning. The $[HCO_3]$ can be directly *measured* using venous blood specimens run by typical laboratory autoanalyzers and can be *calculated* (from the measured pH and $[PCO_2]$) when a blood gas machine is used for these measurements. This has led to a common misconception that $[HCO_3]$ values from a blood gas measurement are not valid and often lead to

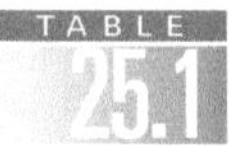

pH Values That Accompany a Wide Physiologic Range of $[H^+]$ Values

$[H^+] = 24\ ([PCO_2]/[HCO_3])$

pH	$[H^+]$	pH	$[H^+]$	pH	$[H^+]$	pH	$[H^+]$	pH	$[H^+]$	pH	$[H^+]$	pH	$[H^+]$
8.00	10	7.80	16	7.59	26	7.39	41	7.19	65	6.99	102	6.79	162
7.99	10	7.79	16	7.58	26	7.38	42	7.18	66	6.98	105	6.78	166
7.98	10	7.78	17	7.57	27	7.37	43	7.17	68	6.97	107	6.77	170
7.97	11	7.77	17	7.56	28	7.36	44	7.16	69	6.96	110	6.76	174
7.96	11	7.76	17	7.55	28	7.35	45	7.15	71	6.95	112	6.75	178
7.95	11	7.75	18	7.54	29	7.34	46	7.14	72	6.94	115	6.74	182
7.94	11	7.74	18	7.53	30	7.33	47	7.13	74	6.93	117	6.73	186
7.93	12	7.73	19	7.52	30	7.32	48	7.12	76	6.92	120	6.72	191
7.92	12	7.72	19	7.51	31	7.31	49	7.11	78	6.91	123	6.71	196
7.91	12	7.70	20	7.50	32	7.30	50	7.10	79	6.90	126	6.70	200
7.90	13	7.69	20	7.49	32	7.29	51	7.09	81	6.89	129	6.69	204
7.89	13	7.68	21	7.48	33	7.28	52	7.08	83	6.88	132	6.68	209
7.88	13	7.67	21	7.47	34	7.27	54	7.07	85	6.87	135	6.67	214
7.87	13	7.66	22	7.46	35	7.26	55	7.06	87	6.86	138	6.66	219
7.86	14	7.65	22	7.45	35	7.25	56	7.05	89	6.85	141	6.65	224
7.85	14	7.64	23	7.44	36	7.24	58	7.04	91	6.84	145	6.64	229
7.84	14	7.63	23	7.43	37	7.23	59	7.03	93	6.83	148	6.63	234
7.83	15	7.62	24	7.42	38	7.22	60	7.02	95	6.82	151	6.62	240
7.82	15	7.61	25	7.41	39	7.21	62	7.01	98	6.81	155	6.61	245
7.81	15	7.60	25	7.40	40	7.20	63	7.00	100	6.80	159	6.60	251

$[H^+]$ values in 10^{-9}.

using only blood chemistry panel determined $[HCO_3]$ values. The reason it is calculated when determined by a blood gas machine is because it does not need to be measured. If you have a *measured* and, therefore, assumed valid $[PCO_2]$ and pH, then H/H allows only one $[HCO_3]$ for that combination of $[PCO_2]$ and pH. If you believe the *measured* $[PCO_2]$ and the *measured* pH, you really have no choice but to believe this *calculated* $[HCO_3]$. Second, venous and arterial $[HCO_3]$ values normally differ, with venous blood values typically being 1 to 2 mmol/L higher than arterial values, so it does not make sense to interpret an *arterial* blood gas using a *venous* $[HCO_3]$. Finally, although the gold standard for measuring systemic pH is from arterial blood, venous blood gas determinations are well correlated with arterial blood specimens, with venous specimens typically having $[HCO_3]$ values approximately 1 mmol/L and $[PCO_2]$ values approximately 4 mm Hg higher and with pH values 0.03 lower than those obtained using simultaneously determined arterial specimens.[1]

GENERAL CONSIDERATIONS IN THE EVALUATION OF THE ACID-BASE STATUS

An abnormal blood pH can exist with any number of combinations of pH, $[HCO_3]$, and $[PCO_2]$ values. Simultaneous metabolic and respiratory acidoses or alkaloses produce the most abnormal pH values, whereas when opposites occur (an acidosis and a simultaneous alkalosis), you may have a near-normal or even normal pH as the effect of one may "cancel" out the effect of the other. A normal pH should thus never be assumed to lack an acid-base disorder. And although the lungs compensate for metabolic disorders and the kidneys for respiratory disorders, neither will compensate to a normal pH, and thus, any abnormal $[HCO_3]$ or $[PCO_2]$ that is associated with a normal pH automatically indicates that there are two *primary* acid-base disorders. Humans increase or decrease minute ventilation to attenuate pH changes brought on by alterations in the $[HCO_3]$, and the kidney can excrete or create HCO_3 to attenuate changes in the $[PCO_2]$. These compensations follow certain rules within limits (**Table 25.2**). Respiratory compensation for metabolic acid-base disorders can be immediate (minutes) as the $[PCO_2]$ can change very quickly by simply increasing or decreasing minute ventilation. The only lag in respiratory response to changes in the $[HCO_3]$ is the lag in time for the cerebrospinal fluid to equilibrate with the systemic pH. In chronic respiratory alkalosis, the kidney can relatively rapidly excrete HCO_3 by simply not reabsorbing it (hours), whereas generating new HCO_3 for a chronic respiratory acidosis can take much longer (days). These timings must be considered when evaluating whether or not an appropriate compensation has or may still occur.

RECOGNIZING AND DETERMINING THE CAUSE OF AN ACID-BASE DISORDER

There are several steps in determining the acid-base status of a patient, including:

1. Is the blood pH abnormal?
2. Is compensation occurring and is the degree of compensation appropriate? (Table 25.2)

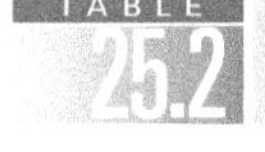

TABLE 25.2 Expected Compensatory Changes for Metabolic and Respiratory Disorders

Disorder	Expected Change[a]
Metabolic acidosis	$[PCO_2] \downarrow = 1.0 - 1.4 \times \Delta[HCO_3]$
Metabolic alkalosis	$[PCO_2] \uparrow = 0.25 - 1.0 \times \Delta[HCO_3]$
Acute respiratory acidosis	$[HCO_3] \uparrow = 0.1 \times \Delta[PCO_2]$ ($\pm$0.3 mmol/L)
Chronic respiratory acidosis	$[HCO_3] \uparrow = 0.4 \times \Delta[PCO_2]$ ($\pm$0.4 mmol/L)
Acute respiratory alkalosis	$[HCO_3] \downarrow = 0.1 - 0.3 \times \Delta[PCO_2]$ (minimum $[HCO_3]$ 18 mmol/L)
Chronic respiratory alkalosis	$[HCO_3] \downarrow = 0.2 - 0.5 \times \Delta[PCO_2]$ (minimum $[HCO_3]$ 14 mmol/L)

[a] $[HCO_3]$ is 24 − $[HCO_3]$ and $\Delta[PCO_2]$ is 40 − $[PCO_2]$.

3. Is there an elevation in the AG?
4. Does the elevation in the AG coincide with the decrease in the [HCO_3]?
5. If the pH is not abnormal, are there two primary disorders present by cancelling each other out?

There is no consensus of what a normal AG [Na] − ([Cl] + [HCO_3]) is, and it ranges in various publications from 6 to 12.[2] The AG will be lower when there is an increase in unmeasured cations as can be seen in hypergammaglobulinemia (and severe hypercalcemia or hypermagnesemia) or when there is a decrease in unmeasured anions, typically seen in hypoalbuminemia. Correction for the latter is commonly necessary in the ICU: for every 1 g/dL drop in serum albumin from 4.0, add 2.5 to the AG. Because a normal AG can vary, the clinician should be careful not to overinterpret mild increases in the AG as they may not represent a clinically significant metabolic acidosis.[2,3]

In an anion gap metabolic acidosis (AGMA), the AG will typically increase approximately 1 for every 1 mmol decrease in the [HCO_3] (the ΔAG = Δ[HCO_3]; **Table 25.3**). Any change in the AG significantly greater than this indicates that the [HCO_3] was initially higher (or is being driven higher) and determines that a simultaneous metabolic alkalosis is present. If the metabolic alkalosis is severe enough, the [HCO_3] could be normal or even elevated above normal and, in doing so, may hide the metabolic acidosis! Because, in lactic acidosis (LA), there may be significant intracellular buffering, the degree of acid production may not be reflected in the [HCO_3]. In order to identify a simultaneous metabolic alkalosis with an LA, the increase in the AG (the ΔAG using a baseline normal AG of 10) should be 1.5 times greater than the change in [HCO_3]. Similarly, if the ΔAG is significantly less than the Δ[HCO_3], a combination of AGMA and nonanion gap metabolic acidosis (NAGMA) is present. With these principles in mind, Table 25.3 summarizes the rules for identifying a hidden metabolic alkalosis or acidosis, or a combination of AGMA and NAGMA.

WHEN TO CONSIDER TREATING A METABOLIC ACIDOSIS

Why is it important to differentiate AGMA from NAGMA, to differentiate respiratory from metabolic acidosis, and to reveal hidden acid-base disorders? A

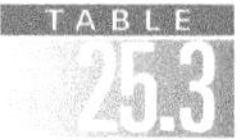

TABLE 25.3 Rules for Determining Complex Acid-Base Disorders Using the Anion Gap

In the Presence of an AGMA
For each 1 mmol/L ↓ in [HCO_3], the AG should ↑ by ~1
Where:

- Δ[HCO_3] = 24 − Patient's [HCO_3]
- ΔAG = Patient's AG − 10

If:

- Δ[HCO_3] > ΔAG = Acidosis is *mixed AG and NAGMA*
- ΔAG > 1.5 × Δ[HCO_3] = *Hidden metabolic alkalosis* in addition to AGMA
- Δ[HCO_3] is zero or negative ([HCO_3] ≥24) = *Hidden metabolic acidosis* in addition to a *hidden metabolic alkalosis*

AG, anion gap; AGMA, anion gap metabolic acidosis; NAGMA, nonanion gap metabolic acidosis.

severe acidemia (acidotic systemic blood pH) adversely affects many physiologic functions but may have its largest impact on hemodynamic stability by causing reduced left ventricular contractility, arterial vasodilation, and impaired responsiveness to catecholamines. A common pH threshold of concern is less than or equal to 7.20. However, it is important to realize that not all pH values of 7.2 have similar clinical implications. To demonstrate this, each of the following four acidemia examples has a pH of 7.2 (using the simplified H/H equation: $[H^+] = 24 ([PCO_2]/[HCO_3])$, and all produce a $[H^+]$ of 63, which from Table 25.1 correlates to a pH of 7.2).

pH	$[HCO_3]$	$[PCO_2]$	Interpretation
(A) 7.20	20	53	Mixed respiratory and metabolic acidosis
(B) 7.20	15	39	Uncompensated metabolic acidosis
(C) 7.20	10	26	Compensated severe metabolic acidosis
(D) 7.20	5	13	Mixed severe metabolic acidosis and respiratory alkalosis

Now let us decrease the $[HCO_3]$ in A to D further by *only* 2 mmol/L more (*keeping the $[PCO_2]$ constant*) and determine the new pH values that correspond to these lower $[HCO_3]$ values (E-H):

$[HCO_3]$		$[HCO_3]$ –2		New pH
(E) 20	→	18	→	7.15
(F) 15	→	13	→	7.14
(G) 10	→	8	→	7.11
(H) 5	→	3	→	6.98

These examples demonstrate that the lower the baseline $[HCO_3]$, any further reduction in the $[HCO_3]$ leads to a greater decrease in the pH, with cases C and D being in a very tenuous acid-base state compared to A and B, despite all having the same baseline pH.

Similarly, let us increase the $[PCO_2]$ by only 5 mm Hg (keeping the $[HCO_3]$ constant) and determine the new pH values for each of these (I-L):

$[PCO_2]$		$[PCO_2]$ +5		New pH
(I) 53	→	58	→	7.16
(J) 39	→	44	→	7.16
(K) 26	→	31	→	7.13
(L) 13	→	18	→	7.06

Again, the lower the baseline $[PCO_2]$, any subsequent increase in the $[PCO_2]$ has a greater effect on the systemic pH. These examples stress the importance of how dissecting the components of a blood gas should be performed to determine whether you need to treat an acidemia and, if so, should the goal be to increase ventilation or to give a source of base ($NaHCO_3$, citrate, acetate). For example, although patients C and D still have a "tolerable" pH of 7.2, you should look past the pH and increase the [HCO_3] so that they have a buffer (no pun intended) to prevent a dangerous fall in pH in the event the [HCO_3] decreases further. Using the simplified H/H equation and Table 25.1 is an extremely useful and easy bedside tool to predict changes in pH based on changes in [HCO_3] and [PCO_2] and can serve as a guide to the required changes in these parameters necessary to achieve a desired pH. Change one, solve for the other!

ANION GAP METABOLIC ACIDOSIS VERSUS NONANION GAP METABOLIC ACIDOSIS IN CONSIDERATION FOR TREATING A METABOLIC ACIDOSIS

The abovementioned examples stress how little changes in [HCO_3] can have a major effect on pH when the [HCO_3] is less than or equal to10 mmol/L. Another consideration in treating a metabolic acidosis is whether or not a patient has an AGMA or NAGMA. The NAGMAs generally are slow to worsen (unless there is massive gastrointestinal HCO_3 loss, such as seen in cholera), and the risk of an acute decrease in [HCO_3] and pH as seen in previous examples is considerably less. Thus, the clinician should be less concerned about "buffering the buffer" if a major component of the acidemic pH is an NAGMA. This is much different than, for example, LA where [HCO_3] levels can decline rapidly and precipitously.

METABOLIC ACIDOSIS: TO TREAT OR NOT TO TREAT?

A mathematical argument has been made to acutely treat specific situations of severe metabolic acidemia. In ICU settings, this is generally achieved by giving intravenous $NaHCO_3$. There are numerous reasons why the administration of $NaHCO_3$ is considered harmful, including increasing intracellular acidosis, decreasing brain pH, increasing CO_2 production, increasing lactic acid production, and Na (extracellular volume) overload.[4-6] In the end, however, concern over the untoward effects of severe acidemia usually wins, and therefore when "push comes to shove," few clinicians let those concerns prevent them from treating a severe metabolic acidemia with $NaHCO_3$, allowing them to "buy time" while simultaneously addressing and treating the underlying cause.

Many textbooks discuss the calculation of the "bicarb deficit": (24 − (patient's [HCO_3]) × 60% to 80% of body weight in kg); however, there is no reason to do this because there is no need to replace the entire deficit. For the same reason as shown in the abovementioned examples that a few mmol/L decrease in [HCO_3] can significantly impact the systemic pH, raising the [HCO_3] by only a few mmol/L can have a similarly positive impact by "buffering the buffer." Given an average patient weighing 80 kg has 60% water, the volume of distribution for calculation of HCO_3 repletion is the total body water at 48 L. And since an ampule of $NaHCO_3$ has 50 mmol of HCO_3, "guestimate" that for an average sized patient, each ampule of $NaHCO_3$ will raise the patient's [HCO_3] by about 1 mmol/L and thus two ampules (100 mmol) may be all that is needed to get a patient "out of the (acidemia) woods." Each ampule has 50 mmol in 50 mL with a concentration of 1 mmol/mL or 1,000 mL/L and a resultant osmolality of 2,000 mOsm/L. This is quite hypertonic and will pull H_2O from the intracellular space to the extracellular space to achieve osmolar equilibrium. The alternative is to use an isotonic $NaHCO_3$ drip typically prepared by adding three ampules of $NaHCO_3$ to 1 L of D5W (final [$NaHCO_3$] = 130 mEq/L). The volume of this drip required to give the same 100 mmol of $NaHCO_3$ is 666 mL, and there is little difference between the expansions of the extracellular space with either method.

LACTIC ACIDOSIS CONSIDERATIONS

The above calculations are meant for a single desired acute increase in [HCO_3] and pH. LA is both the most common and most severe metabolic acid-base abnormality encountered in the ICU. Although it may be related to a finite episode of tissue hypoxia (e.g., a seizure), LA is typically seen in septic patients with multiorgan failure. Lactic acid production can be massive, and $NaHCO_3$ requirements to maintain an acceptable pH will be similarly very high, causing a huge expansion of the extracellular compartment risking clinically dangerous fluid overload. The treatment should focus initially around reversing the cause of the LA. But until this occurs, the patient may require $NaHCO_3$ supplementation to maintain some "acceptable" pH value. However, it is not unusual in LA to require greater than or equal to 100 mmol of $NaHCO_3$/hr (close to 1 L/hr of an isotonic $NaHCO_3$ drip), and this degree of extracellular volume expansion cannot be tolerated indefinitely. Kidney replacement therapy (KRT), on the other hand, may be an improved method to supply $NaHCO_3$ isovolemically. Continuous kidney replacement therapy (CKRT) is ideally designed for the hemodynamically unstable patient that usually accompanies LA. For example, using continuous veno venous hemofiltration with a typical replacement fluid (RF) [$NaHCO_3$] of 35 mmol/L, one can easily see how large quantities of $NaHCO_3$ can be delivered isosmotically and thus isovolemically. If the patient has a [HCO_3] of 5 mmol/L, each liter of hemofiltrate (HF) will remove 5 mmol of $NaHCO_3$. But if that liter of ultrafiltrate is replaced isovolemically using intravenous RF containing 35 mmol/L of $NaHCO_3$, each liter of HF results in a net increase in $35 - 5 = 30$ mmol of $NaHCO_3$. With modern CKRT machines, it is not difficult to achieve an HF rate of 4 to 5 L an hour supplying a net increase (using this example) of 120 to 150 mmol of $NaHCO_3$ per hour without extracellular volume expansion.

OTHER METABOLIC ACIDOSIS CONSIDERATIONS IN THE INTENSIVE CARE UNIT

Propofol infusion syndrome can cause LA as can linezolid.[7,8] Metformin can cause LA when use is accompanied by kidney dysfunction.[9] Propylene glycol is occasionally used as a vehicle in lorazepam, phenobarbital, diazepam, and phenytoin continuous intravenous drips and can similarly cause LA.[10] The new SGLT2 (sodium-glucose cotransporter 2) inhibitors can rarely cause euglycemic diabetic ketoacidosis (see chapter 37).[11]

METABOLIC ALKALOSIS

Severe metabolic alkalosis with a pH greater than or equal to 7.6 is unusual but is associated with cardiac arrhythmias and may need to be treated. Depending on the etiology, a small percentage of these patients may respond to acetazolamide and others to intravenous fluids containing chloride, but many of these patients have simultaneous kidney failure and thus excretion of HCO_3 by the kidneys cannot be expected. This leaves two treatment options: a hydrochloric acid drip and KRT. The former is difficult to obtain and has significant risks of chemical damage to the infusion vein. KRT and specifically hemodialysis using a low bicarbonate dialysate concentration may be ideal. Another option would be to use CKRT with a low or bicarbonate-free dialysate (continuous veno venous hemodialysis or CVVHD) or RF (continuous veno venous hemofiltration or CVVH). The later could be achieved by using normal saline, but if this is done, it is important to pay special attention to the potassium and serum calcium levels because they will drop if not adequately replaced. It is also important to remember that alkalemia already lowers ionized calcium and thus should be monitored frequently. Finally, it is imperative to dissect the entire blood gas to ensure that a respiratory component is not contributing to the alkalosis, as managing that may be a considerably easier maneuver to lowering systemic pH. Sedation and even respiratory paralysis with controlled minute ventilation may be considered in extreme situations.

RESPIRATORY ACID-BASE DISORDERS

Respiratory disorders can cause hypercapnia (respiratory acidosis) and hypocapnia (respiratory alkalosis). Although the [PCO_2] is an equally important component of pH through the H/H equation, these disorders are best handled by ventilation management by a physician well versed in pulmonary physiology. Still, it needs to be stressed that all acid-base disorders need to be broken down into their individual metabolic and respiratory components because it may be easier to improve any abnormal pH by simply "fixing" any respiratory acid-base abnormalities.

References

1. Treger R, Priouz S, Kamangar N, Corry D. Agreement between venous and arterial blood measurements in the intensive care unit. *Clin J Am Soc Nephrol.* 2010;5(3):390-394.
2. Kraut J, Nagami G. The serum anion gap in the evaluation of acid-base disorders: what are its limitations and can its effectiveness be improved? *Clin J Am Soc Nephrol.* 2018;8:2018-2024.
3. Kraut J, Madias N. Serum anion gap: its uses and limitations in clinical medicine. *Clin J Am Soc Nephrol.* 2007;2:162-174.
4. Kraut J, Kurtz I. Use of bicarb in the treatment of severe acidemic states. *Am J Kidney Dis.* 2001;38(4):703-727.
5. Forsythe SM, Schmidt GA. Sodium bicarbonate for the treatment of lactic acidosis. *Chest.* 2000;117(1):260-267.
6. Stacpolle PW. Lactic acidosis: the case against bicarbonate therapy. *Ann Intern Med.* 1986;105(2):276-279.
7. Mirrakhimov A, Voore P, Halytskyy O, Khan M, Ali A. Propofol infusion syndrome in adults: a clinical update. *Crit Care Res Pract.* https://www.hindawi.com/journals/ccrp/2015/260385/
8. Sawyer A, Haley H, Baty S, McGuffey G, Eiland E. Linezolid-induced lactic acidosis corrected with sustained low-efficiency dialysis: a case report. *Am J Kidney Dis.* 2014;64(3): 457-459.
9. Weisberg L. Lactic acidosis in a patient with type 2 diabetes mellitus. *Clin J Am Soc Nephrol.* 2015;10:1476-1483.
10. Zar T, Yusufzai I, Sullivan A, Graeber C. Acute kidney injury, hyperosmolality and metabolic acidosis associated with lorazepam. *Nat Clin Pract Nephrol.* 2007;3(9):515-520.
11. Galaye A, Haidar A, Kassab C, Kazmi S, Sinha P. Severe ketoacidosis associated with canagliflozin (Invokana): a safety concern. *Case Rep Crit Care.* 2016. doi:10.1155/2016/1656182

SECTION VII

Poisonings and Intoxications

26 Drug Dosing in Acute Kidney Injury

Soo Min Jang and Bruce A. Mueller

DRUGS ASSOCIATED WITH ACUTE KIDNEY INJURY

Acute kidney injury (AKI) frequently occurs in the intensive care unit (ICU).[1] It is associated with up to 60% mortality despite considerable advances in clinical practice and kidney replacement therapy (KRT) in the past decades.[2-4] Drug-associated AKI (e.g., aminoglycoside, contrast dye, vancomycin) is common, but nephrotoxins continue to be prescribed regularly in the ICU. In one university hospital's adult ICUs, 23% of the most commonly prescribed drugs were potential nephrotoxins, whereas 40% of commonly prescribed drugs in the pediatric ICUs were potentially nephrotoxic.[5]

Drug-associated nephrotoxicity causes are multifactorial (e.g., age, volume depletion, sepsis, and other comorbidities), yet many cases are preventable. Goldstein et al showed 38% reduction in nephrotoxic medication exposures and a 64% reduction in AKI rates in children through the Nephrotoxic Injury Negated by Just-in-time Action (NINJA) system.[6] This was a prospective quality improvement project implementing a systematic electronic health record screening and decision support process developed in a pediatric hospital. The NINJA study demonstrates that systematic surveillance for nephrotoxic medication exposure and assessing AKI risk can prevent harm. These findings imply that AKI can be preventable by assessing patient's risk for AKI and prescribing alternative medications to limit nephrotoxin exposure. A practical application of this type of approach could be used to prevent aminoglycoside-associated acute tubular necrosis (ATN), which occurs in 11% to 60% of adults.[7] Clinicians in the NINJA study intently monitored for aminoglycoside nephrotoxicity, especially when the patient was receiving prolonged therapy, had elevated aminoglycoside serum concentrations, or had a high nephrotoxin burden[6], and this is a best practice for others to emulate to reduce nephrotoxicity rates. Vancomycin is another antibiotic that has classically been associated with AKI due to ATN, AIN, and even cast nephropathy from vancomycin casts. Though AKI is associated with higher vancomycin levels, some controversy exists whether the high levels are the cause of, or result from the AKI.[8-10]

Piperacillin/tazobactam is commonly used in the ICU and has been associated with kidney injury as well. Evidence is growing, suggesting that concomitant vancomycin and piperacillin/tazobactam increases the risk of nephrotoxicity.[11] Six observational trials involving approximately 1,000 patients were analyzed for this meta-analysis. Nephrotoxicity incidence was substantially increased (2.26, 95% confidence interval [CI]: 1.4-3.6, $p < 0.05$) in the concurrent vancomycin and piperacillin/tazobactam group when compared to the control groups (vancomycin alone or vancomycin/cefepime or meropenem).[11] The combination of vancomycin and piperacillin/tazobactam use also resulted in the highest release of AKI biomarkers (urinary tissue inhibitor of metalloproteinase-2 and insulin-like growth factor binding-protein 7) in approximately 700 ICU patients.[12] AKI developed more frequently in patients who received this drug combination compared to those who received monotherapy of piperacillin/tazobactam ($p = 0.03$) but not vancomycin ($p = 0.29$). Therapeutic drug monitoring and close monitoring of kidney function to adjust drug dosing may be critical in critically ill patients to prevent AKI.[13] Clinicians should be judicious when utilizing known nephrotoxins and choose alternatives when possible in high-risk patients. Increased nephrotoxic medication exposures result in higher risk of AKI, leading to increased hospital stay, hospital costs, and patient morbidity.[14]

PHARMACOKINETIC CHANGES IN ACUTE KIDNEY INJURY

The pharmacokinetic impact of AKI goes beyond simply a reduction in the kidney's ability to provide drug clearance. All aspects of pharmacokinetics can be altered in AKI, including drug hepatic metabolism. Non-renal clearance (CL_{NR}) in AKI patients can be different from that observed in healthy subjects or patients with end-stage kidney disease (ESKD). In AKI, antibiotics such as imipenem, meropenem, and vancomycin have decreased CL_{NR} compared to healthy subjects but higher CL_{NR} than in those with ESRD.[15-17] Given that most drug doses for kidney failure have been generated in stable patients with ESRD, this higher CL_{NR} in AKI suggests that higher doses are needed for these antibiotics in AKI compared to what is recommended for patients with ESRD. This difference in hepatic function in AKI versus ESRD may affect other drugs as well. Indeed, dialysis itself has been reported to alter the liver's metabolic processes.[18] A common drug-metabolizing enzyme, CYP450 3A4, is far more active immediately after a hemodialysis session than immediately before it. KRTs used in the ICU, such as continuous kidney replacement therapy (CKRT), have not been studied in this regard.

Drug absorption and drug distribution are also changed in AKI. Drug absorption may be impaired owing to decreased gastrointestinal motility. The use of vasopressors leads to altered oral drug bioavailability from reduced gut perfusion. Clinicians often do not consider fluid therapy as a "drug therapy," but strong evidence links fluid overload with worsened ICU patient outcome, as discussed in Chapter 10.[19,20] Fluid overload also has substantial influence on pharmacotherapy. For example, fluid resuscitation significantly influences volume of distribution (V_d) of drugs because of changes in extracellular volume from blood loss, fluid resuscitation, fluid shifts, capillary leak, ascites, and so on. Drugs that have small V_d (<0.5 L/kg) and/or water soluble, such as aminoglycosides, are most likely to be affected. For instance, the V_d of gentamicin was reported to be doubled in patients with AKI compared to those with normal kidney function (0.25L/kg versus 0.35L/kg). The clinical application of this is that initial doses would need to be twice as large in AKI patients to achieve the same serum concentration. Given that the efficacy of gentamicin is dependent on achievement of high peak serum concentrations, one could expect that therapeutic outcomes in fluid-overloaded patients would be worse if doses were not increased to account for fluid overload.[21] Protein binding is also altered in patients with AKI because critically ill patients are often hypoalbuminemic. Given that most protein-bound drugs bind to albumin, a reduction in albumin will increase the free fraction of the drug. More unbound (free) drug leads to more available drug to give pharmacologic activity, more drug available to be removed by KRT, and, finally, a greater V_d. The greater V_d again means that a higher initial (loading) dose is needed for many drugs (especially antibiotics) to reach critical serum concentrations in order to fill the larger volume of the patient. Maintenance doses will need to be adjusted for volume changes as kidney function recovers or as kidney replacement therapies remove excess fluid.

DOSING CONSIDERATIONS IN KIDNEY REPLACEMENT THERAPIES

The extent of drug removal can be very different between CKRT, intermittent hemodialysis (IHD), and hybrid KRT, such as prolonged intermittent kidney replacement therapy (PIKRT).[22] A good rule of thumb to remember is that there will be more drug clearance by the KRT with the longer KRT duration, the higher effluent rate, the smaller drug's V_d (<0.8 L/kg), molecular weight (<1000 Da), and protein binding rate. The US Food and Drug Administration does not require pharmaceutical companies to provide drug dosing recommendations for all types of KRT. Preferably, dosing recommendations should arise from published pharmacokinetic trials, yet these studies are rarely conducted.[23] Consequently, many of the published drug dosing tables are based on expert opinions rather than large pharmacokinetic studies conducted in patients who have received each type of KRT. This is challenging for clinicians because therapeutic antibiotic dosing in CKRT depends on pharmacokinetics, pharmacodynamics, CKRT dose, and antibiotic susceptibility. In patients receiving PIKRT or hemodialysis, appropriate dosing also depends on KRT timing relative to the drug's administration time.[22] CKRT drug dosing guidance for new drugs is usually available after the drug has been on the market for a couple of years. Owing to the variability (blood/dialysate flow rates, duration, and frequency) of how PIKRT is performed, dosing recommendations that are broadly applicable are rarely found.[24]

Standard IHD provides 3- to 4-hour bursts of extracorporeal drug clearance in an asymmetric, thrice-weekly timing for most stage 5 chronic kidney disease (CKD5) patients or as often as daily in critically ill patients with AKI.[25] Drug dosing guidelines for IHD are predominantly generated in patients with CKD5, not critically ill patients with AKI. Consequently, there are many reasons why package insert–recommended IHD doses are not appropriate to guide dosing in AKI. Not only is pharmacokinetics different in AKI versus CKD5 patients owing to physiologic differences, but AKI patients may also require more frequent IHD for better metabolic and fluid control. Drug doses that are appropriate for CKD5 patients receiving thrice-weekly hemodialysis are unlikely to be equivalent with AKI patients requiring IHD 5 to 7 times per week. In addition, the drug clearances attained with IHD in the ICU are often less than what can be reached in hemodynamically stable outpatients with better vascular access and higher blood flow rates.

Unlike IHD, CKRT is intended to run 24 hours a day. However, interruptions in CKRT often occur.[26] These interruptions affect drug clearance and should be accounted for when recommending a patient's drug dosing strategy. In contrast to IHD, blood flow is much higher than the effluent (dialysate plus ultrafiltrate) rate in CKRT. Therefore, total delivered effluent rate is the most important determinant of drug clearance by CKRT (CL_{CKRT}). Patients' total drug clearance should equal residual renal clearance plus CL_{NR} plus CL_{CKRT}. Residual kidney function is often not accounted for; however, it is crucial to add residual renal clearance to CL_{NR} to determine total endogenous drug clearance. Changes to any of these will affect overall drug clearance and half-life.

DOSING STRATEGIES

Pharmacodynamic Targets

Antibiotic dosing is based on the pharmacodynamic relationship between antibiotic concentration and antibacterial effects. There are two main types of antibiotic pharmacodynamics: concentration-dependent killing and time-dependent killing. Concentration-dependent antibiotics, such as aminoglycosides and fluoroquinolones, maximize their rate and the extent of bacterial killing at high drug concentrations. The therapeutic goal is to maximize the peak concentration, and it usually occurs when the drug concentration is approximately 10 times the organism's minimum inhibitory concentration (MIC). Major parameters that are correlated with antibiotic efficacy are area under the serum concentration versus time curve (AUC)/MIC and maximum drug concentration (C_{max})/MIC. Time-dependent antibiotics, such as β-lactams (penicillins, cephalosporins, carbapenems), exhibit the maximum rate and extent of bacterial killing when serum concentrations are above minimum bactericidal concentration (MBC) of the organism. Achieving a higher C_{max} does not add additional benefit to drug activity. Thus, the therapeutic goal would be to maximize the time above MBC without having to achieve extremely high C_{max} that may be associated with drug toxicity. Typically, percentage of time above MBC or time above MIC ($T \geq$ MIC) for the dosing interval correlates with the drug's efficacy. For example, meropenem shows very strong bacterial killing effect when its concentration is above MIC for 40% of the dosing interval.[27] This is also the reason that time-dependent antibiotics are often given as an extended or continuous infusion.

Drug Administration

In general, there are four different types of intravenous (IV) drug administration strategies: (1) rapid bolus (push) administration, (2) intermittent infusion, (3) prolonged infusion, and (4) continuous infusion. Bolus administration is when the dose is administered within a minute, intermittent infusion is when the dose is administered within 30 to 60 minutes (as is done for most antibiotics). Prolonged (often called *extended*) infusion occurs when the dose is administered slowly, often over approximately 4 hours or half of the dosing interval. Finally, continuous infusion is, as its name infers, when the dose is given at a continuous rate for the entire time of treatment. When using continuous infusions, a loading dose (LD) should be used to provide initial therapeutic concentrations for concentration-dependent antibiotic medications. For time-dependent antibiotics, it is beneficial to utilize bolus administration or intermittent infusion to avoid initial suboptimal antibiotic exposure, allowing pathogens to develop resistance. Even though bolus administration reaches the peak concentration the fastest, it is avoided in some medications, such as vancomycin, because of side effects (e.g., red man syndrome). Prolonged infusion and continuous infusion can extend the $T \geq$ MIC, but their efficacy has not been extensively studied in patients receiving CKRT. Despite the lack of study, prolonging the β-lactam infusion time is a simple intervention that will increase the $T \geq$ MIC.[28] This intervention should be considered in patients with severe infections who are receiving CKRT and is likely to be effective because the continuous drug clearance from CKRT can be accounted for in the continuous infusion. The best evidence to support prolonged infusions is for cephalosporins, penicillins, and carbapenems. As indicated in **Table 26.1**, these drugs are also good candidates for continuous infusions. Although not often used at most centers, studies evaluating continuous-infusion vancomycin are being published as clinicians try to attain vancomycin pharmacodynamic targets while avoiding large peak concentrations.[29] In IHD or PIKRT, matching a continuous-infusion

TABLE 26.1 Common Antimicrobial Pharmacodynamics and Dosing Considerations

Antimicrobial Pharmacodynamics	Medications	Drug Dosing Strategy Considerations
Time-dependent killing	Acyclovir Penicillins Cephalosporins Clindamycin Fluconazole Carbapenems Vancomycin	1. Continuous or extended infusion in CKRT 2. More frequent administration of smaller doses 3. Supplemental dose during PIKRT and post-IHD 4. Weight-based dosing
Concentration-dependent killing	AMG Colistin Daptomycin Fluoroquinolones Metronidazole	1. Loading dose to achieve PD target goals early 2. Extended dosing interval for AMG 3. Predialytic administration of AMG in IHD or PIKRT 4. Weight-based dosing

AMG, aminoglycosides; CKRT, continuous kidney replacement therapy; IHD, intermittent hemodialysis; PD, pharmacodynamics; PIKRT, prolonged intermittent kidney replacement therapy.

Lewis SJ, Mueller BA. Antibiotic dosing in critically ill patients receiving CKRT: underdosing is overprevalent. *Semin Dial.* 2014;27(5):441-445; Trotman RL, Williamson JC, Shoemaker DM, et al. Antibiotic dosing in critically ill adult patients receiving continuous renal replacement therapy. *Clin Infect Dis.* 2005;41(8):1159-1166.

rate to changing KRT drug clearances can be problematic. Table 26.1 illustrates common antimicrobial pharmacodynamics and dosing strategy considerations.

Other Drug Dosing Implications

Matching drug administration techniques with KRT techniques (Table 26.1) can be an effective way to maximize the ability of reaching pharmacodynamic targets. AKI in the ICU is a dynamic process; as a result, clinicians are challenged to alter drug prescribing as KRT changes are made (changing techniques, administration times, effluent rates). As fluid overload is corrected, dosing may have to change. As kidney function recovers, drugs cleared by the kidneys need to have doses increased. Prescribers can also consider other ways to alter drug therapy besides dosing that may help patients with AKI. For example, clinicians should be mindful of how much of extra fluid they are prescribing when ordering the drug prescription because critically ill patients with AKI are already fluid overloaded, minimizing fluid administration (e.g., avoiding large IV bags when administering medications and nutrition). Pharmacists can assist in developing fluid-restricted drug products when appropriate. Another consideration is to have drug orders with appropriate doses prepared, for instance, when CKRT is stopped unexpectedly owing to filter clotting or access issues. **Table 26.2** discusses dosing considerations for common drug classes in the ICU.

However, in the VA/ATN and RENAL dosing trials (as discussed in Chapter 30), the same antibiotic dosing regimens were used in both effluent intensity groups. Some have suggested that these trials compared differences not only in CKRT intensity but also in antibiotic exposure.[30] A recent Monte Carlo simulation calculated that the influence of antibiotic clearance between two effluent intensity groups in the VA/ATN and RENAL dosing trial was not substantial. Antibiotic target attainment rates

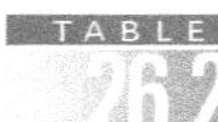

TABLE 26.2 Common Drug Classes in the Intensive Care Unit and Their Dosing Consideration

Medication Class	Drug Dosing Considerations
Antianginal (e.g., isosorbide dinitrate, nitroglycerin, amlodipine, verapamil, propranolol, atenolol, metoprolol)	Dose per effect. You could empirically lower the dose. Monitor the patients' chest pain/Pa_{O_2}/heart rate.
Antiarrhythmic (e.g., amiodarone, procainamide, digoxin, adrenaline, propranolol)	Dose per effect for the most. Digoxin requires dose reduction. Even KRT may not effectively clear digoxin because of high V_d. Monitor the patients' ECG/heart rate.
Antibiotics	Determine whether the drug has time- or concentration-dependent bactericidal activity. Then refer to Table 26.1.
Antiepileptics (e.g., diazepam, phenobarbital, phenytoin, levetiracetam, carbamazepine, lamotrigine)	Highly protein-bound medications should be monitored with caution as there is increased fraction of unbound phenytoin in AKI patients. For example, free phenytoin rather than total phenytoin should be used to monitor concentrations. Levetiracetam, gabapentin, and carbamazepine need dose adjustments based on kidney function. Phenobarbital and lamotrigine may also require dose reduction. Diazepam does not require dose adjustment.
Antifungal	Determine whether the drug has time- or concentration-dependent activity. Then refer to Table 26.1.
Antiplatelet/anticoagulants (e.g., heparin, LMWH, warfarin, ASA, clopidogrel)	LMWH is not recommended in patients with severe kidney dysfunction owing to unpredictable variability in PK response. Heparin is preferred over LMWH. Warfarin, ASA, and clopidogrel do not require dose adjustments based on kidney function. Assess bleeding risk and monitor appropriate lab values (e.g., INR for warfarin).

Antipsychotics (e.g., chlorpromazine, haloperidol, risperidone)	Antipsychotics are generally highly protein bound and not significantly removed by dialysis. Active metabolites may be renally excreted and lead to accumulation. Dose cautiously and monitor patients' response.
Antiviral (e.g., acyclovir, lamivudine, tenofovir, stavudine, zidovudine, nevirapine, efavirenz, ritonavir)	Tenofovir, efavirenz, lamivudine, and emtricitabine are associated with less toxicity compared to stavudine, zidovudine, or nevirapine. Most of the antivirals require dose adjustments based on kidney function. Efavirenz and ritonavir do not need dose adjutments based on kidney function. Acyclovir has been associated with AKI; choose alternatives when possible.
Insulin	Dose per effect. Insulin molecular weight is >5,000 Da and is not cleared by KRT. You could empirically lower the dose or not, monitor the patients' glucose and titrate appropriately.
Pain medications metabolites (e.g., morphine)	Most non-narcotic analgesics are hepatically metabolized, little or no dosage adjustments are needed. Titrate to effective pain management. Metabolites of morphine and meperidine have shown to accumulate in patients with kidney impairment, resulting in serious side effects (prolonged respiratory depression for morphine and neurotoxicity for meperidine).
Paralytics	Dose per effect. You could empirically lower the dose or not, monitor the patients' response.

AKI, acute kidney injury; ASA, aspirin; ECG, electrocardiogram; INR, international normalized ratio; LMWH, low-molecular-weight heparin; Pao_2, partial pressure of oxygen; PD, pharmacodynamics; PK, pharmacokinetics; KRT, kidney replacement therapy; V_d, volume of distribution.

were very similar between high- and low-intensity CKRT in both trials.[31] Nonetheless, finding the optimal antibiotic dose in CKRT is difficult. Studies suggest that we often do not hit antibiotic pharmacokinetic targets with currently recommended doses. For instance, only 53% patients reached the pharmacodynamic target with ceftazidime 2 g every 12 hours and 0% reached the pharmacodynamic target with cefepime 2 g every 12 hours.[32] Consequently, more aggressive dosing should be pursued.[33] Nonetheless, antibiotic toxicity from high doses can occur as well.[34] The RENAL trial investigators reported a wide variability in trough concentrations in five different antibiotics (6.7-fold for meropenem, 3.8-fold for piperacillin, 10.5-fold for tazobactam, 1.9-fold for vancomycin, and 3.9-fold for ciprofloxacin) in the trial.[13] Empiric antibiotic dosing not only failed to achieve predetermined MIC (15%) and higher target concentration (40%) but also showed excessive concentration (10%). This shows the importance of therapeutic drug monitoring (whenever possible) to avoid underdosing and overdosing in critically ill patients. Most drugs in the ICU are not monitored with measured drug concentrations and must be monitored and adjusted in other ways.

CONCLUSION

Drug dosing for patients with AKI receiving any type of KRT can be one of the most challenging endeavors for ICU clinicians. The patient-specific pharmacokinetic factors ensure that critical decisions need to be made on a daily basis. Doses that are therapeutic on the first day in a fluid-overloaded AKI patient will often be incorrect a week later because of changes in volume and KRT. The development of useful clinical decision drug dosing support is being outpaced by the variations in KRTs and introduction of new drugs. Consequently, an understanding of pharmacokinetic and pharmacodynamic principles is essential. Finally, AKI prevention through avoidance of nephrotoxins in high-risk patients may be the most useful intervention that can be made in the ICU.

References

1. Hoste EA, Clermont G, Kersten A, et al. RIFLE criteria for acute kidney injury are associated with hospital mortality in critically ill patients: a cohort analysis. *Crit Care.* 2006;10(3):R73. doi:10.1186/cc4915
2. Chang JW, Jeng MJ, Yang LY, et al. The epidemiology and prognostic factors of mortality in critically ill children with acute kidney injury in Taiwan. *Kidney Int.* 2015;87(3):632-639. doi:10.1038/ki.2014.299
3. Uchino S, Kellum JA, Bellomo R, et al; Beginning and Ending Supportive Therapy for the Kidney (BEST Kidney) Investigators. Acute renal failure in critically ill patients: a multinational, multicenter study. *JAMA.* 2005;294(7):813-818. doi:10.1001/jama.294.7.813
4. Xu X, Nie S, Liu Z, et al. Epidemiology and clinical correlates of AKI in Chinese hospitalized adults. *Clin J Am Soc Nephrol.* 2015;10(9):1510-1518. doi:10.2215/CJN.02140215
5. Taber SS, Mueller BA. Drug-associated renal dysfunction. *Crit Care Clin.* 2006;22(2):357-374, *viii.* doi:10.1016/j.ccc.2006.02.003
6. Goldstein SL, Mottes T, Simpson K, et al. A sustained quality improvement program reduces nephrotoxic medication-associated acute kidney injury. *Kidney Int.* 2016;90(1):212-221. doi:10.1016/j.kint.2016.03.031
7. Awdishu L, Wu SE. Acute kidney injury. In: Boucher BA, Haas CE, eds. *Critical Care Self-Assessment Program.* American College of Clinical Pharmacy; 2017.
8. Luque Y, Louis K, Jouanneau C, et al. Vancomycin-associated cast nephropathy. *J Am Soc Nephrol.* 2017;28(6):1723-1728. doi:10.1681/ASN.2016080867
9. Htike NL, Santoro J, Gilbert B, Elfenbein IB, Teehan G. Biopsy-proven vancomycin-associated interstitial nephritis and acute tubular necrosis. *Clin Exp Nephrol.* 2012;16(2):320-324. doi:10.1007/s10157-011-0559-1
10. Nolin TD. Vancomycin and the risk of AKI: now clearer than Mississippi mud. *Clin J Am Soc Nephrol.* 2016;11(12):2101-2103. doi:10.2215/CJN.11011016
11. Mellen CK, Ryba JE, Rindone JP. Does piperacillin-tazobactam increase the risk of nephrotoxicity when used with vancomycin: a meta-analysis of observational trials. *Curr Drug Saf.* 2017;12(1):62-66. doi:10.2174/1574886311666161024164859

12. Kane-Gill SL, Ostermann M, Shi J, Joyce EL, Kellum JA. Evaluating renal stress using pharmacokinetic urinary biomarker data in critically ill patients receiving vancomycin and/or piperacillin-tazobactam: a secondary analysis of the multicenter sapphire study. *Drug Saf.* 2019. doi:10.1007/s40264-019-00846-x
13. Roberts DM, Roberts JA, Roberts MS, et al. Variability of antibiotic concentrations in critically ill patients receiving continuous renal replacement therapy: a multicentre pharmacokinetic study. *Crit Care Med.* 2012;40(5):1523-1528. doi:10.1097/CCM.0b013e318241e553
14. Moffett BS, Goldstein SL. Acute kidney injury and increasing nephrotoxic-medication exposure in noncritically-ill children. *Clin J Am Soc Nephrol.* 2011;6(4):856-863. doi:10.2215/CJN.08110910
15. Macias WL, Mueller BA, Scarim SK. Vancomycin pharmacokinetics in acute renal failure: preservation of nonrenal clearance. *Clin Pharmacol Ther.* 1991;50(6):688-694. doi:10.1038/clpt.1991.208
16. Mueller BA, Scarim SK, Macias WL. Comparison of imipenem pharmacokinetics in patients with acute or chronic renal failure treated with continuous hemofiltration. *Am J Kidney Dis.* 1993;21(2):172-179. https://www.ncbi.nlm.nih.gov/pubmed/8430678
17. Ververs TF, van Dijk A, Vinks SA, et al. Pharmacokinetics and dosing regimen of meropenem in critically ill patients receiving continuous venovenous hemofiltration. *Crit Care Med.* 2000;28(10):3412-3416. doi:10.1097/00003246-200010000-00006
18. Nolin TD, Appiah K, Kendrick SA, Le P, McMonagle E, Himmelfarb J. Hemodialysis acutely improves hepatic CYP3A4 metabolic activity. *J Am Soc Nephrol.* 2006;17(9):2363-2367. doi:10.1681/ASN.2006060610
19. Foland JA, Fortenberry JD, Warshaw BL, et al. Fluid overload before continuous hemofiltration and survival in critically ill children: a retrospective analysis. *Crit Care Med.* 2004;32(8):1771-1776. https://www.ncbi.nlm.nih.gov/pubmed/15286557
20. Kim IY, Kim JH, Lee DW, et al. Fluid overload and survival in critically ill patients with acute kidney injury receiving continuous renal replacement therapy. *PLoS One.* 2017;12(2):e0172137. doi:10.1371/journal.pone.0172137
21. Petejova N, Zahalkova J, Duricova J, et al. Gentamicin pharmacokinetics during continuous venovenous hemofiltration in critically ill septic patients. *J Chemother.* 2012;24(2):107-112. doi:10.1179/1120009X12Z.0000000006
22. Scoville BA, Mueller BA. Medication dosing in critically ill patients with acute kidney injury treated with renal replacement therapy. *Am J Kidney Dis.* 2013;61(3):490-500. doi:10.1053/j.ajkd.2012.08.042
23. Mueller BA, Smoyer WE. Challenges in developing evidence-based drug dosing guidelines for adults and children receiving renal replacement therapy. *Clin Pharmacol Ther.* 2009;86(5):479-482. doi:10.1038/clpt.2009.150
24. Hoff BM, Maker JH, Dager WE, Heintz BH. Antibiotic dosing for critically ill adult patients receiving intermittent hemodialysis, prolonged intermittent renal replacement therapy, and continuous renal replacement therapy: an update. *Ann Pharmacother.* 2020;54(1):43-55. doi:10.1177/1060028019865873
25. Clark WR, Mueller BA, Alaka KJ, Macias WL. A comparison of metabolic control by continuous and intermittent therapies in acute renal failure. *J Am Soc Nephrol.* 1994;4(7):1413-1420. https://www.ncbi.nlm.nih.gov/pubmed/8161723
26. Claure-Del Granado R, Macedo E, Chertow GM, et al. Effluent volume in continuous renal replacement therapy overestimates the delivered dose of dialysis. *Clin J Am Soc Nephrol.* 2011;6(3):467-475. doi:10.2215/CJN.02500310
27. Drusano GL. Antimicrobial pharmacodynamics: critical interactions of "bug and drug." *Nat Rev Microbiol.* 2004;2(4):289-300. doi:10.1038/nrmicro862
28. Jang SM, Lewis SJ, Mueller BA. Harmonizing antibiotic regimens with renal replacement therapy. *Expert Rev Anti Infect Ther.* 2020;18(9):887-895. doi:10.1080/14787210.2020.1764845
29. Akers KS, Cota JM, Chung KK, Renz EM, Mende K, Murray CK. Serum vancomycin levels resulting from continuous or intermittent infusion in critically ill burn patients with or without continuous renal replacement therapy. *J Burn Care Res.* 2012;33(6):e254-e262. doi:10.1097/BCR.0b013e31825042fa
30. Kielstein JT, David S. Pro: renal replacement trauma or Paracelsus 2.0. *Nephrol Dial Transplant.* 2013;28(11):2728-2731; discussion 2731-2733. doi:10.1093/ndt/gft049
31. Jang SM, Pai MP, Shaw AR, Mueller BA. Antibiotic exposure profiles in trials comparing intensity of continuous renal replacement therapy. *Crit Care Med.* 2019;47(11):e863-e871.
32. Seyler L, Cotton F, Taccone FS, et al. Recommended beta-lactam regimens are inadequate in septic patients treated with continuous renal replacement therapy. *Crit Care.* 2011;15(3):R137. doi:10.1186/cc10257
33. Lewis SJ, Mueller BA. Antibiotic dosing in critically ill patients receiving CRRT: underdosing is overprevalent. *Semin Dial.* 2014;27(5):441-445. doi:10.1111/sdi.12203
34. Lewis SJ, Mueller BA. Antibiotic dosing in patients with acute kidney injury: "Enough but not too much." *J Intensive Care Med.* 2016;31(3):164-176. doi:10.1177/0885066614555490

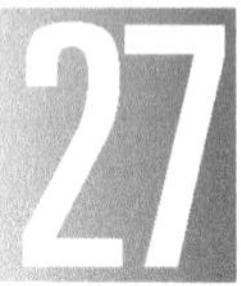

Drugs and Antidotes

Jonathan S. Zipursky and David N. Juurlink

INTRODUCTION

The notion of a universal antidote has captured the minds of physicians and healers since ancient times.[1,2] Today, most acutely poisoned patients are successfully treated with supportive care alone. In 2018, 2.8% of patients who reported to US poison centers received gastrointestinal (GI) decontamination (e.g., activated charcoal, whole bowel irrigation [WBI]), fewer received a specific antidote.[3] From a practical standpoint, because antidotes are sometimes expensive, infrequently used, and prone to expiry, they are not routinely available at all centers.[4] The purpose of this chapter is to review common strategies for decontamination as well as selected antidotes used in the treatment of poisoned patients.

GASTROINTESTINAL DECONTAMINATION

The theory behind GI decontamination is intuitive: if the absorption of an ingested toxic substance can be minimized, the risk of harm should be lessened. Unfortunately, there is very little evidence to support this intuition. There are three main methods of gastric decontamination: single-dose activated charcoal (SDAC), orogastric lavage, and WBI.

When appropriate, GI decontamination should be performed as soon after ingestion as possible. Historically, GI decontamination was recommended within 1 hour of poison ingestion.[5-7] However, longer treatment windows are often justifiable, particularly in the setting of massive ingestions, delayed-release drug preparations, or overdoses involving drugs that can delay gastric emptying such as opioids and anticholinergics. In addition, absorption kinetics differ in overdose relative to therapeutic use, with the drug often remaining in the stomach hours after ingestion.[8,9]

Activated Charcoal

SDAC is the most frequently used method of GI decontamination.[10] Nonionized, organic compounds (i.e., most drugs) bind avidly to charcoal, whereas highly ionized compounds and metals (e.g., lithium, potassium), and liquids (e.g., hydrocarbons) hardly adsorb at all.

Only two randomized controlled trials have examined the efficacy of SDAC in acutely poisoned patients, and neither showed differences in hospital length of stay, intensive care unit (ICU) admission, or mortality.[11,12] For SDAC to be effective, a high ratio of charcoal:drug (based on mass) is optimal. A typical ratio is 10:1, although some have advocated for higher ratios (40:1).[10,13] In most settings, there is little clinical or practical benefit to exceeding a dose of 50 g.[10] There may be utility in administering SDAC later than 1 hour after ingestion in the following scenarios: (a) severe expected toxicity with few other available treatments,

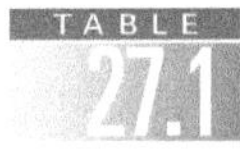

Factors That Cumulatively Increase the Appropriateness of Single-Dose Activated Charcoal

- Recent ingestion
- Serious toxicity anticipated
- Alert, cooperative patient
- Patent airway
- Absence of an available antidote
- Favorable ratio of charcoal:drug
- Ingestion of a modified/extended-release drug preparation
- Substance known to adsorb to activated charcoal
- No ileus or intestinal obstruction

(b) massive ingestion (where there may be formation of a bezoar), and (c) coingestion of drugs that may delay gastric emptying. Factors that cumulatively increase the appropriateness of administering SDAC are listed in **Table 27.1**.

Multidose Activated Charcoal

Activated charcoal is sometimes administered sequentially—"multiple dose activated charcoal (MDAC)"—to enhance elimination of a xenobiotic by interrupting enterohepatic recirculation or enteroenteric recirculation.[2] Multiple doses of charcoal can also be administered in the setting of overdose of a modified-release drug preparation or if a bezoar is suspected. A typical dosing regimen is a charcoal rate of 12.5 g/hr, most commonly given in divided equivalent doses (25 g every 2 hours or 50 g every 4 hours). Potential indications for and contraindications to MDAC are listed in **Table 27.2**.

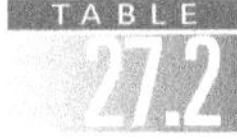

Potential Indications and Contraindications for Multiple Dose Activated Charcoal

Indications

- Ingestion of: *Amanita* sp, amiodarone, amitriptyline, carbamazepine, colchicine, dextropropoxyphene, digitoxin, digoxin, disopyramide, dosulepin, duloxetine, diquat, *Gymnopilus penetrans*, lamotrigine, nadolol, phenobarbital, phenylbutazone, phenytoin, piroxicam, quetiapine, quinine, sotalol, theophylline, valproic acid, verapamil, vinorelbine
- Ingestion of a life-threatening amount of a poison that undergoes enterohepatic recirculation and adsorbs to activated charcoal
- Ingestion of an extended/modified-release drug preparation or in the setting of a massive ingestion where there has been formation of a bezoar

Contraindications

- Intestinal obstruction, ileus, or perforation
- Ingestion of a drug that does not adsorb to activated charcoal
- Unprotected airway, or the activated charcoal could increase the risk of aspiration
- Endoscopy is necessary (e.g., caustics)

Orogastric Lavage

Orogastric lavage (colloquially termed "stomach pumping") involves evacuating stomach contents by aspiration through a large-bore orogastric tube. Although there is a very limited role for gastric lavage in the treatment of acute poisonings, potential indications and contraindications are described in **Table 27.3.**[5] Orogastric lavage should only be attempted by physicians with adequate experience with the procedure. In general, the risks associated with lavage (including aspiration, arrhythmia, esophageal and gastric perforation, and electrolyte imbalances) outweigh the potential benefit for virtually all ingestions.[5]

Whole Bowel Irrigation

WBI refers to the administration of large volumes of osmotically balanced polyethylene glycol (PEG) to promote peristalsis, hastening luminal transit to minimize xenobiotic absorption. Most data to support its use come from volunteer studies, case reports, and case series of patients who have taken extended-release drug formulations, as well as "body packers"—people who swallow or insert rectally multiple packets of illicit drugs (such as cocaine) wrapped in condoms or balloons for the purposes of trafficking.[14,15] No clinical trials have evaluated the use of WBI in acutely poisoned patients.[14]

WBI can be considered for potentially toxic ingestions of sustained-release or enteric-coated drugs, drugs not adsorbed by activated charcoal (e.g., lithium, potassium, iron), and evacuation of illicit drugs in "body packers."[14] Potential indications and contraindications to WBI are found in **Table 27.4.**[2] Because the administration rate of PEG is on the order of 1 to 2 L/hr, compliance may be an issue, and the use of a nasogastric tube is advisable.

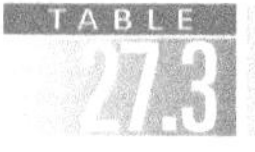

Potential Indications and Contraindications of Orogastric Lavage

Potential Indications	Contraindications
The ingestion is known to cause life-threatening toxicity, or the patient shows evidence of life-threatening toxicity, and: • Reason to believe substantial amounts of xenobiotic still exist in the stomach (based on the timing of ingestion) • The ingested substance: (a) does not adsorb to AC, (b) AC is not available, and (c) the ingestion is so large that the appropriate dose of AC is impractical. • No appropriate antidote or elimination technique exists.	• The ingestion is anticipated to cause limited toxicity. • The xenobiotic adsorbs well to AC and does not exceed the adsorptive capacity of usual doses. • Emesis has occurred. • The patient presents many hours after ingestion and there is little clinical evidence of toxicity. • There is an effective antidote available. • The procedure cannot be performed safely (e.g., lack of equipment or expertise of the operator, airway is unprotected, suspected gastric injury, suspected bezoar).

AC, activated charcoal.

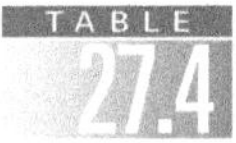

Indications and Contraindications for Whole Bowel Irrigation

Potential Indications	Contraindications
• Ingestion of a toxic amount of a substance, non-amenable to activated charcoal decontamination • Ingestion of toxic amount of extended/modified-release drug • Removal of packets from body packers	• Unprotected airway, or risk of aspiration is high • Evidence of gastrointestinal perforation, ileus, obstruction, hemorrhage • Hemodynamic instability • Uncontrolled vomiting • Signs of xenobiotic/drug leakage from packets of body packers

ANTIDOTES

Antidotes are used to counteract the effects of poisons and often do not impact the systemic absorption or elimination of substances. Common poisonings and available antidotes are listed in **Table 27.5.**[2,16] Specific drugs and commonly used antidotes are discussed in the remainder of the chapter.

Acetaminophen Toxicity

Acetaminophen is one of the most common drugs responsible for accidental overdose and deliberate self-harm worldwide and the most common cause of acute liver failure and hepatotoxicity in the developed world.[17,18] Treatment of acetaminophen toxicity involves one of the most well-studied antidotes: *N*-acetylcysteine (NAC).

At typical therapeutic doses, the majority of acetaminophen is metabolized by sulfation (30%) and glucuronidation (55%).[2,19] In addition, small amounts

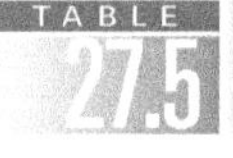

Common Antidotes in Use

Antidote	Poisoning Indication
N-Acetylcysteine	Acetaminophen
Andexanet	Rivaroxaban, apixaban
Antivenom	Snakebite
Atropine	Organophosphate pesticide β-Blocker, calcium channel blocker (CCB)
Benzodiazepines	Stimulants
Calcium salts	CCB Hydrofluoric acid
Carboxypeptidase (glucarpidase)	Methotrexate
Carnitine	Valproic acid
Cyproheptadine	Serotonin syndrome (e.g., SSRIs, SNRIs, MAOIs)

(*continued*)

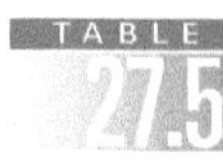

Common Antidotes in Use (*continued*)

Antidote	Poisoning Indication
Dantrolene	Neuroleptic malignant syndrome Malignant hyperthermia
Deferoxamine	Iron, aluminum
DigiFab	Digoxin Other cardiac glycosides (digitoxin-containing plants [oleander, foxglove], toads [bufotoxin])
Dimercaprol	Arsenic
Ethanol	Methanol, ethylene glycol, diethylene glycol
Flumazenil	Benzodiazepines Zopiclone/zolpidem
Folinic acid	Methotrexate
Glucagon	β-Blocker, CCBs
Hydroxocobalamin	Cyanide
Idarucizumab	Dabigatran
Insulin	CCB, β-blocker
Intralipid	Local anesthetics (bupivacaine, lidocaine)
Methylene blue	Methemoglobinemia, refractory shock
Naloxone	Opioids
Octreotide	Sulfonylurea, insulin
Oxygen (hyperbaric)	Carbon monoxide, hydrogen sulfide, cyanide
Physostigmine	Anticholinergic delirium
Pralidoxime	Organophosphate
Protamine	Heparin
Prussian blue	Thallium, cesium
Pyridoxine	Isoniazid, ethylene glycol
Silibinin	*Amanita* sp
Sodium bicarbonate	Sodium channel blocking drugs (e.g., tricyclic antidepressants)
Succimer	Lead, mercury, arsenic
Vitamin K (with prothrombin complex concentration)	Warfarin

MAOI, monoamine oxidase inhibitor; SNRI, serotonin-norepinephrine reuptake inhibitor; SSRI, selective serotonin re-uptake inhibitor.

From Hoffman RS, Howland MA, Lewin NA, Nelson LS, Goldfrank LR. *Goldfrank's Toxicologic Emergencies.* 11th ed. McGraw Hill Education; 2019; Nickson C. Antidotes summary. Life in the fastlane. Accessed October 7, 2019. https://litfl.com/antidotes-summary/; Buckley NA, Dawson AH, Juurlink DN, Isbister GK. Who gets antidotes? Choosing the chosen few. *Br J Clin Pharmacol.* 2016;81(3):402-407. doi:10.1111/bcp.12894

are converted via cytochrome P4502E1 (CYP2E1) to the toxic metabolite *N*-acetyl-*p*-benzoquinoneimine (NAPQI), which is highly reactive and can bind to hepatic macromolecules, resulting in hepatotoxicity (**Figure 27.1**). NAPQI is detoxified via conjugation to glutathione and excreted in the urine. During an acetaminophen overdose, large amounts of NAPQI are produced, overwhelming glutathione stores leading to hepatic cell death.[20]

NAC is used to replenish intracellular glutathione stores. It is hydrolyzed to cysteine, a precursor to glutathione.[21] Acetylcysteine can also supply thiol groups to directly bind NAPQI in the liver.[22] NAC can be given both intravenously and orally. In the setting of acute acetaminophen overdose, a decision to administer NAC is based on a serum acetaminophen concentration drawn at 4 hours or later from the time of ingestion. This value can then be plotted on the Rumack-Matthew nomogram (**Figure 27.2**). A typical NAC regimen is summarized in **Table 27.6**. The Rumack-Matthew curve should not be used to guide treatment in the setting of chronic acetaminophen toxicity or when the time of ingestion is not known. In these scenarios, a decision to treat should be made with expert toxicology consultation and the guidance of a regional poison center. Treatment with NAC within 8 to 10 hours of an acute overdose virtually guarantees a favorable outcome in the setting of acetaminophen toxicity, but does not ensure avoidance of hepatotoxicity.[23]

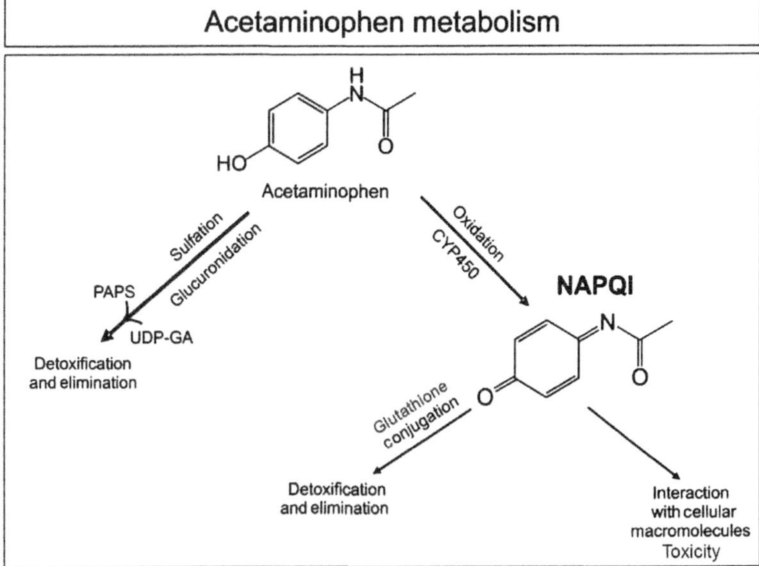

FIGURE 27.1: Acetaminophen metabolism: The majority of acetaminophen is metabolized by sulfation and glucuronidation. In the setting of overdose, a larger portion of acetaminophen is metabolized to NAPQI, which binds to intracellular proteins and causes hepatic damage. NAPQI can be neutralized by conjugation to glutathione. NAPQI, *N*-acetyl-*p*-benzoquinoneimine; PAPS, 3′-Phosphoadenosine 5′-phosphosulfate; UDP-GA, uridine diphosphoglucuronic acid.

From Moyer AM, Fridley BL, Jenkins GD, et al. Acetaminophen-NAPQI hepatotoxicity: a cell line model system genome-wide association study. *Toxicol Sci.* 2011;120(1):33-41. doi:10.1093/toxsci/kfq375

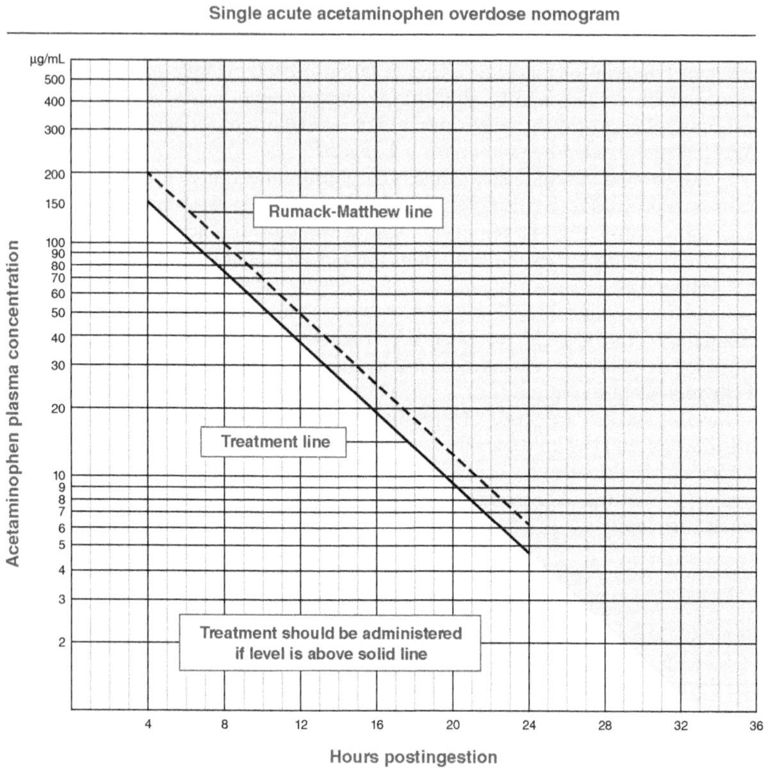

FIGURE 27.2: Rumack-Matthew nomogram: Plot of serial concentrations of acetaminophen versus time since acute ingestion to prognosticate liver toxicity. The nomogram is used to aid treatment decisions—when to start *N*-acetylcysteine—in the setting of acute acetaminophen overdose.

Adapted online from the original publication: Rumack BH, Matthew H. Acetaminophen poisoning and toxicity. *Pediatrics*. 1975;55(6):871-876.

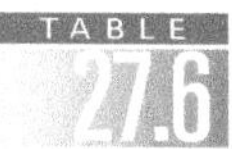

TABLE 27.6 Typical NAC Treatment Protocol

Use 3% NAC solution.
This protocol gives 240 mg/kg of NAC in the first 4 hr and 24 mg/kg in the next 8 hr.
Reassessment should occur at 12 hr.
Maximum lean body mass is 100 kg.

Loading dose	2 mL/kg/hr (to a maximum of 200 mL/hr)
Maintenance dose	0.2 mL/kg/hr (to a maximum of 20 mL/hr) until advised to stop by a toxicologist or regional poison center

NAC, *N*-acetylcysteine.

Naloxone and Flumazenil

Naloxone is a competitive opioid antagonist at μ-, κ-, and δ-opioid receptors and can reverse the effects of both endogenous opioids and xenobiotics.[24,25] Naloxone can be administered intramuscularly, intravenously, intranasally, or through an endotracheal tube.[26] It works rapidly, typically within seconds to minutes, and clinical effects last up to 1 hour. Naloxone can be used both therapeutically and diagnostically in the treatment of respiratory depression from opioid intoxication. Recommended doses are 0.4 to 2 mg, which are usually sufficient to reverse typical opioid doses. However, much higher doses (and even infusions) may be required to treat illicit opioid overdoses, which often involve large amounts of fentanyl or similar clandestinely produced opioids. Care should be exercised when using naloxone in opioid-dependent patients because of the risk of inducing full reversal and, thus, precipitating withdrawal.[27]

Flumazenil is a short-acting negative allosteric modifier at the γ-aminobutyric acid type A ($GABA_A$) receptor and reverses the sedative effects of most benzodiazepines (e.g., lorazepam, midazolam, and diazepam). It can also reverse the effects of other similar non-benzodiazepine drugs that bind the same site on the $GABA_A$ receptor: zopiclone and zolpidem. Flumazenil has no reversal effect on other $GABA_A$ agonists that bind to other sites on the receptor, such as barbiturates, propofol, ethanol, and inhaled anesthetics.[25] Flumazenil is indicated for the diagnosis and treatment of benzodiazepine intoxication/overdose. Most experts agree that the major indication for flumazenil is in the setting of severe benzodiazepine overdose in a patient who is not benzodiazepine dependent. Typical doses are 0.2 mg intravenously every 1 to 2 minutes titrated to clinical effect.

The major risk with flumazenil is the potential to induce benzodiazepine withdrawal, which can lead to seizures and agitation. Therefore, flumazenil should not be used in polysubstance intoxications involving proconvulsant drugs. In clinical practice, flumazenil is used infrequently, because most benzodiazepine overdoses occur in patients expected to be dependent as the result of chronic use, and patients generally do well with supportive care. Flumazenil should only be used in select circumstances where the poisoning is severe and the risk of seizure or withdrawal is felt to be low, ideally in consultation with a toxicologist.

Toxic Alcohols

Methanol, ethylene glycol, and diethylene glycol are relatively nontoxic substances by themselves, but become toxic after metabolism to harmful carboxylic acid metabolites. Methanol and ethylene glycol are commonly found in windshield wiper fluid and antifreeze, respectively. They are by far the most common toxic alcohol exposures worldwide (**Figure 27.3**).

A diagnosis of toxic alcohol ingestion is made by clinical history, characteristic biochemical abnormalities, and quantification of toxic alcohol concentrations by liquid chromatography. Urine microscopy can reveal needle- or envelope-shaped crystals in ethylene glycol toxicity. Patients typically present early after ingestion with an elevated osmolar gap (representing presence of the parent alcohol), with an anion gap developing after conversion to the toxic carboxylic acid metabolite. However, given the heterogeneity of toxic alcohol exposures, not all patients will have an anion or osmolar gap, and the absence of one or the other should never be used to exclude toxic alcohol poisoning.

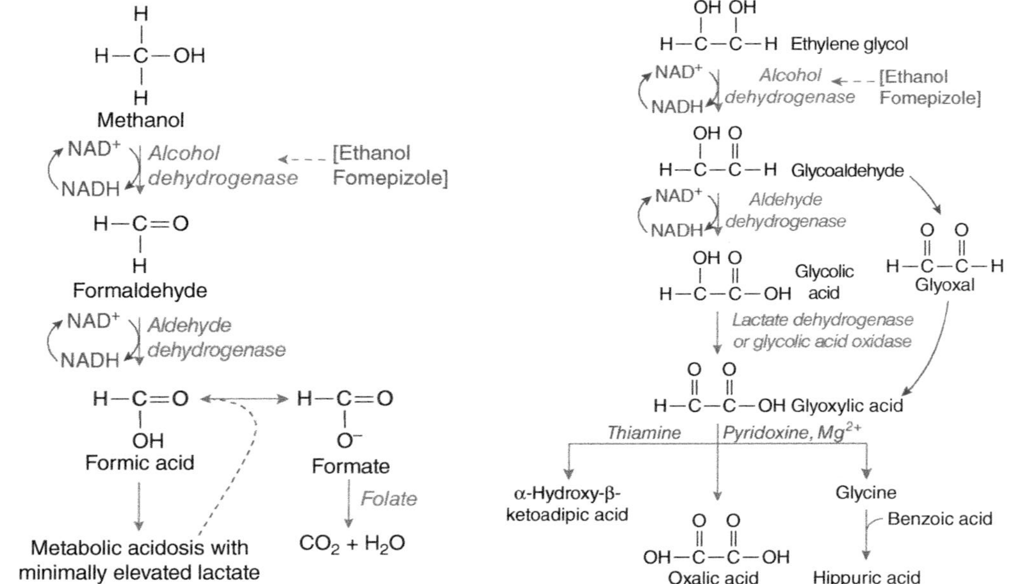

FIGURE 27.3: Metabolism of methanol and ethylene glycol: Parent alcohols are converted to aldehyde intermediates by alcohol dehydrogenase (ADH). The aldehyde intermediates are subsequently converted to carboxylic acid derivatives (formic acid; methanol; oxalic acid; ethylene glycol), which are responsible for the majority of toxicity attributed to toxic alcohols. NAD^+, nicotinamide adenine dinucleotide (oxidized); NADH, nicotinamide adenine dinucleotide (reduced).

From Hoffman RS, Howland MA, Lewin NA, Nelson LS, Goldfrank LR. *Goldfrank's Toxicologic Emergencies*. 11th ed. McGraw Hill Education; 2019.

$$\text{Osmolar gap} = \text{Measured serum osmolality} - \text{Calculated osmolality}$$
$$(2\text{Na} + \text{BUN}/2.8 + \text{Glucose}/18 + [1.25 \times \text{ethanol}/3.7])$$

$$\text{Anion gap} = \text{Na} - (\text{Cl} + \text{HCO}_3)$$

The presence of ethanol can be accounted for when calculating an osmolar gap by multiplying the serum ethanol concentration by a correction factor of 1.25. A normal osmolar gap can range between −9 and +19, which is partly why a normal osmolar gap is an unreliable method to rule out a toxic alcohol ingestion.[28] The osmolar gap is of greatest use when very elevated (typically >30-40) as a clue to the possibility of a recent toxic alcohol ingestion.

Antidote therapy for toxic alcohol involves inhibition of alcohol dehydrogenase (ADH), which should be initiated if poisoning is suspected or if confirmed, and ethylene glycol concentration is 62 mg/dL; methanol concentration is 32 mg/dL (methanol or ethylene glycol concentrations exceed 10 mmol/L) followed by serial acid-base assessments.[29] Two options for antidote treatment exist: inhibition with ethanol (which is transient, because ethanol itself is metabolized by ADH) or competitive inhibition with fomepizole, the preferred antidote. Ethanol competes with other toxic alcohols for ADH (10- and 20-fold higher affinity for ADH compared to methanol and ethylene glycol, respectively).[30,31] A standard protocol is either oral or intravenous administration of ethanol by bolus of 600 mg/kg followed by maintenance doses of 66 to 154 mg/kg/hr.[29] A blood ethanol concentration of 100 mg/dL (22 mmol/L) is generally sufficient for ADH blockade, and blood alcohol concentrations should be checked every 4 to 6 hours.[30] The dose/volume of ethanol given depends on the % ethanol content. A formula to calculate dose of ethanol in mL is:

$$(\text{Dose in mg/kg} \times 0.127 \times \text{bodyweight in kg})/\%\ \text{alcohol by volume}$$

Fomepizole (4-methylpyrazole [4-MP]) is the preferred antidote for ADH blockade. It is a potent ADH inhibitor, with an affinity more than 1,000 times that of methanol or ethylene glycol.[32] A typical dosing regimen is a 15 mg/kg intravenous bolus followed by 10 mg/kg every 12 hours (doses 2-4) and 15 mg/kg every 12 hours (dose 5 and beyond).[29] The dose increase later in the protocol reflects the fact that fomepizole induces its own metabolism through CYP2E1. For patients concurrently receiving dialysis, the dosing frequency needs to be increased (usually to every 4 hours) because as a small molecule, fomepizole is readily cleared by dialysis.

CALCIUM CHANNEL BLOCKER AND β-BLOCKER OVERDOSE

In 2018, calcium channel blockers (CCBs) and β-blockers (BBs) accounted for nearly 10% of poisoning-related deaths reported to US poison centers.[3] BBs antagonize myocardial β1 receptors and, in doing so, limit calcium influx into myocytes and decrease cardiac inotropy and chronotropy.[33] CCBs directly antagonize voltage-gated L-type calcium channels in cardiac myocytes and smooth muscle cells, also leading to decreases in inotropy, chronotropy, and an added effect of peripheral vasodilation. CCBs inhibit release of insulin from islet cells in the pancreas, leading to hyperglycemia and reduced glucose transport into myocardial cells.[33] Therefore, unexplained hyperglycemia can be an important clinical clue that may help distinguish CCB from BB overdose. Toxicity associated with dihydropyridine CCBs (e.g., nifedipine, felodipine, and amlodipine) causes a clinical picture more consistent with vasodilatory shock. In comparison, toxicity with the non-dihydropyridine CCBs (e.g., verapamil, diltiazem) can cause both vasoplegia and decreased inotropy and chronotropy through concomitant atrioventricular node blockade. However, in overdose, drug specificity can be lost, leading to similar clinical pictures with both types of CCBs.

BB and CCB overdose should be managed with GI decontamination and supportive care, including early airway management.[33] The mainstay of treatment for CCB and BB overdoses is high-dose insulin euglycemic therapy (HIET) (**Table 27.7**).[33,34] In the setting of refractory shock, adjunctive treatments can include intra-aortic balloon pumps, intravenous lipid emulsion therapy (Intralipid), methylene blue, and extracorporeal membrane oxygenation (ECMO).[35-40]

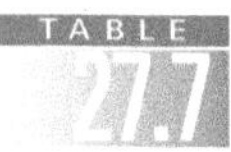

Antidotes for CCB and BB Overdose

Antidote	Comment
Intravenous fluids	There is a risk of volume overload as most patients are euvolemic. Excess fluids can worsen peripheral and pulmonary edema.
Vasopressors	Drugs with both inotropic and chronotropic effects are useful.
Calcium infusions	This is a temporizing measure and tends to be more effective in CCB overdose. There is a risk of hypercalcemia.
Atropine	Unlikely to have sustained benefit and may be counterproductive if WBI is being administered for modified-release ingestions
Glucagon	Often recommended for the treatment of BB overdose because of its ability to increase intracellular cAMP by bypassing the β-receptor. However, it has fallen out of favor due to inconsistent efficacy, short half-life, gastrointestinal side effects (nausea, vomiting, and diarrhea), and high cost given the unusually high doses involved.
HIET	HIET has several postulated mechanisms of action, but the most important has to do with altering myocardial energy utilization. The healthy myocardium uses free fatty acids as a primary energy source, but shifts to glucose in times of stress.[49] HIET facilitates transport of glucose, oxygen, and lactate into myocardium.[49] Insulin can also independently promote calcium-dependent inotropic effects in the myocardium.[49] Typical starting doses are an intravenous insulin load of 0.5-1.0 units/kg—much higher than used for diabetic ketoacidosis—followed by a maintenance infusion of 0.5 to as high as 10 units/kg/hr titrated to hemodynamic parameters. Serum potassium concentrations should be frequently monitored, and supplementation with an intravenous dextrose infusion is also often required.

BB, β-Blocker; cAMP, cyclic adenosine monophosphate; CCB, calcium channel blocker; HIET, high-dose insulin euglycemic therapy; WBI, whole bowel irrigation.

DIGOXIN AND OTHER CARDIAC GLYCOSIDES

Cardiac glycosides represent a diverse group of compounds that encompass xenobiotics (digoxin), but also naturally occurring cardioactive steroids found in plants and animals. They inhibit the cardiac Na^+-K^+-ATPase, increasing intracellular Na^+ and, as a result, intracellular Ca^{2+} (**Figure 27.4**). Digoxin can also cause bradycardia by increasing vagal tone and slowing conduction through the atrioventricular node.

Digoxin has a long elimination half-life (20-50 hours) and is almost entirely cleared through the urine.[41] Early symptoms of acute digoxin toxicity are nausea, vomiting, and diarrhea.[42,43] Other symptoms include malaise, vision changes, and green/yellow vision discolouration.[42,43] Cardiac toxicity is common and may manifest as bradycardia, heart block, or other dysrhythmias (although supraventricular tachycardias are uncommon). Hyperkalemia is one of the hallmarks of acute digoxin poisoning and is often directly related to the severity of poisoning.[44] In the setting of chronic toxicity, hyperkalemia is more likely to have other contributing etiologies, such as the cause of the chronic digoxin toxicity (e.g., kidney injury), and coprescribed medications (renin-angiotensin-aldosterone system [RAAS] inhibitors).[42]

The mainstay of treatment of cardiac glycoside toxicity is anti-digoxin Fab: a monoclonal antibody fragment with a high binding affinity for digoxin that displaces it from the Na^+-K^+-ATPase channel. Antidotes and indications in the setting of cardiac glycoside toxicity are summarized in **Table 27.8.**[45]

SULFONYLUREA AND INSULIN OVERDOSE

Sulfonylurea (SU) and insulin overdoses primarily cause hypoglycemia. People with diabetes can present with symptoms at "normal" blood glucose levels because they are used to higher serum blood glucose levels at baseline, and concomitant treatment with β-blockers can blunt or mask the autonomic response to hypoglycemia.

SUs are insulin secretagogues, stimulating the release of insulin from pancreatic islet cells. They have high oral bioavailability, a rapid onset of action (often within 30 minutes) with peak effects of insulin secretion at 2 to 3 hours, and are

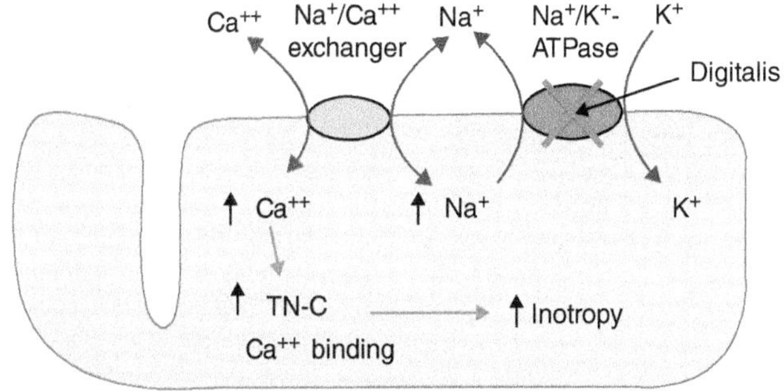

FIGURE 27.4: Mechanisms of digoxin toxicity: Digoxin and other cardiac glycosides exert toxicity by selective blocking of the Na^+-K^+-ATPase. In turn this leads to increases in intracellular Na^+, which leads to accumulation of intracellular Ca^{2+} via the Na^+/Ca^{2+} exchanger. This leads to more Ca^{2+} from the sarcoplasmic reticulum, thereby increasing cardiac contractility. Blocking the Na^+-K^+-ATPase also leads to hyperkalemia.

From Optician. How blood barrier stands up to drug treatments. https://www.opticianonline.net/cet-archive/143

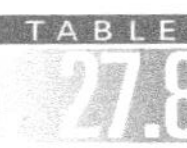
TABLE 27.8

Antidotes for Cardiac Glycoside Toxicity

Antidote	Clinical Indication	Dose	Comment
Anti-digoxin Fab	• Ingested dose of >10 mg digoxin in adult or >4 mg in children (or >0.1 mg/kg) • Dysrhythmia with serum (digoxin) >2 ng/mL (2.6 nmol/L) • Serum K >5 mmol/L • Steady state (digoxin) >7.8 ng/mL (10 mmol/L) • (Digoxin) >11.5 ng/mL (15 nmol/L) • Kidney failure, bradycardia not responding to atropine	Each vial contains 40 mg of anti-digoxin Fab and is capable of neutralizing 0.5 mg of digoxin Acute poisoning: 2 vials Chronic poisoning: 1 vial and repeat if required in 1 hr based on clinical response Cardiac arrest: 5-10 vials over 30 min	Serum digoxin levels are unreliable after administration of anti-digoxin Fab as measuring both free and bound digoxin
Insulin/dextrose	Hyperkalemia	50 mL of 50% dextrose + 10 U of regular insulin IV	
IV calcium	Hyperkalemia	1 amp of calcium gluconate	Intracellular calcium is elevated and giving extra calcium may increase toxicity and lead to sustained cardiac contraction (stone heart). However, this is a theoretical issue, and calcium can be given cautiously in the face of severe hyperkalemia despite cardiac glycoside toxicity.
IV atropine	Bradycardia	0.5-1 mg IV	

IV, intravenous.

primarily excreted by the kidneys.[46] Consequently, they have a narrow therapeutic index and the potential for significant toxicity. Insulin, on the other hand, acts as a direct agonist on transmembrane insulin receptors, leading to downstream effects: increased intracellular glucose uptake and a decrease in hepatic gluconeogenesis and glycogenolysis. Peak effects and duration of action are driven by absorption in subcutaneous tissues, which is primarily dependent on the insulin preparation. However, in the setting of overdose, absorption pharmacokinetics can be altered, leading to prolonged absorption and, consequently, protracted insulin effects.

Treatment of SU and insulin overdoses requires restoring normal glucose levels in part by antagonizing the effects of elevated levels of insulin.[47] Dextrose is generally the initial treatment to increase serum glucose concentrations. However, caution must be exercised after administering dextrose, particularly in SU toxicity or when patients have some innate pancreatic function, because bolus doses of dextrose can cause endogenous insulin secretion, paradoxically worsening hypoglycemia.[48]

Subcutaneous or intravenous octreotide can be given to directly prevent pancreatic insulin release. Octreotide is a somatostatin analog that binds to somatostatin-2 receptors and, by blocking calcium influx into the islet cells, reduces insulin secretion (**Figure 27.5**). It is particularly useful in preventing additional pancreatic insulin secretion following dextrose administration in SU toxicity. Most experts advocate for octreotide to be started as first-line treatment, in particular for SU overdoses. In the setting of insulin overdose, octreotide will

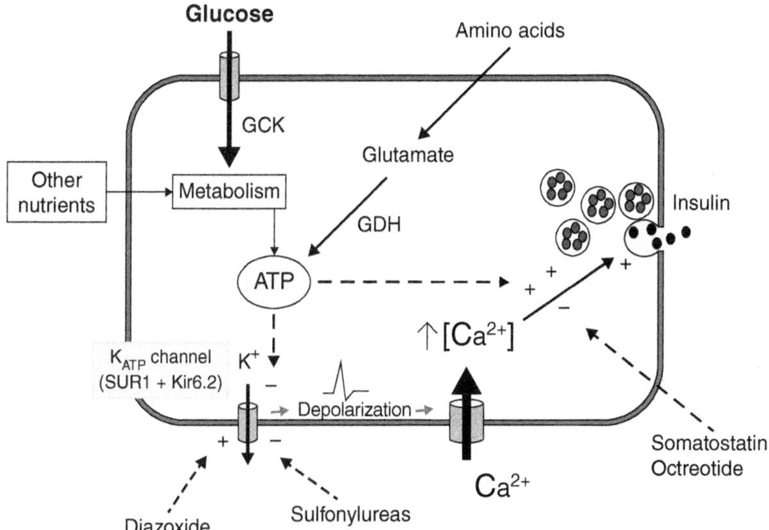

FIGURE 27.5: Mechanism of action of octreotide: Sulfonylureas block voltage-gated K^+ channels on islet cells in the pancreas, leading to higher concentration of intracellular K^+, subsequent increases in intracellular Ca^{2+}, and insulin release via exocytosis. Octreotide binds to somatostatin-2 receptors and blocks Ca^{2+} influx into cells, leading to less insulin secretion. GCK, glucokinase; GDH, glutamate dehydrogenase.

From Klein-Schwartz W, Stassinos GL, Isbister GK. Treatment of sulfonylurea and insulin overdose. *Br J Clin Pharmacol.* 2016;81(3):496-504. doi:10.1111/bcp.12822

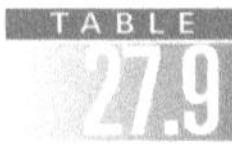

Antidotes for SU and Insulin Overdose

Antidote	Indication	Dose	Potential Adverse Effects
Dextrose (25%-50%)	Initial correction of hypoglycemia Infusions of 5%-20% dextrose can be used for maintenance of euglycemia.	50-100 mL of 25%-50% dextrose solution	Hyperglycemia and paradoxical hypoglycemia (SU overdose), phlebitis at IV site, hyperosmolality
Octreotide	Recurrent hypoglycemia	50-100 μg SC or IV q6-12h	Hyperglycemia, nausea, abdominal pain, diarrhea, bradycardia
Glucagon	*Only to be used if IV access is unavailable*	1 mg IM, IV, SC	Nausea, vomiting, hypokalemia, hyperglycemia

IM, intramuscular; IV, intravenous; SC, subcutaneous; SU, sulfonylurea.

not affect exogenous insulin, but can mitigate further endogenous insulin release. Preferred treatments and antidotes for SU and insulin toxicity are summarized in **Table 27.9**.

CONCLUSIONS

Poisoned patients can present complex management challenges. Many treatment decisions are made based on clinical experience and expert opinion, as most decontamination techniques and antidotes have not been evaluated in rigorous clinical trials. It bears mention that the majority of patients with poisoning exposures can be successfully treated with good supportive care. Antidotes can indeed play a unique role in the treatment of the poisoned patient but, in reality, are only available for a minority of poisonings. High costs, lack of stocking, unfamiliarity with administration, unclear ingestion history and timeline, and potential adverse effects can make administering antidotes fraught with challenges. In addition, the temptation to use an antidote can distract from other aspects of medical care that may be more important for a good clinical outcome. Management advice should always be sought from experts because the care of each poisoned patient must be individualized, and there are often nuances regarding the utility of specialized decontamination techniques and antidotes.

References

1. Thompson C. *Poison and Poisoners.* Harold Shaylor; 1931.
2. Hoffman RS, Howland MA, Lewin NA, Nelson LS, Goldfrank LR. *Goldfrank's Toxicologic Emergencies.* 11th ed. McGraw Hill Education; 2019.
3. Gummin DD, Mowry JB, Spyker DA, et al. 2018 Annual Report of the American Association of Poison Control Centers' National Poison Data System (NPDS): 36th Annual Report. *Clin Toxicol.* 2019;3650:1-194. doi:10.1080/15563650.2019.1677022
4. Juurlink DN, McGuigan MA, Paton TW, Redelmeier DA. Availability of antidotes at acute care hospitals in Ontario. *CMAJ.* 2001;165(1):27-30. http://www.ncbi.nlm.nih.gov/pubmed/11468950

5. Benson BE, Hoppu K, Troutman WG, et al. Position paper update: gastric lavage for gastrointestinal decontamination. *Clin Toxicol (Phila).* 2013;51(3):140-146. doi:10.3109/15563650.2013.770154
6. Chyka PA, Seger D, Krenzelok EP, Vale JA; American Academy of Clinical Toxicology, European Association of Poisons Centres and Clinical Toxicologists. Position paper: single-dose activated charcoal. *Clin Toxicol (Phila).* 2005;43(2):61-87. http://www.ncbi.nlm.nih.gov/pubmed/15822758
7. Vale JA, Kulig K; American Academy of Clinical Toxicology, European Association of Poisons Centres and Clinical Toxicologists. Position paper: gastric lavage. *J Toxicol Clin Toxicol.* 2004;42(7):933-943. http://www.ncbi.nlm.nih.gov/pubmed/15641639
8. Livshits Z, Sampson BA, Howland MA, Hoffman RS, Nelson LS. Retained drugs in the gastrointestinal tracts of deceased victims of oral drug overdose. *Clin Toxicol (Phila).* 2015;53(2):113-118. doi:10.3109/15563650.2014.992528
9. Miyauchi M, Hayashida M, Yokota H. Evaluation of residual toxic substances in the stomach using upper gastrointestinal endoscopy for management of patients with oral drug overdose on admission: a prospective, observational study. *Medicine (Baltimore).* 2015;94(4):e463. doi:10.1097/MD.0000000000000463
10. Juurlink DN. Activated charcoal for acute overdose: a reappraisal. *Br J Clin Pharmacol.* 2016;81(3):482-487. doi:10.1111/bcp.12793
11. Cooper GM, Le Couteur DG, Richardson D, Buckley NA. A randomized clinical trial of activated charcoal for the routine management of oral drug overdose. *QJM.* 2005;98(9):655-660. doi:10.1093/qjmed/hci102
12. Eddleston M, Juszczak E, Buckley NA, et al. Multiple-dose activated charcoal in acute self-poisoning: a randomised controlled trial. *Lancet.* 2008;371(9612):579-587. doi:10.1016/S0140-6736(08)60270-6
13. Olson KR. Activated charcoal for acute poisoning: one toxicologist's journey. *J Med Toxicol.* 2010;6(2):190-198. doi:10.1007/s13181-010-0046-1
14. Thanacoody R, Caravati EM, Troutman B, et al. Position paper update: whole bowel irrigation for gastrointestinal decontamination of overdose patients. *Clin Toxicol (Phila).* 2015;53(1):5-12. doi:10.3109/15563650.2014.989326
15. Kirshenbaum LA, Mathews SC, Sitar DS, Tenenbein M. Whole-bowel irrigation versus activated charcoal in sorbitol for the ingestion of modified-release pharmaceuticals. *Clin Pharmacol Ther.* 1989;46(3):264-271. doi:10.1038/clpt.1989.137
16. Buckley NA, Dawson AH, Juurlink DN, Isbister GK. Who gets antidotes? Choosing the chosen few. *Br J Clin Pharmacol.* 2016;81(3):402-407. doi:10.1111/bcp.12894
17. Larson AM, Polson J, Fontana RJ, et al. Acetaminophen-induced acute liver failure: results of a United States multicenter, prospective study. *Hepatology.* 2005;42(6):1364-1372. doi:10.1002/hep.20948
18. Lancaster EM, Hiatt JR, Zarrinpar A. Acetaminophen hepatotoxicity: an updated review. *Arch Toxicol.* 2015;89(2):193-199. doi:10.1007/s00204-014-1432-2
19. Chiew AL, Isbister GK, Duffull SB, Buckley NA. Evidence for the changing regimens of acetylcysteine. *Br J Clin Pharmacol.* 2016;81(3):471-481. doi:10.1111/bcp.12789
20. Mitchell JR, Jollow DJ, Potter WZ, Gillette JR, Brodie BB. Acetaminophen-induced hepatic necrosis. IV. Protective role of glutathione. *J Pharmacol Exp Ther.* 1973;187(1):211-217. http://www.ncbi.nlm.nih.gov/pubmed/4746329
21. Olsson B, Johansson M, Gabrielsson J, Bolme P. Pharmacokinetics and bioavailability of reduced and oxidized N-acetylcysteine. *Eur J Clin Pharmacol.* 1988;34(1):77-82. doi:10.1007/bf01061422
22. Jones AL. Mechanism of action and value of N-acetylcysteine in the treatment of early and late acetaminophen poisoning: a critical review. *J Toxicol Clin Toxicol.* 1998;36(4):277-285. doi:10.3109/15563659809028022
23. Hendrickson RG, McKeown NJ, West PL, Burke CR. Bactrian ("double hump") acetaminophen pharmacokinetics: a case series and review of the literature. *J Med Toxicol.* 2010;6(3):337-344. doi:10.1007/s13181-010-0083-9
24. Rzasa Lynn R, Galinkin JL. Naloxone dosage for opioid reversal: current evidence and clinical implications. *Ther Adv drug Saf.* 2018;9(1):63-88. doi:10.1177/2042098617744161
25. Sivilotti MLA. Flumazenil, naloxone and the "coma cocktail". *Br J Clin Pharmacol.* 2016;81(3):428-436. doi:10.1111/bcp.12731
26. Wermeling DP. Review of naloxone safety for opioid overdose: practical considerations for new technology and expanded public access. *Ther Adv Drug Saf.* 2015;6(1):20-31. doi:10.1177/2042098614564776
27. Boyer EW. Management of opioid analgesic overdose. *N Engl J Med.* 2012;367(2):146-155. doi:10.1056/NEJMra1202561

28. Aabakken L, Johansen KS, Rydningen EB, Bredesen JE, Ovreb0 S, Jacobsen D. Osmolal and anion gaps in patients admitted to an emergency medical department. *Hum Exp Toxicol.* 1994;13(2):131-134. doi:10.1177/096032719401300212
29. McMartin K, Jacobsen D, Hovda KE. Antidotes for poisoning by alcohols that form toxic metabolites. *Br J Clin Pharmacol.* 2016;81(3):505-515. doi:10.1111/bcp.12824
30. Makar AB, Tephly TR, Mannering GJ. Methanol metabolism in the monkey. *Mol Pharmacol.* 1968;4(5):471-483. http://www.ncbi.nlm.nih.gov/pubmed/4972128
31. Weiss B, Coen G. Effect of ethanol on ethylene glycol oxidation by mammalian liver enzymes. *Enzymol Biol Clin (Basel).* 1966;6(4):297-304. http://www.ncbi.nlm.nih.gov/pubmed/4288711
32. Li TK, Theorell H. Human liver alcohol dehydrogenase: inhibition by pyrazole and pyrazole analogs. *Acta Chem Scand.* 1969;23(3):892-902. http://www.ncbi.nlm.nih.gov/pubmed/4308830
33. Graudins A, Lee HM, Druda D. Calcium channel antagonist and beta-blocker overdose: antidotes and adjunct therapies. *Br J Clin Pharmacol.* 2016;81(3):453-461. doi:10.1111/bcp.12763
34. St-Onge M, Anseeuw K, Cantrell FL, et al. Experts consensus recommendations for the management of calcium channel blocker poisoning in adults. *Crit Care Med.* 2017;45(3):e306-e315. doi:10.1097/CCM.0000000000002087
35. Liang CW, Diamond SJ, Hagg DS. Lipid rescue of massive verapamil overdose: a case report. *J Med Case Rep.* 2011;5:399. doi:10.1186/1752-1947-5-399
36. Young AC, Velez LI, Kleinschmidt KC. Intravenous fat emulsion therapy for intentional sustained-release verapamil overdose. *Resuscitation.* 2009;80(5):591-593. doi:10.1016/j.resuscitation.2009.01.023
37. Baud FJ, Megarbane B, Deye N, Leprince P. Clinical review: aggressive management and extracorporeal support for drug-induced cardiotoxicity. *Crit Care.* 2007;11(2):207. doi:10.1186/cc5700
38. Lo JCY, Darracq MA, Clark RF. A review of methylene blue treatment for cardiovascular collapse. *J Emerg Med.* 2014;46(5):670-679. doi:10.1016/j.jemermed.2013.08.102
39. Jang DH, Nelson LS, Hoffman RS. Methylene blue in the treatment of refractory shock from an amlodipine overdose. *Ann Emerg Med.* 2011;58(6):565-567. doi:10.1016/j.annemergmed.2011.02.025
40. Janion M, Stepień A, Sielski J, Gutkowski W. Is the intra-aortic balloon pump a method of brain protection during cardiogenic shock after drug intoxication? *J Emerg Med.* 2010;38(2):162-167. doi:10.1016/j.jemermed.2007.10.037
41. Bateman DN. Digoxin-specific antibody fragments: how much and when? *Toxicol Rev.* 2004;23(3):135-143. http://www.ncbi.nlm.nih.gov/pubmed/15862081
42. Roberts DM, Gallapatthy G, Dunuwille A, Chan BS. Pharmacological treatment of cardiac glycoside poisoning. *Br J Clin Pharmacol.* 2016;81(3):488-495. doi:10.1111/bcp.12814
43. Kelly RA, Smith TW. Recognition and management of digitalis toxicity. *Am J Cardiol.* 1992;69(18):108-119. doi:10.1016/0002-9149(92)91259-7
44. Pap C, Zacher G, Kárteszi M. Prognosis in acute digitalis poisoning. *Orv Hetil.* 2005;146(11):507-513. http://www.ncbi.nlm.nih.gov/pubmed/15813189
45. Chan BSH, Buckley NA. Digoxin-specific antibody fragments in the treatment of digoxin toxicity. *Clin Toxicol (Phila).* 52(8):824-836. doi:10.3109/15563650.2014.943907
46. Ferner RE, Chaplin S. The relationship between the pharmacokinetics and pharmacodynamic effects of oral hypoglycaemic drugs. *Clin Pharmacokinet.* 1987;12(6):379-401. doi:10.2165/00003088-198712060-00001
47. Klein-Schwartz W, Stassinos GL, Isbister GK. Treatment of sulfonylurea and insulin overdose. *Br J Clin Pharmacol.* 2016;81(3):496-504. doi:10.1111/bcp.12822
48. Henquin JC. Triggering and amplifying pathways of regulation of insulin secretion by glucose. *Diabetes.* 2000;49(11):1751-1760. doi:10.2337/diabetes.49.11.1751
49. Kline JA, Leonova E, Raymond RM. Beneficial myocardial metabolic effects of insulin during verapamil toxicity in the anesthetized canine. *Crit Care Med.* 1995;23(7):1251-1263. doi:10.1097/00003246-199507000-00016

28 Extracorporeal Therapy for Poisonings and Intoxications

Bourne Lewis Auguste and David N. Juurlink

INTRODUCTION

Extracorporeal techniques have been utilized in the management of poisoning since the 1950s.[1,2] However, the lack of large prospective randomized trials, limited evidence from small observational studies, and the relative rarity of poisonings that might warrant such therapies have left clinicians with uncertainty about when to use extracorporeal treatments (ECTRs). In light of this, the EXtracorporeal TReatments In Poisoning (EXTRIP) workgroup was formed in 2010.[3,4] Comprising individuals with expertise in nephrology, pharmacology, toxicology, and evidence synthesis from around the globe, the EXTRIP workgroup has since published several systematic reviews on the use of ECTRs in various poisonings.

In 2016, more than 2.1 million human exposures were reported to poison centers in the United States, with more than 300,000 exposures (or 17.1% of all reported exposures) warranting admission to hospital.[5] Although most cases were managed with supportive care, 0.9% of all hospitalized exposures required ECTR.

Clearance of poisons using ECTR can be classified into four distinct categories based on mechanisms of action. These include diffusive, convective, adsorptive, and centrifugal clearance mechanisms. Diffusive clearance occurs with peritoneal dialysis and hemodialysis, whereas convective clearance occurs with hemofiltration. A combination of both diffusive and convective techniques can be used to further increase clearance with hemodiafiltration. Adsorption occurs with the use of hemoperfusion, whereas centrifugation of blood constituents is used in plasma exchange (PLEX).[6,7] In this chapter, we primarily focus on various types of diffusive and adsorptive clearances in the form of hemodialysis and hemoperfusion for the removal of poisons. We will also provide an overview of the EXTRIP workgroup recommendations regarding the use of ECTR in the management of commonly encountered poisonings.

TYPES OF EXTRACORPOREAL TREATMENT

Hemodialysis and Hemofiltration

Benefits

The countercurrent flow of dialysate and blood during hemodialysis creates a favorable concentration gradient in which poisons can be removed across a semipermeable membrane. Intermittent hemodialysis is most effective for removing poisons that are water soluble, have a low molecular weight and volume of distribution (generally <1 L/kg), and are not highly bound (<80% binding) to plasma proteins.[7,8] Hemodialysis remains the most commonly utilized form of ECTR in the management of poisoning.[9]

Drawbacks

Aside from risks related to the procedure itself, such as infection and hemorrhage, one potential drawback of intermittent hemodialysis treatment is the possibility of "rebound" toxicity after cessation of treatment owing to the redistribution of certain poisons within body compartments. To limit rebound toxicity, continuous kidney replacement therapy (KRT) has been used in clinical practice after intermittent hemodialysis in the forms of continuous venovenous hemofiltration (CVVH), continuous venovenous hemodialysis (CVVHD), or a combined form with continuous venovenous hemodiafiltration (CVVHDF). KRT is primarily used for patients who are hemodynamically unstable.[10] It allows for gentler removal of water and poisons as compared to intermittent hemodialysis, through lower blood and effluent flow rates. These lower flow rates result in a significant (~80%) reduced clearance compared to hemodialysis.[6,10] Consequently, intermittent hemodialysis is preferred over KRT in the management of poisons.

Hemofiltration removes poisons and solvents by use of convective mechanisms and replaces the latter with a physiologic solution. Convection allows for the removal of larger poisons with a molecular weight of up to 25,000 Da.[6] In some instances, mechanisms of convection and diffusion can be combined to optimize clearance in a process termed "hemodiafiltration."

Hemoperfusion

Benefits

In contrast, hemoperfusion involves the circulation of blood through cartridges containing either an anion exchange resin or activated charcoal to remove poisons by adsorption.[7,10-12] Poison clearance by hemoperfusion is not limited by molecular size or protein-binding characteristics, in contrast to the diffusive mechanisms of intermittent hemodialysis.

Drawbacks

Hemoperfusion has major drawbacks, including adsorption of leukocytes, calcium, and platelets.[11,13] Adsorption of the latter can result in thrombocytopenia, impairing primary hemostasis and leading to frequent bleeding in patients receiving hemoperfusion. Additionally, charcoal-coated cartridges may be 10 times costlier than high-efficiency dialyzers.[9] These cartridges need to be changed frequently as they become saturated after a few hours, impairing the efficiency of poison clearance. Cartridges for hemoperfusion also have a short shelf life limited to about 2 years.[14] Overall, hemoperfusion is more challenging to perform than hemodialysis and is associated with greater costs while lacking the ability to correct acid-base and electrolyte abnormalities.

Plasma Exchange

Benefits

PLEX is an alternative method of ECTR for the removal of poisons, particularly those tightly bound to plasma proteins. PLEX involves the removal of plasma (the acellular component of blood) from the circulation, exchanging it with donated plasma, along with albumin and isotonic fluids.[10,15] PLEX can also be considered for poisons with large molecular weights (>50,000 Da).[15]

Drawbacks

The risk-benefit profile for using PLEX for poisons is not as favorable as for other ECTRs, given the possibilities of hypocalcemia and hemorrhage.[16] Citrate used as an anticoagulant for the extracorporeal system in PLEX complexes with free calcium, thereby reducing ionized calcium concentrations, sometimes leading patients to become symptomatic with muscle weakness and paresthesias if calcium is not replaced.[17] PLEX removes platelets and reduces clotting factors, particularly if albumin is used as a replacement rather than fresh frozen plasma.

DIALYZABILITY OF POISONS

Variations in the molecular size, structure, and properties of poisons account for differences in dialyzability. Poison removal is heavily dependent on the amount present in the plasma compartment, and clinical utility is determined by whether its removal will afford a significant reduction in total poison burden. The dialyzability of a poison is dependent on four main factors: (1) endogenous clearance, (2) molecular weight, (3) volume of distribution, and (4) protein binding.[6,7,10]

In cases where the endogenous clearance of a poison or drug is high or is greater than what would be achieved with exogenous clearance, ECTR is rarely indicated. Historically, it has been suggested that extracorporeal clearance should augment total clearance by at least 30% in order to have a meaningful clinical impact.[18] For example, cocaine has a half-life of 0.5 to 1.5 hours and a rapid endogenous clearance. Dialysis is not indicated for cocaine-related toxicity because the incremental effect of extracorporeal clearance on total clearance would be negligible.[3,19]

Molecular weight is another important determinant. Poisons with lower molecular weights are more likely to be dialyzable. Hemodialysis relies on diffusion, and poisons with higher molecular weights are not easily cleared by this method. However, the efficiency of dialyzers has improved substantially over the last few decades. Given the evolution of new high cut-off dialyzers, hemodialysis can be used to clear poisons with molecular weights of up to 15,000 Da.[20] On the other hand, hemofiltration and hemodiafiltration use convection and can enhance clearance of solutes of up to 25,000 Da. Poisons of up to 50,000 Da in size can be removed via adsorption-based techniques such as hemoperfusion.[21]

Poison-protein complexes can be quite large, in some instances exceeding 65,000 Da.[10] These complexes are too large to pass through high cut-off dialyzers or filters. Poisons with more than 80% protein binding are also poorly cleared with hemodialysis.[10] However, protein binding is saturable, and even for highly protein-bound drugs, the free fraction can increase following overdose, allowing the unbound fraction to remove by ECTRs such as hemodialysis or hemofiltration. For example, valproic acid binds avidly to plasma proteins at therapeutic concentrations (80%-94%).[22] In cases of valproic acid toxicity, an increase in free valproic acid concentrations allows its removal with hemodialysis.[10,22,23]

Another important factor determining the dialyzability of a poison is the apparent volume of distribution (V_D).[3,4] Extracorporeal removal of poisons is only effective for poisons within the intravascular compartment.[10] For example, a poison with a small V_D (<1 L/kg) will be much more easily cleared with ECTR as compared to a poison with larger V_D (>2 L/kg). Simply put, as the V_D of a substance increases, its fraction in vascular compartment falls.[24] Poisons with hydrophilic properties tend to distribute into total body water, whereas lipophilic ones preferentially distribute to extravascular compartments such as muscle and adipose tissue, resulting in a larger apparent V_D.[10] Therefore, lipophilic poisons are less easily cleared with dialysis. For example, propranolol is highly lipophilic, with a higher V_D than many other β-blockers, and is removed poorly by dialysis.[25,26]

There may be instances in which the large V_D of a poison may lead to rebound toxicity after intermittent hemodialysis. For example, rebound toxicity may occur with lithium and metformin. Patients should be monitored closely for signs of rebound toxicity after intermittent hemodialysis. Alternatively, KRT following a treatment of hemodialysis can be considered in cases where the risk of rebound toxicity is high. Observational studies have demonstrated that KRT reduces the risk of posttherapy lithium rebound by facilitating gradual lithium removal from intracellular compartments, especially in cases of chronic poisoning.[27]

The EXTRIP workgroup has reviewed the extensive literature and published general guidelines on specific recommendations for ECTR for various poisons.[4,7,28-40] The summaries also provide recommendations against using ECTR for specific agents when the potential adverse effects of treatment are expected to outweigh the potential benefits. Executive summary recommendations are readily available online (https://www.extrip-workgroup.org/recommendations). These recommendations offer practitioners guidance and further clarity as a means to standardize the management of poisonings, particularly in a field where evidence to guide practice is limited.

RECOMMENDED USE OF EXTRACORPOREAL TREATMENT FOR SPECIFIC AGENTS

Analgesics

Analgesic medications in the form of acetaminophen- and salicylate-containing compounds remain leading causes of reported agents to poison centers. These agents are associated with considerable mortality, particularly when diagnosis and timely intervention are delayed. In 2013, 11.8% of all reported fatalities because of poisons in the United States were related to acetaminophen- and salicylate-containing compounds.[41]

Salicylates

Salicylates are present in various forms, with acetylsalicylic acid (ASA; aspirin) the most commonly encountered in clinical practice. It has a molecular weight of 180 Da with a very small V_D (0.2 L/kg).[31,42] Salicylates can also be highly bound to protein (up to 90%), but this can fall to 30% when binding sites are saturated.[43] The features of salicylate poisoning are nonspecific and may delay diagnosis and appropriate management. These include nausea, vomiting, confusion, and dyspnea. If left untreated, salicylate toxicity can rapidly progress to agitation, coma, and eventually death.[31] Initial treatment requires supportive care with intravenous isotonic fluid to treat or avoid intravascular volume contraction. Additional supportive therapy should include intravenous dextrose and bicarbonate administration. Bicarbonate is utilized to promote alkaluria, trapping salicylate (a weak acid) in its ionized form, thereby reducing proximal tubular reabsorption and enhancing elimination by the kidneys.[44] Similarly, maintenance of systemic alkalemia (pH 7.45-7.55) helps minimize the transfer of salicylate across the blood-brain barrier. However, these therapies are often insufficient when the amount of ASA ingested is large or when patients have mental status alterations or acute respiratory distress syndrome.[45] The EXTRIP workgroup recommends ECTR in the form of intermittent hemodialysis for patients with very elevated salicylate concentrations (>7.2 mmol/L [100 mg/dL], with a slightly lower threshold in patients with kidney impairment), salicylate poisoning presenting with altered mental status or hypoxemia requiring supplemental oxygen (**Table 28.1**). The workgroup recommends that hemodialysis continue for at least 6 hours or until there is improvement in symptoms and the serum salicylate concentration is less than 1.4 mmol/L (19 mg/dL).[31] Furthermore, supportive therapy with intravenous bicarbonate should be continued between hemodialysis sessions. Alternative modalities such as KRT or hemoperfusion should only be considered if intermittent hemodialysis is not readily available.

Acetaminophen

Acetaminophen is the most used analgesic worldwide. It is frequently implicated in overdoses and is the leading cause of drug-induced liver failure in North America and the United Kingdom.[32,46,47] Toxicity occurs when acetaminophen glucuronidation and sulfation pathways become saturated, leading to an increase in the synthesis of *N*-acetyl-*p*-benzoquinone imine (NAPQI) by cytochrome P450.[48,49] A highly reactive electrophile, NAPQI is normally reduced by glutathione and eliminated by the kidneys as mercapturic acid and cysteine conjugates.[50] However, as glutathione stores diminish, NAPQI binds to hepatic macromolecules, leading to acute liver injury and, in some instances, fulminant hepatic failure.

Although acetaminophen has characteristics that make it dialyzable such as a small molecular weight of 151 Da, low protein biding, and a low V_D (0.9-1.0 L/kg), first-line therapy is administration of *N*-acetylcysteine (NAC).[32] NAC is used to replenish glutathione stores and to limit the toxic effects of NAPQI, and when given within 10 hours of ingestion is almost universally effective. However, in rare circumstances when NAC is not available or concerns exist about severe allergies, ECTR may be considered as an alternative treatment for acetaminophen toxicity.[32] Additionally, in cases of massive acetaminophen overdose,

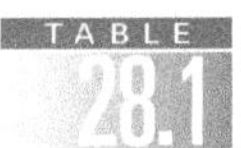

TABLE 28.1 Recommendations for Hemodialysis in Salicylate Poisoning

If any of the following conditions are present, **initiate** extracorporeal treatment:

1. Clinical symptoms:
   a. Altered mental status
   b. Hypoxemia requiring supplemental oxygenation
2. Laboratory features:
   a. Serum salicylate level >7.2 mmol/L (100 mg/dL)
   b. Serum salicylate >6.5 mmol/L (90 mg/dL) with impaired kidney function

If supportive measures fail, then consider initiating extracorporeal treatment if any one of the following conditions are present:

1. Laboratory features:
   a. Serum salicylate >6.5 mmol/L (90 mg/dL)
   b. Serum salicylate >5.8 mmol/L (80 mg/dL) with impaired kidney function
   c. Systemic pH ≤7.20

Juurlink DN, Gosselin S, Kielstein JT, et al; on behalf of EXTRIP Workgroup. Extracorporeal treatment for salicylate poisoning: systematic review and recommendations from the EXTRIP workgroup. *Ann Emerg Med.* 2015;266(2):165-181.

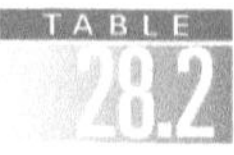

Recommendations for Hemodialysis in Acetaminophen Poisoning

If any of the following conditions are present, **initiate** extracorporeal treatment:

Laboratory and clinical features:

a. Acetaminophen level >1,000 mg/L (6,620 μmol/L) and *N*-acetylcysteine (NAC) is NOT given
b. Acetaminophen level >700 mg/L (4,630 μmol/L) along with patient having altered mental status, metabolic acidosis, an elevated lactate, and NAC is NOT given
c. Acetaminophen level >900 mg/L (5,960 μmol/L) along with patient having altered mental status, metabolic acidosis, an elevated lactate, and NAC is given

Gosselin S, Juurlink DN, Kielstein JT, et al; on behalf of EXTRIP Workgroup. Extracorporeal treatment for acetaminophen poisoning: recommendations from the EXTRIP workgroup. *Clin Toxicol.* 2014;52(8):856-867.

NAC alone may be insufficient to counter extensive mitochondrial impairment caused by NAPQI, which can lead to profound metabolic acidosis and mental status changes. In such patients, ECTR can also be considered to both improve acidemia and enhance removal of acetaminophen.[51] Although there are limited studies examining the pharmacokinetics of NAPQI and its surrogate markers in response to ECTR, the EXTRIP workgroup recommends hemodialysis following massive overdose as a means of removing acetaminophen and correcting metabolic acidosis.[32] The preferred ECTR is intermittent hemodialysis but hemoperfusion or KRT can be considered as alternatives if this is not readily available (**Table 28.2**). If ECTR is utilized, it should be continued until clinical improvement is documented. Furthermore, the workgroup recommends against using ECTR solely on the basis of a reported ingested dose if NAC has not been administered. Importantly, if ECTR is used for massive acetaminophen overdose, NAC dosing should be continued at a higher rate (generally 2-fold), because it too is cleared by ECTR.

Anticonvulsants, Mood Stabilizers, and Sedatives

Valproic Acid

Valproic acid has a high therapeutic index along with broad clinical indications beyond the treatment of partial and generalized seizures.[52] It is also used in the treatment of bipolar disorder and for migraine prophylaxis.[53] Valproic acid has a molecular weight of 166 Da and small V_D (<0.5 L/kg) along with high-protein-binding capacity.[54] However, protein binding decreases significantly with serum concentrations exceeding 1,000 mg/L (700 μmol/L).[23] In patients with acute ingestion of valproic acid, *single-dose* activated charcoal may be considered as the method of gastrointestinal (GI) decontamination.[55] The most common clinical manifestation associated with valproic acid toxicity is central nervous system (CNS) depression, which may initially present as lethargy followed by respiratory depression from cerebral edema.[54,56] If clinical symptoms consistent with cerebral edema or shock are present, then ECTR is recommended (**Table 28.3**). The EXTRIP workgroup states that hemodialys is should be the preferred ECTR in valproic acid poisoning and is continued until either clinical improvement or the serum valproic acid levels are 50 to 100 mg/L (350-700 μmol/L).[36]

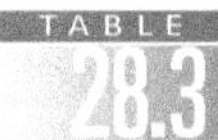

Recommendations for Hemodialysis in Valproic Acid Poisoning

If any of the following conditions are present, **initiate** extracorporeal treatment:

1. Clinical symptoms:
   a. Cerebral edema
   b. Shock
2. Laboratory features:
   a. Serum valproic acid levels >1,300 mg/L (9,000 μmol/L)

Consider extracorporeal treatment if any one of the following conditions are present:

1. Clinical:
   a. Coma or respiratory depression requiring mechanical ventilation
2. Laboratory features:
   a. Serum valproic acid levels >900 mg/L (6,250 μmol/L)
   b. Hyperammonemia present
   c. pH < 7.10

Ghannoum M, Laliberte M, Nolin TD, et al; on behalf of EXTRIP Workgroup. Extracorporeal treatment for valproic acid poisoning: systematic review and recommendations from the EXTRIP workgroup. *Clin Toxicol (Phila)*. 2015;53(5):454-465.

Carbamazepine

An anticonvulsant also used for the treatment of neuropathic pain and bipolar disorder, carbamazepine has a molecular weight of 236 Da, is lipophilic with a variable V_D, and is highly bound to protein.[57] Patients usually develop significant symptoms of toxicity at concentrations exceeding 40 mg/L (169 μmol/L).[33] Carbamazepine toxicity is mainly characterized by CNS symptoms with ataxia, altered level of consciousness, and paradoxical seizures owing to a proconvulsive metabolite. Severe toxicity may manifest as respiratory depression and tricyclic antidepressant (TCA)-like cardiac dysrhythmias, resulting in high-grade cardiac conduction delays and hypotension.[58] Furthermore, carbamazepine exhibits anticholinergic properties at toxic levels, delaying gastric emptying and prolonging absorption[59] (see **Table 28.4** for EXTRIP Recommendations).

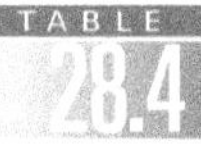

Recommendations for Hemodialysis in Carbamazepine Poisoning

If any of the following conditions are present, **initiate** extracorporeal treatment:

1. Clinical symptoms:
   a. Multiple seizures refractory to medical treatment
   b. Life-threatening dysrhythmias

Consider extracorporeal treatment if any one of the following conditions are present:

1. Clinical:
   a. Coma or respiratory depression requiring mechanical ventilation
2. Laboratory features:
   a. Toxicity persists despite activated charcoal administration and other supportive measures.

Ghannoum M, Yates C, Galvao TF, et al; on behalf of EXTRIP Workgroup. Extracorporeal treatment for carbamazepine poisoning: systematic review and recommendations from the EXTRIP workgroup. *Clin Toxicol (Phila)*. 2014;52(10):993-1004.

Phenytoin

This is a first-line agent in the treatment of generalized tonic-clonic as well as focal seizures. Phenytoin has molecular weight of 252 Da and is 90% protein bound with a V_D of 0.6 to 0.8 L/kg.[60] Although phenytoin has low dialyzability, hemodialysis or hemoperfusion is suggested in select cases where symptoms of severe toxicity in the form of CNS depression are present.[38,60] Patients may also present with hypotension, confusion, respiratory depression, and in unusually severe cases coma (**Table 28.5**). Recommendations from the EXTRIP workgroup discourage ECTR based solely on serum phenytoin concentration or suspected dose.[38]

Barbiturates

The pharmacokinetic properties of barbiturates allow them to be classified into long-acting and short-acting agents. Among this class, phenobarbital is the agent most commonly involved in poisonings.[46] It is a long-acting agent derived from barbituric acid, with a molecular weight of 232 Da. Phenobarbital is 50% protein bound and has a small V_D (0.5 L/kg), making it amenable to clearance via hemodialysis or hemoperfusion.[30,61,62] It is a weak acid and approximately 25% of the drug is cleared in the urine.[62] Urinary alkalinization has been used in cases of moderate phenobarbital poisoning to promote elimination by the kidneys.[30] Multiple-dose activated charcoal (MDAC) is another option to hasten elimination in hemodynamically stable patients.[63,64] However, serum levels of greater than 50 mg/L may lead to coma along with respiratory depression[30]; if these are present, hemodialysis is recommended (**Table 28.6**).

Lithium

Lithium is primarily used for patients with bipolar affective disorder and is currently available in a liquid (lithium citrate) or solid (lithium carbonate) formulation.[65,66] It has a narrow therapeutic index, and the risk of both acute and chronic toxicity is high. Patients with severe toxicity can present with altered level of consciousness and seizures. Lithium has an atomic weight of 7 Da, a small V_D (0.8 L/kg), and 0% of the drug is protein bound.[66-68] Collectively, these properties allow for easy lithium clearance with dialysis. Experts have made strong recommendations for the use of ECTR for the treatment of lithium toxicity in the form of hemodialysis.[37] Hemodialysis should be performed if there is impaired kidney function in the presence of a serum [Li^+] greater than 4.0 mmol/L or in the presence of any of the aforementioned severe symptoms.[37] Weaker indications put forward by the EXTRIP group include serum [Li^+] greater than 5.0 mmol/L, confusion, or if the expected time to a serum [Li^+] less than 1.0 mmol/L exceeds

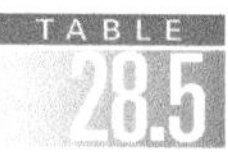

TABLE 28.5 Recommendations for Hemodialysis in Phenytoin Poisoning

Consider extracorporeal treatment if any one of the following conditions are present:
1. Clinical:
   a. Prolonged coma is present or expected.
   b. Prolonged incapacitating ataxia is present or expected.

Anseeuw K, Mowry JB, Burdmann EA, et al; on behalf of EXTRIP Workgroup. Extracorporeal treatment in phenytoin poisoning: systematic review and recommendations from the EXTRIP (Extracorporeal Treatments in Poisoning) workgroup. *Am J Kidney Dis*. 2016;67(2):187-197.

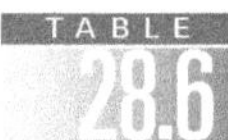

Recommendations for Hemodialysis in Barbiturate Poisoning

If any of the following conditions are present, **initiate** extracorporeal treatment:

1. Clinical symptoms:
   a. Prolonged coma is present or expected.
   b. Shock is present after fluid resuscitation.
   c. Toxicity symptoms persist despite multiple-dose activated charcoal (MDAC) administration.

Consider extracorporeal treatment if any one of the following conditions are present:

1. Clinical:
   a. Respiratory depression requiring mechanical ventilation
2. Laboratory features:
   a. Despite MDAC, serum barbiturate concentration remains elevated or continues to rise

Mactier R, Laliberte M, Mardini J, et al; on behalf of EXTRIP Workgroup. Extracorporeal treatment for barbiturate poisoning: recommendations from the EXTRIP Workgroup. *Am J Kidney Dis.* 2014;64(3):347-358.

36 hours (**Table 28.7**). Hemodialysis or other forms of ECTR may be continued until serum [Li^+] is less than 1.0 mmol/L. Serum [Li^+] often correlates poorly with symptoms of toxicity. Practitioners should rely more on clinical symptoms to determine the need for ECTR. When serum lithium concentrations are not readily available, hemodialysis should be done for a minimum of 6 hours.[37] Given the risk of rebound lithium toxicity (reflecting shift from the intracellular compartment after dialysis), serial measurements of lithium level over a 12-hour period are advisable to ascertain the need, if any, for further hemodialysis. Lastly, KRT modalities may be an appropriate alternative.

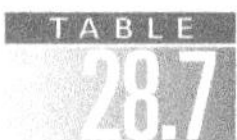

Recommendations for Hemodialysis in Lithium Poisoning

If any of the following conditions are present, **initiate** extracorporeal treatment:

1. Clinical symptoms:
   a. Decreased level of consciousness, seizures, or life-threatening dysrhythmias irrespective of serum [Li^+]
2. Laboratory features:
   a. Impaired kidney function and a serum [Li^+] >4.0 mmol/L

Consider extracorporeal treatment if any one of the following conditions are present:

1. Clinical symptoms:
   a. Confusion is present.
2. Laboratory features:
   a. Serum [Li^+] >5.0 mmol/L
   b. If expected to obtain a serum [Li^+] <1.0 mmol/L with optimal management would exceed 36 hr

Decker BS, Goldfarb DS, Dargan PI, et al; on behalf of EXTRIP Workgroup. Extracorporeal treatment for lithium poisoning: systematic review and recommendations from the EXTRIP Workgroup. *Clin J Am Soc Nephrol.* 2015;10(5):875-887.

Toxic Alcohols

Methanol

Methanol is the simplest primary alcohol, consisting of a methyl group and hydroxyl group. Historically, methanol was produced by distillation of wood, and for this reason it is sometimes referred to as "wood alcohol."[69] Methanol is a major component in several household and industrial products, most notably windshield washer fluid but also paint thinner, solvents, and improperly distilled home alcohol.[70] Methanol toxicity causes CNS depression early after consumption, followed by derangements in acid-base status[71-75] after its successive metabolism by alcohol dehydrogenase and aldehyde dehydrogenase to formic acid, its primary toxic metabolite (**Figure 28.1**). Formic acid causes a high anion gap metabolic acidosis as well as retinal toxicity and visual impairment, which can be severe.[76] In contrast, ethylene glycol is metabolized successively to glycolate (the dominant contributor to the anion gap) and eventually oxalic acid, which leads to deposition of calcium oxalate in the kidneys and acute kidney.[77]

Given their low molecular weights and small V_D, alcohols and their metabolites are easily cleared with hemodialysis. However, preventing oxidative metabolism to toxic metabolites is a critical first step in the management of toxic alcohol ingestion. Fomepizole (Chapter 27) is a competitive inhibitor of alcohol dehydrogenase (ADH) and should be used early in cases of methanol or ethylene glycol ingestion to limit the formation of toxic metabolites (**Table 28.8**).

Where symptoms such as visual impairment or seizures manifest as a result of toxic metabolite accumulation, hemodialysis is warranted. The EXTRIP workgroup has published recommendations guiding the use of ECTR for methanol toxicity, advocating hemodialysis over KRT (**Table 28.9**). The workgroup recommended that hemodialysis could be stopped once the methanol concentration is less than 20 mg/dL (6.2 mmol/L) along with signs of clinical improvement.[39] Furthermore, ADH inhibitors should be continued during hemodialysis, along with supplemental folic acid, the goal of which is to facilitate further metabolism of formic acid to CO_2 and water. Patients who present early with a high methanol serum concentration and who have received an ADH inhibitor should still

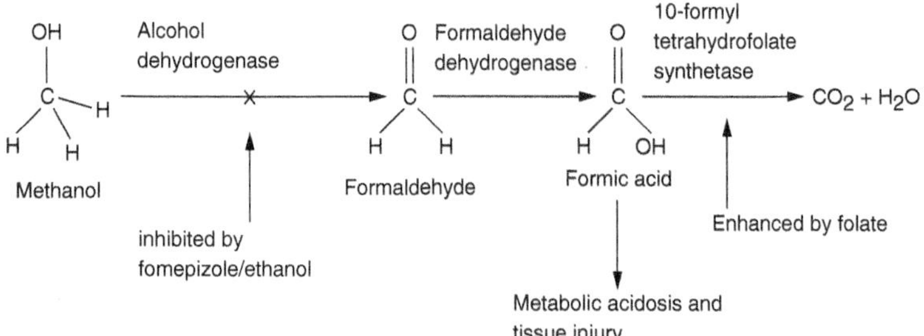

FIGURE 28.1: Metabolic transformation of methanol and associated clinical manifestations with each by-product of methanol. THF, tetrahydrofolate.

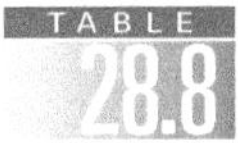

Recommendations for Using Fomepizole or Ethanol in Treating Methanol Toxicity

Load with fomepizole 15 mg/kg *or* ethanol 600 mg/kg[a] if any of the following are present:

1. Plasma methanol level >20 mg/dL (6.2 mmol/L)
2. Confirmed recent ingestion of methanol and osmolar gap >10 mOsm/kg H_2O[b]
3. Strong clinical suspicion of methanol poisoning and at least two of the following criteria:
   a. Arterial pH <7.3
   b. Serum bicarbonate <20 mEq/L (mmol/L)
   c. Osmolar gap >10 mOsm/kg H_2O[b]

[a]Laboratory analysis by freezing point depression method only.

[b]Assumes initial ethanol concentration is zero, dose is independent of chronic drinking status.

Modified from Barceloux DG, Bond GR, Krenzelok EP, Cooper H, Vale JA; American Academy of Clinical Toxicology Ad Hoc Committee on the Treatment Guidelines for Methanol Poisoning. American Academy of Clinical Toxicology practice guidelines on the treatment of methanol poisoning. *J Toxicol Clin Toxicol.* 2002;40:415.

be considered for hemodialysis, as the half-life of methanol in this setting is 40 to 50 hours. Early hemodialysis in such cases, even in the absence of symptoms, is expected to reduce the need for extended fomepizole therapy and prolonged hospitalization. The management principles are similar for poisoning with ethylene glycol, whereas the management of isopropyl alcohol is supportive and does not require ECTR.

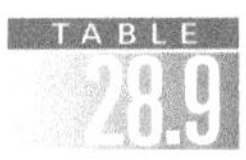

Recommendations for Hemodialysis in Methanol Poisoning

If any of the following conditions are present, initiate extracorporeal treatment:

1. Clinical symptoms:
   a. Coma
   b. Seizures
   c. New visual deficits
2. Laboratory features:
   a. Arterial blood pH ≤7.15
   b. Persistent metabolic acidosis despite antidotes and supportive measures
   c. Anion gap >24 mEq/L (mmol/L)
   d. Serum methanol level >70 mg/dL (21.8 mmol/L) in the context of fomepizole therapy
   e. Serum methanol level >60 mg/dL (18.7 mmol/L) in the context of ethanol treatment
   f. Serum methanol level >50 mg/dL (15.6 mmol/L) in the absence of an alcohol dehydrogenase blocker

Adapted from Roberts DM, Yates C, Megarbane B, et al. Recommendations for the role of extracorporeal treatments in the management of acute methanol poisoning: a systematic review and consensus statement. *Crit Care Med.* 2015;43:461-472.

Other Classes of Agents

Metformin

Metformin is a biguanide antiglycemic agent used in the management of type 2 diabetes mellitus and polycystic ovarian syndrome to augment cellular sensitivity to insulin.[78,79] More than 90% of the drug is eliminated by the kidneys, with active tubular secretion contributing more to clearance by the kidneys than glomerular filtration.[80] Toxicity presents as metformin-associated lactic acidosis (MALA), with serum lactate levels greater than 5 mmol/L and arterial pH less than 7.35 in the context of known metformin exposure and no other attributable cause for lactic acidosis.[81] Although MALA has a reported incidence of less than 0.01 to 0.09 cases/1,000 patient-years, it carries a 30% mortality in patients at risk.[41,82] Metformin has a molecular weight of 129 Da and is nonprotein bound but may have a large V_D of up to 5 L/kg.[83] This large V_D reflects in part the existence of a large compartment within erythrocytes, which is expected to limit removal of the drug with ECTRs such as hemodialysis. Lactic acidosis can be corrected with hemodialysis, and as such the EXTRIP workgroup has recommended that hemodialysis be used as the preferred ECTR in cases of severe acidosis (**Table 28.10**).

Thallium

Thallium is a toxic metal previously used as a component in medicinal agents in the treatment of ringworm infection and as a rodenticide.[84,85] Given the associated risk of toxicity, it is now mostly used in industrial settings for manufacturing high-conductivity electrical equipment along with electrical lighting.[35] However, poisonings continue around the globe where thallium remains used as a rodenticide and may also occur in the context of contaminated drugs of abuse or other herbal products. The accumulation of thallium also accounts for the common clinical manifestations seen with poisoning such as alopecia, painful ascending peripheral neuropathy, and autonomic instability.[35,84,85,86] GI manifestations include nausea, vomiting, and abdominal pain accompanied by either diarrhea or constipation. Severe cases of poisoning have presented with symptoms of altered mental status, respiratory paralysis, and cardiac arrest[87] (see **Table 28.11** for EXTRIP workgroup recommendations for managing thallium poisoning).

Theophylline

Theophylline is used in the treatment of airways disease specifically for bronchospasm related to asthma and chronic obstructive pulmonary disease. It also

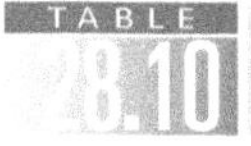

TABLE 28.10 Recommendations for Hemodialysis in Metformin Poisoning

If any of the following conditions are present, initiate extracorporeal treatment:

1. Clinical symptoms:
   a. Shock
   b. Decreased level of consciousness
2. Laboratory features:
   a. Arterial pH <7.0
   b. Serum lactate >20 mmol/L

Calello DP, Liu KD, Wiegand TJ, et al; on behalf of EXTRIP Workgroup. Extracorporeal treatment for metformin poisoning: systematic review and recommendations from the extracorporeal treatments in poisoning workgroup. *Crit Care Med.* 2015;43(8):1716-1730.

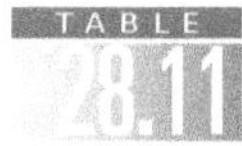

Recommendations for Hemodialysis in Thallium Poisoning

If any of the following conditions are present, **consider** extracorporeal treatment:
1. A combination of a clinical history and symptoms
2. Laboratory features
   Serum thallium level >0.4 mg/dL however, there is stronger evidence supporting the use of dialysis at values >1.0 mg/dL[a]

[a]Assumption that thallium concentrations are readily available at center of practice.

Ghannoum M, Nolin TD, Goldfarb DS, et al; on behalf of EXTRIP Workgroup. Extracorporeal treatment for thallium poisoning: recommendations from the EXTRIP Workgroup. *Clin J Am Soc Nephrol.* 2012;7(10):1682-1690.

has clinical indications in the treatment of neonatal apnea, lethargy, and weight loss.[34] It is a methylxanthine compound with pharmacokinetics similar to caffeine.[88] However, theophylline has a smaller V_D (0.5 L/kg) and a molecular weight of 180 Da with about 40% to 60% of drug being protein bound.[34,88,89] The early clinical symptoms of theophylline poisoning include nausea and vomiting. As serum concentrations rise, cardiovascular features develop, including supraventricular tachycardia; other dysrhythmias and hypotension may manifest.[90] Theophylline also functions as CNS stimulant and may lead to headaches, agitation, and seizures with progressive increases in serum concentrations. The therapeutic range for theophylline is 5 to 15 mg/L (28-83 μmol/L), but symptoms of toxicity tend to occur at concentrations greater than 25 mg/L (>140 μmol/L).[91,92] The mainstay of managing theophylline poisoning is supportive therapy by addressing the underlying features such as hypotension, cardiac dysrhythmias along with correcting electrolyte abnormalities, particularly hypokalemia. Theophylline is highly adsorptive to charcoal, and MDAC can be utilized to enhance elimination; this may be challenging to institute as patients tend to present with intractable vomiting in theophylline toxicity.[93,94] In cases of toxicity where MDAC cannot be effectively administered, ECTR with either hemoperfusion or hemodialysis is recommended.[34] The EXTRIP workgroup has also recommended that ECTR be provided to patients with serum theophylline levels greater than 100 mg/L (555 μmol/L) in acute exposure, with other indications shown in **Table 28.12**. The workgroup also recommends that hemodialysis should be the preferred ECTR for patients and continued until there is either clinical improvement or the serum theophylline level is less than 15 mg/L (83 μmol/L). Provided patients do not have intractable vomiting, MDAC should be continued in conjunction with ECTR.

RECOMMENDATIONS AGAINST THE USE OF EXTRACORPOREAL TREATMENT FOR SPECIFIC AGENTS

Cyclic Antidepressants

Sometimes called TCAs, these drugs have been used in the treatment of depression since their discovery in the 1950s. Although these agents have been largely supplanted by newer classes of antidepressants, namely selective serotonin and norepinephrine reuptake inhibitors, their use in clinical practice remains prevalent. TCAs are also used in the treatment of neuropathic pain, obsessive-compulsive disorders, along with attention deficit hyperactivity disorder.[95-97] TCAs are highly bound to proteins and are extremely lipophilic, resulting in large V_D.[98] These characteristics collectively result in an overall poor dialyzability of this class of

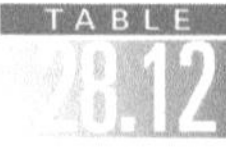

TABLE 28.12 Recommendations for Hemodialysis in Theophylline Poisoning

If any of the following conditions are present, **initiate** extracorporeal treatment:
1. Clinical symptoms:
   a. Seizures
   b. Life-threatening dysrhythmias
   c. Worsening clinical symptoms despite optimal therapy
   d. Shock
2. Laboratory features:
   a. Serum theophylline levels >100 mg/L (555 μmol/L)
   b. Serum theophylline levels continue to rise despite optimal therapy

Consider extracorporeal treatment if any one of the following conditions are present:
1. Clinical:
   a. Gastrointestinal decontamination cannot be administered.
2. Laboratory features:
   a. Serum theophylline levels >60 mg/L (333 μmol/L) in chronic exposure
   b. Patient is <6 mo or >60 yr old and serum theophylline levels are >50 mg/L (278 μmol/L) in chronic exposure

Ghannoum M, Wiegand TJ, Liu KD, et al; on behalf of EXTRIP Workgroup. Extracorporeal treatment for theophylline poisoning: systematic review and recommendations from the EXTRIP workgroup. *Clin Toxicol (Phila)*. 2015;53(4):215-229.

medications. TCAs work primarily by blocking presynaptic reuptake of serotonin and norepinephrine along with muscarinic and α-adrenergic antagonism.[28] Features of an anticholinergic syndrome are often present, including tachycardia, hyperthermia, urinary retention, mydriasis, and flushed skin.[99,100] Given that TCAs also result in cardiac sodium channel blockade, toxicity can result in seizures and wide complex arrhythmias, and cardiac conduction abnormalities are the leading cause of death in TCA poisonings.[101] Measurements of serum drug levels is possible but does not guide management. Intravenous sodium bicarbonate plays an important role in the management of TCA poisoning. It provides sodium loading, which can improve hemodynamics in hypotensive patients and help surmount cardiac sodium channel blockade.[102,103] In light of the poor dialyzability of TCAs, the EXTRIP workgroup does not recommend any form of ECTR for TCA toxicity.[28]

Digoxin

Digoxin, a cardiac glycoside medication first derived from the foxglove plant *Digitalis lanata* in the 1930s, has since been used as an effective agent in the management of atrial fibrillation, atrial flutter, and systolic heart failure.[104] Digoxin has a molecular weight of 781 Da, 20% to 30% of it is bound to protein, and it has very large V_D (~6 L/kg).[29] The highest concentrations of digoxin are found in the heart, kidney, and skeletal muscle with less than 1% of total body composition being present in the plasma.[105] Digoxin is predominantly cleared by the kidneys; therefore, patients with impaired kidney function are at significant risk for developing toxicity. Digoxin toxicity typically occurs at serum concentrations of more than 2.0 ng/mL (2.6 nmol/L); however, toxicity can occur at even lower concentrations in the presence of hypokalemia, hypomagnesemia, or hypercalcemia.[106] The main features of toxicity are cardiac dysrhythmias that may evolve into either ventricular fibrillation or asystole depending on a preexisting history of cardiac disease.[107-109] Digoxin immune Fab (Fab) is the preferred treatment for toxicity as it binds to a rapidly neutralizing free digoxin, preventing it from exerting further inhibition of the myocardial Na^+-K^+-ATPase pump.[110] Fab has an extremely large molecular weight of 46,200 Da and is not easily cleared with most modern-day high cut-off dialyzers. Digoxin-Fab complexes are even more challenging to clear and are removed very slowly by therapeutic PLEX.[111] As a result, the EXTRIP workgroup recommends against using ECTR for the treatment of digoxin toxicity regardless of whether Fab has been administered.[29]

CONCLUSIONS

The majority of poisonings do not require ECTR and can be managed with supportive care, GI decontamination, and, in some instances, enhanced elimination techniques such as MDAC and urinary pH alteration. However, in cases involving poisons that are cleared by ECTR, prompt initiation of extracorporeal clearance may improve outcomes. Additionally, early treatment with ECTR in selected cases may reduce the burden of complications and in turn may shorten hospital length of stay for these patients. Therefore, clinicians must become familiar with various types of poisonings and their toxicokinetic properties that allow them to be removed by ECTR. Clinicians should also have an understanding of the benefits and drawbacks of the various types of ECTR. Hemodialysis is the most common form of ECTR used for the management of poisonings because of its accessibility, lower cost, fewer complications, and concomitant correction of acid-base disturbances. The modernization of dialyzers has also enhanced extracorporeal clearance offered by hemodialysis, making it even more favorable in the management of several poisonings. Although the EXTRIP workgroup recommendations have aimed to standardize practice regarding the use of ECTRs, management of poisonings must be individualized according to patient characteristics and available resources.

References

1. Bywaters EG, Joekes AM. The artificial kidney; its clinical application in the treatment of traumatic anuria. *Proc R Soc Med.* 1948;41(7):420-426.
2. Schreiner GE. The role of hemodialysis (artificial kidney) in acute poisoning. *AMA Arch Intern Med.* 1958;102(6):896-913.
3. Ghannoum M, Nolin TD, Lavergne V, Hoffman RS; EXTRIP Workgroup. Blood purification in toxicology: nephrology's ugly duckling. *Adv Chronic Kidney Dis.* 2011;18(3):160-166.
4. Lavergne V, Nolin TD, Hoffman RS, et al. The EXTRIP (EXtracorporeal TReatments In Poisoning) workgroup: guideline methodology. *Clin Toxicol (Phila).* 2012;50(5):403-413.
5. Gummin DD, Mowry JB, Spyker DA, Brooks DE, Fraser MO, Banner W. 2016 Annual Report of the American Association of Poison Control Centers' National Poison Data System (NPDS): 34th Annual Report. *Clin Toxicol (Phila).* 2017;55(10):1072-1252.
6. Bouchard J, Roberts DM, Roy L, et al. Principles and operational parameters to optimize poison removal with extracorporeal treatments. *Semin Dial.* 2014;27(4):371-380.
7. Ghannoum M, Roberts DM, Hoffman RS, et al. A stepwise approach for the management of poisoning with extracorporeal treatments. *Semin Dial.* 2014;27(4):362-370.
8. Ghannoum M, Lavergne V, Gosselin S, et al. Practice trends in the use of extracorporeal treatments for poisoning in four countries. *Semin Dial.* 2016;29(1):71-80.
9. Bouchard J, Lavergne V, Roberts DM, Cormier M, Morissette G, Ghannoum M. Availability and cost of extracorporeal treatments for poisonings and other emergency indications: a worldwide survey. *Nephrol Dial Transplant.* 2017;32(4):699-706.
10. Ghannoum M, Hoffman RS, Gosselin S, Nolin TD, Lavergne V, Roberts DM. Use of extracorporeal treatments in the management of poisonings. *Kidney Int.* 2018;94(4):682-688.
11. Rahman MH, Haqqie SS, McGoldrick MD. Acute hemolysis with acute renal failure in a patient with valproic acid poisoning treated with charcoal hemoperfusion. *Hemodial Int.* 2006;10(3):256-259.

12. Ouellet G, Bouchard J, Ghannoum M, Decker BS. Available extracorporeal treatments for poisoning: overview and limitations. *Semin Dial.* 2014;27(4):342-349.
13. Shannon MW. Comparative efficacy of hemodialysis and hemoperfusion in severe theophylline intoxication. *Acad Emerg Med.* 1997;4(7):674-678.
14. Shalkham AS, Kirrane BM, Hoffman RS, Goldfarb DS, Nelson LS. The availability and use of charcoal hemoperfusion in the treatment of poisoned patients. *Am J Kidney Dis.* 2006;48(2):239-241.
15. Hastings D, Patel B, Torloni AS, et al. Plasmapheresis therapy for rare but potentially fatal reaction to rituximab. *J Clin Apher.* 2009;24(1):28-31.
16. Perino GC, Grivet V. Hemoperfusion and plasmapheresis complications. *Minerva Urol Nefrol.* 1987;39(2):161-163.
17. Kaplan A. Complications of apheresis. *Semin Dial.* 2012;25(2):152-158.
18. Maher JF, Schreiner GE. The dialysis of poisons and drugs. *Trans Am Soc Artif Intern Organs.* 1968;14:440-453.
19. Jufer RA, Wstadik A, Walsh SL, Levine BS, Cone EJ. Elimination of cocaine and metabolites in plasma, saliva, and urine following repeated oral administration to human volunteers. *J Anal Toxicol.* 2000;24(7):467-477.
20. Kirsch AH, Lyko R, Nilsson LG, et al. Performance of hemodialysis with novel medium cut-off dialyzers. *Nephrol Dial Transplant.* 2017;32(1):165-172.
21. Ghannoum M, Bouchard J, Nolin TD, Ouellet G, Roberts DM. Hemoperfusion for the treatment of poisoning: technology, determinants of poison clearance, and application in clinical practice. *Semin Dial.* 2014;27(4):350-361.
22. Klotz U, Antonin KH. Pharmacokinetics and bioavailability of sodium valproate. *Clin Pharmacol Ther.* 1977;21(6):736-743.
23. van den Broek MP, Sikma MA, Ververs TF, Meulenbelt J. Severe valproic acid intoxication: case study on the unbound fraction and the applicability of extracorporeal elimination. *Eur J Emerg Med.* 2009;16(6):330-332.
24. Oie S. Drug distribution and binding. *J Clin Pharmacol.* 1986;26(8):583-586.
25. Weir MA, Dixon SN, Fleet JL, et al. β-Blocker dialyzability and mortality in older patients receiving hemodialysis. *J Am Soc Nephrol.* 2015;26(4):987-996.
26. Stone WJ, Walle T. Massive propranolol metabolite retention during maintenance hemodialysis. *Clin Pharmacol Ther.* 1980;28(4):449-455.
27. Leblanc M, Raymond M, Bonnardeaux A, et al. Lithium poisoning treated by high-performance continuous arteriovenous and venovenous hemodiafiltration. *Am J Kidney Dis.* 1996;27(3):365-372.
28. Yates C, Galvao T, Sowinski KM, et al. Extracorporeal treatment for tricyclic antidepressant poisoning: recommendations from the EXTRIP Workgroup. *Semin Dial.* 2014;27(4):381-389.
29. Mowry JB, Burdmann EA, Anseeuw K, et al. Extracorporeal treatment for digoxin poisoning: systematic review and recommendations from the EXTRIP Workgroup. *Clin Toxicol (Phila).* 2016;54(2):103-114.
30. Mactier R, Laliberte M, Mardini J, et al. Extracorporeal treatment for barbiturate poisoning: recommendations from the EXTRIP Workgroup. *Am J Kidney Dis.* 2014;64(3):347-358.
31. Juurlink DN, Gosselin S, Kielstein JT, et al. Extracorporeal treatment for salicylate poisoning: systematic review and recommendations from the EXTRIP workgroup. *Ann Emerg Med.* 2015;66(2):165-181.
32. Gosselin S, Juurlink DN, Kielstein JT, et al. Extracorporeal treatment for acetaminophen poisoning: recommendations from the EXTRIP workgroup. *Clin Toxicol (Phila).* 2014;52(8):856-867.
33. Ghannoum M, Yates C, Galvao TF, et al. Extracorporeal treatment for carbamazepine poisoning: systematic review and recommendations from the EXTRIP workgroup. *Clin Toxicol (Phila).* 2014;52(10):993-1004.
34. Ghannoum M, Wiegand TJ, Liu KD, et al. Extracorporeal treatment for theophylline poisoning: systematic review and recommendations from the EXTRIP workgroup. *Clin Toxicol (Phila).* 2015;53(4):215-229.
35. Ghannoum M, Nolin TD, Goldfarb DS, et al. Extracorporeal treatment for thallium poisoning: recommendations from the EXTRIP Workgroup. *Clin J Am Soc Nephrol.* 2012;7(10):1682-1690.
36. Ghannoum M, Laliberte M, Nolin TD, et al. Extracorporeal treatment for valproic acid poisoning: systematic review and recommendations from the EXTRIP workgroup. *Clin Toxicol (Phila).* 2015;53(5):454-465.
37. Decker BS, Goldfarb DS, Dargan PI, et al. Extracorporeal treatment for lithium poisoning: systematic review and recommendations from the EXTRIP workgroup. *Clin J Am Soc Nephrol.* 2015;10(5):875-887.

38. Anseeuw K, Mowry JB, Burdmann EA, et al. Extracorporeal treatment in phenytoin poisoning: systematic review and recommendations from the EXTRIP (extracorporeal treatments in poisoning) workgroup. *Am J Kidney Dis.* 2016;67(2):187-197.
39. Roberts DM, Yates C, Megarbane B, et al. Recommendations for the role of extracorporeal treatments in the management of acute methanol poisoning: a systematic review and consensus statement. *Crit Care Med.* 2015;43(2):461-472.
40. Calello DP, Liu KD, Wiegand TJ, et al. Extracorporeal treatment for metformin poisoning: systematic review and recommendations from the extracorporeal treatments in poisoning workgroup. *Crit Care Med.* 2015;43(8):1716-1730.
41. Mowry JB, Spyker DA, Cantilena LR Jr, McMillan N, Ford M. 2013 Annual Report of the American Association of Poison Control Centers' National Poison Data System (NPDS): 31st Annual Report. *Clin Toxicol (Phila).* 2014;52(10):1032-1283.
42. Levy G. Pharmacokinetics of salicylate elimination in man. *J Pharm Sci.* 1965;54(7):959-967.
43. Lee S, Johnson D, Klein J, Eppler J. Protein binding of acetylsalicylic acid and salicylic acid in porcine and human serum. *Vet Hum Toxicol.* 1995;37(3):224-225.
44. Temple AR. Acute and chronic effects of aspirin toxicity and their treatment. *Arch Intern Med.* 1981;141(3 Spec No):364-369.
45. Fertel BS, Nelson LS, Goldfarb DS. The underutilization of hemodialysis in patients with salicylate poisoning. *Kidney Int.* 2009;75(12):1349-1353.
46. Mowry JB, Spyker DA, Cantilena LR Jr, Bailey JE, Ford M. 2012 Annual Report of the American Association of Poison Control Centers' National Poison Data System (NPDS): 30th Annual Report. *Clin Toxicol (Phila).* 2013;51(10):949-1229.
47. Leise MD, Poterucha JJ, Talwalkar JA. Drug-induced liver injury. *Mayo Clin Proc.* 2014;89(1):95-106.
48. Lee SS, Buters JT, Pineau T, Fernandez-Salguero P, Gonzalez FJ. Role of CYP2E1 in the hepatotoxicity of acetaminophen. *J Biol Chem.* 1996;271(20):12063-12067.
49. Kaplowitz N. Acetaminophen hepatoxicity: what do we know, what don't we know, and what do we do next? *Hepatology.* 2004;40(1):23-26.
50. McGill MR, Jaeschke H. Metabolism and disposition of acetaminophen: recent advances in relation to hepatotoxicity and diagnosis. *Pharm Res.* 2013;30(9):2174-2187.
51. Shah AD, Wood DM, Dargan PI. Understanding lactic acidosis in paracetamol (acetaminophen) poisoning. *Br J Clin Pharmacol.* 2011;71(1):20-28.
52. Mattson RH, Cramer JA, Williamson PD, Novelly RA. Valproic acid in epilepsy: clinical and pharmacological effects. *Ann Neurol.* 1978;3(1):20-25.
53. Kinze S, Clauss M, Reuter U, et al. Valproic acid is effective in migraine prophylaxis at low serum levels: a prospective open-label study. *Headache.* 2001;41(8):774-778.
54. Sztajnkrycer MD. Valproic acid toxicity: overview and management. *J Toxicol Clin Toxicol.* 2002;40(6):789-801.
55. Vale J, Krenzelok EP, Barceloux VD. Position statement and practice guidelines on the use of multi-dose activated charcoal in the treatment of acute poisoning. American Academy of Clinical Toxicology; European Association of Poisons Centres and Clinical Toxicologists. *J Toxicol Clin Toxicol.* 1999;37(6):731-751.
56. Isbister GK, Balit CR, Whyte IM, Dawson A. Valproate overdose: a comparative cohort study of self poisonings. *Br J Clin Pharmacol.* 2003;55(4):398-404.
57. Vree TB, Janssen TJ, Hekster YA, Termond EF, van de Dries AC, Wijnands WJ. Clinical pharmacokinetics of carbamazepine and its epoxy and hydroxy metabolites in humans after an overdose. *Ther Drug Monit.* 1986;8(3):297-304.
58. Hojer J, Malmlund HO, Berg A. Clinical features in 28 consecutive cases of laboratory confirmed massive poisoning with carbamazepine alone. *J Toxicol Clin Toxicol.* 1993;31(3):449-458.
59. Graudins A, Peden G, Dowsett RP. Massive overdose with controlled-release carbamazepine resulting in delayed peak serum concentrations and life-threatening toxicity. *Emerg Med (Fremantle).* 2002;14(1):89-94.
60. Ghannoum M, Troyanov S, Ayoub P, Lavergne V, Hewlett T. Successful hemodialysis in a phenytoin overdose: case report and review of the literature. *Clin Nephrol.* 2010;74(1):59-64.
61. Doenicke A. General pharmacology of barbiturates. Duration of action, metabolism, physicochemical factors. *Acta Anaesthesiol Scand Suppl.* 1965;17:11-16.
62. Roberts DM, Buckley NA. Enhanced elimination in acute barbiturate poisoning—a systematic review. *Clin Toxicol (Phila).* 2011;49(1):2-12.
63. Pond SM, Olson KR, Osterloh JD, Tong TG. Randomized study of the treatment of phenobarbital overdose with repeated doses of activated charcoal. *JAMA.* 1984;251(23):3104-3108.

64. Mohammed Ebid AH, Abdel-Rahman HM. Pharmacokinetics of phenobarbital during certain enhanced elimination modalities to evaluate their clinical efficacy in management of drug overdose. *Ther Drug Monit.* 2001;23(3):209-216.
65. Cade JF. Lithium salts in the treatment of psychotic excitement. *Med J Aust.* 1949;2(10):349-352.
66. Timmer RT, Sands JM. Lithium intoxication. *J Am Soc Nephrol.* 1999;10(3):666-674.
67. Okusa MD, Crystal LJ. Clinical manifestations and management of acute lithium intoxication. *Am J Med.* 1994;97(4):383-389.
68. Geddes JR, Burgess S, Hawton K, Jamison K, Goodwin GM. Long-term lithium therapy for bipolar disorder: systematic review and meta-analysis of randomized controlled trials. *Am J Psychiatry.* 2004;161(2):217-222.
69. Becker CE. Methanol poisoning. *J Emerg Med.* 1983;1(1):51-58.
70. Barceloux DG, Bond GR, Krenzelok EP, Cooper H, Vale JA; American Academy of Clinical Toxicology Ad Hoc Committee on the Treatment Guidelines for Methanol Poisoning. American Academy of Clinical Toxicology practice guidelines on the treatment of methanol poisoning. *J Toxicol Clin Toxicol.* 2002;40(4):415-446.
71. Choi JH, Lee SK, Gil YE, et al. Neurological complications resulting from non-oral occupational methanol poisoning. *J Korean Med Sci.* 2017;32(2):371-376.
72. Chung JY, Ho CH, Chen YC, et al. Association between acute methanol poisoning and subsequent mortality: a nationwide study in Taiwan. *BMC Public Health.* 2018;18(1):985.
73. Jacobsen D, McMartin KE. Methanol and ethylene glycol poisonings. Mechanism of toxicity, clinical course, diagnosis and treatment. *Med Toxicol.* 1986;1(5):309-334.
74. Paasma R, Hovda KE, Tikkerberi A, Jacobsen D. Methanol mass poisoning in Estonia: outbreak in 154 patients. *Clin Toxicol (Phila).* 2007;45(2):152-157.
75. Rostrup M, Edwards JK, Abukalish M, et al. The methanol poisoning outbreaks in Libya 2013 and Kenya 2014. *PLoS One.* 2016;11(3):e0152676.
76. Sullivan-Mee M, Solis K. Methanol-induced vision loss. *J Am Optom Assoc.* 1998;69(1):57-65.
77. Jacobsen D, Hewlett TP, Webb R, Brown ST, Ordinario AT, McMartin KE. Ethylene glycol intoxication: evaluation of kinetics and crystalluria. *Am J Med.* 1988;84(1):145-152.
78. Lashen H. Role of metformin in the management of polycystic ovary syndrome. *Ther Adv Endocrinol Metab.* 2010;1(3):117-128.
79. Maruthur NM, Tseng E, Hutfless S, et al. Diabetes medications as monotherapy or metformin-based combination therapy for type 2 diabetes: a systematic review and meta-analysis. *Ann Intern Med.* 2016;164(11):740-751.
80. Scheen AJ. Clinical pharmacokinetics of metformin. *Clin Pharmacokinet.* 1996;30(5):359-371.
81. Luft D, Deichsel G, Schmulling RM, Stein W, Eggstein M. Definition of clinically relevant lactic acidosis in patients with internal diseases. *Am J Clin Pathol.* 1983;80(4):484-489.
82. Eppenga WL, Lalmohamed A, Geerts AF, et al. Risk of lactic acidosis or elevated lactate concentrations in metformin users with renal impairment: a population-based cohort study. *Diabetes Care.* 2014;37(8):2218-2224.
83. Graham GG, Punt J, Arora M, et al. Clinical pharmacokinetics of metformin. *Clin Pharmacokinet.* 2011;50(2):81-98.
84. Bank WJ, Pleasure DE, Suzuki K, Nigro M, Katz R. Thallium poisoning. *Arch Neurol.* 1972;26(5):456-464.
85. Mulkey JP, Oehme FW. A review of thallium toxicity. *Vet Hum Toxicol.* 1993;35(5):445-453.
86. Moore D, House I, Dixon A. Thallium poisoning. Diagnosis may be elusive but alopecia is the clue. *BMJ.* 1993;306(6891):1527-1529.
87. Desenclos JC, Wilder MH, Coppenger GW, Sherin K, Tiller R, VanHook RM. Thallium poisoning: an outbreak in Florida, 1988. *South Med J.* 1992;85(12):1203-1206.
88. Lelo A, Birkett DJ, Robson RA, Miners JO. Comparative pharmacokinetics of caffeine and its primary demethylated metabolites paraxanthine, theobromine and theophylline in man. *Br J Clin Pharmacol.* 1986;22(2):177-182.
89. Ogilvie RI. Clinical pharmacokinetics of theophylline. *Clin Pharmacokinet.* 1978;3(4):267-293.
90. Shannon M. Life-threatening events after theophylline overdose: a 10-year prospective analysis. *Arch Intern Med.* 1999;159(9):989-994.
91. Greenberg A, Piraino BH, Kroboth PD, Weiss J. Severe theophylline toxicity. Role of conservative measures, antiarrhythmic agents, and charcoal hemoperfusion. *Am J Med.* 1984;76(5):854-860.
92. Shannon M. Predictors of major toxicity after theophylline overdose. *Ann Intern Med.* 1993;119(12):1161-1167.
93. Berlinger WG, Spector R, Goldberg MJ, Johnson GF, Quee CK, Berg MJ. Enhancement of theophylline clearance by oral activated charcoal. *Clin Pharmacol Ther.* 1983;33(3):351-354.
94. Lim TK, Tan CC. Treatment of severe theophylline toxicity with oral activated charcoal and haemodialysis—a case report. *Singapore Med J.* 1988;29(6):601-603.

95. Benbouzid M, Choucair-Jaafar N, Yalcin I, et al. Chronic, but not acute, tricyclic antidepressant treatment alleviates neuropathic allodynia after sciatic nerve cuffing in mice. *Eur J Pain.* 2008;12(8):1008-1017.
96. Koszewska I, Rybakowski JK. Antidepressant-induced mood conversions in bipolar disorder: a retrospective study of tricyclic versus non-tricyclic antidepressant drugs. *Neuropsychobiology.* 2009;59(1):12-16.
97. McQuay HJ, Tramer M, Nye BA, Carroll D, Wiffen PJ, Moore RA. A systematic review of antidepressants in neuropathic pain. *Pain.* 1996;68(2-3):217-227.
98. Jarvis MR. Clinical pharmacokinetics of tricyclic antidepressant overdose. *Psychopharmacol Bull.* 1991;27(4):541-550.
99. Thorstrand C. Clinical features in poisonings by tricyclic antidepressants with special reference to the ECG. *Acta Med Scand.* 1976;199(5):337-344.
100. Trindade E, Menon D, Topfer LA, Coloma C. Adverse effects associated with selective serotonin reuptake inhibitors and tricyclic antidepressants: a meta-analysis. *CMAJ.* 1998;159(10):1245-1252.
101. Bailey B, Buckley NA, Amre DK. A meta-analysis of prognostic indicators to predict seizures, arrhythmias or death after tricyclic antidepressant overdose. *J Toxicol Clin Toxicol.* 2004;42(6):877-888.
102. Blackman K, Brown SG, Wilkes GJ. Plasma alkalinization for tricyclic antidepressant toxicity: a systematic review. *Emerg Med (Fremantle).* 2001;13(2):204-210.
103. Bradberry SM, Thanacoody HK, Watt BE, Thomas SH, Vale JA. Management of the cardiovascular complications of tricyclic antidepressant poisoning: role of sodium bicarbonate. *Toxicol Rev.* 2005;24(3):195-204.
104. Hollman A. Drugs for atrial fibrillation. Digoxin comes from *Digitalis lanata. BMJ.* 1996;312(7035):912.
105. Mooradian AD. Digitalis. An update of clinical pharmacokinetics, therapeutic monitoring techniques and treatment recommendations. *Clin Pharmacokinet.* 1988;15(3):165-179.
106. Young IS, Goh EM, McKillop UH, Stanford CF, Nicholls DP, Trimble ER. Magnesium status and digoxin toxicity. *Br J Clin Pharmacol.* 1991;32(6):717-721.
107. Smith TW, Antman EM, Friedman PL, Blatt CM, Marsh JD. Digitalis glycosides: mechanisms and manifestations of toxicity. Part III. *Prog Cardiovasc Dis.* 1984;27(1):21-56.
108. Smith TW, Antman EM, Friedman PL, Blatt CM, Marsh JD. Digitalis glycosides: mechanisms and manifestations of toxicity. Part II. *Prog Cardiovasc Dis.* 1984;26(6):495-540.
109. Smith TW, Antman EM, Friedman PL, Blatt CM, Marsh JD. Digitalis glycosides: mechanisms and manifestations of toxicity. Part I. *Prog Cardiovasc Dis.* 1984;26(5):413-458.
110. Antman EM, Wenger TL, Butler VP Jr, Haber E, Smith TW. Treatment of 150 cases of life-threatening digitalis intoxication with digoxin-specific Fab antibody fragments. Final report of a multicenter study. *Circulation.* 1990;81(6):1744-1752.
111. Chillet P, Korach JM, Petitpas D, et al. Digoxin poisoning and anuric acute renal failure: efficiency of the treatment associating digoxin-specific antibodies (Fab) and plasma exchanges. *Int J Artif Organs.* 2002;25(6):538-541.

SECTION VIII

Extracorporeal Therapies

Vascular Access for Kidney Replacement Therapy

Ayham Bataineh and Paul M. Palevsky

Vascular access for acute kidney replacement therapy (KRT) is generally achieved using large-bore intravenous catheters. Dialysis catheters generally have two lumens and differ from other vascular catheters in their diameter and length, to provide sufficient blood flow for dialysis or hemofiltration. In general, nontunneled dialysis catheters are used in the acute setting; however, cuffed and tunneled catheters may also be used. This chapter reviews the placement, types, complications, and routine care of catheters for acute KRT.

OPTIMAL CATHETER LOCATION (FEMORAL, SUBCLAVIAN, INTERNAL JUGULAR)

Catheters for KRT can be placed in any vein that is large enough to deliver the blood flows necessary for KRT, including the internal jugular, femoral, and subclavian veins. The optimal site for catheter insertion is uncertain. In general, subclavian dialysis catheters should be avoided owing to the risks of subclavian vein stenosis, which may limit arteriovenous access placement in patients who remain dialysis dependent.[1] In addition, the location of the subclavian vein precludes the ability for direct hemostasis in the event of hemorrhage, particularly in coagulopathic patients. The Kidney Disease Improving Global Outcomes (KDIGO) guidelines recommend the following order for dialysis catheter site selection: right internal jugular vein, femoral veins, left internal jugular vein, and subclavian vein, preferentially using the dominant side to preserve the contralateral side for future dialysis access, if needed.[2] This recommendation was based on a study demonstrating similar rates of infection with jugular and femoral dialysis catheters[3] but progressively higher rates of catheter dysfunction in the femoral (10.3%) and left internal jugular veins (19.5%) as compared to the right internal jugular vein (6.6%)[4] (**Visual Abstracts 29.1** and **29.2**). The external jugular veins may be used as an alternative access to the central veins for catheter placement when other veins are not usable.[5]

Function

Adequate catheter function is critical to achieve adequate blood flow through the extracorporeal circuit, avoid recirculation, and prevent interruptions of treatment. Catheter function will be dependent on a combination of factors, including catheter design and lumen diameter, tip position, the presence of intraluminal obstruction (with blood clot or bacterial contamination), and patient position (e.g., if the patient flexes the hip while femoral line in place). In particular, the use of longer dialyzer catheters to achieve tip placement in the right atrium as compared to the distal superior vena cava is associated with prolongation of circuit patency.[6] Specifically, in a study of 100 patients undergoing continuous KRT randomized to longer (20-24 cm) versus shorter (15-20 cm) catheters inserted into a great thoracic vein, the longer catheters were associated with a prolongation of hemofilter survival by a mean difference of 6.5 hours, improved delivery of dialysis dose, and decreased clotting episodes (2.3 vs 3.6 episodes)[6] (**Visual Abstract 29.3**).

Complications

Dialysis catheters have been associated with higher rates of complications than other central venous catheters, likely related to the larger catheter diameter. In one study, dialysis catheters needed to be removed in more than half of the cases because of complications.[7] These complications can be classified as mechanical, infectious, and thrombotic.[8] Mechanical complications are generally related to the actual placement procedure and include cannulation failure, arterial cannulation, local hematoma, and, in the subclavian or internal jugular position, pneumothorax or hemothorax. In the femoral position, catheter insertion may result in arteriovenous fistula and arterial insufficiency. Catheter-associated thrombus formation may result from the catheter serving as a nidus for clot formation or from mechanical injury to the endothelium, with risk increasing with duration of catheter use. Although catheter-related infections in critically ill patients are generally more common with femoral as compared to internal jugular catheters,[9] rates of infection for dialysis catheters in the femoral and internal jugular position are similar, although rates of femoral catheter infection increased with higher body mass index (BMI).[3] The use of cuffed, tunneled catheters may diminish the risk of infection when the need for KRT is expected to exceed 1 to 3 weeks.[2,9]

OPTIMAL CATHETER TIP POSITION

Optimal positioning of the catheter tip will permit higher blood flows with minimal blood recirculation. For internal jugular vein catheters, the best catheter function is achieved when the catheter tip is in the right atrium or at the junction of the superior vena cava and right atrium, depending on catheter type, rather than, more distally, in the superior vena cava.[6] This catheter position can generally be achieved using a 15- to 20-cm catheter in the right internal jugular vein or a 20- to 24-cm catheter in the left internal jugular vein, depending on patient size and catheter design. When the femoral vein is cannulated, the longest possible catheter (≥24 cm) should be used, with the goal of having the catheter tip in the inferior vena cava (**Table 29.1**).

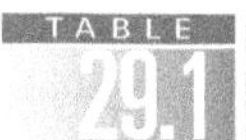

TABLE 29.1 Optimal Catheter Length Based on Insertion Site

Insertion Site	Catheter Length (cm)
Right internal jugular vein[a]	15-20
Left internal jugular vein[a]	20-24
Femoral vein	≥24

[a]Although subclavian catheters should be avoided, optimal subclavian catheter lengths correspond to internal jugular catheter lengths.

TUNNELED VERSUS NONTUNNELED CATHETERS

The KDIGO guidelines recommend initiating KRT using an uncuffed nontunneled dialysis catheter rather than a tunneled dialysis catheter[2]; however, this recommendation is based on minimal data. Tunneled dialysis catheters are associated with a lower risk of infection than nontunneled catheters.[9] Tunneled catheters are generally recommended for patients in whom the duration of dialysis is expected to be prolonged and catheter use is expected to exceed 1 to 3 weeks.

STRATEGIES TO MINIMIZE CATHETER-ASSOCIATED COMPLICATIONS

Mechanical Complications

Real-time ultrasound guidance for catheter insertion is associated with a need for fewer passes to achieve vessel cannulation, a lower rate of arterial puncture, and fewer mechanical complications, including local hematoma, pneumothorax, and hemothorax, than landmark-guided catheter insertion.[2,10]

Catheter-Related Infections

Catheter-related infections may include both exit site infections and catheter-related bloodstream infections (CRBSIs). There have been few studies focused specifically on prevention of dialysis catheter–related infections in the critical care setting, and recommendations for best practices are based on general guidance for central venous catheter insertion and care and from care of dialysis catheters in the chronic dialysis setting.[9]

Use of Catheter Insertion "Bundle" to Avoid Infection

The use of a catheter insertion "bundle" including hand hygiene; full barrier precautions including cap, mask, sterile gown, sterile gloves, and a sterile full-body drape during insertion; and skin antisepsis with chlorhexidine (or 70% alcohol or povidone-iodine if there is a contraindication to chlorhexidine) is associated with decreased risk of CRBSI and should be used for all dialysis catheter insertions[9] (**Table 29.2**).

Catheter Site Care

Catheter site care should follow institutional protocols developed to minimize catheter-associated infections.[9,11] Standard aseptic techniques, including wearing mask, performing hand hygiene, and wearing gloves, should be followed. The catheter exit site should be cleaned with chlorhexidine (or povidone-iodine if skin is sensitive or allergic to chlorhexidine).[12] Either sterile gauze or sterile, transparent, semipermeable dressings should be used to cover the catheter site.[9] The role of topical antibiotics and antiseptic ointments at the catheter exit site is controversial; although generally not recommended for other central venous catheters because of their potential to promote antibiotic resistance and fungal infections, they may reduce the risk of CRBSI associated with dialysis catheters.[9] If used, it is important to ensure that the ointment does not interact with the catheter material as some catheters, particularly if made of polyurethane, may become brittle or crack if exposed to incompatible ointments.[13,14]

Catheter Connection for Kidney Replacement Therapy

A "scrub-the-hub" protocol should be followed whenever accessing the catheter to initiate or disconnect KRT (**Table 29.3**).[15] The use of antibiotic- or antiseptic-impregnated caps may also decrease the risk of CRBSI.[16]

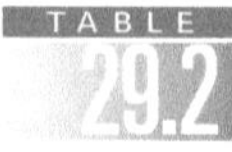

Catheter Insertion Bundle

Hand Hygiene and Aseptic Technique

1. Perform hand hygiene procedures, either by washing hands with conventional soap and water or with alcohol-based hand rubs (ABHRs). Hand hygiene should be performed before and after palpating catheter insertion sites as well as before and after inserting, replacing, accessing, repairing, or dressing a hemodialysis catheter. Palpation of the insertion site should not be performed after the application of antiseptic, unless aseptic technique is maintained.
2. Maintain aseptic technique for the insertion and care of hemodialysis catheters.
3. Sterile gloves should be worn for the insertion of hemodialysis catheters.
4. Use new sterile gloves before handling the new catheter when guidewire exchanges are performed.

Maximal Sterile Barrier Precautions

1. Use maximal sterile barrier precautions, including the use of a cap, mask, sterile gown, sterile gloves, and a sterile full-body drape, for the insertion of or guidewire exchange of dialysis catheters.

Skin Preparation

1. Prepare clean skin with >0.5% chlorhexidine preparation with alcohol before hemodialysis catheter insertion and during dressing changes. If there is a contraindication to chlorhexidine, tincture of iodine, an iodophor, or 70% alcohol can be used as alternatives.
2. Antiseptics should be allowed to dry according to the manufacturer's recommendation prior to placing the catheter.

Catheter Site Dressing Regimens

1. Use either sterile gauze or sterile, transparent, semipermeable dressing to cover the catheter site.
2. If the patient is diaphoretic or if the site is bleeding or oozing, use a gauze dressing until this is resolved.
3. Replace catheter site dressing if the dressing becomes damp, loosened, or visibly soiled.

Source: Adapted from O'Grady NP, Alexander M, Burns LA, et al. Guidelines for the prevention of intravascular catheter-related infections. *Clin Infect Dis.* 2011;52(9):e162-e193.

Catheter "Packing" to Prevent Clotting and Infection

The optimal method for flushing and packing dialysis catheters between use is uncertain. Options include saline, heparinized saline, and sodium citrate.[17-21] In a Cochrane review, there was minimal difference in maintenance of catheter patency with heparin as compared to saline.[17] Four percent of sodium citrate has variably been associated with better catheter patency, lower bleeding risk, and lower rates of catheter infection than heparin or saline[18-21]; however, systemic infusion of concentrated citrate solutions may result in serious hypocalcemia and cardiac arrhythmias.[22] Antibiotic-containing locking solutions should not be routinely used to prevent CRBSI.[9]

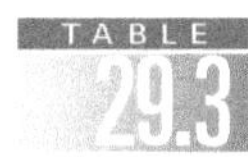

CDC Guidelines for Connection and Disconnection of Dialysis Catheters Including "Scrub-the-Hub" Protocol

Connection Steps

1. Perform hand hygiene and don new clean gloves.
2. Clamp the catheter. (*Note:* **Always** clamp the catheter before removing the cap. Never leave an uncapped catheter unattended.)
3. Disinfect the hub with caps removed using an appropriate antiseptic.
   a. (*Optional*) Prior to cap removal, disinfect the caps and the part of the hub that is accessible and discard the antiseptic pad (i.e., use a separate antiseptic pad for the next step).
   b. Remove the caps and disinfect the hub with a new antiseptic pad for each hub. Scrub the sides (threads) and end of the hub thoroughly with friction, making sure to remove any residue (e.g., blood).
   c. Using the same antiseptic pad, apply antiseptic with friction to the catheter, moving from the hub at least several centimeters toward the body. Hold the limb while allowing the antiseptic to dry.
   d. Use a separate antiseptic pad for each hub/catheter limb. Leave hubs "open" (i.e., uncapped and disconnected) for the shortest time possible.
4. Always handle the catheter hubs aseptically. Once disinfected, do not allow the catheter hubs to touch nonsterile surfaces.
5. Attach sterile syringe, unclamp the catheter, withdraw blood, and flush per facility protocol.
6. Repeat for the other limb (this might occur in parallel).
7. Connect the ends of the blood lines to the catheter aseptically.
8. Remove gloves and perform hand hygiene.

Disconnection Steps

1. Perform hand hygiene and don new clean gloves.
2. Clamp the catheter. (*Note:* **Always** clamp the catheter before disconnecting. Never leave an uncapped catheter unattended.)
3. Disinfect the catheter hub before applying the new cap using an appropriate antiseptic.
   a. (*Optional*) Disinfect the connection prior to disconnection. If this is done, use a separate antiseptic pad for the subsequent disinfection of the hub.
   b. Disconnect the blood line from the catheter and disinfect the hub with a new antiseptic pad. Scrub the sides (threads) and end of the hub thoroughly with friction, making sure to remove any residue (e.g., blood).
   c. Use a separate antiseptic pad for each hub. Leave hubs "open" (i.e., uncapped and disconnected) for the shortest time possible.
4. Always handle the catheter hubs aseptically. Once disinfected, do not allow the catheter hubs to touch nonsterile surfaces. Hold the catheter until the antiseptic has dried.
5. Attach the new sterile caps to the catheter aseptically. Use caution if tape is used to secure caps to the catheter.
6. Ensure that catheter is still clamped.
7. Remove gloves and perform hand hygiene.

CDC, Centers for Disease Control and Prevention.

Source: From Centers for Disease Control and Prevention. Hemodialysis central venous catheter scrub-the-hub protocol. See notes at: https://www.cdc.gov/dialysis/prevention-tools/scrub-protocols.html

References

1. Hernandez D, Diaz F, Rufino M, et al. Subclavian vascular access stenosis in dialysis patients: natural history and risk factors. *J Am Soc Nephrol.* 1998;9(8):1507-1510.
2. Kidney Disease: Improving Global Outcomes (KDIGO) Acute Kidney Injury Work Group. KDIGO clinical practice guideline for acute kidney injury. *Kidney Int.* 2012;2012(Suppl):1-138.
3. Parienti JJ, Thirion M, Megarbane B, et al. Femoral vs jugular venous catheterization and risk of nosocomial events in adults requiring acute renal replacement therapy: a randomized controlled trial. *JAMA.* 2008;299(20):2413-2422.
4. Parienti JJ, Megarbane B, Fischer MO, et al. Catheter dysfunction and dialysis performance according to vascular access among 736 critically ill adults requiring renal replacement therapy: a randomized controlled study. *Crit Care Med.* 2010;38(4):1118-1125.
5. Cho SK, Shin SW, Do YS, Park KB, Choo SW, Choo IW. Use of the right external jugular vein as the preferred access site when the right internal jugular vein is not usable. *J Vasc Interv Radiol.* 2006;17(5):823-829.
6. Morgan D, Ho K, Murray C, Davies H, Louw J. A randomized trial of catheters of different lengths to achieve right atrium versus superior vena cava placement for continuous renal replacement therapy. *Am J Kidney Dis.* 2012;60(2):272-279.
7. Kairaitis LK, Gottlieb T. Outcome and complications of temporary haemodialysis catheters. *Nephrol Dial Transplant.* 1999;14(7):1710-1714.
8. Clark E, Kappel J, MacRae J, et al. Practical aspects of nontunneled and tunneled hemodialysis catheters. *Can J Kidney Health Dis.* 2016;3:2054358116669128.
9. O'Grady NP, Alexander M, Burns LA, et al. Guidelines for the prevention of intravascular catheter-related infections. *Clin Infect Dis.* 2011;52(9):e162-e193.
10. Rabindranath KS, Kumar E, Shail R, Vaux EC. Ultrasound use for the placement of haemodialysis catheters. *Cochrane Database Syst Rev.* 2011;(11):CD005279.
11. Betjes MG. Prevention of catheter-related bloodstream infection in patients on hemodialysis. *Nat Rev Nephrol.* 2011;7(5):257-265.
12. Rosenblum A, Wang W, Ball LK, Latham C, Maddux FW, Lacson E Jr. Hemodialysis catheter care strategies: a cluster-randomized quality improvement initiative. *Am J Kidney Dis.* 2014;63(2):259-267.
13. Rao SP, Oreopoulos DG. Unusual complications of a polyurethane PD catheter. *Perit Dial Int.* 1997;17(4):410-412.
14. Riu S, Ruiz CG, Martinez-Vea A, Peralta C, Oliver JA. Spontaneous rupture of polyurethane peritoneal catheter. A possible deleterious effect of mupirocin ointment. *Nephrol Dial Transplant.* 1998;13(7):1870-1871.
15. Centers for Disease Control and Prevention. Hemodialysis central venous catheter scrub-the-hub protocol. https://www.cdc.gov/dialysis/prevention-tools/scrub-protocols.html; accessed 21 June 2019.
16. Brunelli SM, Van Wyck DB, Njord L, Ziebol RJ, Lynch LE, Killion DP. Cluster-randomized trial of devices to prevent catheter-related bloodstream infection. *J Am Soc Nephrol.* 2018;29(4):1336-1343.
17. Lopez-Briz E, Ruiz Garcia V, Cabello JB, Bort-Marti S, Carbonell Sanchis R, Burls A. Heparin versus 0.9% sodium chloride locking for prevention of occlusion in central venous catheters in adults. *Cochrane Database Syst Rev.* 2018;7:CD008462.
18. Moran JE, Ash SR. Locking solutions for hemodialysis catheters; heparin and citrate—a position paper by ASDIN. *Semin Dial.* 2008;21(5):490-492.
19. Zhao Y, Li Z, Zhang L, et al. Citrate versus heparin lock for hemodialysis catheters: a systematic review and meta-analysis of randomized controlled trials. *Am J Kidney Dis.* 2014;63(3):479-490.
20. Hermite L, Quenot JP, Nadji A, et al. Sodium citrate versus saline catheter locks for non-tunneled hemodialysis central venous catheters in critically ill adults: a randomized controlled trial. *Intensive Care Med.* 2012;38(2):279-285.
21. Weijmer MC, Debets-Ossenkopp YJ, Van De Vondervoort FJ, ter Wee PM. Superior antimicrobial activity of trisodium citrate over heparin for catheter locking. *Nephrol Dial Transplant.* 2002;17(12):2189-2195.
22. Polaschegg HD, Sodemann K. Risks related to catheter locking solutions containing concentrated citrate. *Nephrol Dial Transplant.* 2003;18(12):2688-2690.

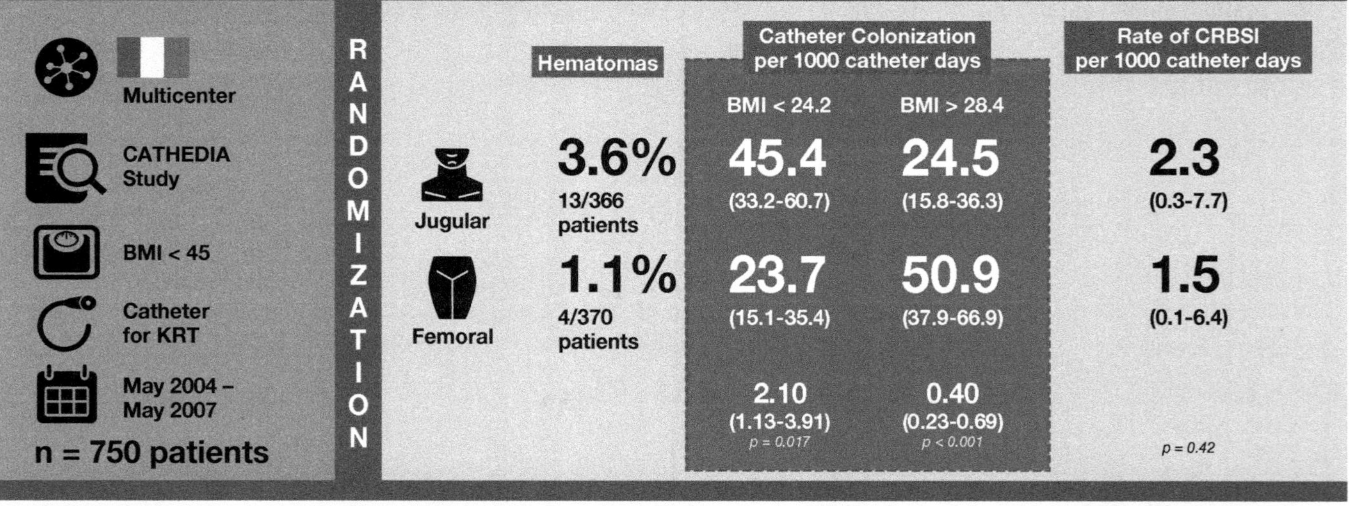

VISUAL ABSTRACT 29.1

Catheter dysfunction and dialysis performance according to vascular access among critically ill adults requiring kidney replacement therapy

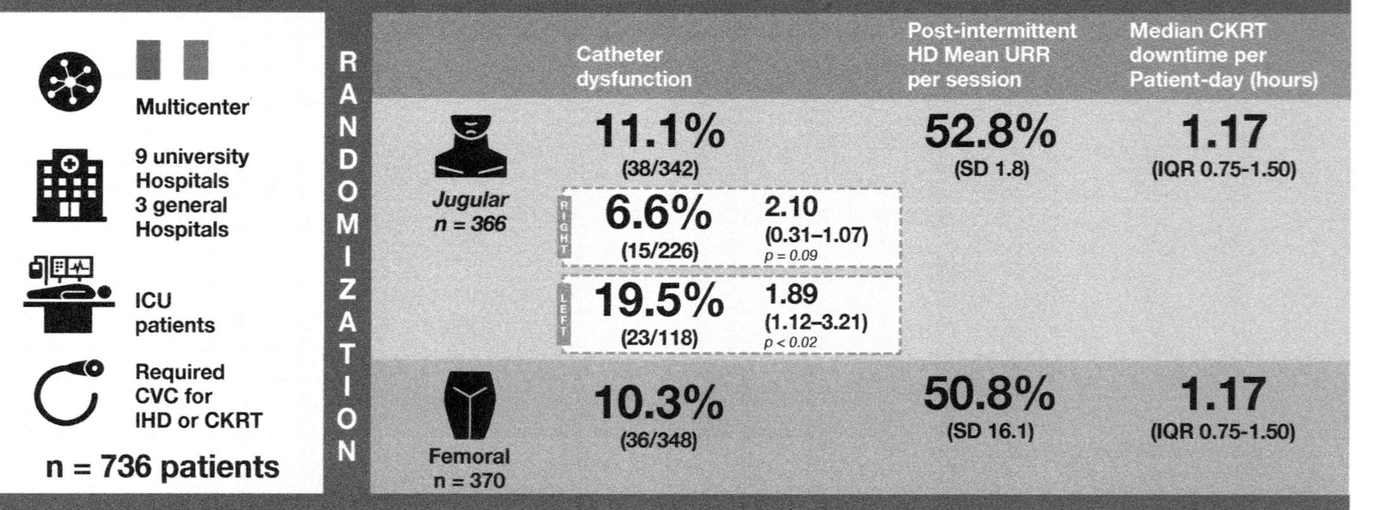

Conclusion: In terms of catheter dysfunction and dialysis performance among critically ill adults requiring acute kidney replacement therapy, jugular site did not significantly outperform femoral site placement.

Parienti JJ, Megarbane B, Fischer MO, Lautrette A, Gazui N, Marin N, et al. ***Catheter dysfunction and dialysis performance according to vascular access among 736 critically ill adults requiring kidney replacement therapy: a randomized controlled study.*** Crit Care Med. 2010;38(4):1118-25.

Does the length and location of catheter tip improve the life span of the dialyzer circuit used for CKRT ?

Unblinded

Single center Study design

31-bed Multi-disciplinary ICU

Continuous Kidney Replacement Therapy

RANDOMIZATION

	Average Dialyzer Life Span (hours) PRIMARY OUTCOME	Delivered Dialysis Dose (%)	# of clotted dialyzers	# of circuits taken down due to access	Atrial arrhythmias
Long Catheter 20-24 cms n = 47	6.5 (11-32)	91% (85-100)	2.3	0.19	28%
Short Catheter 15-20 cms n = 47	17.5 (8-23)	81% (72-97)	3.6	0.53	21%
(25th-75th percentile)	$p = 0.001$	$p < 0.001$	$p = 0.04$	$p = 0.04$	$p = 0.60$

Conclusion: The use of longer soft silicone short-term dialysis catheters targeting right atrial placement appeared to be safe and could improve dialyzer life span and daily dialysis dose of CKRT delivered compared with the use of shorter catheters targeting superior vena cava placement.

Morgan D, Ho K, Murray C, Davies H, Louw J. ***A randomized trial of catheters of different lengths to achieve right atrium versus superior vena cava placement for continuous kidney replacement therapy.*** Am J Kidney Dis. 2012;60(2):272-9.

Dosing of Kidney Replacement Therapy

Huiwen Chen and Paul M. Palevsky

Kidney replacement therapy (KRT) is the primary means of support in critically ill patients with kidney failure because of acute kidney injury (AKI). Although acute hemodialysis and other forms of KRT have been routinely utilized for more than a half century, rigorous evaluation of the optimal prescription of therapy has only been undertaken since the turn of the millennium.[1-7] If the delivered dose of KRT is inadequate, removal of toxins and control of electrolytes and acid-base status may not be sufficient to control uremic symptoms and other complications of kidney failure. Conversely, excessive dose may be associated with micronutrient depletion; contribute to inadequate dosing of medications, particularly antibiotics; and result in increased costs.[8-10]

WHAT IS KIDNEY REPLACEMENT DOSE?

There are multiple dimensions to assessment of the "dose" of KRT. These include clearance of small water-soluble solutes such as urea that are readily removed by diffusion; clearance of larger ("middle-molecular-weight") solutes such as beta-2-microglobulin and cytokines that are less well removed by diffusion; volume management; and even duration of treatment within each modality of KRT.[11] With this caveat, most studies of the intensity of delivery of KRT have quantified the delivered dose of therapy based on the clearance of urea, used as a surrogate marker for clearance of low-molecular-weight uremic toxins.[12-14] During intermittent hemodialysis, urea removal is commonly quantified based on the fractional reduction in blood urea concentration (urea reduction ratio or URR) or as the unitless index Kt/V_{urea}, where K is the effective dialyzer urea clearance, t is the duration of dialysis, and V is the volume of distribution of urea. Assumptions underlying standard methods for the assessment of Kt/V_{urea}, including stability of nitrogen balance and urea generation rates and consistency of volume status over repetitive treatment cycles, may not apply in the acute setting. Alterations in regional blood flow in hemodynamically unstable patients may result in disequilibrium between body fluid compartments, violating assumptions of single-pool kinetic models.[15] In addition, the volume of distribution of urea may be expanded and exceed estimates of total body water.[16,17] Despite these limitations, and in the absence of better indices of dialysis dose, URR and Kt/V_{urea} have been successfully applied for dose quantification in critically ill patients undergoing acute hemodialysis.[5,15] Although the concept of Kt/V_{urea} can also be applied to continuous modalities of KRT,[14] dose quantification of small-solute clearance for these modalities is more commonly assessed based on effluent flow rate normalized to body weight (mL/kg/hr).[1,5,6]

INTERMITTENT HEMODIALYSIS

The delivered dose of intermittent hemodialysis can be varied by increasing the solute clearance on a fixed dialysis treatment schedule or by increasing the frequency of treatment. No randomized controlled trials have evaluated the appropriate dose per treatment on a fixed 3 times per week or every-other-day treatment schedule. In a trial that assigned 160 patients in an alternating manner to daily versus every-other-day hemodialysis, daily dialysis was associated with lower mortality (28% vs 46%; $p = 0.01$).[2] Although the study targeted a Kt/V_{urea} of 1.2 per treatment, the actual delivered dose was substantially lower (0.94 ± 0.11 in the alternated-day arm vs 0.92 ± 0.16 in the daily dialysis arm), resulting in a relatively high time-averaged blood urea nitrogen (BUN) (104 ± 18 mg/dL) in the alternate-day arm, especially considering the cohort's high rates of sepsis, respiratory failure, and altered mental status. In contrast, in the Acute Renal Failure Trial Network (ATN) study, in which patients randomized to more intensive KRT received intermittent hemodialysis on a 6 day/week schedule (daily, except Sunday) when hemodynamically stable, whereas those randomized to less intensive KRT received intermittent hemodialysis 3 times per week (every other day, except Sunday), there was no difference in mortality associated with more intensive KRT,[5] even in analyses limited to patients who remained hemodynamically stable throughout the duration of the study[18] (**Visual Abstract 30.1**). In the ATN study, however, the delivered dose of intermittent hemodialysis was carefully monitored, with a target Kt/V of 1.2 to 1.4 per treatment, resulting in delivery of a mean Kt/V_{urea} of 1.3 per treatment in both treatment arms.

Based on these data, the Kidney Disease Improving Global Outcomes (KDIGO) Clinical Practice Guidelines for AKI recommend delivering "...a Kt/V_{urea} of 3.9 per week when using intermittent or extended KRT in AKI."[19] This recommendation is somewhat misleading, as Kt/V_{urea} is not an arithmetic function and the weekly dose cannot be derived by simply summing the delivered Kt/V_{urea} for each treatment during the week.[20] The European Renal Best Practice position statement advocates against using Kt/V_{urea} as a measure of the dose intermittent or extended KRT in AKI, recommending instead that the duration of dialysis should be adapted to allow maintenance of metabolic and volume status.[21] Given the frequent inability to deliver the actually prescribed dose of intermittent dialysis, we recommend monitoring predialysis and postdialysis blood urea concentrations. Based on the results of the ATN study, we do not believe that there is a benefit to increasing the frequency of therapy beyond 3 times per week so long as an adequate degree of small-solute control, such as a Kt/V_{urea} more than 1.2 per treatment, is achieved, and there is adequate control of electrolyte, acid-base status, and volume status. More frequent treatment may be needed if the target solute clearance cannot be achieved, for control of electrolyte and acid-base status, particularly in hypercatabolic patients, or for volume management. In addition, it is important to note that in the ATN study, despite strict dosing guidelines, the mean achieved Kt/V for the first treatment was only 1.1, demonstrating the need for monitoring to ensure achievement of the target delivered dose. Given the issues with assessment of Kt/V_{urea}, assessment of URR may provide a reasonable alternative in the acute setting, with a URR greater than or equal to 0.67 serving as a reasonable surrogate for a Kt/V_{urea} greater than or equal to 1.2 (**Table 30.1**).[22]

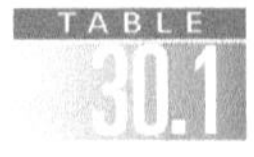

Target Dose of Kidney Replacement Therapy (KRT) in Acute Kidney Injury

Modality of KRT	Typical Target Dose
Intermittent hemodialysis (delivered on a 3×/wk schedule)	Kt/V_{urea} >1.2 per treatment; or URR > 0.67
Continuous kidney replacement therapy	Total effluent flow of 20-25 mL/kg/hr

URR, urea reduction ratio.

CONTINUOUS KIDNEY REPLACEMENT THERAPY

During continuous hemofiltration, the concentration of low-molecular-weight solutes in the ultrafiltrate will generally approximate their concentration in plasma water. During continuous hemodialysis, the dialysate flow rate is usually much lower than blood flow, permitting nearly complete equilibration between plasma and dialysate. Thus, regardless of continuous kidney replacement therapy (CKRT) modality (e.g., continuous venovenous hemofiltration [CVVH], continuous venovenous hemodialysis [CVVHD], or continuous venovenous hemodiafiltration [CVVHDF]), the concentration of low-molecular-weight solutes such as urea in the effluent (consisting of spent dialysate plus ultrafiltrate) will approximate that in plasma, and effluent flow rate will equal clearance. Dosing of solute control during CKRT is, therefore, based on effluent flow rate, normalized to total body weight.

Although several studies suggested that higher delivered doses of CKRT were associated with improved survival,[1,3] these results were not confirmed in the two largest multicenter randomized controlled trials.[5,6] In the ATN study, 1,124 critically ill patients with severe AKI in the United States were randomized to strategies of more intensive and less intensive KRT[5] (Visual Abstract 30.1). Within each treatment strategy, patients who were hemodynamically stable received conventional intermittent hemodialysis (every other day, except Sunday, in the less intensive arm; and daily, except Sunday, in the more intensive arm) and either prolonged intermittent KRT (PIKRT) or CVVHDF when they were hemodynamically unstable (with CVVHDF dosed at 20 mL/kg/hr in the less intensive arm and 35 mL/kg/hr in the more intensive arm). Overall mortality at 60 days was not different between the two treatment arms (53.6% in the intensive arm vs 51.5% in the less intensive arm; $p = 0.47$). Similarly, the Randomized Evaluation of Normal versus Augmented Level (RENAL) replacement therapy study randomized 1,508 critically ill patients with severe AKI in Australia and New Zealand to CVVHDF at either 25 or 40 mL/kg/hr[6] (**Visual Abstract 30.2**). All-cause mortality 90 days after randomization was 44.7% in both treatment arms ($p = 0.99$). In patients with sepsis-associated AKI, even higher doses of hemofiltration were not associated with any additional benefit.[23] Meta-analysis of patient-level data from multiple randomized controlled trials confirms the lack of benefit associated with higher doses of CKRT and raises concern that these higher doses may be associated with impaired recovery of kidney function[24] (**Visual Abstract 30.3**). The KDIGO Clinical Practice Guidelines for AKI recommend "...delivering an effluent volume of 20-25 mL/kg/hr for CKRT in AKI"[19] (Table 30.1). The guidelines note that this will usually require a higher prescription of effluent volume; however, if careful attention is provided to minimizing time off of therapy, this may not be necessary, and we generally do not prescribe doses more than 25 mL/kg/hr. In addition, prescription of therapy needs to be individualized to ensure that the delivered therapy achieves adequate control of all aspects of electrolyte, acid-base, and fluid balance and is not merely focused on clearance of urea and other low-molecular-weight solutes. In hypercatabolic patients, more intensive CKRT may be required for adequate control of acidosis, hyperkalemia, and other electrolytes.

SUMMARY

The dose of KRT in AKI comprises multiple dimensions, and KRT in AKI should be prescribed to meet the multiple goals of electrolyte, acid-base, and fluid balance in addition to clearance of small solutes such as urea. When intermittent hemodialysis is used, there is no additional benefit to increasing small-solute clearance beyond a Kt/V_{urea} of 1.2 per treatment (corresponding to a URR of at least 0.67) on a thrice-weekly schedule. More frequent treatments may be required if the target solute clearance cannot be achieved, for control of electrolytes and acid-base status in markedly hypercatabolic patients and for volume management in the setting of marked volume overload. When CKRT is used, delivery of an effluent flow of 20 to 25 mL/kg/hr is generally sufficient; however, dosing should be individualized for each patient.

References

1. Ronco C, Bellomo R, Homel P, et al. Effects of different doses in continuous veno-venous haemofiltration on outcomes of acute renal failure: a prospective randomised trial. *Lancet.* 2000;356(9223):26-30.
2. Schiffl H, Lang SM, Fischer R. Daily hemodialysis and the outcome of acute renal failure. *N Engl J Med.* 2002;346(5):305-310.
3. Saudan P, Niederberger M, De Seigneux S, et al. Adding a dialysis dose to continuous hemofiltration increases survival in patients with acute renal failure. *Kidney Int.* 2006;70(7):1312-1317.
4. Tolwani AJ, Campbell RC, Stofan BS, Lai KR, Oster RA, Wille KM. Standard versus high-dose CVVHDF for ICU-related acute renal failure. *J Am Soc Nephrol.* 2008;19(6):1233-1238.
5. Palevsky PM, Zhang JH, O'Connor TZ, et al; VA/NIH Acute Renal Failure Trial Network. Intensity of renal support in critically ill patients with acute kidney injury. *N Engl J Med.* 2008;359(1):7-20.
6. Bellomo R, Cass A, Cole L, et al; The RENAL Replacement Therapy Study Investigators. Intensity of continuous renal-replacement therapy in critically ill patients. *N Engl J Med.* 2009;361(17):1627-1638.
7. Faulhaber-Walter R, Hafer C, Jahr N, et al. The Hannover Dialysis Outcome Study: comparison of standard versus intensified extended dialysis for treatment of patients with acute kidney injury in the intensive care unit. *Nephrol Dial Transplant.* 2009;24(7):2179-2186.
8. Mueller BA, Pasko DA, Sowinski KM. Higher renal replacement therapy dose delivery influences on drug therapy. *Artif Organs.* 2003;27(9):808-814.
9. Lewis SJ, Mueller BA. Antibiotic dosing in critically ill patients receiving CRRT: underdosing is overprevalent. *Semin Dial.* 2014;27(5):441-445.
10. Sigwalt F, Bouteleux A, Dambricourt F, Asselborn T, Moriceau F, Rimmele T. Clinical complications of continuous renal replacement therapy. *Contrib Nephrol.* 2018;194:109-117.
11. Vijayan A, Palevsky PM. Dosing of renal replacement therapy in acute kidney injury. *Am J Kidney Dis.* 2012;59(4):569-576.
12. Clark WR, Mueller BA, Kraus MA, Macias WL. Renal replacement therapy quantification in acute renal failure. *Nephrol Dial Transplant.* 1998;13(Suppl 6):86-90.
13. Garred L, Leblanc M, Canaud B. Urea kinetic modeling for CRRT. *Am J Kidney Dis.* 1997;30(5 Suppl 4):S2-S9.
14. Clark WR, Leblanc M, Ricci Z, Ronco C. Quantification and dosing of renal replacement therapy in acute kidney injury: a reappraisal. *Blood Purif.* 2017;44(2):140-155.

15. Kanagasundaram NS, Greene T, Larive AB, et al. Dosing intermittent haemodialysis in the intensive care unit patient with acute renal failure—estimation of urea removal and evidence for the regional blood flow model. *Nephrol Dial Transplant.* 2008;23(7):2286-2298.
16. Himmelfarb J, Evanson J, Hakim RM, Freedman S, Shyr Y, Ikizler TA. Urea volume of distribution exceeds total body water in patients with acute renal failure. *Kidney Int.* 2002;61(1):317-323.
17. Ikizler TA, Sezer MT, Flakoll PJ, et al. Urea space and total body water measurements by stable isotopes in patients with acute renal failure. *Kidney Int.* 2004;65(2):725-732.
18. Vijayan A, Delos Santos RB, Li T, Goss CW, Palevsky PM. Effect of frequent dialysis on renal recovery: results from the acute renal failure trial network study. *Kidney Int Rep.* 2018;3(2):456-463.
19. KDIGO Clinical Practice Guidelines for Acute Kidney Injury. Section 5: dialysis interventions for treatment of AKI. *Kidney Int Suppl (2011).* 2012;2(1):89-115.
20. Gotch FA, Sargent JA, Keen ML. Whither goes Kt/V? *Kidney Int Suppl.* 2000;76:S3-S18.
21. Jorres A, John S, Lewington A, et al. A European Renal Best Practice (ERBP) position statement on the Kidney Disease Improving Global Outcomes (KDIGO) Clinical Practice Guidelines on Acute Kidney Injury: part 2: renal replacement therapy. *Nephrol Dial Transplant.* 2013;28(12):2940-2945.
22. Liang KV, Zhang JH, Palevsky PM. Urea reduction ratio may be a simpler approach for measurement of adequacy of intermittent hemodialysis in acute kidney injury. *BMC Nephrol.* 2019;20(1):82.
23. Joannes-Boyau O, Honore PM, Perez P, et al. High-volume versus standard-volume haemofiltration for septic shock patients with acute kidney injury (IVOIRE study): a multicentre randomized controlled trial. *Intensive Care Med.* 2013;39(9):1535-1546.
24. Wang Y, Gallagher M, Li Q, et al. Renal replacement therapy intensity for acute kidney injury and recovery to dialysis independence: a systematic review and individual patient data meta-analysis. *Nephrol Dial Transplant.* 2018;33(6):1017-1024.

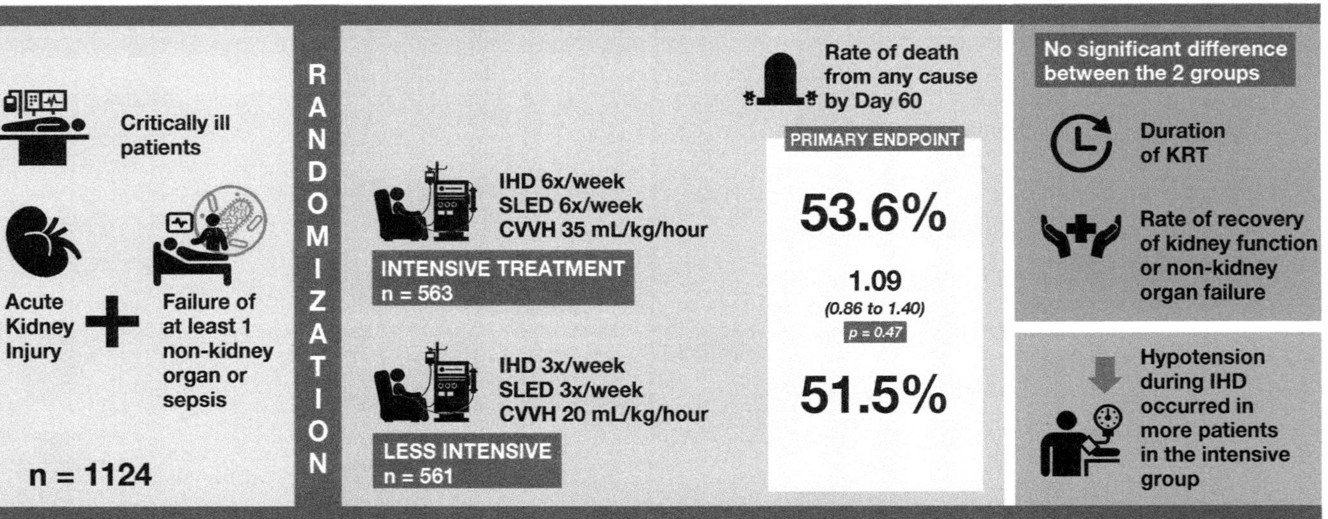

Conclusion: Intensive kidney support in critically ill patients with acute kidney injury did not decrease mortality, improve recovery of kidney function, or reduce the rate of nonrenal organ failure as compared with less-intensive therapy involving a defined dose of intermittent hemodialysis three times per week and continuous kidney-replacement therapy at 20 ml per kilogram per hour.

VA/NIH Acute Kidney Failure Trial Network, Palevsky PM, Zhang JH, O'Connor TZ, Chertow GM, Crowley ST, et al. ***Intensity of kidney support in critically ill patients with acute kidney injury.*** N Engl J Med. 2008;359(1):7-20.

VISUAL ABSTRACT 30.1

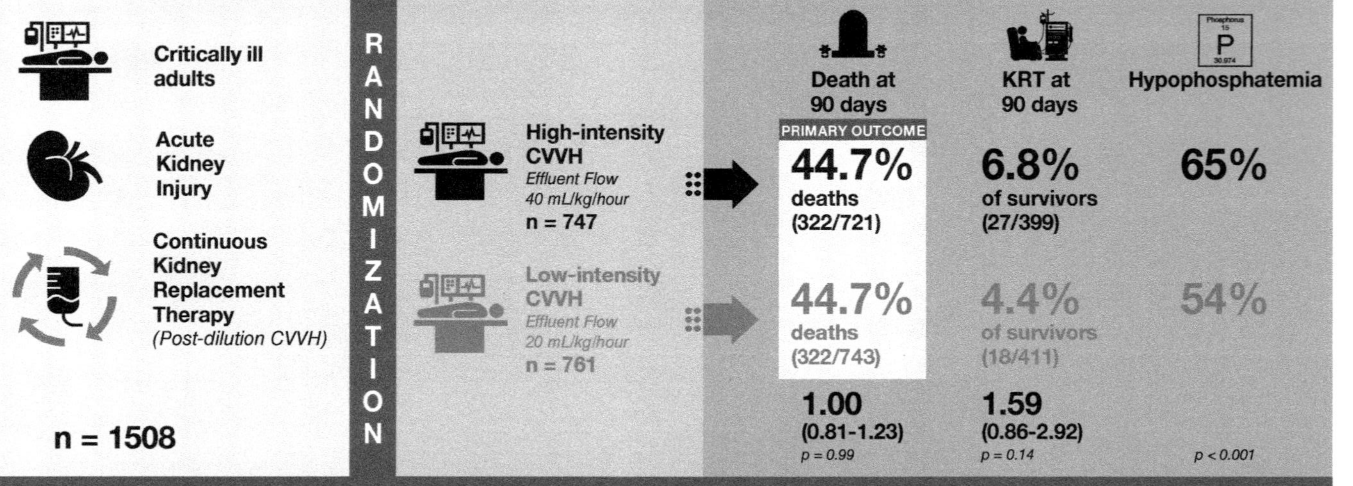

VISUAL ABSTRACT 30.2

Is higher intensity dose kidney replacement therapy (KRT) associated with survival benefit and better kidney recovery in acute kidney injury (AKI)?

META-ANALYSIS

ICU patients

Severe Acute Kidney Injury (AKI)

8 prospective Randomized Controlled Trials

n = 3682

	High Intensity	Low Intensity	
PRIMARY OUTCOME Mortality at Day 28	40.8% (769/1184)	41.4% (744/1798)	0.93 (1.80–1.09) *p* = 0.40
SECONDARY OUTCOME KRT dependence at Day 28	29.7% (292/983)	24.9% (235/943)	1.15 (1.00–1.33) *p* = 0.05

Time to cessation of KRT through 28 days was longer in patients receiving higher intensity KRT (log-rank test p = 0.02) and when CKRT was used as the initial modality of KRT (log-rank test p = 0.03).

Conclusion: In severe AKI patients, higher intensity KRT does not affect mortality but appears to delay kidney recovery.

Wang Y, Gallagher M, Li Q, Lo S, Cass A, Finfer S, et al. ***Kidney replacement therapy intensity for acute kidney injury and recovery to dialysis independence: a systematic review and individual patient data meta-analysis.*** Nephrol Dial Transplant. 2018;33(6): 1017-24.

VISUAL ABSTRACT 30.3

31 Timing of Kidney Replacement Therapy

Alejandro Y. Meraz-Muñoz,
Sean M. Bagshaw, and Ron Wald

INTRODUCTION

Acute kidney injury (AKI) is a frequent complication of critical illness affecting up to two-thirds of patients admitted to the intensive care unit (ICU).[1,2] Patients who receive KRT for their AKI are at high risk of death with short-term mortality exceeding 50%.[3,4] However, even patients who survive the acute phase of illness continue to be at risk of persistent chronic kidney disease, with some progressing to long-term dialysis dependence.[5-8] Previous studies have reported that 16% and 22% of patients with severe AKI remained dialysis dependent at 90 days and 1 year, respectively, after kidney replacement therapy (KRT) initiation.[3,9] The KRT prescription in critically ill patients with AKI is informed by high-quality evidence in regard to small molecule clearance,[10,11] the choice of KRT modality,[12] and anticoagulation.[13] However, the more fundamental question of when to commence KRT has been a source of debate for decades.

SCOPE OF THE PROBLEM

In critically ill patients with complications of AKI that pose an unequivocal threat to life (e.g., severe hyperkalemia, acidemia, and fluid overload that are refractory to medical measures), there is no debate about the need to urgently initiate KRT,[14] assuming this is consistent with the patient's goals of care. However, observational data have suggested that these "emergency" indications are not the most common triggers for starting KRT in usual practice.[2,15,16] It would appear that for most patients, the decision to start KRT tends to be more nuanced and incorporates trends in markers of kidney function and nonkidney organ dysfunction. The inherent subjectivity that guides the initiation of KRT in the setting of AKI is highlighted by the diversity in clinical practice, as demonstrated by epidemiologic studies[15,16] and self-reported practice surveys.[17-20] The justification for commencing KRT in the absence of an AKI-related emergency is predicated on the rationale that earlier or preemptive KRT initiation will proactively lead to more effective volume control as well as the maintenance of electrolyte and acid-base homeostasis. Furthermore, earlier initiation of KRT will hasten the clearance of uremic solutes that accumulate in the setting of AKI and that possibly mediate systemic toxicity. However, the precise identity of these putative toxins has not been delineated, making this component of acute KRT much more difficult to objectively evaluate. A "preemptive" or "early" approach is supported by several observational studies[21-25] and one randomized controlled trial (RCT).[26]

Enthusiasm for preemptive KRT should be tempered by the well-established risks of KRT, including iatrogenic complications occurring during catheter insertion, catheter-related bloodstream infections, iatrogenic hemodynamic instability, hypophosphatemia, and compromised therapeutic levels of vital drugs. In addition, lowering the threshold for KRT initiation would likely lead to increased health care costs, at least in the short term. The adjusted incremental cost of a hospitalization on which a patient received KRT for AKI is 10,000-15,000 USD.[27,28]

Decisions regarding the timing of KRT initiation are further complicated by the fact that many patients with severe AKI may experience spontaneous recovery of kidney function. Thus, a policy of preemptively commencing KRT could lead to its delivery to some individuals who are destined to recover kidney function irrespective of the receipt of KRT. Currently, there are no prediction scores that accurately anticipate the need of KRT in critically ill patients with AKI. Although several biomarkers have shown promise, a recent meta-analysis concluded that the strength of evidence prevents their routine use[29] (see Chapters 16 and 17). Finally, as discussed in Chapter 16, the furosemide stress test is a tool that accurately predicts patients at risk of progression to more severe AKI and may help guide decision-making around KRT initiation.

RECENT RANDOMIZED CONTROLLED TRIALS

The quality of evidence on the topic of KRT initiation has been greatly enhanced since 2016 with the publication of four large RCTs that compared different strategies for KRT initiation in critically ill patients with AKI (**Table 31.1**).

The Early versus Late Initiation of Renal Replacement Therapy in Critically Ill Patients with Acute Kidney Injury (ELAIN) trial was a single-center RCT conducted in Germany (**Visual abstract 31.1**).[26] It enrolled 231 critically ill patients of whom the vast majority had a recent surgery (50% cardiac surgery), with Kidney Disease Improving Global Outcomes (KDIGO) stage 2 (doubling of serum creatinine from baseline or 12 hours of oliguria) and at least one of the following: sepsis, refractory fluid overload, worsening sequential organ failure assessment (SOFA) score, or requiring vasoactive support. Participants were randomized to two groups: early KRT initiation (KRT to be started within 8 hours of KDIGO stage 2 AKI criteria being met, $n = 112$) or delayed initiation (KRT to be started if patient progressed to KDIGO stage 3 AKI or in the event of a traditional clinical indication supervening, $n = 119$). Continuous kidney replacement therapy (CKRT) was the mandated modality for all patients commencing KRT in both arms of the trial. All patients in the early initiation arm received KRT as did 91% in the delayed initiation arm. The median intergroup difference in time to KRT initiation from randomization was 21 hours (interquartile range, 18-24). Early initiation of KRT conferred a reduction in 90-day mortality compared with delayed initiation (39% vs 55%; $p = 0.03$).

The Artificial Kidney Initiation in Kidney Injury (AKIKI) trial was a multicenter RCT conducted at 31 centers in France that was designed to test the hypothesis that delayed initiation of KRT would confer lower morality in critically ill patients with severe AKI (**Visual Abstract 31.2**).[30] The trial enrolled 620 patients with KDIGO stage 3 AKI who required mechanical ventilation, catecholamine infusion, or both and did not have a life-threatening complication related to AKI. Approximately two-thirds of the patients in this mixed medical-surgical cohort had septic shock. Participants were randomized to a strategy of early initiation (within 6 hours of KDIGO stage 3 AKI, $n = 311$) or delayed initiation

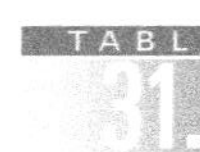

TABLE 31.1 Summary of Recent Randomized Controlled Trials Examining the Timing of KRT Initiation in Critically Ill Patients With AKI

	ELAIN (n = 231)	**AKIKI (n = 620)**	**IDEAL-ICU (n = 488)**	**STARRT-AKI (n = 3,019)**
Setting and population	Single center in Germany; 95% surgical patients (47% cardiac surgery)	31 centers in France; 80% medical patients	24 centers in France; 100% septic shock patients	168 centers in 15 countries; 67% medical patients
Key inclusion criteria	KDIGO stage 2 AKI, plus NGAL >150 ng/mL and sepsis, vasopressors, volume overload	KDIGO stage 3 AKI plus mechanical ventilation and/or catecholamine use	RIFLE stage F, AKI within 48 hr of vasopressor initiation	KDIGO stage 2-3 AKI
Key exclusion criteria	Emergency indications for KRT. Preexisting eGFR <30 mL/min/1.73 m^2	Emergency indications for KRT. Preexisting CrCl <30 mL/min	Emergency indications for KRT.	Emergency indications for KRT. Previous KRT, preexisting eGFR <20 mL/min/1.73 m^2. Clinician perception of mandated need for KRT or imminent kidney recovery
SOFA score (early vs delayed)	15.6 vs 16.0	10.9 vs 10.8	12.2 vs 12.4	11.6 vs 11.8
Window for KRT initiation in early arm	Within 8 hr of stage 2 AKI	Within 6 hr of stage 3 AKI	Within 12 hr of stage F AKI	Within 12 hr of full trial eligibility

Triggers for KRT initiation in delayed arm	Within 12 hr of progression to stage 3 AKI, BUN >100 mg/dL, K >6 MEq/L, or edema resistant to diuretics	If BUN >112 mg/dL, K >6 mmol/L, pH <7.1, oliguria >72 hr, acute pulmonary edema	48 hr after inclusion, unless recovery of kidney function, or if K >6 mmol/L, pH <7.1, fluid overload	$K \geq 6.0$ mmol/L, pH ≤ 7.20, $HCO_3 \leq 12$ mmol/L, severe hypoxia ($PaO_2/FiO_2 \leq 200$) due to volume overload, or persistent AKI ≥ 72 hr
Percentage of patients in the delayed group that received KRT	91% at a median of 25 hr postrandomization	51% at a median of 57 hr postrandomization	62% at a median of 51 hr postrandomization	62% at median of 31 hr postrandomization
Initial KRT modality	CKRT (CVVHDF)	Mixed (CKRT 45%)	Mixed (CKRT 56%)	Mixed (CKRT 70%)
Primary outcome (early vs delayed)	90-d mortality: 39% vs 54% ($p = 0.03$)	60-d mortality: 49% vs 50% ($p = 0.79$)	90-d mortality: 58% vs 54% ($p = 0.38$)	90-d mortality: 44% vs 44% ($p = 0.92$)

AKI, acute kidney injury; BUN, blood urea nitrogen; CrCl, creatinine clearance; CKRT, continuous kidney replacement therapy; CVVHDF, continuous venovenous hemodiafiltration; eGFR, estimated glomerular filtration rate; KDIGO, Kidney Disease Improving Global Outcomes; KRT, kidney replacement therapy; NGAL, neutrophil gelatinase–associated lipocalin; PaO_2/FiO_2, Ratio of arterial oxygen partial pressure in mmHg to fractional inspired oxygen; RIFLE, Risk, Injury, Failure, Loss, End stage kidney disease; SOFA, sequential organ failure assessment.

(KRT initiated in the presence of oliguria persisting for >72 hours, blood urea nitrogen [BUN] >112 mg/dL, hyperkalemia, metabolic acidosis, and/or pulmonary edema because of fluid overload, n = 308). The delivered KRT modality was left to the discretion of the clinical team and the majority of participants who commenced KRT received intermittent therapy. Nearly all patients in the early strategy received KRT, whereas only about half of those in the delayed arm initiated KRT. Among participants who commenced KRT, those randomized to the delayed-strategy arm started KRT 55 hours later than those in the early arm. Mortality at 60 days did not differ between the early and delayed strategies (48.5% in the early strategy vs 49.7% in the delayed strategy, hazard ratio [HR] 1.03, 95% confidence interval [CI]: 0.82-1.29, p = 0.79). Patients randomized to early KRT initiation had fewer dialysis-free days (17 vs 19 days, $p < 0.001$) and a higher risk of iatrogenic complications, notably central venous catheter–associated infections and hypophosphatemia.

The Initiation of Dialysis Early versus Delayed in the Intensive Care Unit (IDEAL-ICU) trial was conducted at 29 centers in France and tested the hypothesis that earlier initiation of KRT would confer a 10% absolute reduction in 90-day all-cause mortality in critically ill patients with septic shock and severe AKI (**Visual Abstract 31.3**).[31] Patients in the early-strategy group were to receive KRT within 12 hours after documentation of stage 3 AKI, whereas those randomized to the delayed arm were mandated to commence KRT if an emergent indication developed or after 48 hours of persistent AKI. The investigators planned to recruit 864 patients, but recruitment ceased after the randomization of 488 participants because of perceived futility. Nearly all patients (97%) assigned to the early-strategy group received KRT, whereas 62% in the delayed-strategy group received KRT. Among patients in the delayed arm who did not commence KRT, the majority had spontaneous recovery of kidney function. The primary outcome of 90-day all-cause mortality was not reduced by a strategy of earlier KRT initiation (58% vs 54% in the early and delayed initiation arms, respectively, p = 0.38).

The Standard versus Accelerated initiation of Renal Replacement Therapy in Acute Kidney Injury (STARRT-AKI) trial was conducted at 168 centers in 15 countries and tested whether an accelerated strategy of KRT initiation would confer a reduction in 90-day all-cause mortality as compared to a standard strategy (**Visual Abstract 31.4**).[32] Patients with stage 2 or 3 AKI were included but unlike previous trials, eligibility was not predicated on the duration of AKI. Key exclusions included overt indications for KRT initiation (i.e., hyperkalemia, severe metabolic acidosis), lack of commitment to offer KRT, and preexisting advanced chronic kidney disease. Once patients met core inclusion criteria and the preliminary exclusions were eliminated, patients were provisionally eligible. Final eligibility depended on clinicians' equipoise: specifically, attending physicians were asked to exclude patients whom they felt either needed immediate KRT initiation or mandatory deferral of KRT because of the anticipation of imminent recovery of kidney function. This approach helped ensure that the trial only enrolled patients for whom the question of whether and when to commence KRT was a matter of genuine clinical uncertainty. Once clinicians confirmed the presence of equipoise, patients were declared to be fully eligible and were randomized to an accelerated strategy (KRT to be commenced within 12 hours of full eligibility criteria) or a standard strategy, which discouraged clinicians from commencing KRT unless one or more of the following criteria supervened: serum potassium 6.0 mmol/L or more, pH less than or equal to

7.20, serum bicarbonate 12 mmol/L or less, or severe respiratory failure with a ratio of the partial pressure of arterial oxygen to the fraction of inspired oxygen less than or equal to 200 perceived to be the result of volume overload. If AKI persisted for more than 72 hours, the decision to initiate KRT or not was transferred to the discretion of the clinician. Unlike the previous trials, the standard strategy did not come with an obligation to commence KRT even if one of the aforementioned conditions was met.

Among the 3,019 randomized patients, 2,927 (1,465 and 1,462 in the accelerated and standard strategies, respectively) were eligible for the modified intention-to-treat analysis. The majority of patients randomized to the accelerated-strategy arm commenced KRT a median of 6 hours from meeting eligibility, whereas 62% of the standard-strategy participants started KRT a median of 31 hours from the time of eligibility. The primary outcome of 90-day all-cause mortality was 43.9% in the accelerated arm versus 43.7% in the standard arm (relative risk [RR] 1.00; 0.93-1.09). These findings were consistent across all prespecified subgroups, including those with and without sepsis and preexisting chronic kidney disease, respectively. There was no evidence of heterogeneity of treatment effect across categories of illness acuity. Among survivors, there was a significantly higher likelihood of persistent dialysis dependence at 90 days in patients randomized to the accelerated strategy (10.4% vs 6.0% in the standard arm; RR 1.74, 95% CI: 1.24-2.43). Adverse events were more common in the accelerated arm (23% vs 16.5%), mainly driven by hypotension and hypophosphatemia.

Notwithstanding the differences in study design among the various RCTs that have studied timing strategies for KRT initiation, the preponderance of evidence does not favor the preemptive initiation of KRT prior to the emergence of objective triggers. Moreover, an early approach comes at the cost of a variety of adverse effects and a higher likelihood of persistent KRT dependence, possibly because of the hemodynamic instability conferred by the delivery of KRT.

REMAINING AREAS OF UNCERTAINTY

Though clinical trials show that earlier initiation of KRT does not improve outcomes and may be harmful, it is unclear how long it is safe to delay KRT in the face of severe persistent AKI even if a conventional indication for KRT does not emerge. The recently completed AKIKI-2 trial, which evaluated the effect of further delaying KRT beyond the threshold for KRT initiation in the delayed arm of the original AKIKI trial, will hopefully shed light on this (ClinicalTrials.gov Identifier: NCT03396757). Furthermore, as highlighted by the substantial number of patients who did not receive KRT in the delayed/standard arms of AKIKI, IDEAL-ICU, and STARRT-AKI, the identification and validation of biomarkers that anticipate AKI progression may help inform the precise delivery of KRT.

SUMMARY AND CONCLUSIONS

For critically ill patients with AKI whose philosophy of care includes the escalation of treatment with the addition of organ support therapy, KRT should be started immediately in the presence of any life-threatening AKI complication that can be remedied by KRT. The initiation of KRT in the absence of such a complication has not resulted in improved patient survival and exposes patients to a higher risk of adverse events. In the face of severe AKI that is unaccompanied by metabolic or volume complications, clinicians are advised to defer the initiation of KRT with close monitoring for kidney recovery.

References

1. Hoste EA, Clermont G, Kersten A, et al. RIFLE criteria for acute kidney injury are associated with hospital mortality in critically ill patients: a cohort analysis. *Crit Care.* 2006;10(3):R73.
2. Hoste EAJ, Bagshaw SM, Bellomo R, et al. Epidemiology of acute kidney injury in critically ill patients: the multinational AKI-EPI study. *Intensive Care Med.* 2015;41(8):1411-1423.
3. Bagshaw SM, Laupland KB, Doig CJ, et al. Prognosis for long-term survival and renal recovery in critically ill patients with severe acute renal failure: a population-based study. *Crit Care.* 2005;9(6):R700.
4. Uchino S, Bellomo R, Goldsmith D, et al. An assessment of the RIFLE criteria for acute renal failure in hospitalized patients. *Crit Care Med.* 2006;34(7):1913-1917.
5. Hoste EAJ, Kellum JA, Selby NM, et al. Global epidemiology and outcomes of acute kidney injury. *Nat Rev Nephrol.* 2018;14:607-625.
6. Wald R, Quinn RR, Luo J, et al; for the University of Toronto Acute Kidney Injury Research Group. Chronic dialysis and death among survivors of acute kidney injury requiring dialysis. *JAMA.* 2009;302(11):1179.
7. Wald R, Shariff S, Adhikari NK, et al. The association between renal replacement therapy modality and long-term outcomes among critically ill adults with acute kidney injury: a retrospective cohort study. *Crit Care Med.* 2014;42(4):868-877.
8. Chua H-R, Wong W-K, Ong VH, et al. Extended mortality and chronic kidney disease after septic acute kidney injury. *J Intensive Care Med.* 2020;35(6):527-535.
9. Wald R, McArthur E, Adhikari NKJ, et al. Changing incidence and outcomes following dialysis-requiring acute kidney injury among critically ill adults: a population-based cohort study. *Am J Kidney Dis.* 2015;65(6):870-877.
10. Palevsky PM, Zhang JH, O'Connor TZ, et al. Intensity of renal support in critically ill patients with acute kidney injury. The VA/NIH Acute Renal Failure Trial Network. *N Engl J Med.* 2008;359(1):7-20.
11. The RENAL Replacement Therapy Study Investigators, Bellomo R, Cass A. Intensity of continuous renal-replacement therapy in critically ill patients. *N Engl J Med.* 2009;361(17):1627-1638.
12. Vinsonneau C, Camus C, Combes A, et al. Continuous venovenous haemodiafiltration versus intermittent haemodialysis for acute renal failure in patients with multiple-organ dysfunction syndrome: a multicentre randomised trial. *The Lancet.* 2006;368(9533):379-385.
13. Kutsogiannis DJ, Gibney RTN, Stollery D, et al. Regional citrate versus systemic heparin anticoagulation for continuous renal replacement in critically ill patients. *Kidney Int.* 2005;67(6):2361-2367.
14. Kellum JA, Lameire N, Aspelin P, et al. Kidney disease: improving global outcomes (KDIGO) Acute Kidney Injury work group. KDIGO clinical practice guideline for acute kidney injury. *Kidney Int.* 2012;2(1):1-138.
15. Bagshaw SM, Wald R, Barton J, et al. Clinical factors associated with initiation of renal replacement therapy in critically ill patients with acute kidney injury—a prospective multicenter observational study. *J Crit Care.* 2012;27(3):268-275.
16. Clark E, Wald R, Levin A, et al. Timing the initiation of renal replacement therapy for acute kidney injury in Canadian intensive care units: a multicentre observational study. *Can J Anesth Can Anesth.* 2012;59(9):861-870.
17. RENAL Study Investigators. Renal replacement therapy for acute kidney injury in Australian and New Zealand intensive care units: a practice survey. *Crit Care Resusc.* 2008;10(3):225-230.
18. Mehta RL, Letteri JM. Current status of renal replacement therapy for acute renal failure. *Am J Nephrol.* 1999;19(3):377-382.
19. Uchino S, Bellomo R, Morimatsu H, et al. Continuous renal replacement therapy: a worldwide practice survey. *Intensive Care Med.* 2007;33(9):1563-1570.
20. Clark E, Wald R, Walsh M, et al. Timing of initiation of renal replacement therapy for acute kidney injury: a survey of nephrologists and intensivists in Canada. *Nephrol Dial Transplant.* 2012;27(7):2761-2767.
21. Sugahara S, Suzuki H. Early start on continuous hemodialysis therapy improves survival rate in patients with acute renal failure following coronary bypass surgery. *Hemodial Int.* 2004;8(4):320-325.
22. Bagshaw SM, Uchino S, Bellomo R, et al. Timing of renal replacement therapy and clinical outcomes in critically ill patients with severe acute kidney injury. *J Crit Care.* 2009;24(1):129-140.

23. Shiao C-C, Wu V-C, Li W-Y, et al. Late initiation of renal replacement therapy is associated with worse outcomes in acute kidney injury after major abdominal surgery. *Crit Care.* 2009;13(5):R171.
24. Carl DE, Grossman C, Behnke M, et al. Effect of timing of dialysis on mortality in critically ill, septic patients with acute renal failure. *Hemodial Int.* 2010;14(1):11-17.
25. Vaara ST, Reinikainen M, Wald R, et al. Timing of RRT based on the presence of conventional indications. *Clin J Am Soc Nephrol.* 2014;9(9):1577-1585.
26. Zarbock A, Kellum JA, Schmidt C, et al. Effect of early vs delayed initiation of renal replacement therapy on mortality in critically ill patients with acute kidney injury: the ELAIN randomized clinical trial. *JAMA.* 2016;315(20):2190.
27. Collister D, Pannu N, Ye F, et al. Health care costs associated with AKI. *Clin J Am Soc Nephrol.* 2017;12(11):1733-1743.
28. Silver SA, Long J, Zheng Y, et al. Cost of acute kidney injury in hospitalized patients. *J Hosp Med.* 2017;12(2):70-76.
29. Klein SJ, Brandtner AK, Lehner GF, et al. Biomarkers for prediction of renal replacement therapy in acute kidney injury: a systematic review and meta-analysis. *Intensive Care Med.* 2018;44(3):323-336.
30. Gaudry S, Hajage D, Schortgen F, et al. Initiation strategies for renal-replacement therapy in the intensive care unit. *N Engl J Med.* 2016;375(2):122-133.
31. Barbar SD, Clere-Jehl R, Bourredjem A, et al. Timing of renal-replacement therapy in patients with acute kidney injury and sepsis. *N Engl J Med.* 2018;379(15):1431-1442.
32. The STARRT-AKI Investigators, Canadian Critical Care Trials Group, Australian and New Zealand Intensive Care Society Clinical Trials Group, et al. Timing of initiation of renal-replacement therapy in acute kidney injury. *N Engl J Med.* 2020;383(3):240-251.

Effect of Early vs Delayed Initiation of Kidney Replacement Therapy on Mortality in Critically Ill Patients With Acute Kidney Injury: ELAIN

Single center

Critically ill patients

Criteria for initiation of KRT in early group
KDIGO AKI 2 *within 8 hours*

NGAL > 150 ng/mL

Aug 2013 thru June 2015

n = 231

RANDOMIZATION

	Mortality at Day 90 (PRIMARY ENDPOINT)	Recovered kidney function at Day 90	Duration of KRT	Length of Hospital stay
EARLY KRT *within 8 hours of diagnosis of AKI 2* n = 112 *** 112 received KRT**	39% (44/112)	54% (60/112)	9 days [Q1, Q3: 4, 44]	51 days [Q1, Q3: 31, 74]
DELAYED KRT *within 12 hours of diagnosis of AKI 3* n = 119 *** 108 received KRT**	55% (65/119)	39% (46/119)	25 days [Q1, Q3: 7, >90]	82 days [Q1, Q3: 67, >90]
Difference	-15.4% (-28.1,-2.6) *p = 0.03*	14.9% (2.2,27.6) *p = 0.02*	-18 days (-41,4)	-37 days (-∞,-19.5)

Conclusions: Among critically ill patients with AKI, early initiation of KRT reduced 90-day all-cause mortality, as compared to a strategy of delayed initiation.

Zarbock A, Kellum JA, Schmidt C, Van Aken H., et al. ***Effect of Early vs Delayed Initiation of Kidney Replacement Therapy on Mortality in Critically Ill Patients With Acute Kidney Injury: The ELAIN Randomized Clinical Trial.*** JAMA 2016 May 24-31;315(20):2190-9

VISUAL ABSTRACT 31.1

Initiation Strategies for Kidney-Replacement Therapy in the Intensive Care Unit: AKIKI

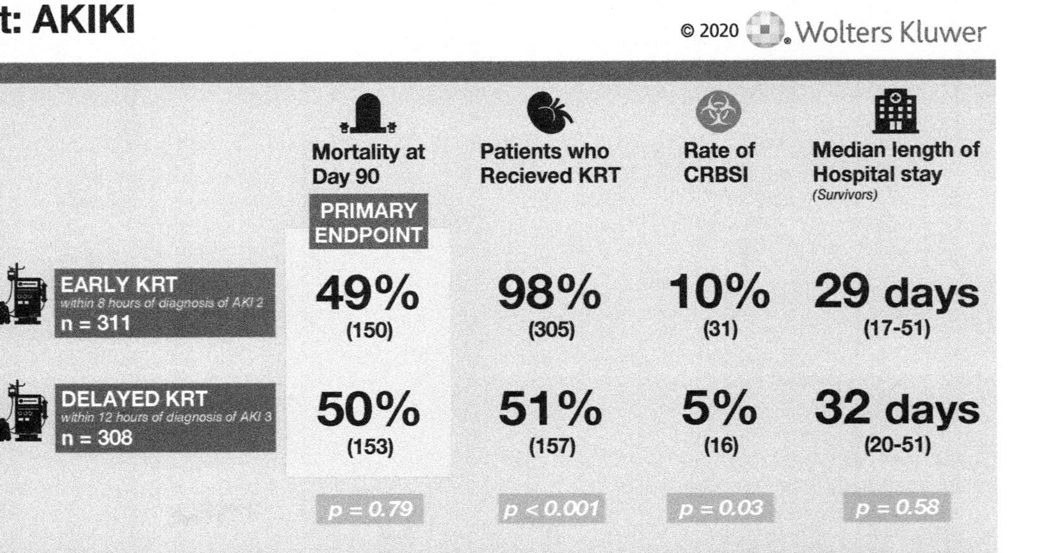

Conclusion: Among critically ill patients with severe acute kidney injury, there was no significant difference in mortality between an early and delayed strategies of KRT initiation.

Gaudry S, Hajage D, Schortgen F, Martin-Lefevre L, et al. ***Initiation Strategies for Kidney-Replacement Therapy in the Intensive Care Unit.*** N Engl J Med 2016 Jul 14;375(2):122-33.

VISUAL ABSTRACT 31.2

Timing of Kidney-Replacement Therapy in Patients with Acute Kidney Injury and Sepsis: IDEAL-ICU

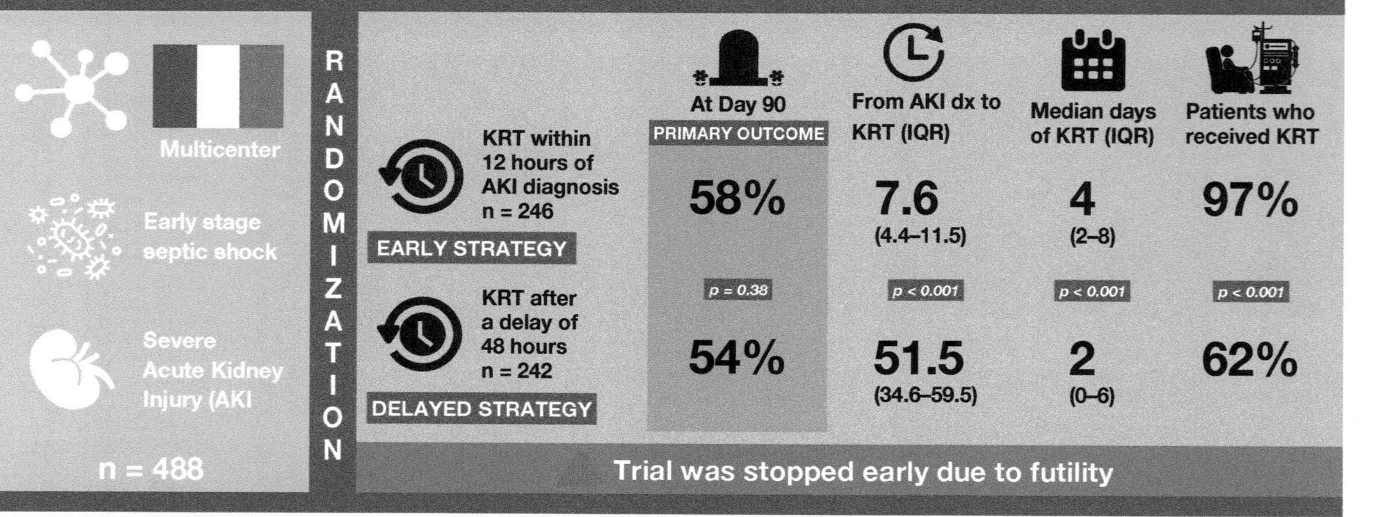

Conclusion: Among patients with acute kidney injury and septic shock, there was no significant difference in overall mortality at 90 days between patients who were assigned to an early KRT initiation strategy and those who were assigned to a delayed strategy.

Barbar SD, Clere-Jehl R, Bourredjem A, Hernu R, et al. ***Timing of Kidney-Replacement Therapy in Patients With Acute Kidney Injury and Sepsis.*** N Engl J Med 2018 Oct 11;379(15):1431-1442.

VISUAL ABSTRACT 31.3

Timing of Initiation of Kidney-Replacement Therapy in Acute Kidney Injury: STARRT-AKI

Multinational RCT
168 hospitals
15 countries

Critically ill Patients

Severe AKI criteria
KDIGO AKI 2 or 3

Oct 2015 thru Sept 2019

n = 3019 (2927 in final analysis)

RANDOMIZATION

	@ Day 90 (PRIMARY ENDPOINT)	Patients who received KRT	Dependence @ 90 days	≥1 adverse event(s)
ACCELERATED-STRATEGY *within 12 hours of meeting eligibility criteria* n = 1465	44% (643/1465)	97% (1418/1465)	10% (85/814)	23% (346/1503)
STANDARD-STRATEGY *Conventional indications or AKI ≥72h* n = 1462	44% (639/1462)	62% (903/1462)	6% (49/815)	17% (245/1489)
	RR 1.00 (0.93-1.09)		RR 1.74 (1.24-2.43)	*p* < 0.001

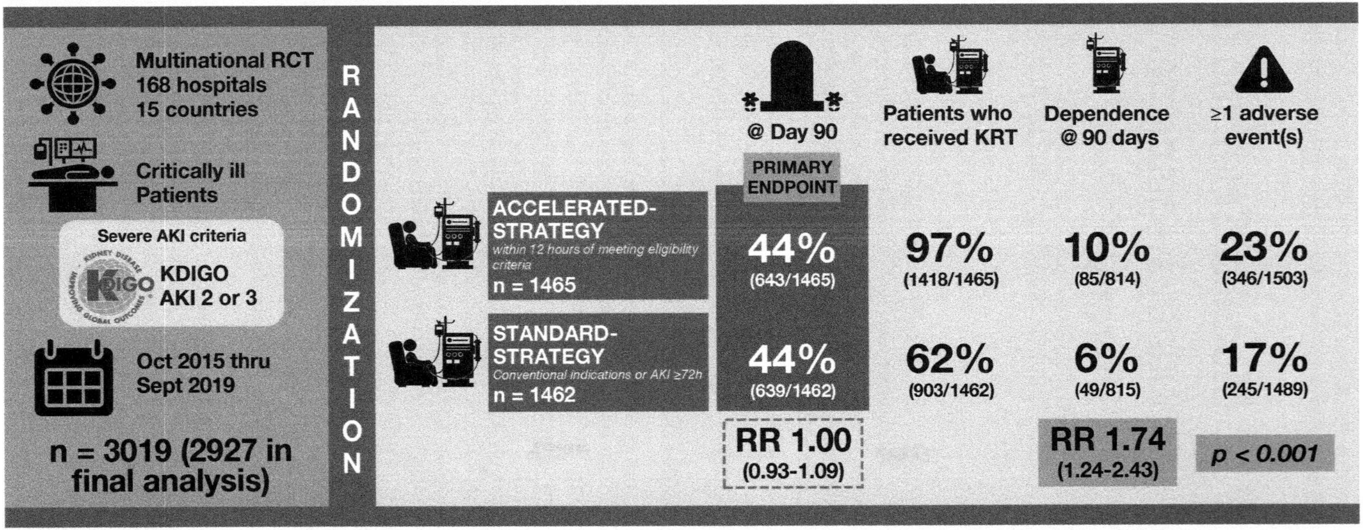

Conclusion: Among critically ill patients with acute kidney injury, an accelerated kidney replacement strategy did not confer a lower risk of death at 90 days than a standard strategy.

STARRT-AKI Investigators. ***Timing of Initiation of Kidney-Replacement Therapy in Acute Kidney Injury.*** N Engl J Med. 2020;383(3):240-251.

VISUAL ABSTRACT 31.4

Modality Selection of Kidney Replacement Therapy

Madhuri Ramakrishnan and Anitha Vijayan

INTRODUCTION

Providing safe and effective kidney replacement therapy (KRT) for patients with acute kidney injury (AKI) in the intensive care unit (ICU) is critical to improving patient outcomes. There are various types of modalities of KRT available for use, and selection of a particular modality depends on patient factors, physician preferences, and institutional resources. The available modalities of KRT include continuous kidney replacement therapy (CKRT), prolonged intermittent kidney replacement therapy (PIKRT), intermittent hemodialysis (IHD), and peritoneal dialysis (PD). In this chapter, we compare and contrast the various modalities of KRT used in the management of AKI.

CONTINUOUS KIDNEY REPLACEMENT THERAPY

Solute clearance during CKRT transpires via convection (solvent drag), diffusion, or a combination of the two mechanisms. Adsorption (adherence of molecules to the filter membrane) does not play a major role in solute clearance during CKRT. Continuous venovenous hemofiltration (CVVH), continuous venovenous hemodialysis (CVVHD), and continuous venovenous hemodiafiltration (CVVHDF) are the three modalities of CKRT for solute clearance and ultrafiltration. In addition, slow continuous ultrafiltration (SCUF) can be prescribed when the sole purpose of extracorporeal support is volume removal. CKRT is the recommended modality for hemodynamically unstable, critically ill patients with AKI.[1] CKRT is also the preferred modality in patients with AKI who have acute brain injury or cerebral edema, because hemodynamic fluctuations during IHD can potentially increase ICP and increase the risk for neurologic impairment.[1-3] The recommended dose for CKRT is an effluent flow rate of 20 to 25 mL/kg/hr.[1] The various modalities of CKRT are described further. **Table 32.1** outlines the dialysate, replacement fluid, ultrafiltration, and blood flow rates among the three modalities.

Continuous venovenous hemofiltration: CVVH utilizes convective clearance for solute removal. The movement of fluid across the membrane, driven by transmembrane pressure gradient (TMP), will move solutes through the membrane. Solute clearance is determined by the rate of ultrafiltration, which has to be high to allow effective solute removal. Replacement fluid (a solution with electrolyte composition similar to extracellular fluid) is added back to circulation, to prevent hypovolemia and maintain homeostasis. Therefore, the net ultrafiltration rate or net fluid removal rate is the difference between the applied ultrafiltration flow

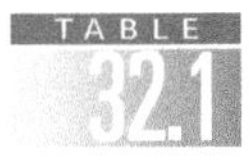

Characteristics of CKRT Modalities

Parameter	CVVH	CVVHD	CVVHDF
Solute transport	Convection	Diffusion	Convection + Diffusion
Blood flow rate [Q_B] (mL/min)	150-300	150-300	150-300
Dialysate flow rate [Q_D] (mL/kg/hr)	0	20-25	10-12.5
Replacement fluid rate [Q_R] (mL/kg/hr)	20-25	0	10-12.5
Ultrafiltration rate [Q_{UF}] (mL/kg/hr)[a]	20-31	0-6	10-18.5
Net ultrafiltration rate [Q_{NET}]	$Q_{UF} - Q_R$	Q_{UF}	$Q_{UF} - Q_R$
Effluent flow rate [Q_{EFF}]	Q_{UF}	$Q_D + Q_{NET}$	$Q_{UF} + Q_D$

CKRT, continuous kidney replacement therapy; CVVH, continuous venovenous hemofiltration; CVVHD, continuous venovenous hemodialysis; CVVHDF, continuous venovenous hemodiafiltration; UF, ultrafiltration.

[a]Displayed UF rates are an example. Exact UF rates may vary depending on hourly UF targets.

rate and replacement fluid flow rate. Convective clearance is efficient in removing both small (<100 Da) and middle molecules (100-5,000 Da) such as cytokines. Replacement fluid can be administered either prefilter or postfilter (**Figure 32.1A** and **B**). Prefilter dilution results in approximately 15% reduction in solute clearance.[4] Postdilution will increase filtration fraction and is associated with reduced filter life because of clotting.[5]

Continuous venovenous hemodialysis: CVVHD uses diffusive clearance for removal of molecules across a semipermeable membrane. Dialysate solution runs countercurrent to the blood, and molecules move across the membrane from high to low concentration (**Figure 32.1C**). CVVHD is ideal for small molecular clearance, but does not provide significant clearance of middle molecules.[4] Ultrafiltration allows for fluid removal; however, compared to continuous hemofiltration, the ultrafiltration rate is lower and limited to net fluid removal alone.

Continuous venovenous hemodiafiltration: CVVHDF combines diffusive and convective clearance for solute removal. The net ultrafiltration, similar to CVVH, is the difference between the applied ultrafiltration rate and replacement fluid rate. Similar to CVVH, replacement fluid can be administered pre- or postfilter (**Figure 32.1D** and **E**).

Slow continuous ultrafiltration: SCUF is the application of ultrafiltration alone for removal of plasma water. The ultrafiltration rate is low, and there is no effective solute clearance. Therefore, SCUF is recommended only when the sole purpose for initiating KRT is fluid removal.

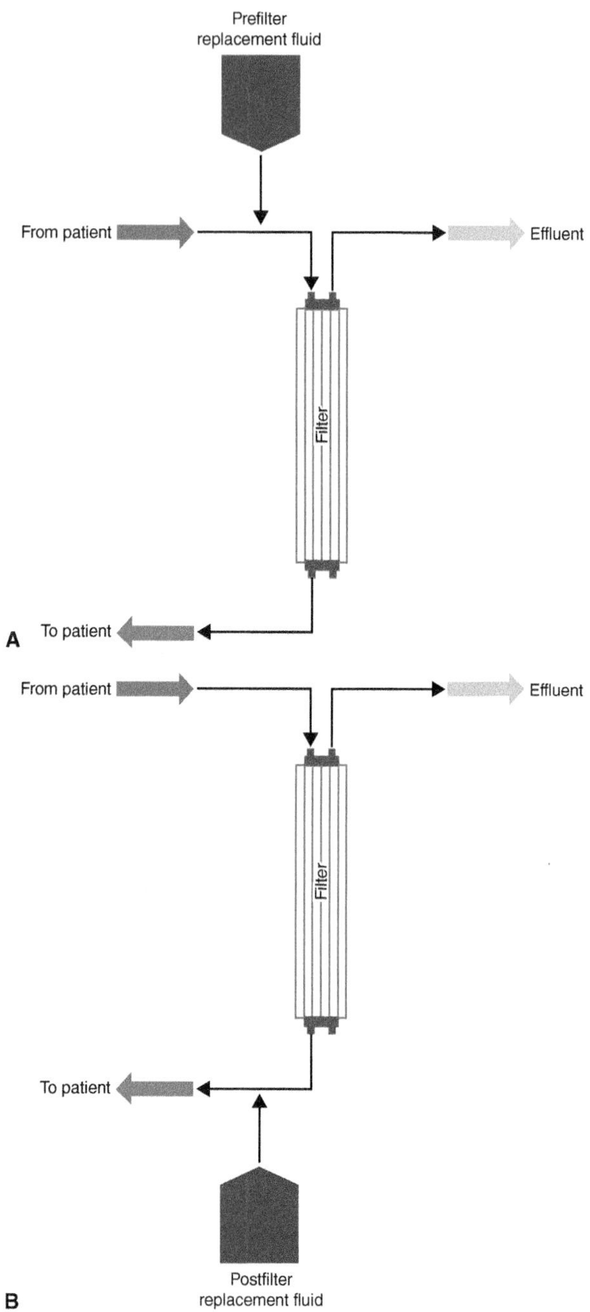

FIGURE 32.1: **A:** Schematic of continuous venovenous hemofiltration (CVVH) with prefilter administration of replacement fluid. **B:** Schematic of CVVH with postfilter administration of replacement fluid.

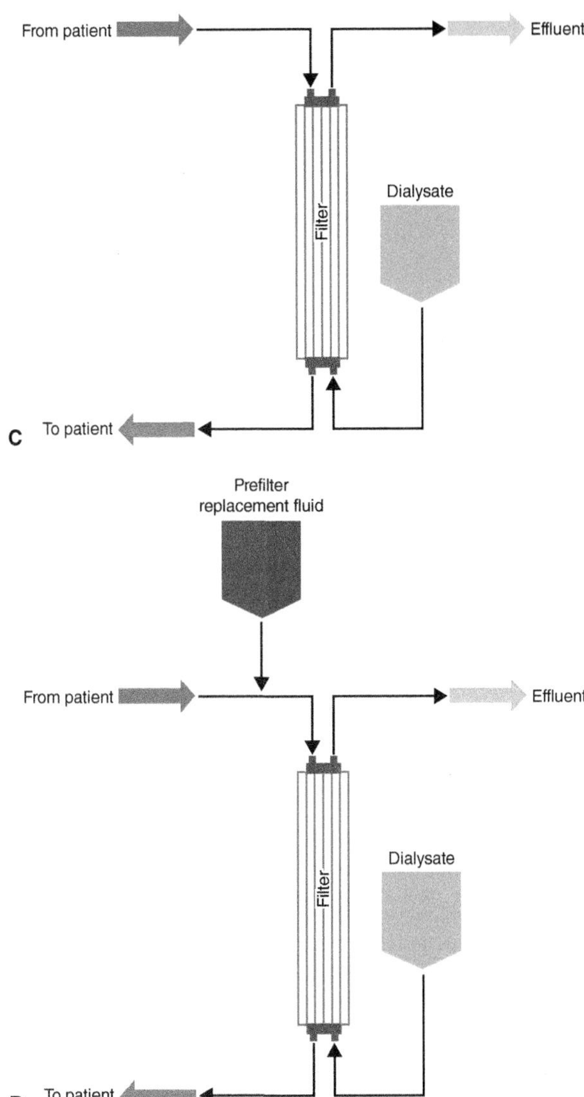

FIGURE 32.1: (*continued*) **C:** Schematic of continuous venovenous hemodialysis (CVVHD). **D:** Schematic of continuous venovenous hemodiafiltration (CVVHDF) with prefilter administration of replacement fluid.

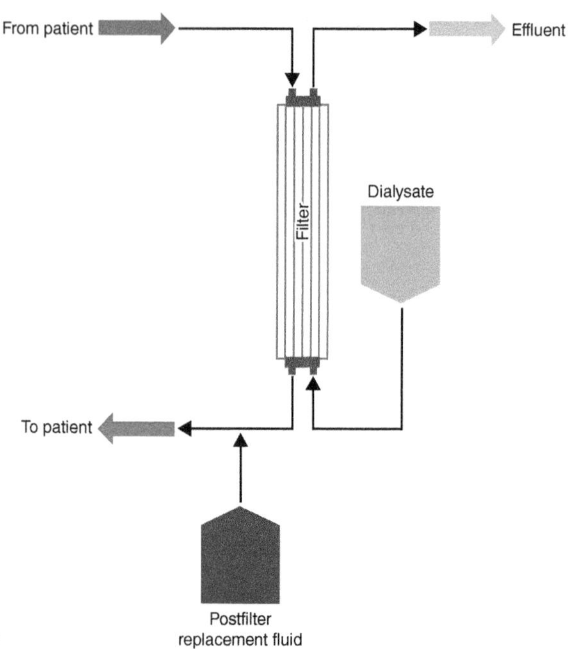

FIGURE 32.1: (*continued*) **E:** Schematic of CVVHDF with postfilter administration of replacement fluid.

CONVECTION VERSUS DIFFUSION IN CONTINUOUS KIDNEY REPLACEMENT THERAPY

There is no difference for small molecular clearance between diffusive and convective modalities.[4] Some studies have suggested that convective clearance reduces mediators of inflammation in systemic inflammatory response syndrome.[6] However, a decrease in the level of plasma cytokines and other inflammatory mediators with CVVH[6,7] has not consistently translated to a difference in patient outcomes.[8] In the Optimal Mode of Clearance in critically ill patients with AKI (OMAKI) study by Wald and colleagues, CVVH, as compared to CVVHD, was associated with a decrease in vasopressor requirements, but there was no improvement in survival (**Visual Abstract 32.1**).[8] In a single-center study of 371 patients with AKI, CVVHDF was associated with improved 28-day survival, when compared to CVVH (59% vs 39%, respectively).[9] However, it must be noted that dose of KRT was significantly higher in the CVVHDF group (42 vs 25 mL/kg/hr) and therefore the benefit seen with CVVHDF cannot be explained solely based on the difference in the mechanism of solute clearance. A meta-analysis of 19 randomized controlled studies comparing CVVH to CVVHD demonstrated no difference in mortality or other clinical outcomes.[10]

INTERMITTENT HEMODIALYSIS

IHD is used primarily for the management of AKI in hemodynamically stable patients. IHD is an ideal choice when rapid clearance of a solute (e.g., life-threatening hyperkalemia), prompt correction of severe metabolic acidosis, or immediate

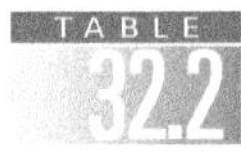

TABLE 32.2 Advantages and Disadvantages of CKRT and IHD

	CKRT	IHD
Hemodynamic stability	++	–
Fluid balance achievement	+	–
Continuous metabolic control	+	–
Stable intracranial pressure	++	–
Unlimited nutrition	+	–
Need for intensive care nursing support	+	–
Rapid removal of toxins	–	+
Limited anticoagulation	–	+
Need for hemodialysis nursing support	±	+
Patient mobility	–	+

CKRT, continuous kidney replacement therapy; IHD, intermittent hemodialysis.

clearance of a dialyzable toxin (e.g., lithium overdose) is required, even in hemodynamically unstable patients. Current recommendation is to prescribe IHD to deliver a single-pool Kt/V_{urea} of 1.3 (**Table 32.2**), three times per week.[11-13] Additional IHD treatments can be provided as needed for hypervolemia, hyperkalemia, or other indications. Routinely increasing the frequency of IHD to greater than three treatments per week has not demonstrated improvement in outcomes and may impair kidney recovery.[11,14]

COMPARISON OF INTERMITTENT HEMODIALYSIS TO CONTINUOUS KIDNEY REPLACEMENT THERAPY

Prospective observational and randomized controlled trials, after adjusting for severity of illness, have not demonstrated improved patient survival with CKRT compared to IHD (**Visual Abstract 32.2**) (**Table 32.3**).[15-22] In addition, data do not show that one modality may be superior to another in terms of kidney recovery. One meta-analysis suggested that initial treatment with IHD may be associated with higher rates of dialysis dependence, but this conclusion was based on 16 observational studies.[23] Randomized controlled trials have not demonstrated any difference in the rate of kidney recovery between patients with AKI initiated on IHD and CKRT (Visual Abstract 32.2).[15,20,21] In patients with AKI who have traumatic brain injury, other causes of raised intracranial pressure (ICP), or end-stage liver disease with encephalopathy, CKRT is associated with stabilization of ICP and improved cerebral perfusion when compared to IHD.[24] Cerebral hypoperfusion and sudden fluctuations in serum osmolality may be some of the factors associated with changes in ICP during IHD.[2,3] Patients with hemodynamic instability, especially because of sepsis, may benefit from a continuous modality as it offers the option for slower solute removal and ultrafiltration, which are not feasible during a 4-hour IHD session.

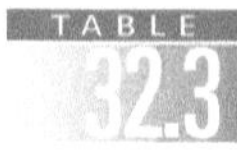

Prospective Trials Comparing CKRT to IHD

Investigator/Year of Publication	Number of Patients	Study Design	IHD % Mortality	CKRT % Mortality	*p* Value
Guerin et al (2002)[17,a]	587	IHD/CVVH or CVVHDF	58.8	79.4	<0.001
Mehta et al (2001)[41]	166	IHD vs CVVHDF[b]	47.6	65.5	<0.02
Gasparovic et al (2003)[16]	104	IHD vs CVVH	59.6	71.1	ns
Augustine et al (2004)[15]	80	IHD vs CVVHD	70	67.5	ns
Uehlinger et al (2005)[20]	125	IHD vs CVVHDF	51	47	0.72
Vinsonneau et al (2006)[21]	259	IHD vs CVVHDF	68.5	67.4	0.98
Lins et al. (2009)[18]	316	IHD vs CVVH	62.5	58.1	0.43
Schefold et al (2014)[19]	252	IHD vs CVVH	60.5	56.1	0.5
Truche et al (2016)[22,a]	1360	IHD vs CVVH or CVVHD	35	46.5	ns

Mortality reported as in-hospital mortality, 14-day mortality, 30-day mortality, or 60-day mortality in different studies. CKRT, continuous Kidney replacement therapy; CVVH, continuous venovenous hemofiltration; CVVHD, continuous venovenous hemodialysis; CVVHDF, continuous venovenous hemodiafiltration; IHD, intermittent hemodialysis.
[a]Prospective multicenter observational trials.
[b]15.5% of CKRT were treated with CVVHDF.

PROLONGED INTERMITTENT KIDNEY REPLACEMENT THERAPY

The term PIKRT encompasses a wide array of hybrid KRTs that do not fall into the traditional realm of continuous or intermittent procedures. In one of the early descriptions of PIKRT, a modified IHD machine was used to deliver diffusive clearance over 6 to 8 hours overnight, with a blood flow rate of 200 mL/min and dialysate flow rate of 300 mL/min to critically ill patients with AKI.[25] Subsequently, numerous publications have described hybrid therapies using various equipment and modalities of clearance.[26] The most commonly used term, sustained low-efficiency dialysis (SLED), in which there is slow diffusive clearance over a prolonged period, is utilized. Although majority of publications reported diffusive clearance during PIKRT, a few have reported convective clearance or combination of both.[27-30] Most centers have used a modified IHD machine, but our center and others utilize a traditional CKRT machine to deliver PIKRT.[26,28] PIKRT can be used as a substitute for CKRT or IHD, or as a transition therapy from continuous to intermittent KRT. In the majority of the institutions worldwide, PIKRT is used as a substitute for CKRT and not as a substitute for IHD.[31] When compared to IHD, PIKRT offers longer duration of therapy, with lower dialysate and blood flow rates and therefore more hemodynamic stability. PIKRT also can negate the need for one-on-one dialysis nursing which is normally required during IHD in the ICU.[25,32] In contrast to CKRT, PIKRT does not subject the patient to KRT for 24 hours; at the same time, PIKRT allows for adequate small molecular clearance and ultrafiltration without significant hemodynamic fluctuations.[26] PIKRT allows the hemodynamically unstable patient to go for radiologic and surgical procedures and perform physical therapy while receiving sufficient KRT for solute clearance and metabolic control. In our center, PIKRT is performed at night, leaving the daytime for various procedures and physical therapy. The key differences between IHD, CKRT, and PIKRT are highlighted in **Table 32.4**. Unlike IHD and CKRT, there is no consensus regarding the dosing and frequency of PIKRT treatments.

COMPARISON OF PROLONGED INTERMITTENT KIDNEY REPLACEMENT THERAPY WITH CONTINUOUS KIDNEY REPLACEMENT THERAPY

PIKRT is considered an alternative to CKRT for hemodynamically unstable patients.[12] In the largest randomized controlled trial comparing SLED (using batched dialysate) to CVVH in 232 critically ill patients with AKI, there was no difference in the primary outcome of 90-day mortality (49.6% and 55.6%, respectively) (**Visual Abstract 32.3**).[32] There was no difference in hemodynamic parameters between the two groups, but the SLED group demonstrated decreased duration of mechanical ventilation, ICU stay, and shorter time to kidney recovery. SLED was also associated with reduced nursing time. It should be noted that this was a single-center study and CVVH patients were prescribed an effluent flow rate of 35 mL/kg/hr, and achieved an effluent flow rate of almost 31 mL/kg/hr, which is higher than recommended effluent flow rates of 20 to 25 mL/kg/hr. Solute clearance (e.g., urea clearance) was not measured and therefore it is difficult to ascertain whether delivered dose of therapy was similar between the two groups. A pooled analysis of observational studies demonstrated lower mortality risk with PIKRT compared with CKRT, but this probably reflected selection bias as PIKRT may have been chosen specifically for the less sick patients.[33] In the same paper, meta-analysis of seven randomized controlled trials showed no difference in mortality between SLED and CKRT.[33]

PERITONEAL DIALYSIS

PD was the earliest modality of KRT used in AKI, but its use decreased with the advent of IHD. PD continued to be utilized for hemodynamically unstable patients until technologic advancements led to the development of CKRT in the 1980s. However, the most recent guidelines from the International Society of Peritoneal Dialysis (ISPD) recommend that PD should be considered as a suitable alternative to blood-based therapies for AKI.[34] PD is used more frequently in the pediatric population and in adults in resource-poor settings.[34] In resource-poor settings, manual PD offers advantage over blood-based KRT in that it does not require electricity. Other advantages of PD include less potential for dialysis disequilibrium, avoidance of blood contact with a synthetic membrane, and lack of requirement of anticoagulation. Disadvantages include unpredictable ultrafiltration and solute clearance, risk for peritonitis, and inability to perform PD in those with abdominal surgeries and/or peritoneal injury.

Delivering PD in the ICU is similar to those in the outpatient settings and can be either as automated PD via cycler or as manual exchanges. Access for PD requires the

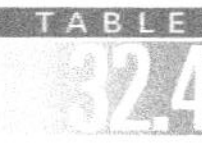

TABLE 32.4 Comparison of Different Modalities of Extracorporeal KRT

	IHD	CKRT	PIKRT
Clearance	Diffusion	Diffusion, convection, or both	Diffusion, convection, or both[a]
Type of machine	Standard IHD machine	Standard CKRT machine	Either IHD or CKRT machine[b]
Q_b (mL/min)	400-500	100-200	150-400
Q_d (mL/min)	600-800	25-30	100-200
Duration	3-4 hr	Continuous	6-12 hr
Frequency	3 d/wk	Continuous	3-7 d/wk
Timing of procedure	Usually daytime	Continuous	Daytime or night
Anticoagulation	Can be performed without anticoagulation	Usually requires anticoagulation	Can be performed without anticoagulation
Vascular access	AVF/AVG/CVC	CVC[c]	CVC[c]
Usual UF rate	0-5,000 mL/3-4 hr	0-200 mL/hr	0-4,000 mL/6-12 hr
Required dialysis nursing time	High	Low	Low to moderate
Patient location	ICU, ward, step-down unit	ICU	ICU or step-down unit
Cost	$	$$$	$$

$ = estimate of cost; AVF, arteriovenous fistula; AVG, arteriovenous graft; CKRT, continuous kidney replacement therapy; CVC, central venous catheter; ICU, intensive care unit; IHD, intermittent hemodialysis; PIKRT, prolonged intermittent kidney replacement therapy; Q_b, blood flow rate; Q_d, dialysate flow rate; KRT, kidney replacement therapy; UF, ultrafiltration.

[a]Majority of PIKRT trials have reported a diffusive modality.

[b]Majority of PIKRT trials have used an IHD machine.

[c]One center has reported safely using AVF and AVG for CKRT.[42]

Table adapted from Edrees F, Li T, Vijayan A. Prolonged intermittent kidney replacement therapy. *Adv Chronic Kidney Dis.* 2016;23(3):195-202, with permission from Elsevier.

placement of either a flexible or a rigid catheter, and ISPD guidelines recommend that tunneled catheters be placed to avoid leaks and reduce infection rates.[34] Similar to outpatient PD, a closed Y connection delivery system is recommended, but this may not be feasible in low-resource areas. The standard outpatient PD utilizes a lactate buffered solution. However, similar to CKRT, bicarbonate-based solution may be preferable in critically ill patients as this has been associated with more rapid improvement in metabolic acidosis in one small study.[35] The dose of PD for the management of AKI is undetermined, although a systematic review recommended a standard Kt/V_{urea} of 2.1, based on extrapolation from extracorporeal therapies.

COMPARISON OF PERITONEAL DIALYSIS TO INTERMITTENT HEMODIALYSIS AND CONTINUOUS KIDNEY REPLACEMENT THERAPY

Data regarding the use of PD in the management of AKI are limited. Observational studies have suggested that PD can be a safe alternative to IHD and CKRT for AKI in the ICU.[36] Few randomized trials have compared PD to extracorporeal KRT for the management of AKI and have shown conflicting results.[37-40] A systematic review of 24 studies, including 4 randomized controlled studies, concluded that there is no evidence to suggest any significant difference in mortality between PD and the extracorporeal methods of KRT.[36]

SUMMARY

KRT plays a vital supportive role in the management of critically ill patients with AKI. KRT can be performed using any of the modalities—CKRT, PIKRT, IHD, and PD—depending on available equipment, personnel, and resources. Certain patient factors and clinical situations may dictate the use of one modality over another at initiation of KRT. However, selection of modality of KRT should be considered as a dynamic process, and a patient's clinical condition may warrant the transition from one modality to another depending on hemodynamic status and other factors. Future studies should be directed toward optimizing the prescription of the various modalities, with respect to standardizing the dose of KRT, addressing dosing of medications with each modality, and standardizing the terminology and equipment used for KRT.

References

1. KDIGO. Section 5: dialysis interventions for treatment of AKI. *Kidney Int Suppl.* 2012;2(1):89-115.
2. Lund A, Damholt MB, Wiis J, Kelsen J, Strange DG, Moller K. Intracranial pressure during hemodialysis in patients with acute brain injury. *Acta Anaesthesiol Scand.* 2019;63(4):493-499.
3. Regolisti G, Maggiore U, Cademartiri C, et al. Cerebral blood flow decreases during intermittent hemodialysis in patients with acute kidney injury, but not in patients with end-stage renal disease. *Nephrol Dial Transplant.* 2013;28(1):79-85.
4. Brunet S, Leblanc M, Geadah D, Parent D, Courteau S, Cardinal J. Diffusive and convective solute clearances during continuous renal replacement therapy at various dialysate and ultrafiltration flow rates. *Am J Kidney Dis.* 1999;34(3):486-492.
5. Uchino S, Fealy N, Baldwin I, Morimatsu H, Bellomo R. Pre-dilution vs. post-dilution during continuous veno-venous hemofiltration: impact on filter life and azotemic control. *Nephron Clin Pract.* 2003;94(4):c94-c98.
6. Kellum JA, Johnson JP, Kramer D, Palevsky P, Brady JJ, Pinsky MR. Diffusive vs. convective therapy: effects on mediators of inflammation in patient with severe systemic inflammatory response syndrome. *Crit Care Med.* 1998;26(12):1995-2000.
7. Morgera S, Slowinski T, Melzer C, et al. Renal replacement therapy with high-cutoff hemofilters: impact of convection and diffusion on cytokine clearances and protein status. *Am J Kidney Dis.* 2004;43(3):444-453.

8. Wald R, Friedrich JO, Bagshaw SM, et al. Optimal mode of clearance in critically ill patients with acute kidney injury (OMAKI)—a pilot randomized controlled trial of hemofiltration versus hemodialysis: a Canadian Critical Care Trials Group project. *Crit Care.* 2012;16(5):R205.
9. Saudan P, Niederberger M, De Seigneux S, et al. Adding a dialysis dose to continuous hemofiltration increases survival in patients with acute renal failure. *Kidney Int.* 2006;70(7):1312-1317.
10. Friedrich JO, Wald R, Bagshaw SM, Burns KE, Adhikari NK. Hemofiltration compared to hemodialysis for acute kidney injury: systematic review and meta-analysis. *Crit Care.* 2012;16(4):R146.
11. Palevsky PM, Zhang JH, O'Connor TZ, et al; VA/NIH Acute Renal Failure Trial Network. Intensity of renal support in critically ill patients with acute kidney injury. *N Engl J Med.* 2008;359(1):7-20.
12. Palevsky PM, Liu KD, Brophy PD, et al. KDOQI US commentary on the 2012 KDIGO clinical practice guideline for acute kidney injury. *Am J Kidney Dis.* 2013;61(5):649-672.
13. Vijayan A, Palevsky PM. Dosing of renal replacement therapy in acute kidney injury. *Am J Kidney Dis.* 2012;59(4):569-576.
14. Vijayan A, Delos Santos RB, Li T, Goss CW, Palevsky PM. Effect of frequent dialysis on renal recovery: results from the acute renal failure trial network study. *Kidney Int Rep.* 2018;3(2):456-463.
15. Augustine JJ, Sandy D, Seifert TH, Paganini EP. A randomized controlled trial comparing intermittent with continuous dialysis in patients with ARF. *Am J Kidney Dis.* 2004;44(6):1000-1007.
16. Gasparovic V, Filipovic-Grcic I, Merkler M, Pisl Z. Continuous renal replacement therapy (CRRT) or intermittent hemodialysis (IHD)—what is the procedure of choice in critically ill patients? *Ren Fail.* 2003;25(5):855-862.
17. Guerin C, Girard R, Selli JM, Ayzac L. Intermittent versus continuous renal replacement therapy for acute renal failure in intensive care units: results from a multicenter prospective epidemiological survey. *Intensive Care Med.* 2002;28(10):1411-1418.
18. Lins RL, Elseviers MM, Van der Niepen P, et al; SHARF Investigators. Intermittent versus continuous renal replacement therapy for acute kidney injury patients admitted to the intensive care unit: results of a randomized clinical trial. *Nephrol Dial Transplant.* 2009;24(2):512-518.
19. Schefold JC, von Haehling S, Pschowski R, et al. The effect of continuous versus intermittent renal replacement therapy on the outcome of critically ill patients with acute renal failure (CONVINT): a prospective randomized controlled trial. *Crit Care.* 2014;18(1):R11.
20. Uehlinger DE, Jakob SM, Ferrari P, et al. Comparison of continuous and intermittent renal replacement therapy for acute renal failure. *Nephrol Dial Transplant.* 2005;20(8):1630-1637.
21. Vinsonneau C, Camus C, Combes A, et al. Continuous venovenous haemodiafiltration versus intermittent haemodialysis for acute renal failure in patients with multiple-organ dysfunction syndrome: a multicentre randomised trial. *Lancet.* 2006;368(9533):379-385.
22. Truche AS, Darmon M, Bailly S, et al. Continuous renal replacement therapy versus intermittent hemodialysis in intensive care patients: impact on mortality and renal recovery. *Intensive Care Med.* 2016;42(9):1408-1417.
23. Schneider AG, Bellomo R, Bagshaw SM, et al. Choice of renal replacement therapy modality and dialysis dependence after acute kidney injury: a systematic review and meta-analysis. *Intensive Care Med.* 2013;39(6):987-997.
24. Davenport A, Will EJ, Davison AM. Continuous vs. intermittent forms of haemofiltration and/or dialysis in the management of acute renal failure in patients with defective cerebral autoregulation at risk of cerebral oedema. *Contrib Nephrol.* 1991;93:225-233.
25. Kumar VA, Craig M, Depner TA, Yeun JY. Extended daily dialysis: a new approach to renal replacement for acute renal failure in the intensive care unit. *Am J Kidney Dis.* 2000;36(2):294-300.
26. Edrees F, Li T, Vijayan A. Prolonged intermittent renal replacement therapy. *Adv Chronic Kidney Dis.* 2016;23(3):195-202.
27. Abe M, Okada K, Suzuki M, et al. Comparison of sustained hemodiafiltration with continuous venovenous hemodiafiltration for the treatment of critically ill patients with acute kidney injury. *Artif Organs.* 2010;34(4):331-338.
28. Gashti CN, Salcedo S, Robinson V, Rodby RA. Accelerated venovenous hemofiltration: early technical and clinical experience. *Am J Kidney Dis.* 2008;51(5):804-810.
29. Marshall MR, Ma T, Galler D, Rankin AP, Williams AB. Sustained low-efficiency daily diafiltration (SLEDD-f) for critically ill patients requiring renal replacement therapy: towards an adequate therapy. *Nephrol Dial Transplant.* 2004;19(4):877-884.
30. Naka T, Baldwin I, Bellomo R, Fealy N, Wan L. Prolonged daily intermittent renal replacement therapy in ICU patients by ICU nurses and ICU physicians. *Int J Artif Organs.* 2004;27(5):380-387.

31. Marshall MR, Creamer JM, Foster M, et al. Mortality rate comparison after switching from continuous to prolonged intermittent renal replacement for acute kidney injury in three intensive care units from different countries. *Nephrol Dial Transplant.* 2011;26(7):2169-2175.
32. Schwenger V, Weigand MA, Hoffmann O, et al. Sustained low efficiency dialysis using a single-pass batch system in acute kidney injury—a randomized interventional trial: the Renal Replacement Therapy Study in Intensive Care Unit Patients. *Crit Care.* 2012;16(4):R140.
33. Zhang L, Yang J, Eastwood GM, Zhu G, Tanaka A, Bellomo R. Extended daily dialysis versus continuous renal replacement therapy for acute kidney injury: a meta-analysis. *Am J Kidney Dis.* 2015;66(2):322-330.
34. Cullis B, Abdelraheem M, Abrahams G, et al. Peritoneal dialysis for acute kidney injury. *Perit Dial Int.* 2014;34(5):494-517.
35. Thongboonkerd V, Lumlertgul D, Supajatura V. Better correction of metabolic acidosis, blood pressure control, and phagocytosis with bicarbonate compared to lactate solution in acute peritoneal dialysis. *Artif Organs.* 2001;25(2):99-108.
36. Chionh CY, Soni SS, Finkelstein FO, Ronco C, Cruz DN. Use of peritoneal dialysis in AKI: a systematic review. *Clin J Am Soc Nephrol.* 2013;8(10):1649-1660.
37. Phu NH, Hien TT, Mai NT, et al. Hemofiltration and peritoneal dialysis in infection-associated acute renal failure in Vietnam. *N Engl J Med.* 2002;347(12):895-902.
38. Al-Hwiesh A, Abdul-Rahman I, Finkelstein F, et al. Acute kidney injury in critically ill patients: a prospective randomized study of tidal peritoneal dialysis versus continuous renal replacement therapy. *Ther Apher Dial.* 2018;22(4):371-379.
39. George J, Varma S, Kumar S, Thomas J, Gopi S, Pisharody R. Comparing continuous venovenous hemodiafiltration and peritoneal dialysis in critically ill patients with acute kidney injury: a pilot study. *Perit Dial Int.* 2011;31(4):422-429.
40. Gabriel DP, Caramori JT, Martim LC, Barretti P, Balbi AL. High volume peritoneal dialysis vs daily hemodialysis: a randomized, controlled trial in patients with acute kidney injury. *Kidney Int Suppl.* 2008(108):S87-S93.
41. Mehta RL, McDonald B, Gabbai FB, et al; Collaborative Group for Treatment of ARF in the ICU. A randomized clinical trial of continuous versus intermittent dialysis for acute renal failure. *Kidney Int.* 2001;60(3):1154-1163.
42. Al Rifai A, Sukul N, Wonnacott R, Heung M. Safety of arteriovenous fistulae and grafts for continuous renal replacement therapy: the Michigan experience. *Hemodial Int.* 2018;22(1):50-55.

Can CVVH be feasibly compared to CVVHD in critically ill patients with acute kidney injury requiring CKRT?

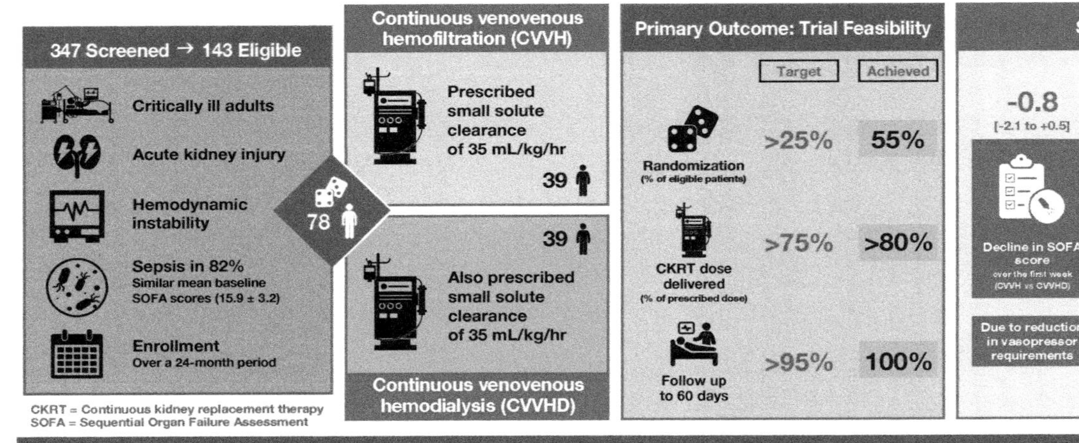

Conclusion: A large trial comparing CVVH to CVVHD would be feasible. There is a trend toward improved vasopressor requirements among CVVH-treated patients over the first week of treatment.

Wald R, Friedrich JO, Bagshaw SM, et al. ***Optimal Mode of clearance in critically ill patients with Acute Kidney Injury (OMAKI)--a pilot randomized controlled trial of hemofiltration versus hemodialysis: a Canadian Critical Care Trials Group project.*** Crit Care. 2012;16(5): R205.

VISUAL ABSTRACT 33.1

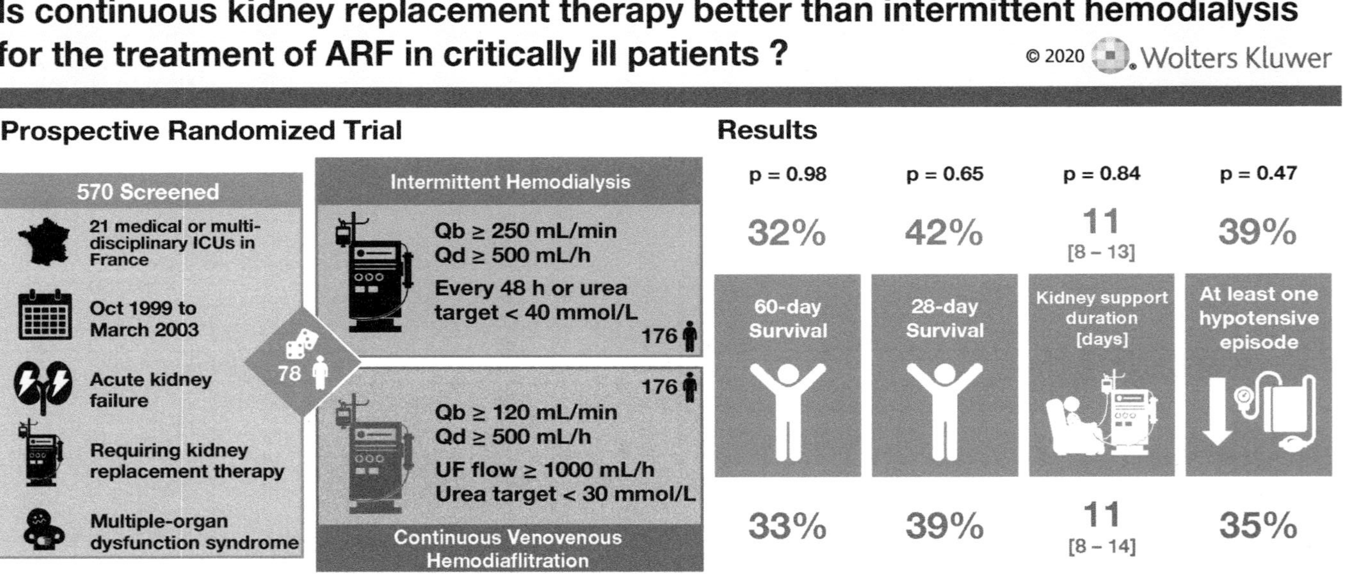

Conclusion: In this randomised study comparing continuous venovenous hemodiafiltration with intermittent hemodialysis for ARF in MODS, there was no difference in survival at any time.

Vinsonneau C, Camus C, Combes A, et al. ***Continuous venovenous haemodiafiltration versus intermittent haemodialysis for acute kidney failure in patients with multiple-organ dysfunction syndrome: a multicentre randomised trial.*** Lancet. 2006;368(9533):379-85.

VISUAL ABSTRACT 32.2

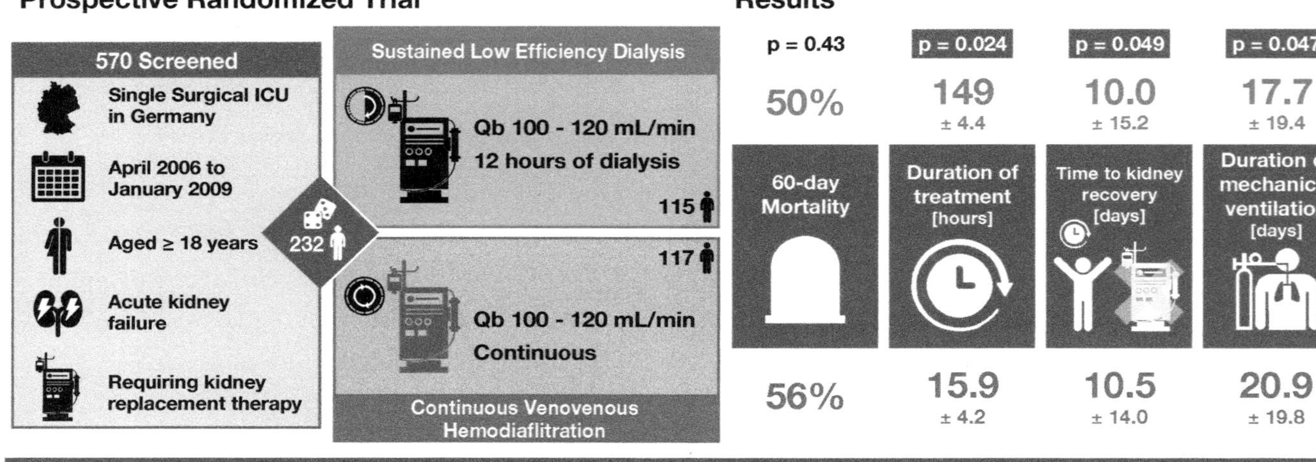

VISUAL ABSTRACT 32.3

Anticoagulation and Kidney Replacement Therapy

Andrew B. Barker and Ashita J. Tolwani

INTRODUCTION

Continuous kidney replacement therapy (CKRT) is the preferred form of dialysis in hemodynamically unstable critically ill patients with acute kidney injury (AKI) and often requires anticoagulation to prevent clotting of the extracorporeal circuit. Contact of blood with the foreign surface of the extracorporeal circuit results in activation of both the intrinsic and extrinsic pathways of coagulation and activation of platelets.[1] Although CKRT is intended to run for 24 hours a day, average daily therapy has been reported to be closer to 16 hours because of interruptions, including circuit clotting.[2,3] Circuit clotting can markedly decrease the effectiveness of CKRT.[4] Adequate CKRT hemofilter survival without anticoagulation has been described in critically ill patients at high bleeding risk because of coagulopathy and liver dysfunction.[5-8] When blood flow, hematocrit, and total effluent flow rates are held constant, purely convective modes of therapy, such as continuous venovenous hemofiltration (CVVH), always have a higher filtration fraction compared with diffusive therapies. Maintaining a filtration fraction less than 20% to 25% can prolong hemofilter patency. Hemofilter survival without anticoagulation can also be prolonged by a well-functioning vascular access, higher blood flow rates, using predilution replacement fluid to reduce the filtration fraction in convective CKRT, decreasing the blood-air contact in the bubble trap, and ensuring prompt reaction to alarms.[9,10]

Despite these measures, most patients on CKRT require some form of anticoagulation (**Table 33.1**). This chapter will discuss the most common

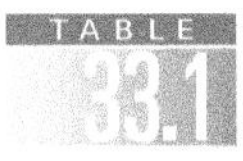

TABLE 33.1 Selection of Anticoagulant for CKRT

	Choice of Anticoagulant for CKRT	
Clinical Condition	**No Liver Failure**	**Severe Liver Failure**
Low risk of bleeding	RCA, UFH	UFH, no anticoagulation
High risk of bleeding	RCA	No anticoagulation
Heparin-induced thrombocytopenia	RCA, argatroban	Bivalirudin

CKRT, continuous kidney replacement therapy; RCA, regional citrate anticoagulation; UFH, unfractionated heparin.

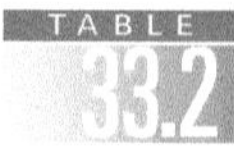

Dosing of Common Anticoagulants for Continuous Kidney Replacement Therapy

Anticoagulant	Loading Dose	Rate	Monitoring
Heparin 500 U/mL	2,000-5,000 U	5-10 U/kg/hr	Target aPTT in the circuit 45-60 s or anti-Xa activity 0.3-0.6 IU/mL
Regional heparin with protamine	N/A	Heparin prefilter: 1,000-1,500 U/hr Protamine postfilter: 10-12 mg/hr	Patient aPTT <45 s and circuit aPTT 50-80 s
Regional citrate anticoagulation	N/A	Infused to achieve a citrate blood concentration 3-4 mmol/L	Target postfilter iCa^{++} <0.35 mmol/L
Enoxaparin	0.15 mg/kg	0.05 mg/kg/hr	Target anti-Xa 0.25-0.35
Dalteparin	15-25 U/kg	5 U/kg/hr	Target anti-Xa 0.25-0.35
Argatroban	100 µg/kg	1 µg/kg/min	Target aPTT 1.5-2 times baseline Reduce initial dose to 0.5 µg/kg/min in the setting of liver failure
Prostacyclin	N/A	2-8 ng/kg/min infused prefilter	N/A

aPTT, activated partial thromboplastin time; iCa, ionized calcium.

anticoagulation options available for CKRT: unfractionated heparin (UFH) and regional citrate anticoagulation (RCA). Less common options include UFH with protamine reversal, low-molecular-weight heparin (LMWH), thrombin antagonists (argatroban and bivalirudin), heparinoids, and platelet-inhibiting agents. **Table 33.2** summarizes dosing of anticoagulants for CKRT.

UNFRACTIONATED HEPARIN

UFH is widely used for CKRT.[11] UFH potentiates antithrombin III by a 1,000-fold, resulting in inhibition of factors IIa (thrombin) and Xa.[12] The molecular weight of UFH ranges from 5,000 to 30,000 Da. The larger heparin fragments have mainly anti-IIa activity, whereas the smaller fragments principally inhibit Xa. The larger fragments are cleared more rapidly than the smaller fragments. As a result, an anticoagulant effect from the inhibited Xa can occur in the setting of a normal activated partial thromboplastin time (aPTT) because of the delayed clearance of the smaller fragments.[13-15] The plasma half-life of UFH is approximately 90 minutes but can increase up to 3 hours in the presence of kidney insufficiency. There are many existing CKRT protocols for systemic heparin anticoagulation; however, an ideal regimen for heparin anticoagulation with CKRT has not been identified. Usually, heparin is administered as an initial bolus of 25 to 50 U/kg or 2,000 to 5,000 IU followed by a continuous infusion of 5 to 10 IU/kg/hr into the arterial limb of the dialysis circuit. The optimal aPTT (i.e., the level at which there is minimal clotting of the filter, with little or no increase in the risk of hemorrhage) is not known with certainty.[6,7,15-20] Typical protocols target the aPTT in the extracorporeal circuit between 45 and 60 seconds or anti-Xa activity between 0.3 and 0.6 IU/mL.

The advantages of UFH are that it is inexpensive, widely available and familiar to physicians and nurses, easy to administer, simple to monitor, and reversible with protamine. Disadvantages include the unpredictable and complex pharmacokinetics of UFH (resulting in dosing variability), the development of heparin-induced thrombocytopenia (HIT), heparin resistance because of low patient antithrombin levels, and the increased risk of hemorrhage.[15] van de Wetering et al[16] demonstrated that the efficacy of UFH for prolonging filter life was proportional to the aPTT and not to the heparin dose. Hemofilter clotting occurred less frequently when the aPTT was increased by 10 seconds, but coincided with a 50% increase in the incidence of intracranial or retroperitoneal bleeding. Considering all the administration methods of heparin, the incidence of bleeding episodes ranges from 10% to 50%, with mortality because of bleeding as high as 15%.[16-18] To minimize the systemic effects of heparin, regional heparin anticoagulation has been attempted by administering UFH prefilter and protamine sulfate postfilter, thus restricting anticoagulation to the circuit. However, protamine sulfate is associated with hypotension and anaphylaxis, and the protocols utilizing heparin and protamine are difficult to standardize.[21,22] An initial ratio between prefilter heparin (in units) and postfilter protamine (in mg) of 100 has been recommended, with subsequent adjustment according to the aPTT. The ratio is adjusted to achieve a patient aPTT less than 45 seconds and a circuit aPTT between 50 and 80 seconds. The amount of protamine required to achieve a target aPTT can vary substantially because the heparin-protamine complex is taken up by the reticuloendothelial system and broken down, thus releasing free heparin and protamine into the circulation.[23] In practice, UFH at 1,000 to 1,500 units/hr is infused prefilter and neutralized with postfilter protamine at 10 to 12 mg/hr. If this approach is used, both circuit and patient aPTT should be closely monitored. Importantly, regional heparinization can still result in HIT.

REGIONAL CITRATE ANTICOAGULATION

Citrate was first reported as an anticoagulant for hemodialysis in the 1960s by Morita et al[24] and for CKRT in 1990 by Mehta et al.[25] Citrate is infused into the blood at the beginning of the extracorporeal circuit and provides anticoagulation by chelating ionized calcium (iCa^{++})[26-28] (**Figure 33.1**). Ionized magnesium is also chelated by citrate but to a lesser extent. Optimal regional anticoagulation occurs when the iCa^{++} concentration in the extracorporeal circuit is below 0.35 mmol/L (measured as the postfilter iCa^{++} level), which corresponds to approximately 3 to 4 mmol of citrate per liter of blood.[29] Because citrate is a small molecule, the majority of the calcium-citrate complex is removed across the hemofilter. Any calcium-citrate complex that remains postfilter is returned to the patient and metabolized to bicarbonate by the liver, kidney, and skeletal muscle. Each citrate molecule potentially yields three bicarbonate molecules: 3Na citrate + $3H_2CO_3 \leftrightarrow$ citric acid + $3NaHCO_3$.[26-28] Calcium released from the calcium-citrate complex helps restore normal iCa^{++} concentrations, although a systemic calcium infusion

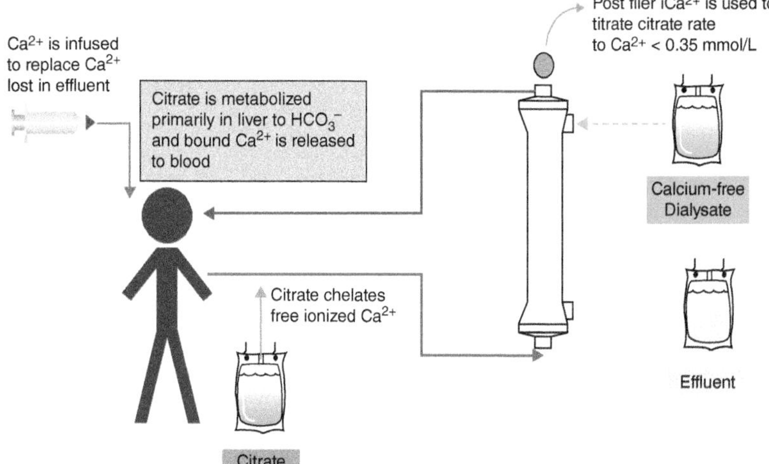

FIGURE 33.1: Regional citrate anticoagulation circuit.

is required to replace the calcium that is lost in the effluent. RCA is reversed by the infusion of a calcium chloride or calcium gluconate into the end of the circuit or directly through a separate intravenous line.[26-28] This rate is constantly adjusted according to frequent measurements of plasma calcium concentration to prevent hypocalcemia or hypercalcemia. Advantages of citrate anticoagulation include the avoidance of systemic anticoagulation and HIT. The disadvantage is that citrate adds complexity and labor intensity to CKRT.

Although RCA has several advantages, potential complications include hypernatremia from the use of commercially available hypertonic citrate solutions (such as 4% trisodium citrate [TSC] and 2.2% anticoagulant citrate dextrose [ACD] solution), hypocalcemia, hypercalcemia, and acid-base disorders.[26-28] It is therefore necessary to frequently monitor acid-base status, electrolytes, and ionized calcium in the systemic circulation. Metabolic alkalosis can result because of excessive citrate load. Strategies to reduce the risk of alkalosis include decreasing the blood flow and thereby decreasing the amount of citrate needed to maintain therapeutic level, or increasing the effluent flow rate.[30,31] Patients with severe liver failure and lactic acidosis may have difficulty with citrate metabolism and develop citrate accumulation, which is characterized by low systemic iCa^{++}, elevated total serum calcium, metabolic acidosis, and an increased anion gap.[32-35] The accumulation of citrate causes the systemic iCa^{++} concentration to fall, whereas the bound fraction of calcium rises. If the calcium infusion is increased to correct the low iCa^{++}, most of the calcium is bound to citrate. A disproportional rise in total calcium occurs, whereas iCa^{++} remains low. As a result, the calcium gap (total calcium − iCa^{++}) or the calcium ratio (total calcium/iCa^{++}) increases. Citrate accumulation is likely when the ratio of total serum calcium to iCa^{++} concentration exceeds 2.5. Citrate accumulation can be managed by decreasing the blood flow, increasing the effluent rate, decreasing the target citrate concentration in the hemofilter, or changing to an alternate form of anticoagulation.[30,31] Metabolic acidosis can also result if the delivery of citrate is insufficient to adequately buffer the acidosis. This can be corrected by increasing the blood flow or decreasing the effluent rate.[30,31] If properly monitored, regional citrate-related complications are uncommon, and RCA has been used safely in patients with advanced liver disease as well as in perioperative liver transplant patients.[36-38]

Because of the potential for electrolyte abnormalities, the patient's electrolytes should be monitored at least every 6 hours and should include iCa^{++}, magnesium, and calculation of the anion gap. At least twice-daily, total blood calcium concentration should be monitored to calculate the calcium ratio or calcium gap. The need for monitoring anticoagulation efficacy in the circuit depends on the method of citrate delivery. If the dose of citrate is fixed in relation to the blood flow, frequent monitoring of circuit iCa^{++} levels (i.e., postfilter iCa^{++} levels) is not necessary as long as blood flow is constant. If the citrate dose is not fixed to a constant blood flow rate, postfilter iCa^{++} levels should be measured at least every 6 hours and the infusion of citrate titrated for an iCa^{++} of less than 0.35 mmol/L. Once steady state is reached after 48 to 72 hours and the patient remains stable, monitoring of electrolytes can be decreased to every 12 hours.

A variety of methods of RCA are described in the literature.[39-56] Citrate is administered either as a separate citrate solution or added to a calcium-free predilution replacement fluid. The anticoagulant effect of citrate can be measured by the postfilter iCa and citrate titrated to maintain the circuit iCa^{++} less than 0.35 mmol/L, or the amount of citrate needed to maintain a concentration of 3 to 4 mmol/L in the blood can be calculated and fixed to the blood flow rate without measurement of postfilter iCa^{++} levels. **Table 33.3** lists the fixed citrate rate needed for various blood flow rates using the most common citrate solutions, 4% TSC and 2.2% ACD-A. The use of citrate anticoagulation may require modification of the dialysate composition, depending on the citrate formulation used. Use of 4% TSC or other hypertonic citrate solutions results in a very significant sodium

TABLE 33.3 Dose of Common Formulations of Citrate for Fixed Blood Flow Rate

QB (mL/min)	4% TSC (mL/hr)	ACD-A (mL/hr)
Amount of Citrate Delivered to Achieve Blood Citrate Concentration of 3 mmol/L		
100	132	159
125	165	200
150	199	239
200	265	319
Amount of Citrate Delivered to Achieve Blood Citrate Concentration of 4 mmol/L		
100	175	210
125	218	262
150	262	315
200	350	420

ACD-A, anticoagulant citrate dextrose A; QB, blood flow rate; TSC, trisodium citrate.

load to the patient (420 mmol/L in a 4% TCA solution), and compensatory hyponatremic replacement and/or dialysate solutions may be required to prevent the development of electrolyte abnormalities. Because citrate provides an alkali load, buffers (e.g., bicarbonate, lactate) may need to be reduced in concentration or deleted from the dialysate and replacement fluids. The dialysate and replacement fluids usually are calcium free to prevent reversal of the citrate effect in the extracorporeal circuit, although calcium-containing solutions have been used successfully.[57,58]

Multiple randomized trials[39-43,59-62] and three meta-analyses[63-65] have suggested that RCA is better than heparin at preserving filter patency and decreases the risk of adverse events, including bleeding. There does not appear to be a survival benefit of either heparin or RCA (See **Visual Abstracts 33.1**, **33.2** and **33.3**).[63-65] The largest meta-analysis (11 randomized trials, 992 patients) compared RCA with either systemic (9 trials) or regional (2 trials) heparin.[65] The risk of circuit loss was lower with RCA compared with regional heparin (hazard ratio [HR] 0.52, 95% confidence interval [CI] 0.35-0.77, $p = 0.001$) and systemic heparin (HR 0.76, 95% CI 0.59-0.98, $p = 0.04$). The risk of bleeding was lower with RCA compared with systemic heparin (relative risk [RR] 0.36, 95% CI 0.21-0.60, $p < 0.001$) and similar between RCA and regional heparin. The authors reported a higher incidence of HIT in the heparin groups, whereas hypocalcemia was increased in citrate groups. No significant survival difference was observed between the groups. They concluded that RCA should be considered as a better anticoagulant than heparin for CKRT in AKI patients who have no contraindications to citrate.

ARGATROBAN

Argatroban is a second-generation direct thrombin inhibitor used in patients with HIT. It is the preferred CKRT anticoagulant in patients with HIT. For argatroban, the most recent literature suggests a bolus of 100 μg/kg followed by a starting infusion of 1 μg/kg/min, or dosing based on the degree of critical illness. A formula proposed to determine the argatroban infusion rate in μg/kg/min is as follows: 2.15 − (0.06 × acute physiology and chronic health evaluation [APACHE] II score) or 2.06 − (0.03 × simplified acute physiology score [SAPS] II score).[66] Dose reduction is required in hepatic failure. The target aPTT is 1.5 to 2 times baseline. If the patient has severe liver disease, the argatroban infusion is decreased to 0.5 μg/kg/min.

CONCLUSION

The choice of anticoagulant for CKRT should be determined by availability, patient characteristics, physician and nursing expertise, and ease of monitoring. Although systemic heparinization has been considered the standard of care for CKRT in the past, multiple randomized controlled trials (RCTs) suggest that RCA is superior in hemofilter survival and bleeding risk when compared to heparin-based systemic anticoagulation. Metabolic complications with RCA can be avoided by the use of strict protocols, appropriate training, and availability of safer citrate solutions and integrated CKRT citrate software. Recent studies show that citrate can even be used in patients with liver failure with increased monitoring and adjustment of citrate dose. For these reasons, the Kidney Disease Improving Global Outcomes (KDIGO) clinical practice guidelines for AKI have recommended RCA as the preferred anticoagulation modality for CKRT in critically ill patients in whom it is not contraindicated.[67]

References

1. Schetz M. Anticoagulation in continuous renal replacement therapy. *Contrib Nephrol.* 2001;(132):283-303.
2. Venkataraman R, Kellum JA, Palevsky P. Dosing patterns for continuous renal replacement therapy at a large academic medical center in the United States. *J Crit Care.* 2002;17:246-250.
3. Luyckx VA, Bonventre JV. Dose of dialysis in acute renal failure. *Semin Dial.* 2004;17:30-36.
4. Tolwani A. Continuous renal-replacement therapy for acute kidney injury. *N Engl J Med.* 2012;367:2505-2514.
5. Bellomo R, Parkin G, Love J, Boyce N. Use of continuous haemodiafiltration: an approach to the management of acute renal failure in the critically ill. *Am J Nephrol.* 1992;12:240-245.
6. Morabito S, Guzzo I, Solazzo A, et al. Continuous renal replacement therapies: anticoagulation in the critically ill at high risk of bleeding. *J Nephrol.* 2003;16:566-571.
7. Tan HK, Baldwin I, Bellomo R. Continuous veno-venous hemofiltration without anticoagulation in high-risk patients. *Intensive Care Med.* 2000;26:1652-1657.
8. Uchino S, Fealy N, Baldwin I, et al. Continuous venovenous hemofiltration without anticoagulation. *ASAIO J.* 2004;50:76-80.
9. Davies H, Leslie G. Maintaining the CRRT circuit: non-anticoagulant alternatives. *Aust Crit Care.* 2006;19:133-138.
10. Joannidis M, Oudemans-van Straaten HM. Clinical review: patency of the circuit in continuous renal replacement therapy. *Crit Care.* 2007;11:218.
11. Uchino S, Bellomo R, Morimatsu H, et al. Continuous renal replacement therapy: a worldwide practice survey. The beginning and ending supportive therapy for the kidney (B.E.S.T. kidney) investigators. *Intensive Care Med.* 2007;33:1563-1570.
12. Damus PS, Hicks M, Rosenberg RD. Anticoagulant action of heparin. *Nature.* 1973;246: 355-357.
13. Baker BA, Adelman MD, Smith PA, Osborn JC. Inability of the activated partial thromboplastin time to predict heparin levels. Time to reassess guidelines for heparin assays. *Arch Intern Med.* 1997;157:2475-2479.
14. Greaves M, Control of Anticoagulation Subcommittee of the Scientific and Standardization Committee of the International Society of Thrombosis and Haemostasis. Limitations of the laboratory monitoring of heparin therapy. Scientific and Standardization Committee Communications: on behalf of the Control of Anticoagulation Subcommittee of the Scientific and Standardization Committee of the International Society of Thrombosis and Haemostasis. *Thromb Haemost.* 2002;87:163-164.
15. Hirsh J, Warkentin TE, Shaughnessy SG, et al. Heparin and low-molecular-weight heparin: mechanisms of action, pharmacokinetics, dosing, monitoring, efficacy, and safety. *Chest.* 2001;119:64S-94S.
16. van de Wetering J, Westendorp RG, van der Hoeven JG, et al. Heparin use in continuous renal replacement procedures: the struggle between filter coagulation and patient hemorrhage. *J Am Soc Nephrol.* 1996;7:145-150.
17. Davenport A, Will EJ, Davison AM. Comparison of the use of standard heparin and prostacyclin anticoagulation in spontaneous and pump-driven extracorporeal circuits in patients with combined acute renal and hepatic failure. *Nephron.* 1994;66:431-437.
18. Martin PY, Chevrolet JC, Suter P, et al. Anticoagulation in patients treated by continuous venovenous hemofiltration: a retrospective study. *Am J Kidney Dis.* 1994;24:806-816.
19. Bellomo R, Teede H, Boyce N. Anticoagulant regimens in acute continuous hemodiafiltration: a comparative study. *Intensive Care Med.* 1993;19:329-332.
20. Leslie GD, Jacobs IG, Clarke GM. Proximally delivered dilute heparin does not improve circuit life in continuous venovenous haemodiafiltration. *Intensive Care Med.* 1996;22:1261-1264.
21. Kaplan AA, Petrillo R. Regional heparinization for continuous arterio-venous hemofiltration (CAVHV). *ASAIO Trans.* 1987;33:312-315.
22. Horrow JC. Protamine: a review of its toxicity. *Anesth Analg.* 1985;64:348-361.
23. Blaufox MD, Hampers CL, Merrill JP. Rebound anticoagulation occurring after regional heparinization for hemodialysis. *Trans Am Soc Artif Intern Organs.* 1966;12:207-209.
24. Morita Y, Johnson RW, Dorn RE, et al. Regional anticoagulation during hemodialysis using citrate. *Am J Med Sci.* 1961;242:32-43.
25. Mehta RL, McDonald BR, Aguilar MM, et al. Regional citrate anticoagulation for continuous arteriovenous hemodialysis in critically ill patients. *Kidney Int.* 1990;38:976-981.
26. Oudemans-van Straaten HM, Ostermann M. Bench-to-bedside review: citrate for continuous renal replacement therapy, from science to practice. *Crit Care.* 2012;16:249.
27. Tolwani A, Wille KM. Advances in continuous renal replacement therapy. Citrate anticoagulation update. *Blood Purif.* 2012;34:88-93.

28. Davenport A, Tolwani A. Citrate anticoagulation for continuous renal replacement therapy (CRRT) in patients with acute kidney injury admitted to the intensive care unit. *NDT Plus* 2009;2:439-447.
29. Calatzis A, Toepfer M, Schramm W, et al. Citrate anticoagulation for extracorporeal circuits: effects on whole blood coagulation activation and clot formation. *Nephron.* 2001;89:233-236.
30. Morabito S, Pistolesi V, Tritapepe L, et al. Regional citrate anticoagulation for RRTs in critically ill patients with AKI. *Clin J Am Soc Nephrol.* 2014;9:2173-2188.
31. Schneider AG, Journois D, Rimmelé T. Complications of regional citrate anticoagulation: accumulation or overload? *Crit Care.* 2017;21(1):281.
32. Apsner R, Schwarzenhofer M, Derfler K, et al. Impairment of citrate metabolism in acute hepatic failure. *Wien Klin Wochenschr.* 1997;109:123-127.
33. Kramer L, Bauer E, Joukhadar C, et al. Citrate pharmacokinetics and metabolism in cirrhotic and noncirrhotic critically ill patients. *Crit Care Med.* 2003;31:2450-2455.
34. Meier-Kriesche HU, Gitomer J, Finkel K, DuBose T. Increased total to ionized calcium ratio during continuous venovenous hemodialysis with regional citrate anticoagulation. *Crit Care Med.* 2001;29:748-752.
35. Bakker AJ, Boerma EC, Keidel H, et al. Detection of citrate overdose in critically ill patients on citrate-anticoagulated venovenous haemofiltration: use of ionised and total/ionised calcium. *Clin Chem Lab Med.* 2006;44:962-966.
36. Saner FH, Treckmann JW, Geis A, et al. Efficacy and safety of regional citrate anticoagulation in liver transplant patients requiring post-operative renal replacement therapy. *Nephrol Dial Transplant.* 2012;127:1651-1657.
37. Slowinski T, Morgera S, Joannidis M, et al. Safety and efficacy of regional citrate anticoagulation in continuous venovenous hemodialysis in the presence of liver failure: the liver citrate anticoagulation threshold (L-CAT) observational study. *Crit Care.* 2015;19:349.
38. Zhang W, Bai M, Yu Y, et al. Safety and efficacy of regional citrate anticoagulation for continuous renal replacement therapy in liver failure patients: a systematic review and meta-analysis. *Crit Care.* 2019;23:22.
39. Monchi M, Berghmans D, Ledoux D, et al. Citrate vs. heparin for anticoagulation in continuous venovenous hemofiltration: a prospective randomized study. *Intensive Care Med.* 2004;30:260-265.
40. Hetzel GR, Schmitz M, Wissing H, et al. Regional citrate versus systemic heparin for anticoagulation in critically ill patients on continuous venovenous haemofiltration: a prospective randomized multicentre trial. *Nephrol Dial Transplant.* 2011;26:232-239.
41. Oudemans-van Straaten HM, Bosman RJ, Koopmans M, et al. Citrate anticoagulation for continuous venovenous hemofiltration. *Crit Care Med.* 2009;37:545-552.
42. Gattas DJ, Rajbhandari D, Bradford C, et al. A randomized controlled trial of regional citrate versus regional heparin anticoagulation for continuous renal replacement therapy in critically ill adults. *Crit Care Med.* 2015;43:1622-1629.
43. Stucker F, Ponte B, Tataw J, et al. Efficacy and safety of citrate-based anticoagulation compared to heparin in patients with acute kidney injury requiring continuous renal replacement therapy: a randomized controlled trial. *Crit Care.* 2015;19:91.
44. Tolwani AJ, Prendergast MB, Speer RR, et al. A practical citrate anticoagulation continuous venovenous hemodiafiltration protocol for metabolic control and high solute clearance. *Clin J Am Soc Nephrol.* 2006;1:79-87.
45. Mehta RL, McDonald BR, Ward DM. Regional citrate anticoagulation for continuous arteriovenous hemodialysis. An update after 12 months. *Contrib Nephrol.* 1991;93:210-214.
46. Gabutti L, Marone C, Colucci G, et al. Citrate anticoagulation in continuous venovenous hemodiafiltration: a metabolic challenge. *Intensive Care Med.* 2002;28:1419-1425.
47. Bagshaw SM, Laupland KB, Boiteau PJ, Godinez-Luna T. Is regional citrate superior to systemic heparin anticoagulation for continuous renal replacement therapy? A prospective observational study in an adult regional critical care system. *J Crit Care.* 2005;20:155-161.
48. Thoenen M, Schmid ER, Binswanger U, et al. Regional citrate anticoagulation using a citrate-based substitution solution for continuous venovenous hemofiltration in cardiac surgery patients. *Wien Klin Wochenschr.* 2002;114:108-114.
49. Hofmann RM, Maloney C, Ward DM, Becker BN. A novel method for regional citrate anticoagulation in continuous venovenous hemofiltration (CVVHF). *Ren Fail.* 2002;24:325-335.
50. Mitchell A, Daul AE, Beiderlinden M, et al. A new system for regional citrate anticoagulation in continuous venovenous hemodialysis (CVVHD). *Clin Nephrol.* 2003;59:106-114.
51. Morgera S, Scholle C, Melzer C, et al. A simple, safe and effective citrate anticoagulation protocol for the genius dialysis system in acute renal failure. *Nephron Clin Pract.* 2004;98:c35-c40.
52. Swartz R, Pasko D, O'Toole J, Starmann B. Improving the delivery of continuous renal replacement therapy using regional citrate anticoagulation. *Clin Nephrol.* 2004;61:134-143.

53. Cointault O, Kamar N, Bories P, et al. Regional citrate anticoagulation in continuous venovenous haemodiafiltration using commercial solutions. *Nephrol Dial Transplant.* 2004;19:171-178.
54. Egi M, Naka T, Bellomo R, et al. A comparison of two citrate anticoagulation regimens for continuous veno-venous hemofiltration. *Int J Artif Organs.* 2005;28:1211-1218.
55. Bihorac A, Ross EA. Continuous venovenous hemofiltration with citrate-based replacement fluid: efficacy, safety, and impact on nutrition. *Am J Kidney Dis.* 2005;46:908-918.
56. Naka T, Egi M, Bellomo R, et al. Low-dose citrate continuous veno-venous hemofiltration (CVVH) and acid-base balance. *Int J Artif Organs.* 2005;28:222-228.
57. Ong SC, Wille KM, Speer R, Tolwani AJ. A continuous veno-venous hemofiltration protocol with anticoagulant citrate dextrose formula A and a calcium-containing replacement fluid. *Int J Artif Organs.* 2014;37:499-502.
58. Kirwan CJ, Hutchison R, Ghabina S, et al. Implementation of a simplified regional citrate anticoagulation protocol for post-dilution continuous hemofiltration using a bicarbonate buffered, calcium containing replacement solution. *Blood Purif.* 2016;42:349-355.
59. Kutsogiannis DJ, Gibney RT, Stollery D, et al. Regional citrate versus systemic heparin anticoagulation for continuous renal replacement in critically ill patients. *Kidney Int.* 2005;67:2361-2367.
60. Betjes MG, van Oosterom D, van Agteren M, et al. Regional citrate versus heparin anticoagulation during venovenous hemofiltration in patients at low risk for bleeding: similar hemofilter survival but significantly less bleeding. *J Nephrol.* 2007;20:602-608.
61. Fealy N, Baldwin I, Johnstone M, et al. A pilot randomized controlled crossover study comparing regional heparinization to regional citrate anticoagulation for continuous venovenous hemofiltration. *Int J Artif Organs.* 2007;30:301-307.
62. Schilder L, Nurmohamed SA, Bosch FH, et al. Citrate anticoagulation versus systemic heparinisation in continuous venovenous hemofiltration in critically ill patients with acute kidney injury: a multi-center randomized clinical trial. *Crit Care.* 2014;18:472.
63. Zhang Z, Hongying N. Efficacy and safety of regional citrate anticoagulation in critically ill patients undergoing continuous renal replacement therapy. *Intensive Care Med.* 2012;38:20-28.
64. Wu MY, Hsu YH, Bai CH, et al. Regional citrate versus heparin anticoagulation for continuous renal replacement therapy: a meta-analysis of randomized controlled trials. *Am J Kidney Dis.* 2012;59:810-818.
65. Bai M, Zhou M, He L, et al. Citrate versus heparin anticoagulation for continuous renal replacement therapy: an updated meta-analysis of RCTs. *Intensive Care Med.* 2015;41:2098-2110.
66. Link A, Girndt M, Selejan S, Mathes A, Bohm M, Rensing H. Argatroban for anticoagulation in continuous renal replacement therapy. *Crit Care Med.* 2009;37(1):105-110.
67. Kidney Disease: Improving Global Outcomes (KDIGO) Acute Kidney Injury Work Group. KDIGO clinical practice guideline for acute kidney injury. *Kidney Int Suppl.* 2012;2:1.

Is regional citrate superior to regional heparin for circuit anticoagulation in CKRT?

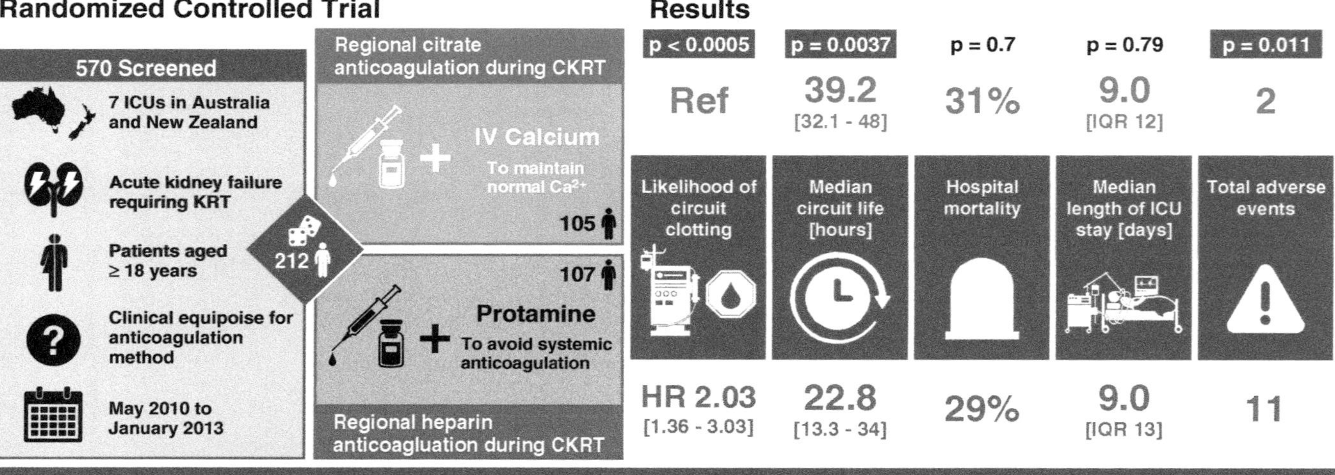

Conclusion: In this randomized trial comparing regional citrate with regional heparin anticoagulation during CKRT, there was longer circuit life with regional citrate anticoagulation.

Gattas DJ, Rajbhandari D, Bradford C, Buhr H, Lo S, Bellomo R. ***A Randomized Controlled Trial of Regional Citrate Versus Regional Heparin Anticoagulation for Continuous Kidney Replacement Therapy in Critically Ill Adults.*** Crit Care Med. 2015;43(8):1622-9.

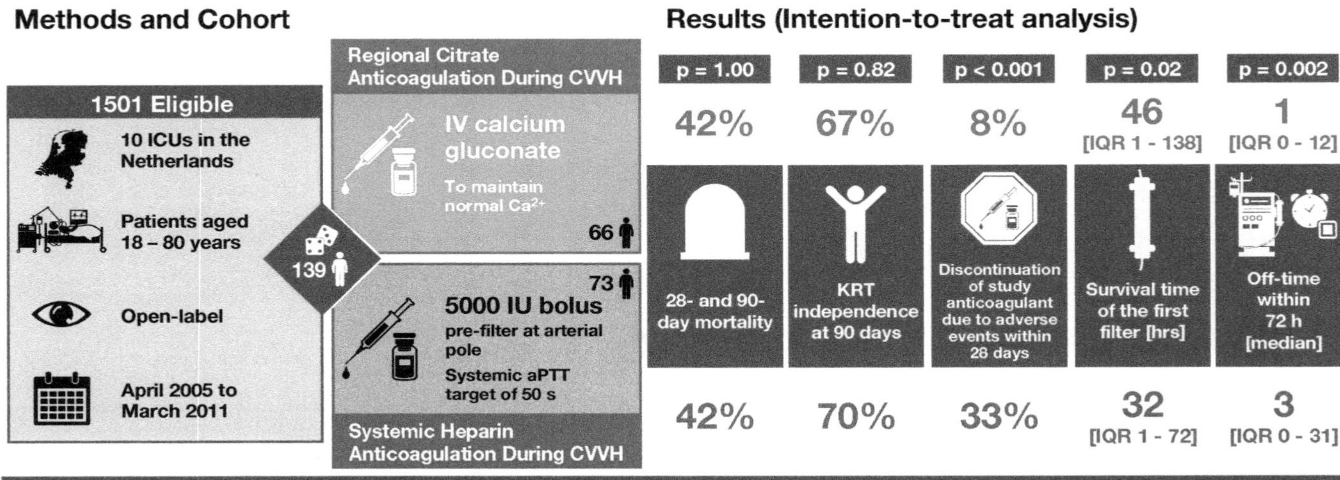

Conclusion: This multi-centre randomized controlled trial showed that regional anticoagulation with citrate for CVVH had benefits compared to heparin in terms of safety and efficacy, but not in terms of kidney and patient outcomes.

Schilder L, Nurmohamed SA, Bosch FH, et al. ***Citrate anticoagulation versus systemic heparinisation in continuous venovenous hemofiltration in critically ill patients with acute kidney injury: a multi-center randomized clinical trial.*** Crit Care. 2014;18(4):472.

VISUAL ABSTRACT 33.2

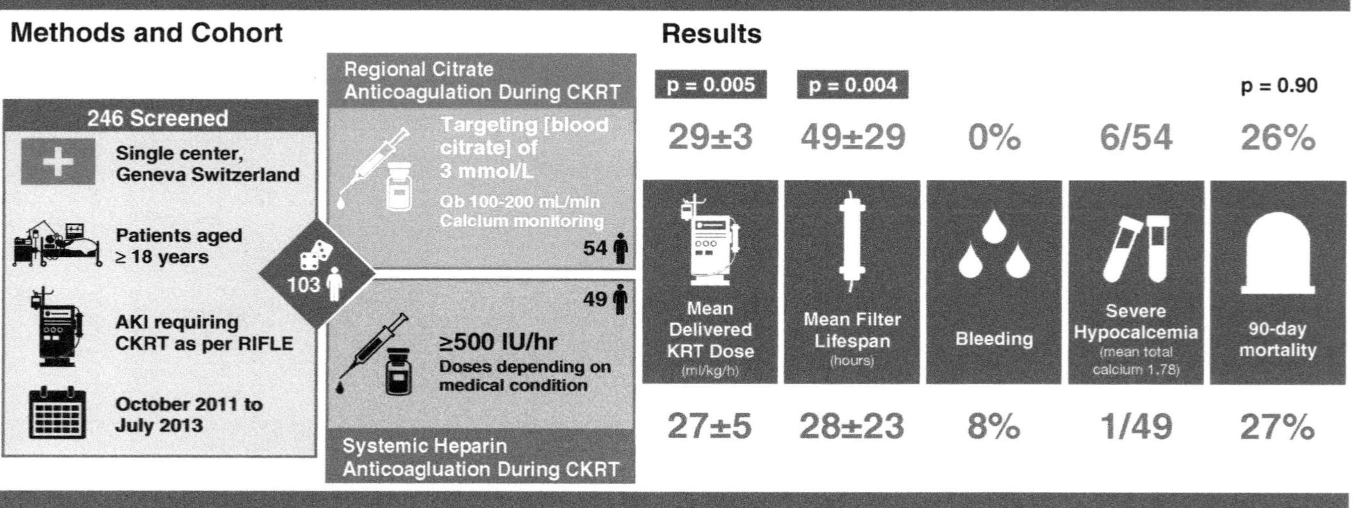

VISUAL ABSTRACT 33.3

34 Blood Purification in the Intensive Care Unit

Aron Jansen and Peter Pickkers

INTRODUCTION

Sepsis, defined as a life-threatening organ dysfunction caused by a dysregulated host response to infection, is one of the leading causes of organ failure, including acute kidney injury (AKI), and death in patients in the intensive care unit (ICU).[1] Despite advances in supportive care over the past couple of decades, there is no targeted therapy specifically for sepsis as of yet and mortality rates still exceed 30%.[2] Therefore, there is an unmet medical need for specific interventions that may improve clinical outcome for sepsis patients.

In sepsis pathophysiology, circulating pathogen-associated molecular patterns (PAMPs), including endotoxins (lipopolysaccharides, LPS), are recognized by immune cells and trigger a rapid and overwhelming inflammatory cascade. In turn, the excessive production of proinflammatory cytokines may lead to hemodynamic instability and end-organ failure, whereas the equally excessive release of anti-inflammatory cytokines may severely suppress the immune system and render the host susceptible to secondary infections.[3] Correspondingly, elevated plasma levels of LPS and cytokines are associated with higher incidence and severity of AKI and an increased mortality in sepsis patients.[4-6] Therefore, the removal of excess cytokines and endotoxins from the circulation seems like a plausible treatment option that may improve sepsis outcome.

Over the past decades, several blood purification instruments with different binding capacities have been developed. These instruments can be categorized into different groups on the basis of their mechanism of action: LPS-binding devices (e.g., the polymyxin B hemoperfusion [PMX] device; Toraymyxin, Toray Medical Co., Ltd, Tokyo, Japan), extracorporeal cytokine hemoadsorption devices (e.g., CytoSorb, Cytosorbents Co., NJ, USA), a combination of LPS and cytokine capturing devices (e.g., oXiris, Baxter, Meyzieu, France), and therapeutic plasma exchange (TPE). A graphical overview of the differences and similarities between these devices is depicted in **Figure 34.1**.

The Toraymyxin device consists of a hemoperfusion column that contains polymyxin B–immobilized fibers that selectively bind endotoxins in patients' blood but does not capture endogenous inflammatory mediators. Moreover, as it does not offer any solute clearance, PMX treatment cannot serve as kidney replacement therapy (KRT).[7] The hollow-fiber purification device oXiris has an acrylonitrile and methanesulfonate (AN69) membrane that captures both endotoxins and cytokines and can be used simultaneously as a form of KRT, whereas CytoSorb, a porous adsorbent polymer bead device, does not allow simultaneous KRT or binding of endotoxins, but selectively removes circulating cytokines with

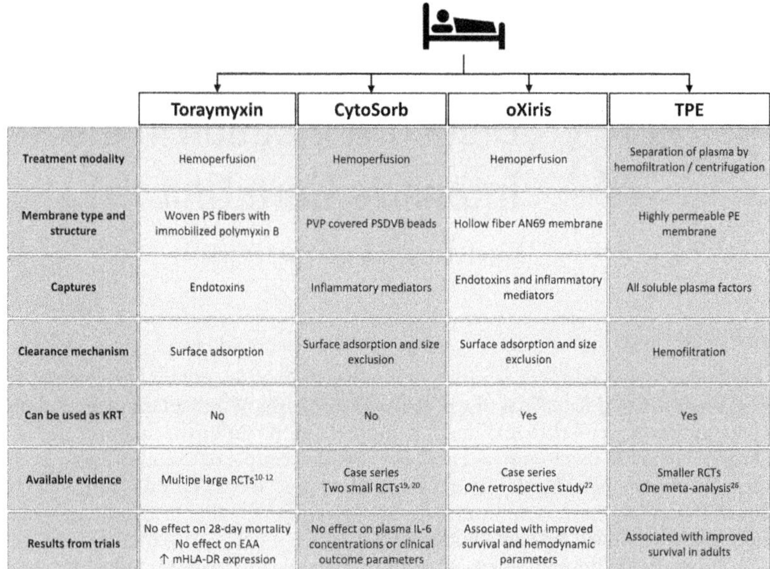

	Toraymyxin	CytoSorb	oXiris	TPE
Treatment modality	Hemoperfusion	Hemoperfusion	Hemoperfusion	Separation of plasma by hemofiltration / centrifugation
Membrane type and structure	Woven PS fibers with immobilized polymyxin B	PVP covered PSDVB beads	Hollow fiber AN69 membrane	Highly permeable PE membrane
Captures	Endotoxins	Inflammatory mediators	Endotoxins and inflammatory mediators	All soluble plasma factors
Clearance mechanism	Surface adsorption	Surface adsorption and size exclusion	Surface adsorption and size exclusion	Hemofiltration
Can be used as KRT	No	No	Yes	Yes
Available evidence	Multipe large RCTs[10-12]	Case series Two small RCTs[19, 20]	Case series One retrospective study[22]	Smaller RCTs One meta-analysis[26]
Results from trials	No effect on 28-day mortality No effect on EAA ↑ mHLA-DR expression	No effect on plasma IL-6 concentrations or clinical outcome parameters	Associated with improved survival and hemodynamic parameters	Associated with improved survival in adults

FIGURE 34.1: Differences and similarities between the currently available extracorporeal blood purification techniques. AN69, acrylonitrile and methanesulfonate; EAA, endotoxin activity essay; HLA, human leukocyte antigen; IL-6, interleukin 6; PE, polyethylene; PS, polystyrene; PSDVB, porous polystyrene divinylbenzene; PVP, polyvinylpyrrolidone; RCT, randomized controlled trial; KRT, kidney replacement therapy; TPE, therapeutic plasma exchange.

a molecular weight up to 60 kDa (e.g., interleukin [IL]-1β, IL-6, IL-8, IL-10, and tumor necrosis factor [TNF]-α) by surface adsorption and size exclusion.[7] TPE is based on the principle of the separation of contaminated plasma from whole blood and replacing it with fresh frozen plasma (FFP), albumin, or saline, thereby removing endotoxins, cytokines, and other potentially harmful substances from the circulation. Moreover, potentially depleted beneficial substances, such as coagulation factors, can be replenished using TPE. Over the years, several studies have been performed to evaluate the clinical efficacy of the different blood purification techniques. This chapter reflects on the relevant literature on blood purification techniques and will provide clinicians with advice on the use of these techniques in clinical practice.

POLYMYXIN B HEMOPERFUSION

Polymyxin B hemoperfusion, developed since 1981 and approved for the treatment of endotoxemia by the Japanese Health Insurance system in 1994,[8] is one of the earliest and best researched forms of blood purification we know today. The technique is based on the selective binding of circulating endotoxins by polymyxin B, an antibiotic derived from the bacterium *Bacillus polymyxa* with strong bactericidal activity against gram-negative microorganisms and LPS-binding properties. It was discovered in 1947 and was used effectively to combat infections with gram-negative bacteria. However, early systemic administration of polymyxins was associated with high incidences of kidney adverse events, such as kidney dysfunction, hematuria, proteinuria, and acute tubular necrosis.[9] The proposed mechanism is that polymyxins, because of their D-amino acid content and fatty acid component, may increase membrane permeability, eventually leading to cell swelling and lysis. In addition, polymyxins may interact with neurons, which have high lipid contents, and can thereby cause neurologic side effects such as dizziness, paresthesia, (partial) deafness, and even neuromuscular blockade resulting in muscle weakness and respiratory failure.[9] Given these strong nephrotoxic and neurotoxic effects, systemic administration of polymyxin B is restricted. To enable selective adsorption of circulating endotoxins, polymyxin B was covalently immobilized on the surface of polystyrene-derived carrier fibers in the Toraymyxin hemoperfusion column.

RESULTS FROM RANDOMIZED CLINICAL TRIALS

Three major trials have investigated the clinical efficacy of PMX in sepsis patients.[10-12] The Early Use of Polymyxin B Hemoperfusion in Abdominal Septic Shock (EUPHAS) trial,[10] published in 2009, was an open-label randomized controlled trial (RCT) in ten Italian tertiary care ICUs (**Visual Abstract 34.1**). Sixty-four postoperative abdominal septic shock patients were randomized to either standard care (n = 30) or standard care plus two 2-hour PMX sessions on consecutive days (n = 34). The EUPHAS trial, originally planned to include 60 patients in each group, was terminated prematurely after an interim analysis demonstrated a survival benefit in the PMX group. Moreover, physiologic endpoints such as mean arterial pressure (MAP), inotropic score, vasopressor dependency index, and sequential organ failure assessment (SOFA) scores were reported to improve significantly over time within the PMX group, whereas these parameters did not change in the control group. Although these results seem very promising at first glance, the EUPHAS trial received criticism because of several limitations in the statistical analysis. First, although clinical parameters improved significantly within the PMX group and not in the control group, changes over time were not significantly different between the two groups. Second, the reported difference in mortality, expressed as a hazard ratio of 0.36 (95% confidence interval [CI] 0.16-0.80), illustrates a significant improvement in survival time, whereas the absolute 28-day mortality did not differ significantly between the two groups (11/34 patients [32%] in the PMX group vs 16/30 patients [53%] in the control group, $\chi^2(1) = 2.88, p = 0.09$). Third, the primary endpoint of this study was change in hemodynamic parameters and the study was not powered to demonstrate a difference in mortality. Last, with a high mortality rate of 53% in the control group, selection bias may limit the generalizability of these results to other patient populations.

The Effects of Hemoperfusion With a Polymyxin B Membrane in Peritonitis With Septic Shock (ABDO-MIX) trial[11], published in 2015, was the second large European multicenter randomized trial to evaluate the clinical efficacy of PMX in abdominal sepsis patients (**Visual Abstract 34.2**). In this French open-label trial, standard care was compared with standard care plus two cycles of PMX for 2 hours in 243 patients. PMX failed to demonstrate a survival benefit, or an effect on resolution of organ dysfunction or inflammatory biomarkers. Incomplete PMX sessions were reported in 38% of patients. In a post hoc per-protocol analysis, adjusting for baseline differences and confounding factors, no differences in mortality or other clinical outcomes between the two groups were demonstrated. However, with an observed mortality of 23% and a median score of 59 points on the Simplified Acute Physiologic Score (SAPS)-II 2 of 59 in the control group, the selected patient population was less severely ill than expected and may therefore have benefited less from PMX treatment. Furthermore, because circulating endotoxin levels were not assessed, patients with low endotoxin levels may have been enrolled, theoretically diluting the efficacy of PMX treatment.

In 2018 the evaluating the Use of Polymyxin B Hemoperfusion in a Randomized controlled trial of Adults Treated for Endotoxemia and Septic Shock (EUPHRATES) trial was published (**Visual Abstract 34.3**).[12] In contrast to the EUPHAS and ABDOMIX trial, only patients with confirmed endotoxemia (defined as an endotoxin activity assay [EAA] >0.6) were enrolled ($n = 244$). Moreover, a detailed sham procedure was used as a treatment-blinding mechanism. PMX treatment did not result in improvements in 28-day mortality or other clinical endpoints, nor did it have any effect in a selected group of patients with a Multiple Organ Dysfunction Score (MODS) greater than 9. Interestingly, changes in EAA over time did not differ between the PMX and sham treatment groups, suggesting that the current treatment regimen of 2-hour PMX sessions might be too short to sufficiently remove endotoxin from the circulation in patients with continuous endotoxemia.

In a post hoc analysis, the authors report a significant adjusted survival benefit in PMX-treated patients in the subgroup with an "addressable" EAA level (defined as an EAA between 0.6 and 0.89) who completed two complete PMX sessions.[13] No therapeutic benefit in patients with a higher EAA level was observed. Several methodological limitations undermine the credibility of these post hoc results, as is described comprehensively elsewhere.[14]

In conclusion, despite the sound pathophysiologic theory behind polymyxin B hemoperfusion current evidence does not support use of PMX in sepsis patients and should therefore be limited to research settings only.

EXTRACORPOREAL CYTOKINE HEMOADSORPTION

Because circulating cytokines are key drivers of the systemic inflammatory response in sepsis, associated with organ dysfunction and mortality,[17] devices that capture and clear cytokines from the circulation might improve outcome for sepsis patients. Another possible benefit of targeting cytokines instead of endotoxins is that these devices could also be used in hyperinflammatory syndromes other than sepsis, such as autoimmune disease, (surgical) trauma, burns, or cytokine release syndrome associated with chimeric antigen receptor (CAR) T-cell therapy. As of today, two such devices are available. However, being relatively new, they have not yet been tested extensively in large RCTs, and available evidence is limited to smaller trials or case series.

CytoSorb is a hemoadsorption device that can easily be built into extracorporeal blood pump circuits. It consists of a hemoperfusion column containing highly porous polystyrene divinylbenzene (PSDVB) copolymer beads covered with polyvinylpyrrolidone (PVP) that remove cytokines and other mid-molecular-weight molecules (up to 60 kDa) by surface adsorption and size exclusion. Although its cytokine-adsorbing capacities have been demonstrated in several preclinical studies,[7,18] treatment with CytoSorb (placed in the cardiopulmonary bypass circuit) did not alter plasma levels of IL-6 and other cytokines in 19 cardiac surgery patients, nor did it affect clinical outcome parameters compared with the control group ($n = 18$).[19] Correspondingly, adding 6 hours of CytoSorb hemoperfusion per day for up to 7 days to standard of care therapy did not alter plasma levels of IL-6 or other inflammatory cytokines in 47 mechanically ventilated patients with septic shock, compared with 51 patients in the control group.[20] Interestingly, IL-6 elimination rates over the filter ranged from 5% to 18% throughout the entire 6-hour hemoperfusion period, so there was demonstrated clearance of cytokines in these patients. Although these findings might seem contradictory, they are not unusual in the light of the cytokinetic theory.[21] Because cytokines are produced primarily by resident macrophages in the tissues, plasma cytokine levels may remain stable during CytoSorb hemoperfusion because of a cytokine shift from the interstitium into the circulation. The circulation acts as a sink, thereby draining the tissues.

The hollow-fiber AN69 membrane device oXiris had similar cytokine-adsorbing capacities as CytoSorb in a closed-loop circulation model.[7] In contrast to CytoSorb, however, oXiris also captures endotoxins and can be used simultaneously as a form of KRT. Although only case series and no prospective clinical trials are available, use of the oXiris filter was associated with improved survival and hemodynamic status in a retrospective cohort study in 31 patients with septic shock.[22] A trial is currently being planned to see if these results can be reproduced in a prospective manner (NCT03914586).

THERAPEUTIC PLASMA EXCHANGE

TPE is an extracorporeal treatment modality that is based on the principle of separating plasma containing harmful substances, such as endotoxins and inflammatory mediators, from whole blood and replenishing it with FFPs, thereby restoring deficient plasma proteins such as coagulation factors. Given its mechanism of action, TPE has traditionally been tested in diseases that are characterized by the presence of excessive plasma solutes. In myeloma patients, for instance, elevated plasma levels of monoclonal light chains are filtered in the kidney and form obstructive casts in the distal tubule, causing "cast nephropathy" and, eventually, kidney failure. Although current evidence does not support routine use of TPE for the treatment of kidney failure in myeloma patients,[23] there are signals that it may be effective when used only in patients with biopsy-confirmed cast nephropathy and when the dosing of TPE is guided by a target reduction in serum light chains.[24]

As for the use of TPE in sepsis patients, high-quality data on its efficacy are sparse and many trials were either of a preclinical nature or had low recruiting numbers, as is described extensively elsewhere.[25] In a meta-analysis, including four trials (one in adults, two in children, and one in both) enrolling a total of 194 critically ill patients with sepsis and septic shock, use of TPE was not associated with a significant reduction in all-cause mortality.[26] In a subgroup analysis, however, plasma exchange was associated with a lower mortality rate in adults (relative risk [RR] 0.63, 95% confidence interval [CI] 0.42-0.96; I^2 0%), but not in children (RR 0.96, 95% CI 0.28-3.38; I^2 60%). A prospective RCT is currently being planned to evaluate the use of TPE in sepsis (NCT03065751). Until results from large trials suggest otherwise, use of TPE for the treatment of sepsis is not recommended.

COMPLICATIONS OF BLOOD PURIFICATION TECHNIQUES

Clinicians should be aware that the application of blood purification techniques is not free of risk. The potential risks associated with blood purification techniques can be roughly demarcated into two domains: risks that are common to any extracorporeal treatment and risks that are associated with blood purification specifically.

Common adverse events of extracorporeal therapies in general are catheter-related complications (such as bleeding from the puncture site or thromboembolism), clot formation within the extracorporeal circuit, hemolysis, hypothermia, hypotension, or allergic responses to device materials.

The most prevalent side effect of hemoperfusion is thrombocytopenia, although platelet counts usually restore within 1 or 2 days following hemoperfusion.[28] Other common side effects are hypocalcemia, hypoglycemia, neutropenia, and hypothermia, although these side effects are usually minor and either correct spontaneously or can easily be corrected. Coating absorbents with a polymer solution can reduce the frequency of these side effects by impairing platelet adhesion and complement activation. Another important consideration for clinicians is that most hemoperfusion treatments remove their target molecules in a nonspecific manner and other, potentially beneficial substances (such as antibiotics or vasoactive agents) may also be removed from the circulation. These risks may be reduced by postponing the administration of these drugs until after each session in intermittent hemoperfusion regimens, whereas therapeutic drug monitoring and dosage adjustments may improve drug efficacy during continuous hemoperfusion.

The frequency and types of complications of TPE depend on the total volume that is replaced and on the type of replacement fluid that is used. Citrate-induced hypocalcemia (and associated symptoms such as paresthesias or QT-prolongation) and inadvertent removal of medication can occur with any replacement fluid. Replacement with nonplasma fluids specifically may lead to depletion of immunoglobulins, and monitoring of immunoglobulin G (IgG) levels is recommended for patients undergoing aggressive TPE.[29] Use of donor plasma as replacement fluid may trigger allergic reactions, and urticaria and wheezing, for example, are common side effects.[30] Anaphylaxis and transfusion-related acute lung injury (TRALI) are rare but potentially lethal adverse effects of replacement with donor plasma, and continuous monitoring of vital signs during TPE should be performed.

CONCLUSION

In conclusion, blood purification techniques can roughly be divided into three major categories on the basis of their mechanism of action: LPS-binding devices, cytokine-adsorbing devices, and TPE. Although the rationale behind these different techniques is based on valid pathophysiologic theories, none of these therapies have been shown to improve patient outcomes. At this moment, the quality of some of the available evidence is contestable because of small trial sample sizes and flaws in methodology. Nevertheless, there are signals that blood purification might be beneficial for certain patient subgroups and for endpoints other than mortality, such as hemodynamic stabilization and immunologic parameters. This should be further explored in future trials. Importantly, blood purification techniques are not free of risk and can result in serious complications related to the needed procedures or their capturing properties. Therefore, on the basis of current evidence, blood purification techniques should be viewed as an experimental therapy to be used in research settings only.

References

1. Zarjou A, Agarwal A. Sepsis and acute kidney injury. *JASN.* 2011;22:999-1006.
2. Fleischmann C, Scherag A, Adhikari NKJ, et al. Assessment of global incidence and mortality of hospital-treated sepsis. Current estimates and limitations. *Am J Respir Crit Care Med.* 2016;193:259-272.
3. Osuchowski MF, Welch K, Siddiqui J, Remick DG. Circulating cytokine/inhibitor profiles reshape the understanding of the SIRS/CARS continuum in sepsis and predict mortality. *J Immunol.* 2006;177:1967-1974.
4. Kellum JA, Kong L, Fink MP, et al. Understanding the inflammatory cytokine response in pneumonia and sepsis: results of the Genetic and Inflammatory Markers of Sepsis (GenIMS) study. *Arch Inter Med.* 2007;167:1655-1663.
5. Opal SM, Scannon PJ, Vincent JL, et al. Relationship between plasma levels of lipopolysaccharide (LPS) and LPS-binding protein in patients with severe sepsis and septic shock. *J Infect Dis.* 1999;180:1584-1589.
6. Payen D, Lukaszewicz AC, Legrand M, et al. A multicentre study of acute kidney injury in severe sepsis and septic shock: association with inflammatory phenotype and HLA genotype. *PLoS One.* 2012;7:e35838.
7. Malard B, Lambert C, Kellum JA. In vitro comparison of the adsorption of inflammatory mediators by blood purification devices. *Intensive Care Med Exp.* 2018;6:12.
8. Shimizu T, Miyake T, Tani M. History and current status of polymyxin B-immobilized fiber column for treatment of severe sepsis and septic shock. *Ann Gastroenterol Surg.* 2017;1:105-113.
9. Falagas ME, Kasiakou SK. Toxicity of polymyxins: a systematic review of the evidence from old and recent studies. *Crit Care.* 2006;10:R27.
10. Cruz DN, Antonelli M, Fumagalli R, et al. Early use of polymyxin B hemoperfusion in abdominal septic shock: the EUPHAS randomized controlled trial. *JAMA.* 2009;301:2445-2452.
11. Payen DM, Guilhot J, Launey Y, et al. Early use of polymyxin B hemoperfusion in patients with septic shock due to peritonitis: a multicenter randomized control trial. *Intensive Care Med.* 2015;41:975-984.
12. Dellinger RP, Bagshaw SM, Antonelli M, et al. Effect of targeted polymyxin B hemoperfusion on 28-day mortality in patients with septic shock and elevated endotoxin level: the EUPHRATES randomized clinical trial. *JAMA.* 2018;320:1455-1463.
13. Klein DJ, Foster D, Walker PM, et al. Polymyxin B hemoperfusion in endotoxemic septic shock patients without extreme endotoxemia: a post hoc analysis of the EUPHRATES trial. *Intensive Care Med.* 2018;44:2205-2212.
14. Pickkers P, Russell JA. Treatment with a polymyxin B filter to capture endotoxin in sepsis patients: is there a signal for therapeutic efficacy? *Intensive Care Med.* 2019;45:282-283.
15. Chang T, Tu YK, Lee CT, et al. Effects of polymyxin B hemoperfusion on mortality in patients with severe sepsis and septic shock: a systemic review, meta-analysis update, and disease severity subgroup meta-analysis. *Crit Care Med.* 2017;45:e858-e864.
16. Srisawat N, Tungsanga S, Lumlertgul N, et al. The effect of polymyxin B hemoperfusion on modulation of human leukocyte antigen DR in severe sepsis patients. *Crit Care.* 2018;22: 279.
17. Schulte W, Bernhagen J, Bucala R. Cytokines in sepsis: potent immunoregulators and potential therapeutic targets—an updated view. *Mediators Inflamm.* 2013;2013:165974.
18. Kellum JA, Song M, Venkataraman R. Hemoadsorption removes tumor necrosis factor, interleukin-6, and interleukin-10, reduces nuclear factor-kappaB DNA binding, and improves short-term survival in lethal endotoxemia. *Crit Care Med.* 2004;32:801-805.
19. Bernardi MH, Rinoesl H, Dragosits K, et al. Effect of hemoadsorption during cardiopulmonary bypass surgery—a blinded, randomized, controlled pilot study using a novel adsorbent. *Crit Care.* 2016;20:96.
20. Schadler D, Pausch C, Heise D, et al. The effect of a novel extracorporeal cytokine hemoadsorption device on IL-6 elimination in septic patients: a randomized controlled trial. *PLoS One.* 2017;12:e0187015.
21. Honoré PM, Matson JR. Extracorporeal removal for sepsis: acting at the tissue level—the beginning of a new era for this treatment modality in septic shock. *Crit Care Med.* 2004;32:896-897.

22. Schwindenhammer V, Girardot T, Chaulier K, et al. oXiris® use in septic shock: experience of two French centres. *Blood Purif.* 2019; 47:29-35. https://www.karger.com/Article/FullText/499510
23. Clark WF, Stewart AK, Rock GA, et al. Plasma exchange when myeloma presents as acute renal failure: a randomized, controlled trial. *Ann Intern Med.* 2005;143:777-784.
24. Leung N, Gertz MA, Zeldenrust SR, et al. Improvement of cast nephropathy with plasma exchange depends on the diagnosis and on reduction of serum free light chains. *Kidney Int.* 2008;73:1282-1288.
25. Rimmelé T, Kellum JA. Clinical review: blood purification for sepsis. *Crit Care.* 2011;15:205.
26. Rimmer E, Houston BL, Kumar A, et al. The efficacy and safety of plasma exchange in patients with sepsis and septic shock: a systematic review and meta-analysis. *Crit Care.* 2014;18:699.
27. Knaup H, Stahl K, Schmidt BMW. Early therapeutic plasma exchange in septic shock: a prospective open-label nonrandomized pilot study focusing on safety, hemodynamics, vascular barrier function, and biologic markers. *Crit Care.* 2018;22:285.
28. Weston MJ, Langley PG, Rubin MH, et al. Platelet function in fulminant hepatic failure and effect of charcoal haemoperfusion. *Gut.* 1977;18:897-902.
29. Keller AJ, Urbaniak SJ. Intensive plasma exchange on the cell separator: effects on serum immunoglobulins and complement components. *Br J Haematol.* 1978;38:531-540.
30. Reutter JC, Sanders KF, Brecher ME, Jones HG, Bandarenko N. Incidence of allergic reactions with fresh frozen plasma or cryo-supernatant plasma in the treatment of thrombotic thrombocytopenic purpura. *J Clin Apher.* 2001;16:134-138.

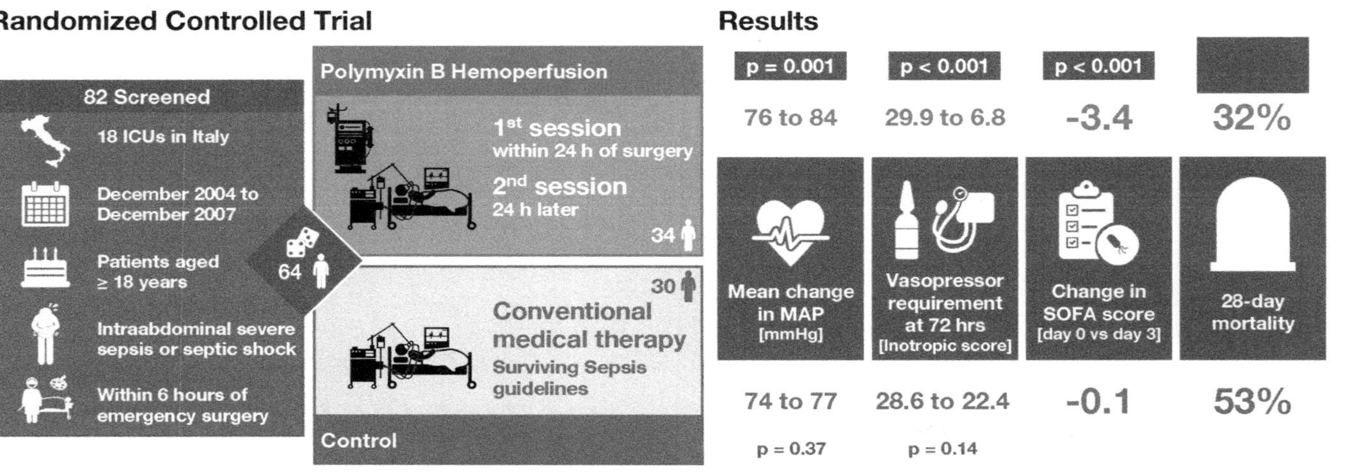

VISUAL ABSTRACT 34.1

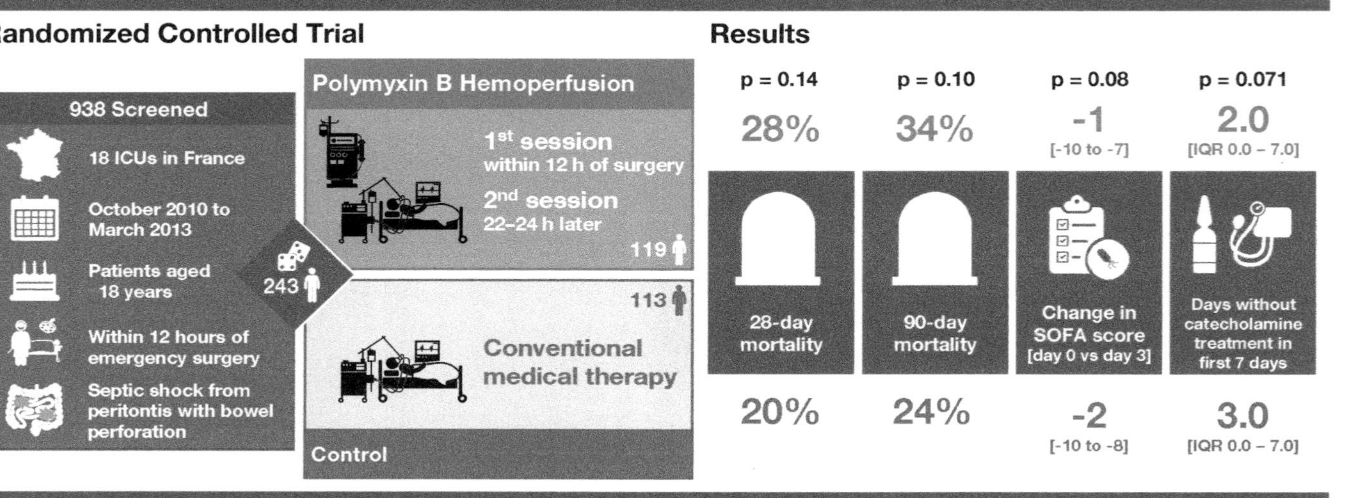

VISUAL ABSTRACT 34.2

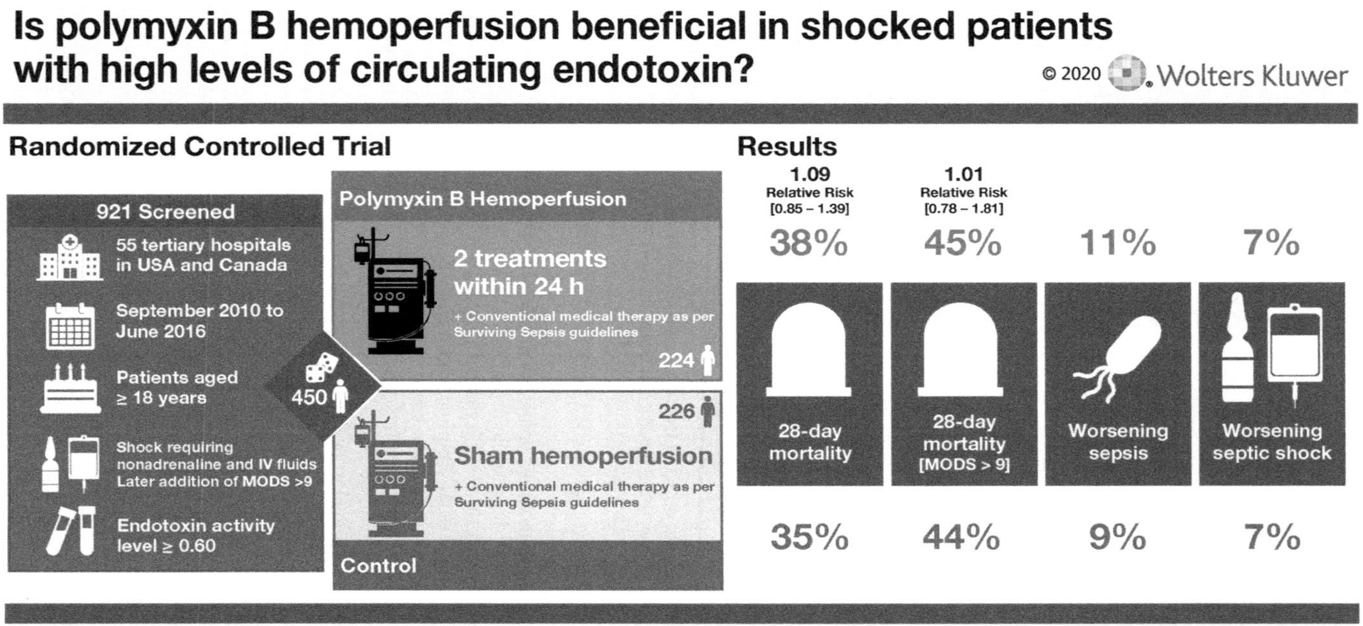

Is polymyxin B hemoperfusion beneficial in shocked patients with high levels of circulating endotoxin?

 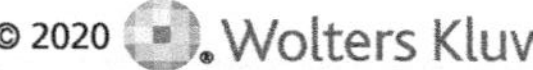

Randomized Controlled Trial

921 Screened

- 55 tertiary hospitals in USA and Canada
- September 2010 to June 2016
- Patients aged ≥ 18 years
- Shock requiring nonadrenaline and IV fluids
  Later addition of MODS >9
- Endotoxin activity level ≥ 0.60

450

Polymyxin B Hemoperfusion

2 treatments within 24 h

+ Conventional medical therapy as per Surviving Sepsis guidelines

224

Control

Sham hemoperfusion

+ Conventional medical therapy as per Surviving Sepsis guidelines

226

Results

	28-day mortality	28-day mortality [MODS > 9]	Worsening sepsis	Worsening septic shock
Relative Risk	1.09 [0.85 – 1.39]	1.01 [0.78 – 1.81]		
Polymyxin B Hemoperfusion	38%	45%	11%	7%
Control	35%	44%	9%	7%

Conclusion: In this randomized trial of patients with septic shock and high circulating endotoxin activity, polymyxin B hemoperfusion did not decrease 28-day mortality when compared to sham hemoperfusion.

Dellinger RP, Bagshaw SM, Antonelli M, et al. ***Effect of Targeted Polymyxin B Hemoperfusion on 28-Day Mortality in Patients With Septic Shock and Elevated Endotoxin Level: The EUPHRATES Randomized Clinical Trial.*** JAMA. 2018;320(14): 1455-1463.

VISUAL ABSTRACT 34.3

Extracorporeal Membrane Oxygenation in the Intensive Care Unit

Danielle Laufer and Kevin C. Thornton

INTRODUCTION

ECMO (extracorporeal membrane oxygenation) is an advanced form of temporary cardiopulmonary life support for patients with severe cardiac and/or respiratory failure. Since its development in the 1970s, ECMO technology has continued to change and improve, but the basic concept remains the same: continuous extracorporeal circulation of blood to a device that provides gas exchange and perfusion to the body. In short, the ECMO circuit drains blood from the venous system, pumps it through an artificial lung where carbon dioxide is removed and oxygen is added, and returns it to the body. There are two main forms of ECMO, which can be differentiated on the basis of the vessels cannulated: either two venous vessels in the venovenous (V-V) configuration or a venous and an arterial vessel in the venoarterial (V-A) configuration. V-V ECMO is indicated in isolated respiratory failure in patients with adequate cardiac output, and V-A ECMO is indicated in patients with cardiac or mixed cardiopulmonary failure.

HISTORY

Numerous scientific advances including the discovery of heparin and the development of the artificial heart-lung machine preceded the first successful use of ECMO in an adult trauma patient in 1971.[1,2] This patient survived respiratory failure after being supported on ECMO for 3 days.[3] Another pivotal moment came in 1975 with the first successful use of ECMO to support an infant with respiratory distress syndrome.[2]

In 1979, a randomized controlled trial compared ECMO with conventional mechanical ventilation in adults with severe acute respiratory failure. The results were grim with poor survival in both groups and a high complication rate.[4] Despite poor outcomes in adults at this time, results for the use of ECMO in newborns were more promising and ECMO became a well-established therapy in the treatment of respiratory failure in neonates.[3]

The use of ECMO in adults did not become more common until the late 2000s. In 2009, a multicenter randomized trial compared conventional ventilatory support with ECMO in patients with severe acute respiratory distress syndrome (ARDS) (**Visual Abstract 35.1**). This study showed a survival benefit in patients that were treated at an ECMO center.[5] Also in 2009, the H1N1 pandemic led to an increase in adults with severe, rapidly progressing ARDS that was successfully treated with ECMO (**Visual Abstract 35.2** and **Visual Abstract 35.3**).[6,7] Published in 2018, a large randomized trial, ECMO to Rescue Lung Injury in Severe ARDS (EOLIA), evaluated early initiation of ECMO in patients with ARDS compared with standard care (**Visual Abstract 35.4**). While they found no statistically significant difference in 60-day mortality between the two groups, ECMO proved to be superior for several secondary endpoints. Notably, patients in the ECMO group had significantly more days without kidney replacement therapy (KRT) than those in the control group at 60 days (50 vs 32 days; 95% confidence interval [CI], 0 to 51).[8] Despite these recent trials, there is still a need for more data to better define the role of ECMO as well as optimal management strategies.

INDICATIONS

The primary indication for ECMO is severe cardiac and/or respiratory failure.

Respiratory Failure

ECMO is a rescue therapy for select patients with severe respiratory failure when more conventional therapies (e.g., pharmacologic paralysis, pulmonary vasodilators, prone ventilation) have failed. Common disease processes treated with ECMO are listed in **Table 35.1** and include conditions that lead to both hypoxemic and hypercarbic respiratory failure. ARDS is the most common of these indications.[9] ECMO is also a management option for patients with decompensated pulmonary vascular disease, including pulmonary hypertension and acute, massive pulmonary embolism. ECMO is frequently used as a bridge to lung transplantation although the duration of pretransplant support varies greatly between centers.[10]

Cardiac Failure

The use of ECMO in the setting of cardiac failure is well established and common indications are listed in **Table 35.2**. The most common cardiac indication

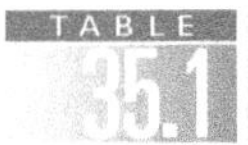

TABLE 35.1 Indications for ECMO in Respiratory Failure

Indications for ECMO in Respiratory Failure
Acute respiratory distress syndrome
Pneumonia
Trauma
COPD exacerbation
Status asthmaticus
Pulmonary vascular disease
Bridge to lung transplantation

COPD, chronic obstructive pulmonary disease; ECMO, extracorporeal membrane oxygenation.

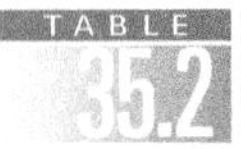

TABLE 35.2 Indications for ECMO in Cardiac Failure

Indications for ECMO in Cardiac Failure
Inability to wean off CPB after heart surgery
High-risk cardiac surgery
Cardiogenic shock after MI
Myocarditis
Dilated cardiomyopathy
Heart failure secondary to drug toxicity
Primary graft failure after heart transplant
Bridge to ventricular assist device or transplantation
Extracorporeal cardiopulmonary resuscitation

CPB, cardiopulmonary bypass; ECMO, extracorporeal membrane oxygenation; MI, myocardial infarction.

is the inability to wean from cardiopulmonary bypass following cardiac surgery.[11] Patients with irreversible cardiac conditions may also be ECMO candidates as a bridge to ventricular assist device (VAD) implantation, high-risk cardiac surgery, or heart transplantation.[12,13] More recently, ECMO has been used to reestablish circulation after cardiac arrest refractory to standard therapies, called "extracorporeal cardiopulmonary resuscitation" (eCPR). There are some early promising studies, but ECMO is not yet an established therapy in this setting.[14]

CONTRAINDICATIONS

The initiation of ECMO is a major decision that should be made by a multidisciplinary team of pulmonologists, cardiologists, cardiac surgeons, and intensivists. Absolute contraindications to ECMO include irreversible cardiac or pulmonary disease in patients who are not candidates for VAD implantation and/or transplantation, terminal illness such as widespread metastatic disease, and uncontrolled active hemorrhage.[15] Relative contraindications include significant brain injury, conditions precluding use of anticoagulation, advanced age (often >65 years old), multiorgan failure, severe aortic incompetence, aortic dissection, and mechanical ventilation for more than 5 to 10 days.[11]

EXTRACORPOREAL MEMBRANE OXYGENATION CONFIGURATIONS

Venovenous Extracorporeal Membrane Oxygenation

V-V ECMO traditionally involves two venous cannulation sites, one for venous drainage and the other for return of oxygenated blood. Most commonly, one cannula is placed in the femoral vein and the other in the right internal jugular vein. Disadvantages of this cannulation strategy include patient immobility because of the femoral cannula and recirculation of oxygenated blood into the circuit if the cannulas are in close proximity.[16] A newer cannulation system, using a dual-lumen single-stage cannula, allows for only one venous puncture site. This double-lumen cannula is placed in the right internal jugular vein, drains blood from the superior vena cava (SVC) and inferior vena cava (IVC), and reinfuses oxygenated blood into the right atrium directed toward the tricuspid valve. This allows for increased mobility and less recirculation. A disadvantage of this technique is that echocardiographic or fluoroscopic guidance is needed during cannulation to ensure that the cannula is properly positioned.

Venoarterial Extracorporeal Membrane Oxygenation

Vascular access for V-A ECMO is most commonly via the femoral vessels. One cannula is placed via the femoral vein into the right atrium and removes blood from the body. This deoxygenated blood travels to the ECMO machine and is then returned via a cannula placed in the femoral artery. Oxygenated blood travels retrograde through the aorta to supply the coronary arteries and aortic arch branches including the cerebral circulation. Most patients will have some degree of cardiac function with blood from patient's lungs being ejected through the aortic valve. This blood meets the retrograde oxygenated blood from the ECMO circuit at some point in the aorta depending on the relative flows in each direction. This area is called the "mixing zone." In the context of coexisting respiratory failure, the blood exiting the heart may not be well oxygenated. As cardiac function changes or ECMO flow is altered, this "zone" may move more proximal or distal in the aorta. For this reason, arterial lines are often placed on the right upper extremity and cerebral oximeters may be useful to ensure adequate cerebral oxygenation. Strategies to manage this issue include increasing ventilator support to improve oxygenation or increasing flow through the femoral arterial cannula to move the mixing zone more proximal into the ascending aorta. Other sites for arterial cannulation include the axillary/subclavian artery or carotid artery, although these techniques increase the risk of limb ischemia or neurologic injury, repectively.[17]

Central V-A ECMO involves cannulating the right atrium (venous cannula) and aorta (arterial cannula). This is performed through a median sternotomy and is most commonly used in the setting of postcardiotomy failure.[17] This technique uses larger cannulas allowing increased flow rates and hemodynamic support. Disadvantages include increased risk of bleeding, infection, and cardiac thrombosis.[18]

COMPONENTS

The ECMO circuit is composed of five main components.

Tubing and Cannulas

The tubing is responsible for transporting blood out of the patient to the membrane oxygenator and pump and then back into the patient. The maximum flow obtained by the pump is often dependent on the size of the cannulae, which is dependent on the location and size of the vessel cannulated. Typical adult flow rates are between 60 and 80 mL/kg/min.[19] The tubing is often heparin coated, reducing the risk of thrombosis and minimizing the inflammatory response as the blood is exposed to foreign materials.[20]

The Pump

The pump is responsible for the flows obtained by the circuit. There are two types of blood pumps: roller pumps and centrifugal pumps. Centrifugal pumps are most commonly employed in modern ECMO platforms as they cause less hemolysis, thereby minimizing the need for frequent transfusions.[20]

Pressures in the venous line are continuously measured. A normal pressure in the venous line is −50 to −80 mm Hg, and values below −100 mm Hg imply impaired venous drainage.[21] If there is negative pressure buildup in the line, "chattering" or shaking of the cannula can occur. This can usually be improved by decreasing the pump flow or volume administration.

Membrane Oxygenator

There are two types of membranes: silicone membranes and hollow-fiber membranes, with silicone membranes being more popular in the United States.[11] Blood passes on one side of the membrane, and "sweep" gas flow passes in the opposite direction on the other side of the membrane. An air-oxygen mixture is delivered to the membrane and maintains a diffusion gradient for oxygen delivery and carbon dioxide extraction. In simple terms, a set FiO_2 determines the percentage of oxygen added to the blood, and the sweep flow rate determines the rate of carbon dioxide extraction. Membrane function is monitored by measuring the difference in pre- and postmembrane pressures (called transmembrane pressures) as well as postoxygenator blood gases. A decrease in the partial pressure of O_2 or increase in CO_2 in sampling blood after the oxygenator indicates oxygenator failure. Likewise, an increase in transmembrane pressure, usually because of thrombus, is also an indicator of oxygenator failure.[20] Changing an oxygenator involves replacing the ECMO circuit in a controlled fashion. This is done by temporarily decreasing flows, clamping the circuit, cutting the connecting tubing, and quickly reconnecting to a new primed circuit in a sterile fashion.

Heat Exchanger

The heat exchanger prevents blood from losing heat as it flows within the ECMO circuit. Warming is achieved by circulating warm water around the oxygenator or tubing. The water is usually heated to 37°C to 40°C, but not more than 42°C to avoid overheating.[11]

Console

The pump console displays the pump speed (RPM) and flow rate (L/min). A few safety mechanisms are present in the case of an electrical failure. These include a stand-alone battery in the console as well as an emergency hand crank to power the pump.

WEANING

Weaning should be attempted once the underlying disease process has improved, although little evidence exists to guide this process. A proposed strategy for weaning from V-V ECMO[22] is as follows:

- Circuit flows are reduced (typically by 0.5 to 1.0 L/min) to less than 2.5 L/min.
- Ventilator is adjusted to lung-protective settings: tidal volumes to less than or equal to 6 mL/kg, peak airway pressures to less than 30 mm H_2O, FiO_2 decreased to maintain oxygen saturation greater than 90%.
- Sweep decreased incrementally to less than 1 L/min.

If blood gases remain stable on these lowered settings, the patient is ready for decannulation. A trial of decannulation can be done by disconnecting the sweep flow from the oxygenator. Blood will circulate through the ECMO circuit without additional gas exchange. The sweep can be reinitiated if the patient does not tolerate the trial.

To assess readiness for weaning from V-A ECMO, both heart and lung function must be considered. A proposed strategy for weaning from V-A ECMO[23] is as follows:

- Recovery of pulsatile arterial flow and mean arterial pressure (MAP) greater than 60 on minimal inotropic support
- Pulmonary function must not be severely impaired as evidenced by PaO_2/FiO_2 greater than 100 mm Hg with the ECMO FiO_2 set low. If not, consider bridging from V-A to V-V ECMO.
- Cardiac function and hemodynamics must be monitored in real time as ECMO flow rates are reduced gradually to a minimum of 1.5 to 1 L/min. Predictors of successful weaning during a turn-down trial include adequate pulse pressure and echocardiography showing improved left ventricular and right ventricular ejection fractions.[23]

COMPLICATIONS

The most common complication of ECMO is bleeding at cannulation sites, which is increased because of the need for systemic anticoagulation.[15] Other hematologic complications include thrombosis, hemolysis, thrombocytopenia, and disseminated vascular coagulopathy.[16] Stroke, typically hemorrhagic, is one of the most feared complications leading to increased mortality.[24] Patients are at risk of limb ischemia and compartment syndrome when cannulated via an arterial cannula, which may compromise distal perfusion. Insertion of a distal perfusion cannula that provides forward flow to the cannulated limb can decrease this risk.[25] Infectious complications occur at varying rates and depend on the number of days on ECMO, length of mechanical ventilation, and hospital length of stay.[26]

EXTRACORPOREAL MEMBRANE OXYGENATION AND THE KIDNEY

Acute kidney injury (AKI) is commonly seen in ECMO patients, with approximately 50% requiring KRT.[27] It has been reported that AKI during ECMO therapy can increase mortality 4-fold.[28] Possible causes of AKI during ECMO therapy include decreased kidney perfusion because of nonpulsatile flow, hemolysis, hypercoagulable state, hormonal factors such as disruption of the renin-angiotensin-aldosterone axis, and strong inflammatory response.[25,26,29] KRT allows for optimization of fluid balance, electrolytes, and acid-base status in these patients.

Continuous kidney replacement therapy (CKRT) is the most common treatment for AKI while supported by ECMO because of its hemodynamic stability, although combining these two techniques has unique challenges.[28] Specifically, the need for additional large vascular access is difficult when the ECMO circuit already occupies one to two sites. Pressures in the ECMO circuit are often incompatible with CKRT pressure limits and can cause the machine to stop. Most CKRT machines are designed to be connected to venous pressures ranging from 0 to 20 mm Hg. Pressure in the ECMO circuit can range from very negative in prepump segments (<-100 mm Hg) to very positive in postpump segments ($>+300$ mm Hg).[19,30]

There are three techniques for combining ECMO and CKRT.

1. **Separate ECMO and CKRT Circuits**

   This technique involves two independent circuits and vascular access sites. Advantages of this technique include no influence of ECMO flows on CKRT functionality, and the ultrafiltration rate is controlled purely by the CKRT machine. Obtaining additional large vascular access for CKRT is not without risk in the setting of systemic anticoagulation. Furthermore, the negative pressure applied to the venous limb of the ECMO circuit increases the risk of air entrainment during venous cannulation. This can be avoided by temporarily placing a clamp onto the ECMO tubing and decreasing the flows during venous puncture.
2. **Inline Technique**

   A hemofilter is placed in the high-pressure, postpump portion of the ECMO circuit and blood can be returned pre- or postpump **(Figure 35.1)**. Advantages of this technique include economic efficiency and smaller priming volume. The main disadvantage of this technique is that it requires external infusion pumps that can lead to large measurement errors in fluid balance (>800 mL).[29]
3. **Combining the ECMO and CKRT Circuits**

   A CKRT machine can be connected to the ECMO circuit in a variety of configurations **(Figure 35.2A-D)**. Risks when joining a CKRT machine to a preexisting ECMO circuit include substantial blood loss when connecting to a high-pressure part of the circuit and air entrapment when connecting to a low-pressure part of the circuit.[29] In Figure 35.2C, the CKRT machine is connected via the pre- and postoxygenator access ports. The benefits of this configuration include ease of connection to preexisting ports, oxygenator acting as a bubble and clot trap, and ease of measuring pre- and postoxygenator pressures.

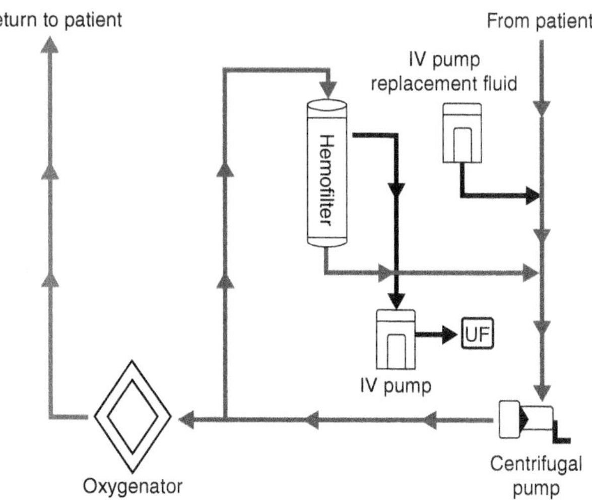

FIGURE 35.1: Inline technique. The hemofilter inflow is connected after the centrifugal pump and blood returns to the circuit before the pump. Alternately, blood can be returned after the pump. IV, intravenous; UF, ultrafiltrate.

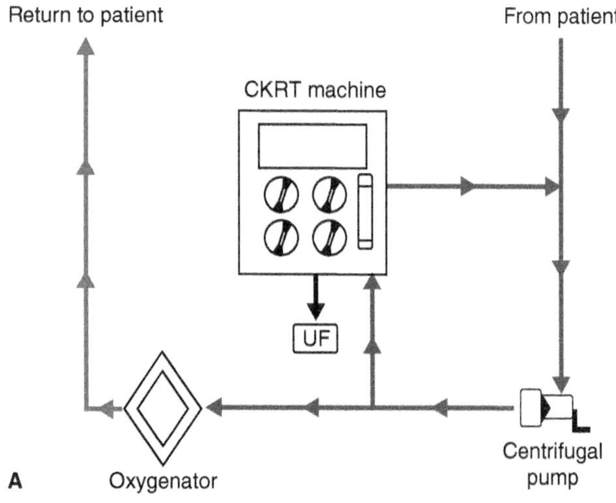

FIGURE 35.2: Four configurations for connecting a CKRT machine to an ECMO circuit. **A:** The CKRT inflow is connected after the pump and outflow is before the pump. **B:** The CKRT machine is connected between the pump and the oxygenator. **C:** The CKRT machine is connected via pre- and postoxygenator access ports. **D:** The CKRT inflow is connected distal to the membrane oxygenator and the outflow is connected proximal to the centrifugal pump. CKRT, continuous kidney replacement therapy; ECMO, extracorporeal membrane oxygenation.

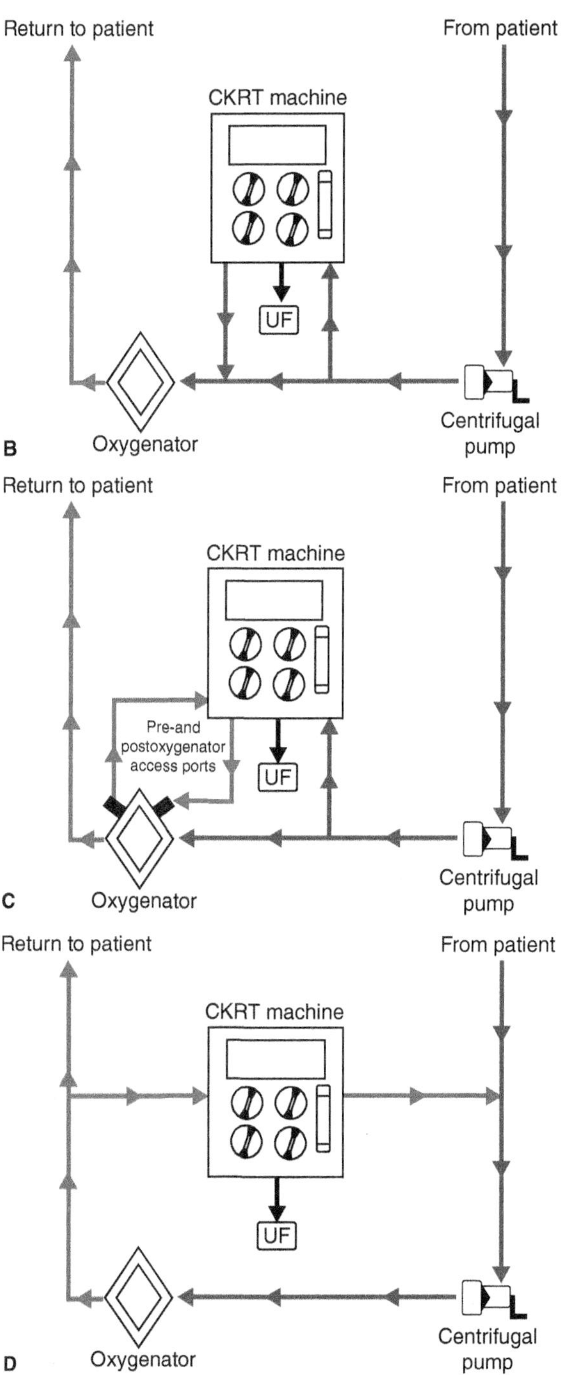

FIGURE 35.2: (*continued*)

MANAGING KIDNEY REPLACEMENT THERAPY ON EXTRACORPOREAL MEMBRANE OXYGENATION

ECMO results in a strong systemic inflammatory response that can lead to leaky capillaries.[27] For this reason, many patients do not tolerate significant fluid removal early in their ECMO course. Over time, filtration can be increased to remove larger volumes of fluid and help aid lung/cardiac recovery. Excessive ultrafiltration rates may also contribute to decreased ECMO flows. Chattering in the cannula may signify depleted intravascular volume and it would be advisable to decrease the ultrafiltration rate in this scenario. Systemic anticoagulation used in ECMO is usually sufficient to prevent clotting within the KRT circuit. If ECMO is achieved without anticoagulation, it is important to use typical KRT circuit anticoagulants such as citrate.[27]

CONCLUSIONS

ECMO continues to be an expanding treatment option for patients with refractory cardiopulmonary failure. With advancements in technology and clinical trials evaluating its efficacy, ECMO has become safer and more commonly used in the ICU setting. Due to its complexity, patients requiring ECMO should be referred to centers with expertise in this technology. Acute kidney injury is a common complication in the ECMO patient and often requires KRT. Initiating and managing KRT while on ECMO is complex and requires critical care nephrologists to have in-depth knowledge of this growing modality.

References

1. Rashkind WJ, Freeman A, Klein D, et al. Evaluation of a disposable plastic, low volume, pumpless oxygenator as a lung substitute. *J Pediatr.* 1965;66:94-102.
2. Chauhan S, Subin S. Extracorporeal membrane oxygenation, an anesthesiologist's perspective: physiology and principles. Part 1. *Ann Card Anaesth.* 2011;14:218-229.
3. Wolfson PJ. The development and use of extracorporeal membrane oxygenation in neonates. *Ann Thorac Surg.* 2003;76(6):S2224-S2229.
4. Zapol WM, Snider MT, Hill JD, et al. Extracorporeal membrane oxygenation in severe acute respiratory failure. A randomized prospective study. *JAMA.* 1979;242:2193-2196.
5. Peek GJ, Mugford M, Tiruvoipati R, et al. Efficacy and economic assessment of conventional ventilatory support versus extracorporeal membrane oxygenation for severe adult respiratory failure (CESAR): a multicentre randomised controlled trial. *Lancet.* 2009;374(9698):1351-1363.
6. Davies A, Jones D, Bailey M, et al. Extracorporeal membrane oxygenation for 2009 influenza A(H1N1) acute respiratory distress syndrome. *JAMA.* 2009;302:1888-1895.
7. Noah MA, Peek GJ, Finney SJ, et al. Referral to an extracorporeal membrane oxygenation center and mortality among patients with severe 2009 influenza A(H1N1). *JAMA.* 2011;306(15):1659-1668.
8. Combes A, Hajage D, Capellier G, et al. Extracorporeal membrane oxygenation for severe acute respiratory distress syndrome. *New Eng J Med.* 2018;378(21):1965-1975.
9. Abrams D, Brodie D. Extracorporeal membrane oxygenation for adult respiratory failure. *Chest.* 2017;152(3):639-649.
10. Tsiouris A, Budev M, Yun J. Extracorporeal membrane oxygenation as a bridge to lung transplantation in the United States: a multicenter survey. *ASAIO J.* 2018;64(5):689-693.
11. Allen S, Holena D, McCunn M, et al. A review of the fundamental principles and evidence base in the use of extracorporeal membrane oxygenation (ECMO) in critically ill adult patients. *J Intensive Care Med.* 2011;26(1):13-26.
12. Napp L, Kühn C, Bauersachs J. ECMO in cardiac arrest and cardiogenic shock. *Herz.* 2017;42(1):27-44.
13. Dobrilovic N, Lateef O, Michalak L, et al. Extracorporeal membrane oxygenation bridges inoperable patients to definitive cardiac operation. *ASAIO J.* 2019;65(1):43-48.
14. Chen Y, Lin J, Yu H, et al. Cardiopulmonary resuscitation with assisted extracorporeal life-support versus conventional cardiopulmonary resuscitation in adults with in-hospital cardiac arrest: an observational study and propensity analysis. *Lancet.* 2008;372(9638):554-561.

15. Kulkarni T, Sharma NS, Diaz-Guzman E. Extracorporeal membrane oxygenation in adults: a practical guide for internists. *Cleve Clin J Med.* 2016;83(5):373-384.
16. Abrams D, Brodie D. Respiratory extracorporeal membrane oxygenation in the cardiothoracic intensive care unit. In: Valchanov K, Jones N, Hogue CW, eds. *Core Topics in Cardiothoracic Critical Care.* 2nd ed. Cambridge University Press; 2018:202-209.
17. Ali J, Jenkins D. Cardiac extracorporeal membrane oxygenation. In: Valchanov K, Jones N, Hogue CW, eds. *Core Topics in Cardiothoracic Critical Care.* 2nd ed. Cambridge University Press; 2018:193-201.
18. Pavlushkov E, Berman M, Valchanov K. Cannulation techniques for extracorporeal life support. *Ann Trans Med.* 2017;5(4):70.
19. ELSO Guidelines for Cardiopulmonary Extracorporeal Life Support. Extracorporeal Life Support Organization, Version 1.4. 2017.
20. Vuylsteke A, Brodie D, Combes A, et al. The ECMO circuit. In: *ECMO in the Adult Patient (Core Critical Care).* Cambridge University Press; 2017:25-57.
21. Miller, RD ed. *Miller's Anesthesia.* 7th ed. Elsevier; 2015.
22. Vuylsteke A, Brodie D, Combes A, et al. Liberation from ECMO. In: *ECMO in the Adult Patient (Core Critical Care).* Cambridge University Press; 2017:165-170.
23. Ortuno S, Delmas C, Diehl J, et al. Weaning from veno-arterial extra-corporeal membrane oxygenation: which strategy to use? *Ann Cardiothorac Surg.* 2019;8(1):E1-E8.
24. Fletcher-Sandersjöö A, Thelin EP, Bartek J, et al. Incidence, outcome, and predictors of intracranial hemorrhage in adult patients on extracorporeal membrane oxygenation: a systematic and narrative review. *Front Neurol.* 2018;9:548.
25. Madershahian N, Nagib R, Wippermann J, et al. A simple technique of distal limb perfusion during prolonged femoro-femoral cannulation. *J Card Surg.* 2006;21(2):168-169.
26. Schmidt M, Bréchot N, Hariri S, et al. Nosocomial infections in adult cardiogenic shock patients supported by venoarterial extracorporeal membrane oxygenation. *Clin Infect Dis.* 2012;55(12):1633-1641.
27. Vuylsteke A, Brodie D, Combes A, et al. Specifics of intensive care management. In: *ECMO in the Adult Patient (Core Critical Care).* Cambridge University Press; 2017:171-196.
28. Villa G, Katz N, Ronco C. Extracorporeal membrane oxygenation and the kidney. *Cardiorenal Med.* 2015;6(1):50–60.
29. Seczyńska B, Królikowski W, Nowak I, et al. Continuous renal replacement therapy during extracorporeal membrane oxygenation in patients treated in medical intensive care unit: technical considerations. *Ther Apher Dial.* 2014;18(6):523-534.
30. Tymowski CD, Augustin P, Houissa H, et al. CRRT connected to ECMO: managing high pressures. *ASAIO J.* 2017;63(1):48-52.

What effect and cost is there to using ECMO in patients with severe respiratory failure?

Randomized Controlled Trial

766 Screened

- 103 hospitals in the UK
- Aged 18 – 65 years
- Severe respiratory failure
  Murray score >3.0/pH <7.20
- July 2001 to August 2006

180 randomized

Consideration for ECMO

Transferred to ECMO center

Venovenous ECMO commenced
if no response to treatment per ARDS protocol within 12 h

90 → Received ECMO → 68

Control

90 → Received treatment as assigned → 90

Intermittent positive-pressure ventilation and/or
High-frequency oscillatory ventilation

Results (Intention-to-treat analysis)

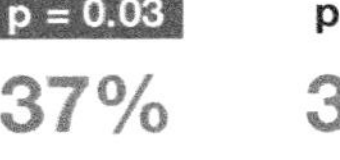

	Death or severe disability at 6 months	Death at 6 months	Severe disability	Mean cost of treatment
	p = 0.03	p = 0.07		
Consideration for ECMO	37%	37%	0%	£73,979
Control	53%	45%	1%	£33,435

Conclusion: There was a significant improvement in survival without severe disability at 6 months in patients transferred for consideration for ECMO treatment compared with continued conventional ventilation.

Peek GJ, Mugford M, Tiruvoipati R, et al. ***Efficacy and economic assessment of conventional ventilatory support versus extracorporeal membrane oxygenation for severe adult respiratory failure (CESAR): a multicentre randomised controlled trial.*** Lancet. 2009; 374(9698):1351-63.

VISUAL ABSTRACT 25.1

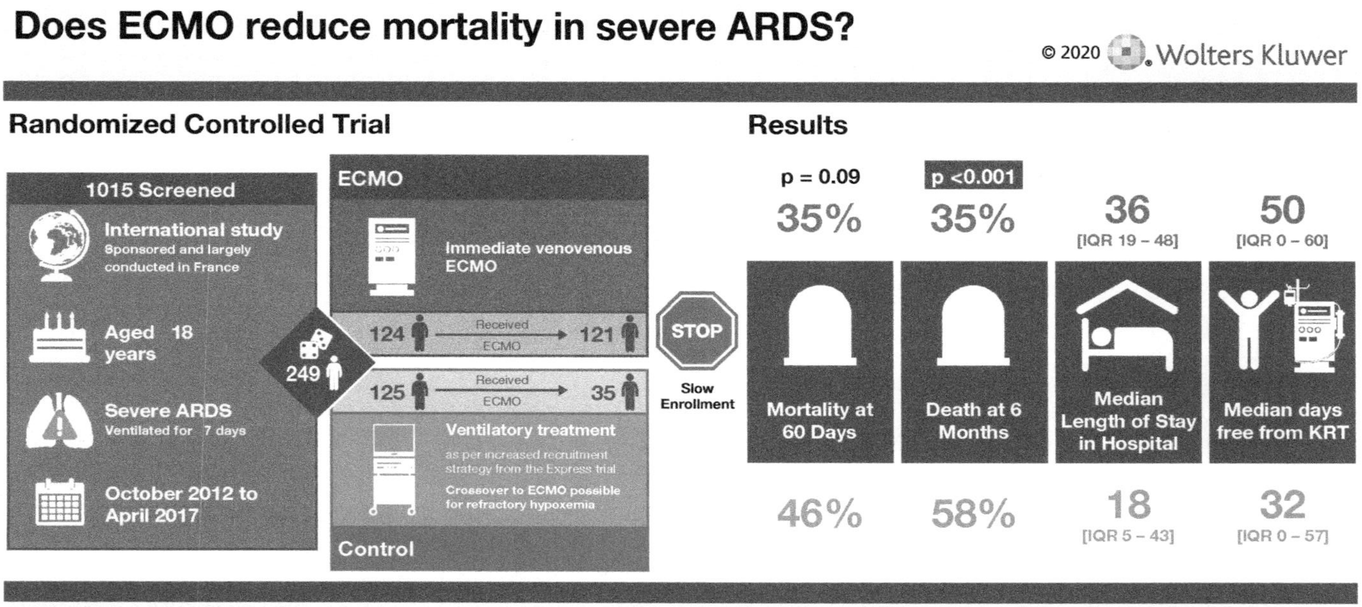

Does ECMO reduce mortality in severe ARDS?

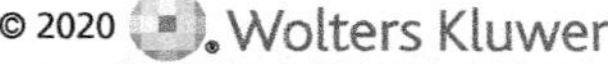

Randomized Controlled Trial

1015 Screened

International study
Sponsored and largely conducted in France

Aged 18 years

Severe ARDS
Ventilated for 7 days

October 2012 to April 2017

249

ECMO

Immediate venovenous ECMO

124 — Received ECMO → 121

125 — Received ECMO → 35

Ventilatory treatment
as per increased recruitment strategy from the Express trial
Crossover to ECMO possible for refractory hypoxemia

Control

STOP

Slow Enrollment

Results

	Mortality at 60 Days	Death at 6 Months	Median Length of Stay in Hospital	Median days free from KRT
p	p = 0.09	p <0.001		
ECMO	35%	35%	36 [IQR 19 – 48]	50 [IQR 0 – 60]
Control	46%	58%	18 [IQR 5 – 43]	32 [IQR 0 – 57]

Conclusion: In this randomized trial involving patients with very severe ARDS, there was no reduction in mortality at 60 days with early application of ECMO compared to control.

Combes A, Hajage D, Capellier G, et al. ***Extracorporeal Membrane Oxygenation for Severe Acute Respiratory Distress Syndrome.*** N Engl J Med. 2018;378(21):1965-1975.

VISUAL ABSTRACT 35.2

Does ECMO reduce mortality in H1N1-related ARDS?

Matched Cohort Study

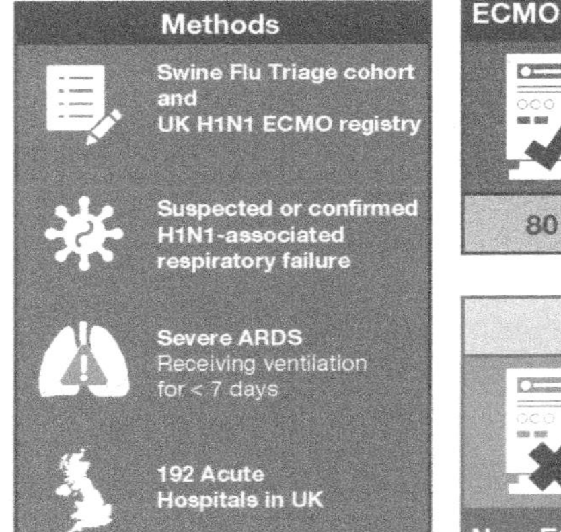

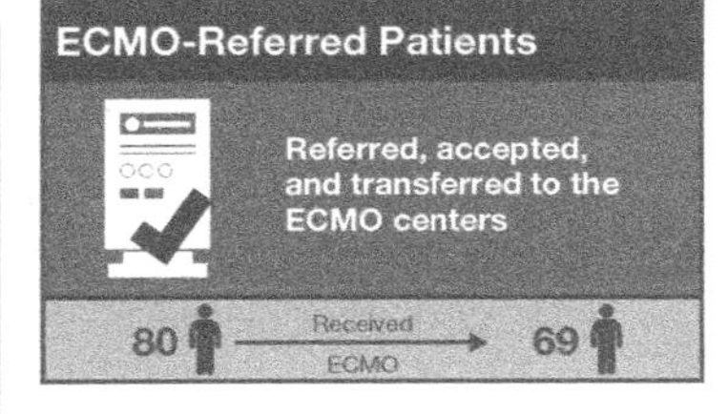

Results

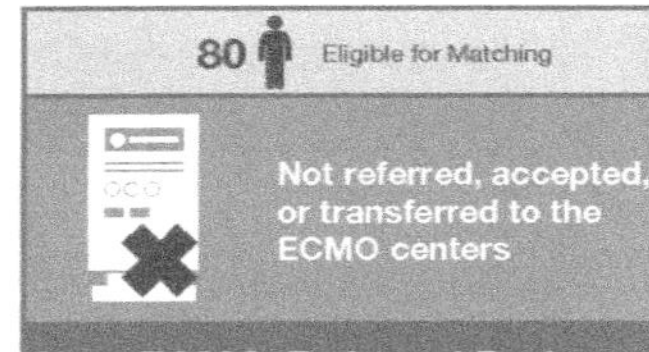

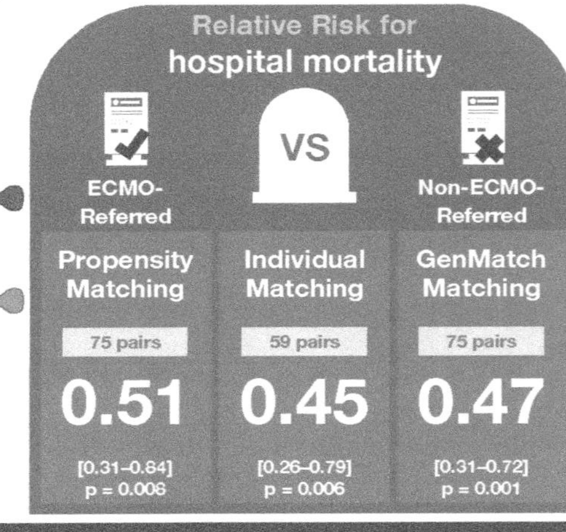

Conclusion: Compared to a cohort of patients with severe H1N1-related ARDS and referred, accepted, and transferred to UK ECMO centers, the hospital mortality for matched non–ECMO-referred patients was approximately double.

Noah MA, Peek GJ, Finney SJ, et al. ***Referral to an extracorporeal membrane oxygenation center and mortality among patients with severe 2009 influenza A(H1N1).*** JAMA. 2011;306(15):1659-68.

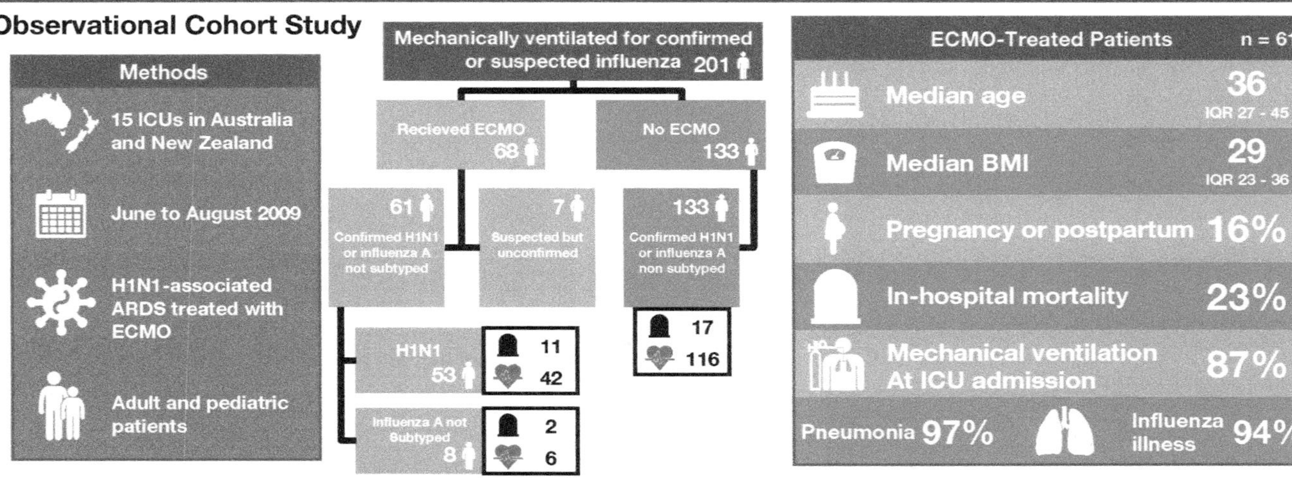

Conclusion: One-third of patients received ECMO during the 2009 influenza A (H1N1) winter pandemic in Australia and New Zealand. These patients were often young adults with severe hypoxemia. The mortality rate at the end of the study period was 21%.

Davies A, Jones D, Bailey M, et al. ***Extracorporeal Membrane Oxygenation for 2009 Influenza A(H1N1) Acute Respiratory Distress Syndrome.*** JAMA. 2009;302(17):1888-95.

VISUAL ABSTRACT 35.4

SECTION IX

Specific Conditions

Sepsis-Associated Acute Kidney Injury

Steven D. Pearson, Neal R. Klauer, and Jason T. Poston

INTRODUCTION

Sepsis is a syndrome defined by organ dysfunction because of a dysregulated host response to infection. Septic shock is a subset of sepsis defined by hypotension requiring vasopressors to maintain a mean arterial pressure (MAP) of 65 mm Hg or above and serum lactate above 2 mmol/L after resuscitation (**Table 36.1**).[1] Both the definition and management of sepsis have been refined over several decades as our understanding of the underlying pathophysiology has evolved, resulting in a decrease in sepsis-associated mortality. The mainstays of treatment for sepsis and septic shock remain largely supportive and include early antibiotics, judicious fluid resuscitation, appropriate selection of vasopressors, and lung protective strategies for mechanical ventilation.[2] Acute kidney injury (AKI) is a common complication, with up to 60% of sepsis cases associated with AKI.[3] This chapter summarizes sepsis-associated AKI (SA-AKI) definitions, risk factors, pathophysiology, and treatment.

DEFINITIONS

Sepsis has long been recognized as a significant cause of morbidity and mortality, yet it was not until the late 20th century that consensus definitions existed to guide clinical practice and research. The first consensus definitions introduced the systemic inflammatory response syndrome (SIRS), with *sepsis* defined as the presence of SIRS in addition to a confirmed infectious process. *Severe sepsis* was defined as sepsis with organ dysfunction and septic shock as sepsis with persistent hypotension, emphasizing a continuum of physiologic and laboratory abnormalities resulting from the inflammatory response and resultant organ failure.[4] These definitions, with modest revision in 2001, went on to guide clinical practice and sepsis research for nearly 25 years.[5] While facilitating critical advancements, the limitations of these definitions and the SIRS criteria were exposed by clinical experience over the subsequent decades. SIRS was found to be nonspecific and overly sensitive and failed to predict meaningful clinical outcomes.[6,7] In 2016, the Sepsis-3 definitions were introduced as an empirically based response to these shortcomings. SIRS and severe sepsis were eliminated, with *sepsis* being redefined as "life-threatening organ dysfunction caused by the dysregulated host response to infection." The presence of organ dysfunction is detected by a change of at least two points on the Sequential Organ Failure Assessment (SOFA), which is associated with a mortality of 10%.[1,8] *Septic shock* is defined as sepsis with hypotension requiring vasopressors to maintain an MAP of 65 mm Hg or above and serum lactate above 2 mmol/L after adequate resuscitation and is associated with a mortality above 40%.[9] Screening

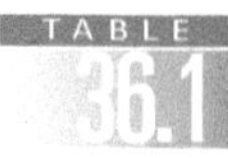

The Sequential Organ Failure Assessment Score

SOFA Score	**1**	**2**	**3**	**4**
Respiration[a]				
PaO_2/FiO_2 (mm Hg)	<400	<300	<220	<100
SaO_2/FiO_2	221-301	142-220	67-141	<67
Coagulation				
Platelets $\times 10^3/mm^3$	<150	<100	<50	<20
Liver				
Bilirubin (mg/dL)	1.2-1.9	2.0-5.9	6.0-11.9	>12.0
Cardiovascular[b]				
Hypotension	MAP < 70	Dopamine ≤ 5 or dobutamine (any)	Dopamine > 5 or norepinephrine ≤ 0.1	Dopamine > 15 or norepinephrine > 0.1
CNS				
Glasgow Coma Score	13-14	10-12	6-9	<6
Kidney				
Creatinine (mg/dL) or urine output (mL/d)	1.2-1.9	2.0-3.4	3.5-4.9 or <500	>5.0 or <200

[a]PaO_2/FiO_2 ratio was used preferentially. If not available, the SaO_2/FiO_2 ratio was used.
[b]Vasoactive mediations administered for at least 1 hr (dopamine and norepinephrine μg/kg/min).

CNS, central nervous system; MAP, mean arterial pressure; SaO_2, peripheral arterial oxygen saturation; SOFA, Sequential Organ Failure Assessment.

From Jones AE, Trzeciak S, Kline JA. The Sequential Organ Failure Assessment score for predicting outcome in patients with severe sepsis and evidence of hypoperfusion at the time of emergency department presentation. *Crit Care Med.* 2009;37(5):1649-1654.

for sepsis in patients with infection can be done at the bedside with the quick SOFA (qSOFA), where meeting two or more of the three criteria is suggestive of sepsis.[5] Although widely adopted, the diagnostic and predictive performance of the Sepsis-3 definitions are variable across clinical settings (emergency department, ward, intensive care unit [ICU]), and newer prediction models may offer both superior diagnostic accuracy and prognostication ability.[10-12]

Criteria for identifying AKI in the presence of sepsis are the same as those used for AKI of other forms. Similar to sepsis, these definitions have undergone frequent revision. The current standard is the Kidney Disease Improving Global Outcomes (KDIGO) guidelines,[13] which were preceded by the Acute Kidney Injury Network (AKIN) and RIFLE (Risk, Injury, Failure, Loss, End-Stage Kidney Disease) classifications.[14,15] Chapter 5 provides further details on these definitions. Many patients meeting consensus criteria for sepsis or septic shock also meet established criteria for AKI and are considered to have SA-AKI.[3] Importantly, patients with sepsis complicated by AKI have a higher mortality rate than septic patients without AKI, and SA-AKI is associated with a higher mortality rate than AKI of other etiologies.[16]

EPIDEMIOLOGY

The incidence of sepsis appears to be on the rise, whereas mortality seems to be decreasing. In the United States from 1979 through 2000, the incidence of sepsis increased from 82.7 to 240.4 per 100,000 population, whereas the in-hospital mortality rate decreased from 28% to 18%, with a net increase in total number of sepsis-related deaths.[17] Data from England, New Zealand, and Australia confirm these trends of increasing incidence with decreasing mortality.[2,18-20] Although AKI is commonly seen in patients with sepsis, obtaining accurate information regarding the incidence and trends of SA-AKI remains difficult because of the many confounding factors commonly encountered in an ICU population. From the available data, AKI can be seen in up to 60% of patients with septic shock and is associated with an increased mortality.[3]

PATHOPHYSIOLOGY

Organ dysfunction in sepsis had long been thought to be primarily driven by hypoperfusion and resulting tissue hypoxia and ischemic injury. Recent advances, however, have shown that organ dysfunction during sepsis develops even in the absence of decreased oxygen delivery. Other mechanisms that contribute to organ dysfunction include microvascular dysfunction, endothelial injury, alterations of cellular metabolism, and immune system dysregulation.[21] Similarly, renal hypotension and ischemic injury are not the sole cause of SA-AKI, with inflammatory, vascular, and metabolic changes playing a role.[22-24] Variations in renal microcirculation, diffusion limitation from edema and inflammation, production of reactive oxygen species, and damage to the endothelial barrier and glycocalyx likely contribute to the structural and functional changes seen in SA-AKI.[25,26] Recently, research has suggested that mitochondrial dysregulation may also play an important role.[27] Though these mechanisms are not currently fully understood, further investigation will improve our understanding of the inflammatory cascade of sepsis as well as their effects on changes in kidney histology, microcirculation, and macrocirculation and may provide insight on potential new therapies for the prevention and treatment of SA-AKI.

DETECTION OF SEPSIS-ASSOCIATED ACUTE KIDNEY INJURY

As AKI accompanying sepsis is independently associated with increased morbidity and mortality, early detection is imperative to ensure appropriate supportive care and therapy. Current classification systems for identifying and diagnosing AKI remain limited by a reliance on urine output and serum creatinine and the inherent challenges related to these measures, as discussed in Chapter 5.[13] Urinalysis and urine microscopy offer a potential tool for the early identification of AKI, specifically in patients with sepsis, as SA-AKI results in greater microscopic evidence of tubular injury when compared to AKI of other etiologies.[28] Furthermore, the presence of new albuminuria has been associated with the development of AKI in critically ill patients with sepsis and may predict AKI before functional impairment in these patients.[29] Serum biomarkers and their potential for predicting development of AKI are discussed in detail in Chapters 16 and 17.

PREVENTION AND MEDICAL TREATMENT

Table 36.2 highlights select randomized controlled clinical trials, informing current management strategies for patients with SA-AKI.

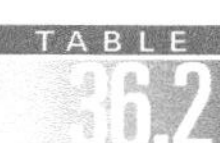

TABLE 36.2 Randomized Controlled Clinical Trial Summaries

Study	Trial Design	Number of Subjects	Patient Population	Intervention and Control	Primary Outcome	Major Conclusion
Balanced crystalloids vs saline in critically ill patients[51]	Cluster randomized, multiple crossover trial	Total: 15,802 Balanced crystalloid: 7,942 (50.2%) 0.9% saline: 7,860 (49.8%)	Single-academic-center ICU population	0.9% saline vs balance crystalloid solution (lactated Ringer or plasma-Lyte A)	Composite outcome within 30 d (all-cause mortality, new KRT, or persistent kidney dysfunction defined as elevation in Cr > 200% baseline)	Use of balanced crystalloid fluids was associated with a significant 1% absolute reduction in the composite outcome
Timing of KRT in patients with acute kidney injury[75]	Randomized controlled trial	Total: 477 Early intervention: 239 (50.1%) Delayed intervention: 238 (49.9%)	Multicenter ICU population with septic shock	Early intervention (KRT within 12 hr of kidney failure) vs delayed intervention (KRT at 48 hr after kidney failure). Dialysis started early if acute indication was met for either group	All-cause mortality at 90 d	No significant difference in 90 d mortality for patients with septic shock with early or delayed KRT

Trial of early, goal-directed resuscitation for septic shock[92]	Randomized controlled trial	Total: 1,260 Early goal-directed therapy: 623 (49.4%) Usual care: 620 (49.2%)	Multicenter ICU population with septic shock	Early goal-directed therapy (i.e., protocol-driven resuscitation utilizing $ScvO_2$ monitoring) vs usual care	All-cause mortality at 90 d	No significant difference in 90 d mortality between goal-directed resuscitation and usual care
Goal-directed resuscitation for patients with early septic shock[93]	Randomized controlled trial	Total: 1,600 Early goal-directed therapy: 796 (49.8%) Usual care: 804 (50.3%)	Multicenter ICU population with septic shock	Early goal-directed therapy (i.e., protocol-driven resuscitation utilizing $ScvO_2$ monitoring) vs usual care	All-cause mortality at 90 d	No significant difference in 90 d mortality between goal-directed resuscitation and usual care
A randomized trial of protocol-based care for early septic shock[94]	Randomized controlled trial	Total: 1,341 Early goal-directed therapy: 439 (32.7%) Protocol-based standard therapy: 446 (33.2%) Usual care: 456 (34%)	Multicenter ED population with septic shock	Early goal-directed therapy (i.e., protocol-driven resuscitation utilizing $ScvO_2$ monitoring) vs protocol-based standard care (i.e., less aggressive early resuscitation) vs usual care	In-hospital death from any cause at 60 d	No significant difference in in-hospital death from any cause at 60 d between any intervention groups

Cr, creatinine; ED, emergency department; ICU, intensive care unit; KRT, kidney replacement therapy.

Resuscitation

Endothelial dysfunction, increased capillary permeability, and decreased venomotor tone resulting from the inflammatory cascade of sepsis lead to relative hypovolemia and decreased systemic vascular resistance. These initial hemodynamic changes result in hypotension requiring prompt resuscitation of circulation with intravenous fluids followed by vasoactive medications if required. Intravenous fluids should be administered in a judicious manner, however, because over-resuscitation and higher cumulative fluid balance in patients with sepsis and septic shock are associated with increased mortality.[30] Multiple studies have demonstrated the harms of excessive fluid administration and fluid accumulation during and after the development of AKI and have shown positive fluid balance to be an independent risk factor for death.[31-34] Exactly how much resuscitation is required while avoiding the harms of excess fluid administration is still an area of debate and discussion. Protocol-based resuscitation targeting normalization of static physiologic parameters, such as central venous pressure, MAP, and central venous oxygen saturation, showed promise initially.[35] More recent studies, however, have shown that protocol-based resuscitation results in higher cumulative fluid administration without a reduction in mortality or AKI when compared with standard care, though this may be in part due to improvements in standard care.[36,37] Likewise, a more conservative transfusion threshold of 7 g/dL (compared to 9 g/dL) improved mortality and was not associated with an increased need for kidney replacement therapy (KRT).[38] Current clinical guidelines recommend a modest initial intravenous fluid bolus of 30 mL/kg within 3 hours followed by frequent assessment of fluid responsiveness using dynamic measures (e.g., arterial pulse pressure variation, passive leg raise) to guide additional fluid resuscitation or initiation of vasoactive medications.[39] Recent research has attempted to reconcile these discrepancies by identifying various sepsis phenotypes hypothesized to have different responses to goal-directed therapy.[40]

Fluid Selection

Multiple studies have shown that the use of hyperoncotic starch solutions (pentastarch and hydroxyethyl starch) for resuscitation in sepsis results in increased risk of AKI, need for KRT, and death. These solutions should be avoided in patients with sepsis and all patients at risk for developing AKI.[41-44] Robust data on the use of albumin versus crystalloid solutions have failed to show an improvement in renal outcomes or mortality, and therefore, albumin cannot be recommended over less costly crystalloid solutions for resuscitation in sepsis.[45-47] Selection of crystalloid solution appears to be of importance, with a growing body of evidence comparing the use of balanced crystalloids with isotonic saline solutions[48,49] Most, but not all, studies have shown the use of balanced crystalloids results in improved kidney outcomes and suggests a mortality benefit, particularly in the subset of critically ill patients with sepsis; none have demonstrated improved outcomes with isotonic saline solutions.[50-53] Taken as a whole, this body of evidence suggests that balanced crystalloid solutions should be utilized as a resuscitation fluid in sepsis in the absence of contraindications.

Vasoactive Medications

Norepinephrine has been generally favored as the first-line agent of choice in septic shock, as the available data largely suggest either improved outcomes or lower rates of adverse events when compared to other vasopressors. Low-dose dopamine for the prevention and treatment of AKI has been shown to be ineffective,[54] and when compared with norepinephrine for shock, dopamine use leads to higher rates of arrhythmias and increased mortality.[55,56] Epinephrine has also been shown to have higher rates of adverse events compared to norepinephrine.[57] Phenylephrine has not been found to be superior to norepinephrine in septic shock,[58] and its use as a first-line vasopressor was associated with increased sepsis-related mortality during a national US norepinephrine shortage.[59] When compared to norepinephrine, vasopressin has been shown to have similar rates of adverse events as well as similar outcomes in terms of both kidney failure and mortality and can be considered a viable first-line alternative to norepinephrine.[60-62] Recently, angiotensin II has emerged as a novel and effective vasoactive agent for the management of vasodilatory shock, though it has not yet been compared directly to other vasopressors.[63] Initial data also suggest a benefit specifically in the subgroup of patients with vasodilatory shock and AKI treated with angiotensin II compared with placebo.[64]

When titrating dose of vasopressors, MAP targets above 65 mm Hg resulted in lower rates of KRT in the subset of patients with a history of hypertension, but did not show a mortality benefit and resulted in increased arrhythmias.[65] Consensus guidelines recommend norepinephrine and vasopressin as first-line vasopressors with a target MAP goal of 65 mm Hg, although individual patient characteristics should also guide these treatment decisions.[66]

Corticosteroids

The use of adjuvant corticosteroids in septic shock remains controversial owing to decades of conflicting data. Whereas some large randomized controlled clinical trials have demonstrated a mortality benefit,[67] others have shown no improvement in outcomes.[68] In addition, multiple large meta-analyses have shown either a small mortality benefit or shortened duration of shock without a mortality benefit, and no trials have shown an improvement in either AKI or need for KRT.[69,70] Current expert guidelines recommend against the routine use of corticosteroids in sepsis and suggest their use be reserved for those with refractory shock with persistent hemodynamic instability despite adequate fluid resuscitation and vasopressors.[66]

Mechanical Ventilation

Patients with sepsis and septic shock often require invasive mechanical ventilation with positive pressure because of the hypoxemia and acidosis resulting from multisystem organ failure. Invasive mechanical ventilation is a known independent risk factor for the development of AKI, with the mechanism likely being related to deleterious hemodynamic, neurohormonal, and inflammatory changes.[71,72] Whereas some studies have shown less kidney failure with low tidal volume ventilation, others have shown no difference in renal outcomes with different mechanical ventilation strategies.[73,74] The optimal strategy of mechanical ventilation for preventing kidney injury without compromising support of the respiratory system is unknown, and best practices for a lung protective ventilation strategy should be followed, as discussed in Chapter 3.

Kidney Replacement Therapy

Most of the data regarding KRT in the setting of sepsis are pulled from studies of heterogeneous ICU patient populations, although several studies have investigated KRT specifically in SA-AKI. The timing of KRT initiation has been an area of great practical interest. The available data generally show no benefit, and one study suggests potential harm with early initiation; in the largest of these studies, close to 60% of enrolled patients had sepsis at randomization.[75-79] The dose of KRT administered in the specific setting of SA-AKI has been studied as well, with multiple trials showing no benefit of continuous KRT at higher doses (70 to 80 mL/kg/hr) compared to conventional doses (35 to 40 mL/kg/hr).[80,81] These results agree with the larger trials done in all critically ill patients with kidney failure, which inform current dosing guidelines, and Chapter 30 provides more details on this topic.[82,83] In addition, no studies have shown improved outcomes with either continuous KRT or intermittent hemodialysis when compared to each other.[84] Regardless of the timing, dose, or modality, a recent retrospective analysis showed a trend of improving mortality in patients receiving KRT in the ICU over the past decade. The specific mechanisms to account for these observations, however, are unclear.[85]

Emerging Therapies

Although no specific pharmacologic therapy has yet proven effective for the treatment of SA-AKI, several novel and established agents have been and are currently undergoing study. In animal sepsis models, alkaline phosphatase blunted the systemic inflammatory response and reduced organ dysfunction. However, it failed to improve kidney function in critically ill patients with established SA-AKI, though all-cause mortality was lower in the alkaline phosphatase group.[86] In a secondary post hoc analysis of a randomized controlled trial of thiamine in patients with septic shock, patients who received thiamine had lower serum creatinine levels and less need for KRT than the placebo group, although these results have yet to be replicated in a primary analysis.[87] Given the preliminary findings of improved outcomes of patients with AKI requiring KRT in a subgroup analysis of the ATHOS-3 trial, angiotensin II offers to be a promising choice of vasoactive medication that may have additional benefits in patients with sepsis and AKI, though further prospective study is needed.[64] Vitamin C has also gained much attention after an observational study reported a significant decrease in mortality for patients with septic shock treated with a combination of vitamin C, thiamine, and corticosteroids.[88] Subsequent randomized controlled studies, however, have been unable to replicate those results.[89,90] Though further studies are currently ongoing, the potential benefit of vitamin C should be balanced against the known risk of calcium oxalate nephropathy associated with high intravenous doses.[91]

References

1. Singer M, Deutschman CS, Seymour CW, et al. The Third International Consensus Definitions for Sepsis and Septic Shock (Sepsis-3). *JAMA.* 2016;315:801-810.
2. Gotts JE, Matthay MA. Sepsis: pathophysiology and clinical management. *BMJ.* 2016;353:i1585.
3. Bagshaw SM, Lapinsky S, Dial S, et al. Acute kidney injury in septic shock: clinical outcomes and impact of duration of hypotension prior to initiation of antimicrobial therapy. *Intensive Care Med.* 2009;35:871-881.
4. Bone RC, Balk RA, Cerra FB, et al. Definitions for sepsis and organ failure and guidelines for the use of innovative therapies in sepsis. *Chest.* 1992;101:1644-1655.
5. Levy MM, Fink MP, Marshall JC, et al. 2001 SCCM/ESICM/ACCP/ATS/SIS International Sepsis Definitions Conference. *Intensive Care Med.* 2003;29:530-538.
6. Alberti C, Brun-Buisson C, Goodman SV, et al. Influence of systemic inflammatory response syndrome and sepsis on outcome of critically ill infected patients. *Am J Respir Crit Care Med.* 2003;168:77-84.
7. Sprung CL, Sakr Y, Vincent J-L, et al. An evaluation of systemic inflammatory response syndrome signs in the sepsis occurrence in acutely ill patients (SOAP) study. *Intensive Care Med.* 2006;32:421-427.

8. Ferreira FL, Bota DP, Bross A, et al. Serial evaluation of the SOFA score to predict outcome in critically ill patients. *JAMA.* 2001;286:1754-1758.
9. Shankar-Hari M, Phillips GS, Levy ML, et al. Developing a new definition and assessing new clinical criteria for septic shock: for the Third International Consensus Definitions for Sepsis and Septic Shock (Sepsis-3). *JAMA.* 2016;315:775-787.
10. Churpek MM, Snyder A, Han X, et al. Quick sepsis-related organ failure assessment, systemic inflammatory response syndrome, and early warning scores for detecting clinical deterioration in infected patients outside the intensive care unit. *Am J Respir Crit Care Med.* 2017;195:906-911.
11. Freund Y, Lemachatti N, Krastinova E, et al. Prognostic accuracy of Sepsis-3 criteria for in-hospital mortality among patients with suspected infection presenting to the emergency department. *JAMA.* 2017;317:301-308.
12. Seymour CW, Liu VX, Iwashyna TJ, et al. Assessment of clinical criteria for sepsis: for the Third International Consensus Definitions for Sepsis and Septic Shock (Sepsis-3). *JAMA.* 2016;315:762-774.
13. Kellum JA, Lameire N; KDIGO AKI Guideline Work Group. Diagnosis, evaluation, and management of acute kidney injury: a KDIGO summary (Part 1). *Crit Care.* 2013;17:204.
14. Joannidis M, Metnitz B, Bauer P, et al. Acute kidney injury in critically ill patients classified by AKIN versus RIFLE using the SAPS 3 database. *Intensive Care Med.* 2009;35:1692-1702.
15. Thakar CV, Christianson A, Freyberg R, et al. Incidence and outcomes of acute kidney injury in intensive care units: a veterans administration study. *Crit Care Med.* 2009;37:2552-2558.
16. Bagshaw SM, Uchino S, Bellomo R, et al. Septic acute kidney injury in critically ill patients: clinical characteristics and outcomes. *Clin J Am Soc Nephrol.* 2007;2:431-439.
17. Martin GS, Mannino DM, Eaton S, et al. The epidemiology of sepsis in the United States from 1979 through 2000. *N Engl J Med.* 2003;348:1546-1554.
18. Kaukonen K-M, Bailey M, Suzuki S, et al. Mortality related to severe sepsis and septic shock among critically ill patients in Australia and New Zealand, 2000-2012. *JAMA.* 2014;311:1308-1316.
19. McPherson D, Griffiths C, Williams M, et al. Sepsis-associated mortality in England: an analysis of multiple cause of death data from 2001 to 2010. *BMJ Open.* 2013;3:e002586.
20. Kadri SS, Rhee C, Strich JR, et al. Estimating ten-year trends in septic shock incidence and mortality in United States academic medical centers using clinical data. *Chest.* 2017;151:278-285.
21. Pool R, Gomez H, Kellum JA. Mechanisms of organ dysfunction in sepsis. *Crit Care Clin.* 2018;34:63-80.
22. Gómez H, Kellum JA. Sepsis-induced acute kidney injury. *Curr Opin Crit Care.* 2016;22:546-553.
23. Langenberg C, Gobe G, Hood S, et al. Renal histopathology during experimental septic acute kidney injury and recovery. *Crit Care Med.* 2014;42:e58-e67.
24. Maiden MJ, Otto S, Brealey JK, et al. Structure and function of the kidney in septic shock. A prospective controlled experimental study. *Am J Respir Crit Care Med.* 2016;194:692-700.
25. Post EH, Kellum JA, Bellomo R, et al. Renal perfusion in sepsis: from macro-to microcirculation. *Kidney Int.* 2017;91:45-60.
26. Chelazzi C, Villa G, Mancinelli P, et al. Glycocalyx and sepsis-induced alterations in vascular permeability. *Crit Care.* 2015;19:26.
27. Sun J, Zhang J, Tian J, et al. Mitochondria in sepsis-induced AKI. *J Am Soc Nephrol.* 2019;30:1151-1161.
28. Bagshaw SM, Haase M, Haase-Fielitz A, et al. A prospective evaluation of urine microscopy in septic and non-septic acute kidney injury. *Nephrol Dial Transplant.* 2011;27:582-588.
29. Neyra JA, Manllo J, Li X, et al. Association of de novo dipstick albuminuria with severe acute kidney injury in critically ill septic patients. *Nephron Clin Pract.* 2014;128:373-380.
30. Neyra JA, Li X, Canepa-Escaro F, et al. Cumulative fluid balance and mortality in septic patients with or without acute kidney injury and chronic kidney disease. *Crit Care Med.* 2016;44:1891-1900.
31. Grams ME, Estrella MM, Coresh J, et al. Fluid balance, diuretic use, and mortality in acute kidney injury. *Clin J Am Soc Nephrol.* 2011;6:966-973.
32. Liu KD, Thompson BT, Ancukiewicz M, et al. Acute kidney injury in patients with acute lung injury: impact of fluid accumulation on classification of acute kidney injury and associated outcomes. *Crit Care Med.* 2011;39:2665-2671.
33. Payen D, de Pont AC, Sakr Y, et al. A positive fluid balance is associated with a worse outcome in patients with acute renal failure. *Crit Care.* 2008;12:R74.
34. Bouchard J, Soroko SB, Chertow GM, et al. Fluid accumulation, survival and recovery of kidney function in critically ill patients with acute kidney injury. *Kidney Int.* 2009;76:422-427.
35. Rivers E, Nguyen B, Havstad S, et al. Early goal-directed therapy in the treatment of severe sepsis and septic shock. *N Engl J Med.* 2001;345:1368-1377.

36. Rowan K, Angus D, Bailey M, et al. Early, goal-directed therapy for septic shock—a patient-level meta-analysis. *N Engl J Med.* 2017;376:2223-2234.
37. Kellum JA, Chawla LS, Keener C, et al. The effects of alternative resuscitation strategies on acute kidney injury in patients with septic shock. *Am J Respir Crit Care Med.* 2016; 193:281-287.
38. Holst LB, Haase N, Wetterslev J, et al. Lower versus higher hemoglobin threshold for transfusion in septic shock. *N Engl J Med.* 2014;371:1381-1391.
39. Howell MD, Davis, AM. Management of sepsis and septic shock. *JAMA.* 2017;317:847-848.
40. Seymour CW, Kennedy JN, Wang S, et al. Derivation, validation, and potential treatment implications of novel clinical phenotypes for sepsis. *JAMA.* 2019;321:2003-2017.
41. Brunkhorst FM, Engel C, Bloos F, et al. Intensive insulin therapy and pentastarch resuscitation in severe sepsis. *N Engl J Med.* 2008;358:125-139.
42. Myburgh JA, Finfer S, Bellomo R, et al. Hydroxyethyl starch or saline for fluid resuscitation in intensive care. *N Engl J Med.* 2012;367:1901-1911.
43. Perner A, Haase N, Guttormsen AB, et al. Hydroxyethyl starch 130/0.42 versus Ringer's acetate in severe sepsis. *N Engl J Med.* 2012;367:124-134.
44. Zarychanski R, Abou-Setta AM, Turgeon AF, et al. Association of hydroxyethyl starch administration with mortality and acute kidney injury in critically ill patients requiring volume resuscitation: a systematic review and meta-analysis. *JAMA.* 2013;309:678-688.
45. Caironi P, Tognoni G, Masson S, et al. Albumin replacement in patients with severe sepsis or septic shock. *N Engl J Med.* 2014;370:1412-1421.
46. The SAFE Study Investigators. Impact of albumin compared to saline on organ function and mortality of patients with severe sepsis. *Intensive Care Med.* 2011;37:86-96.
47. Xu J-Y, Chen Q-H, Xie J-F, et al. Comparison of the effects of albumin and crystalloid on mortality in adult patients with severe sepsis and septic shock: a meta-analysis of randomized clinical trials. *Crit Care.* 2014;18:702.
48. Raghunathan K, Bonavia A, Nathanson BH, et al. Association between initial fluid choice and subsequent in-hospital mortality during the resuscitation of adults with septic shock. *Anesthesiology.* 2015;123:1385-1393.
49. Raghunathan K, Shaw A, Nathanson B, et al. Association between the choice of IV crystalloid and in-hospital mortality among critically ill adults with sepsis. *Crit Care Med.* 2014;42:1585-1591.
50. Self WH, Semler MW, Wanderer JP, et al. Balanced crystalloids versus saline in noncritically ill adults. *N Engl J Med.* 2018;378:819-828.
51. Semler MW, Self WH, Wanderer JP, et al. Balanced crystalloids versus saline in critically ill adults. *N Engl J Med.* 2018;378:829-839.
52. Young P, Bailey M, Beasley R, et al. Effect of a buffered crystalloid solution vs saline on acute kidney injury among patients in the intensive care unit: the SPLIT randomized clinical trial. *JAMA.* 2015;314:1701-1710.
53. Yunos NaM, Bellomo R, Hegarty C, et al. Association between a chloride-liberal vs chloride-restrictive intravenous fluid administration strategy and kidney injury in critically ill adults intravenous strategy for kidney injury in adults. *JAMA.* 2012;308:1566-1572.
54. Kellum JA, Decker JM. Use of dopamine in acute renal failure: a meta-analysis. *Crit Care Med.* 2001;29:1526-1531.
55. De Backer D, Biston P, Devriendt J, et al. Comparison of dopamine and norepinephrine in the treatment of shock. *N Engl J Med.* 2010;362:779-789.
56. De Backer D, Aldecoa C, Njimi H, et al. Dopamine versus norepinephrine in the treatment of septic shock: a meta-analysis. *Crit Care Med.* 2012;40:725-730.
57. Myburgh JA, Higgins A, Jovanovska A, et al. A comparison of epinephrine and norepinephrine in critically ill patients. *Intensive Care Med.* 2008;34:2226-2234.
58. Morelli A, Ertmer C, Rehberg S, et al. Phenylephrine versus norepinephrine for initial hemodynamic support of patients with septic shock: a randomized, controlled trial. *Crit Care.* 2008;12:R143.
59. Vail E, Gershengorn HB, Hua M, et al. Association between US norepinephrine shortage and mortality among patients with septic shock. *JAMA.* 2017;317:1433-1442.
60. Gordon AC, Mason AJ, Thirunavukkarasu N, et al. Effect of early vasopressin vs norepinephrine on kidney failure in patients with septic shock: the VANISH randomized clinical trial. *JAMA.* 2016;316:509-518.
61. Lauzier F, Lévy B, Lamarre P, et al. Vasopressin or norepinephrine in early hyperdynamic septic shock: a randomized clinical trial. *Intensive Care Med.* 2006;32:1782-1789.
62. Russell JA, Walley KR, Singer J, et al. Vasopressin versus norepinephrine infusion in patients with septic shock. *N Engl J Med.* 2008;358:877-887.
63. Khanna A, English SW, Wang XS, et al. Angiotensin II for the treatment of vasodilatory shock. *N Engl J Med.* 2017;377:419-430.

64. Tumlin JA, Murugan R, Deane AM, et al. Outcomes in patients with vasodilatory shock and renal replacement therapy treated with intravenous angiotensin II. *Crit Care Med.* 2018;46:949-957.
65. Asfar P, Meziani F, Hamel J-F, et al. High versus low blood-pressure target in patients with septic shock. *N Engl J Med.* 2014;370:1583-1593.
66. Rhodes A, Evans LE, Alhazzani W, et al. Surviving sepsis campaign: international guidelines for management of sepsis and septic shock: 2016. *Crit Care Med.* 2017;45:486-552.
67. Annane D, Renault A, Brun-Buisson C, et al. Hydrocortisone plus fludrocortisone for adults with septic shock. *N Engl J Med.* 2018;378:809-818.
68. Venkatesh B, Finfer S, Cohen J, et al. Adjunctive glucocorticoid therapy in patients with septic shock. *N Engl J Med.* 2018;378:797-808.
69. Rochwerg B, Oczkowski SJ, Siemieniuk RAC, et al. Corticosteroids in sepsis: an updated systematic review and meta-analysis. *Crit Care Med.* 2018;46:1411-1420.
70. Rygård SL, Butler E, Granholm A, et al. Low-dose corticosteroids for adult patients with septic shock: a systematic review with meta-analysis and trial sequential analysis. *Intensive Care Med.* 2018;44:1003-1016.
71. Koyner JL, Murray PT. Mechanical ventilation and lung–kidney interactions. *Clin J Am Soc Nephrol.* 2008;3:562-570.
72. Kuiper JW, Groeneveld ABJ, Slutsky AS, et al. Mechanical ventilation and acute renal failure. *Crit Care Med.* 2005;33:1408-1415.
73. Brower RG, Matthay MA, Morris A, et al. Ventilation with lower tidal volumes as compared with traditional tidal volumes for acute lung injury and the acute respiratory distress syndrome. *N Engl J Med.* 2000;342:1301-1308.
74. van den Akker JP, Egal M, Groeneveld AJ. Invasive mechanical ventilation as a risk factor for acute kidney injury in the critically ill: a systematic review and meta-analysis. *Crit Care.* 2013;17:R98.
75. Barbar SD, Clere-Jehl R, Bourredjem A, et al. Timing of renal-replacement therapy in patients with acute kidney injury and sepsis. *N Engl J Med.* 2018;379:1431-1442.
76. Gaudry S, Hajage D, Schortgen F, et al. Timing of renal support and outcome of septic shock and acute respiratory distress syndrome. A post hoc analysis of the AKIKI randomized clinical trial. *Am J Respir Crit Care Med.* 2018;198:58-66.
77. Payen D, Mateo J, Cavaillon JM, et al. Impact of continuous venovenous hemofiltration on organ failure during the early phase of severe sepsis: a randomized controlled trial. *Crit Care Med.* 2009;37:803-810.
78. Zarbock A, Kellum JA, Schmidt C, et al. Effect of early vs delayed initiation of renal replacement therapy on mortality in critically ill patients with acute kidney injury: the ELAIN randomized clinical trial. *JAMA.* 2016;315:2190-2199.
79. STARRT-AKI Investigators. Timing of initiation of renal-replacement therapy in acute kidney injury. *N Engl J Med.* 2020;383:240-251.
80. Joannes-Boyau O, Honoré PM, Perez P, et al. High-volume versus standard-volume haemofiltration for septic shock patients with acute kidney injury (IVOIRE study): a multicentre randomized controlled trial. *Intensive Care Med.* 2013;39:1535-1546.
81. Park JT, Lee H, Kee YK, et al. High-dose versus conventional-dose continuous venovenous hemodiafiltration and patient and kidney survival and cytokine removal in sepsis-associated acute kidney injury: a randomized controlled trial. *Am J Kidney Dis.* 2016;68:599-608.
82. Bellomo R, Cass A, Cole L, et al. Intensity of continuous renal-replacement therapy in critically ill patients. *N Engl J Med.* 2009;361:1627-1638.
83. Palevsky P, Zhang JH, O'Connor TZ, et al. Intensity of renal support in critically ill patients with acute kidney injury. *N Engl J Med.* 2008;359:7-20.
84. Schefold JC, von Haehling S, Pschowski R, et al. The effect of continuous versus intermittent renal replacement therapy on the outcome of critically ill patients with acute renal failure (CONVINT): a prospective randomized controlled trial. *Crit Care.* 2014;18:R11.
85. Miyamoto Y, Iwagami M, Aso S, et al. Temporal change in characteristics and outcomes of acute kidney injury on renal replacement therapy in intensive care units: analysis of a nationwide administrative database in Japan, 2007–2016. *Crit Care.* 2019;23:172.
86. Pickkers P, Mehta RL, Murray PT, et al. Effect of human recombinant alkaline phosphatase on 7-day creatinine clearance in patients with sepsis-associated acute kidney injury: a randomized clinical trial. *JAMA.* 2018;320:1998-2009.
87. Moskowitz A, Andersen LW, Cocchi MN, et al. Thiamine as a renal protective agent in septic shock. a secondary analysis of a randomized, double-blind, placebo-controlled trial. *Ann Am Thorac Soc.* 2017;14:737-741.
88. Marik PE, Khangoora V, Rivera R, et al. Hydrocortisone, vitamin C, and thiamine for the treatment of severe sepsis and septic shock: a retrospective before-after study. *Chest.* 2017;151:1229-1238.

89. Fowler AA, III, Truwit JD, Hite RD, et al. Effect of vitamin c infusion on organ failure and biomarkers of inflammation and vascular injury in patients with sepsis and severe acute respiratory failure: the CITRIS-ALI randomized clinical trial. *JAMA.* 2019;322:1261-1270.
90. Fujii T, Luethi N, Young PJ, et al. Effect of vitamin c, hydrocortisone, and thiamine vs hydrocortisone alone on time alive and free of vasopressor support among patients with septic shock: the VITAMINS randomized clinical trial. *JAMA.* 2020;323:423-431.
91. Cossey LN, Rahim F, Larsen CP. Oxalate nephropathy and intravenous vitamin C. *Am J Kidney Dis.* 2013;61:1032-1035.
92. Mouncey PR, Osborn TM, Power GS, et al. Trial of early, goal-directed resuscitation for septic shock. *N Engl J Med.* 2015;372:1301-1311.
93. The ARISE Investigators, the ANZICS Clinical Trials Group. Goal-directed resuscitation for patients with early septic shock. *N Engl J Med.* 2014;371:1496-1506.
94. The ProCESS Investigators. A randomized trial of protocol-based care for early septic shock. *N Engl J Med.* 2014;370:1683-1693.

Diabetic Ketoacidosis

Joel M. Topf, Nirali Ramani, Claudia Rodriguez Rivera, and Andrew Kowalski

INTRODUCTION

Uncontrolled diabetes can result in severe acute illness requiring critical care called hyperglycemic crisis. The syndrome is divided into two conditions depending on the presence of ketoacidosis. Hyperglycemic hyperosmolar state (HHS) is severe, uncontrolled diabetes because of a relative lack of insulin that results in severe hyperglycemia, hyperosmolality, and altered mental status ranging from lethargy to coma. In diabetic ketoacidosis (DKA), an absolute lack of insulin causes the body to switch from glucose to ketones as the primary fuel, leading to a severe anion gap metabolic acidosis. Both of these syndromes have a host of metabolic abnormalities that require careful monitoring and management.

PATHOLOGY

Hyperglycemic crises begin with a lack of insulin, either relative or absolute. This results in intracellular hypoglycemia despite extracellular hyperglycemia and triggers release of counterregulatory hormones (glucagon, catecholamines, cortisol, growth hormone) in an attempt to increase intracellular glucose. If there is an absolute lack of insulin, the body shifts from glucose, as the primary carbohydrate, to ketones (e.g., 3-β-hydroxybutyrate, acetoacetate, or acetone); this is the road to DKA. Otherwise, a small amount of insulin keeps ketosis in check despite being unable to correct the hyperglycemia. This leads to HHS.

The lack of insulin along with increased glucagon causes lipolysis in the adipocytes, releasing triglycerides that are metabolized to glycerol and free fatty acids. The liver takes these up and converts the glycerol to glucose via gluconeogenesis and converts the fatty acids to acetyl coenzyme A (CoA) via beta oxidation. Acetyl CoA can enter the tricarboxylic acid (TCA) cycle to produce adenosine triphosphate (ATP) for the hepatocyte, but to provide energy for the rest of the body it is converted to ketones via ketogenesis (see **Figure 37.1**).

β-Hydroxybutyrate and acetoacetate are strong acids and are responsible for the anion gap metabolic acidosis characteristic of DKA. β-Hydroxybutyrate accumulates early in disease and is the dominant ketone until late in the disease when acetoacetate predominates.

In HHS, the counterregulatory hormones increase glucose. The insulin that is available is inadequate to control the hyperglycemia but is sufficient to suppress ketoacidosis. Precipitating events for HHS are conditions that stimulate the release of counterregulating hormones and promote dehydration.

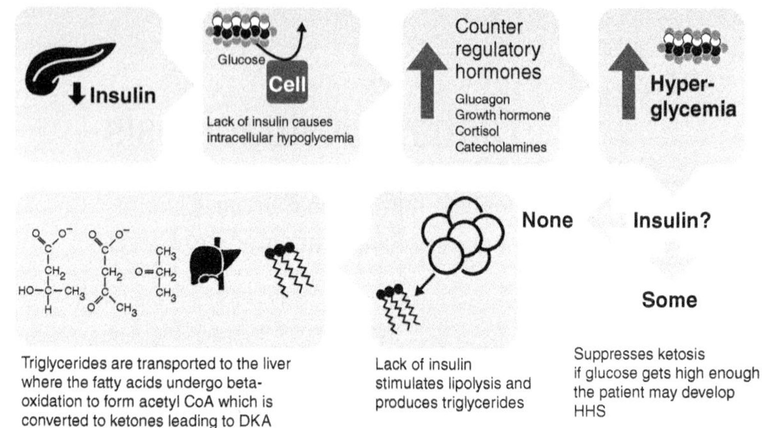

FIGURE 37.1: The roads to DKA and HHS. CoA, coenzyme A; DKA, diabetic ketoacidosis; HHS, hyperglycemic hyperosmolar state.

EPIDEMIOLOGY

Between 2009 and 2014 the rate of DKA increased from 19.5 to 30.2 per 1,000 persons. Thankfully, the case fatality rate has fallen from 1.1% in 2000 to 0.4% in 2014.[1] Overall, the mortality rate in adults with DKA is less than 1%, but can rise to over 5% in the elderly.[2] Because the etiology of DKA requires an absolute lack of insulin, it is more common in patients with type 1 diabetes mellitus, so the average age tends to be younger than with HHS. Despite this stereotype, fully a third of patients with DKA have type 2 diabetes.[2]

HHS is less well studied. The mortality from HHS is quite a bit higher than found in DKA, probably in part because of the increased age of patients. In a review of case series, Fadini et al reported an average hospital mortality of 17%.[3]

DIAGNOSIS

Laboratory Evaluation

The diagnosis of DKA and HHS depends primarily on biochemical parameters. For DKA, patients should have ketones in the blood or urine, acidosis (pH < 7.3), and hyperglycemia. The latter can be quite variable, with some patients presenting with euglycemic DKA, that is, blood sugars less than 200 to 300.

In HHS, patients have hyperglycemia without the ketoacidosis, so the pH is more than 7.3 and serum bicarbonate is more than 18. Compared with DKA, the glucose tends to be higher with HHS ($>$650 mg/dL). Serum osmolality will typically be over 350 mOsm/kg.[4] There is a positive linear correlation between osmolality and mental status changes.[5] If patients have significant stupor with an osmolality less than 320, an alternative etiology should be considered.[2]

Schwab et al retrospectively looked at nearly 700 people presenting to the hospital with acute illness and hyperglycemia. Urinary ketones had a sensitivity of 99% with a negative predictive value of 100% for the diagnosis of DKA.[6] Another clue to the diagnosis is the presence of an abnormally elevated anion gap. An anion gap greater than 16 had a sensitivity of 92%.

In assessing patients with DKA, venous blood gases are as accurate as arterial blood gases.[7] Other electrolyte findings include hyponatremia because of the hyperglycemia causing a movement of intracellular water to the extracellular compartment diluting the serum sodium. Hyperkalemia is found despite patients generally presenting with total body potassium depletion.

Signs and Symptoms

The primary symptoms for both DKA and HHS are fatigue, polyuria, polydipsia, and mental status changes. On physical exam, patients appear dehydrated with signs of volume depletion, including tachycardia, dry mucous membranes, and hypotension. Kussmaul respirations can be seen in DKA as patients hyperventilate to compensate for metabolic acidosis. Nausea, vomiting, and diffuse abdominal pain are more common in DKA. More severe neurologic symptoms including coma and seizure as well as focal findings (hemianopia and hemiparesis) are more common with HHS.

Pancreatitis is a known cause of DKA, and patients with DKA often have gastrointestinal (GI) symptoms including vomiting as well as abdominal pain, so pancreatitis is often considered an instigating etiology, but in some cases the pancreatitis may be due to the DKA. The elevated triglycerides and acidemia of DKA may trigger acute pancreatitis. Lipase is often elevated in DKA. In some cases, this is due to acute pancreatitis, but in others it is simply an epiphenomenon of DKA.[8] Yadav et al looked at 150 consecutive cases of DKA and found that a third had elevated lipase.[9]

TREATMENT

Hyperglycemic crises are primarily characterized by hyperglycemia, which drives osmotic diuresis leading to loss of water, sodium, and potassium. From that, one can deduce the three most important medications for the treatment of hyperglycemic crisis:

1. Volume
2. Insulin
3. Potassium

The rest is commentary.

Volume

Patients with DKA and HHS typically present with profound fluid deficits. This can be up to 5 L in DKA and as high as 9 to 12 L in HHS.

In moderate disease, the initial fluid resuscitation should be a bolus of 20 mL/kg (approximately 1 L) followed by 500 mL/hr for the first 4 hours, after which the rate can be decreased to 250 mL/hr. In mild cases, patients may not need a bolus and can just start with 250 mL/hr of isotonic crystalloids. In severe disease, fluids should be given "wide open" until perfusion is improved. The goal of intravenous (IV) fluids is to restore perfusion and replace fluid deficits; higher fluid rates can wash out serum ketones, resulting in a prolonged phase of non-anion gap metabolic acidosis after correcting the ketosis.[10]

The standard resuscitation fluid is normal saline (NS) but given the side effect of non–anion gap metabolic acidosis induced by NS, this may not be the ideal resuscitation fluid. However, randomized controlled trials have found no advantage to balanced solutions in DKA. The only adult trial of NS versus lactated Ringer's (LR) in DKA was underpowered for its primary outcome, the normalization of pH, and found no difference. However, patients randomized to LR took longer to get their blood sugars below 250 than patients randomized to NS (410 vs 300 minutes).[11] A small trial ($N = 66$) of NS versus the balanced solution Plasma-Lyte in pediatric DKA similarly found no difference in the incidence of new or progressive AKI, in time to resolution of DKA, need for kidney replacement therapy (KRT), mortality, or lengths of pediatric intensive care unit (PICU) and hospital stay.[12]

Osmotic diuresis typically causes loss of more water than sodium, pushing osmolality and sodium concentration up. The serum sodium, however, is usually normal or low on presentation because of dilution from the osmotic movement of water from the intracellular to the extracellular compartment. The Katz conversion allows the doctor to see what the sodium would be with a normal serum glucose[13] (see **Equation 37.1**).

$$\text{Adjusted sodium} = \text{measured sodium} + (0.016 \times [\text{glucose} - 100]) \quad \text{(Eq 37.1)}$$

If the adjusted serum sodium is elevated (and some say high normal), consideration should be made for switching IV fluids from NS to a hypotonic solution like 0.45% NaCl.[4] Note: the adjusted sodium should not be used to calculate the anion gap, it is only used to give a sense of where the sodium will be after correction of the glucose, to orient providers on any underlying dysnatremia.

Insulin

In patients with severe volume depletion, which is more common in HHS, insulin should not be initiated until fluid resuscitation has at least partially been corrected. Insulin moves glucose into the cell, which can rapidly lower the extracellular osmolality resulting in extracellular fluid moving back into the cells which can worsen extracellular volume depletion and precipitate cardiovascular collapse. The recommendations from the American Diabetes Association (ADA) are the same for both conditions:

- IV insulin
- Initiate treatment with a bolus of 0.1 units/kg
- Followed by a drip at 0.1 units/kg/hr

Alternatively

- No bolus
- IV infusion of insulin at 0.16 units/kg

A retrospective study revealed no difference in outcomes with bolus or no bolus therapy for DKA with equivalent episodes of hypoglycemia, rate of glucose change, and length of stay.[14] Though IV insulin is the standard of care because of its short half-life and easy titration, it is possible to manage mild to moderate DKA with subcutaneous insulin with hourly injections of regular or similar rapid-onset insulins. A Cochrane systematic review and meta-analysis of subcutaneous insulin reviewed five randomized controlled trials and found the data to be of low to very low quality, and they could not find any advantages or disadvantages compared to IV regular insulin for treating mild or moderate DKA.[15]

In DKA, IV insulin is used not just to lower the serum glucose, but, importantly, to reverse the ketosis. It is essential that the insulin drip be continued until the glucose is less than 200 *and* at least two of the following conditions are met:

1. pH > 7.3
2. Serum bicarbonate > 15
3. Anion gap < 12

Hyperglycemia is usually corrected in the first 6 hours of admission, but ketosis typically persists for 12 hours, so insulin needs to be continued far longer than needed to just correct hyperglycemia. Patients should be started on dextrose infusions to prevent hypoglycemia during this period.

In HHS, IV insulin should be continued until the osmolality and mental status return to normal. Subcutaneous insulin should be started 2 hours prior to stopping the IV insulin.

Potassium

Patients with hyperglycemic crisis have significant potassium deficits (3–5 mmol/kg) as potassium is lost because of the osmotic diuresis.[16] Despite these potassium deficits, patients typically present with hyperkalemia. Once insulin begins, potassium may correct quickly, revealing the underlying potassium deficit. Potassium should be started as soon as the serum potassium is in the normal range. If the potassium is above 3.3 mEq/L, 20 to 30 mEq of KCl can be added to each liter of resuscitation fluids. If the potassium is below 3.2 mEq/L, insulin should be delayed until the potassium is normalized to prevent potentially lethal cardiac arrhythmias.[4] Before giving potassium to any patient, physicians should evaluate kidney function.

OTHER ISSUES IN MANAGEMENT

Bicarbonate

The evidence to support bicarbonate in DKA is not only absent, but when it has been investigated, the trend is toward harm. A 2011 systematic review of bicarbonate in DKA, found only two studies showed a short-term (at 2 hours) increase in pH with bicarbonate.[17] Five other studies that looked for early improvements in pH were unable to find any. More concerning were the signals of harm from bicarbonate therapy. Three studies found prolonged ketosis associated with the use of bicarbonate. Three other studies showed increased potassium supplementation with alkali use. The current ADA guideline does not recommend bicarbonate for pH greater than 7.1, values where studies have shown harm without evidence of benefit. For patients with pH below 6.9, the ADA recommends giving 50 mmol of isotonic bicarbonate an hour until the pH is over 7.0.[2]

Phosphorus

Patients with DKA often have hyperphosphatemia at presentation, but like potassium this hyperphosphatemia is just disguising decreased total body phosphorus. Insulin quickly shifts phosphorus back into cells and often reveals the underlying hypophosphatemia. There is some evidence that treating hypophosphatemia can improve respiration and cardiac function (see Chapter 23); however, the evidence in DKA shows no clinical benefit and some harm (hypocalcemia and hypomagnesemia).[18,19] If the phosphorus is below 1 mmol/L, it can be treated by adding 20 to 30 mmol of sodium phosphorus to the resuscitation fluids. Average phosphorus deficit in DKA is 1 mmol/kg.[2] There are no data on the treatment of hypophosphatemia in HHS.

Hypercoagulable State

Both DKA and HHS are thought to be hypercoagulable states with numerous case reports of arterial and venous thrombotic events.[20-21] Currently, patients should get standard prophylactic anticoagulation as there are no studies or recommendations for full anticoagulation.

The Primary Initiating Event

HHS and DKA usually follow an inciting event. These events can be severe medical problems, including sepsis, trauma, acute pancreatitis, and myocardial infarction. Nonadherence with insulin is an important inciting event. The nature of the inciting event likely drives much of the morbidity of the disease. New-onset diabetes is a common cause of DKA and HHS.

Acute Kidney Injury

Acute kidney injury (AKI) is common in DKA; however, it is largely hemodynamic and much of it resolves with fluid resuscitation. In a retrospective case series of DKA admitted to the ICU, Orban et al found that 50% had at least a 50% increase in creatinine from baseline on admission. By 24 hours, half of that AKI had fully recovered. Acute dialysis was used in 3% of patients in the first 24 hours.[23] As has been found with AKI in general, following recovery from AKI because of DKA, patients have faster loss of glomerular filtration rate (GFR) and worse kidney and survival outcomes compared to DKA patients without AKI.[24]

SPECIAL CASES

Euglycemic Diabetic Ketoacidosis

Euglycemic DKA is defined as DKA with a glucose less than 250 mg/dL. It is not the same as starvation or alcoholic ketosis. In starvation and alcoholic ketosis, hypoglycemia suppresses endogenous insulin and stimulates glucagon, triggering lipolysis and ketosis. The acidosis tends to be more mild than found in DKA, but the key difference is that starvation and alcohol respond to glucose infusions where patients quickly release endogenous insulin, suppressing the ketosis. Unless the patient has concurrent diabetes, no insulin infusions should be needed to reverse the ketosis in alcoholic or starvation ketosis (see **Table 37.1**). Euglycemic DKA was first described by Munro who reported DKA with a blood sugar less than 300 mg/dL in 37 of 311 cases.[25] It is currently much less common than that. Possible causes of euglycemic DKA include sodium glucose cotransporter 2 inhibitors (SGLT2i), insulin administration prior to coming to the hospital, concurrent food restriction, vomiting, and other inhibition of gluconeogenesis (Table 37.1).

SGLT2i were introduced in 2013 as a novel class of antihyperglycemic medications. Since then they have been found to have powerful cardiovascular and kidney protective activity in patients with and without diabetes. Their primary mechanism of action is blocking glucose reabsorption in the proximal tubule resulting in glucosuria. Fralick et al did a propensity-matched study of patients with type 2 diabetes and found patients initiated on SGLT2i had 4.9 episodes of DKA per 1,000 person-years versus 2.3 events per 1,000 person-years in patients

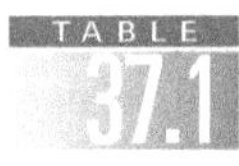

Different Causes of Anion Gap Metabolic Acidosis

	DKA	HHS	Starvation Ketosis	Uremic Acidosis	Alcohol Ketosis	Lactic Acidosis	Toxic Alcohol Ingestion
pH	↓	Normal	Normal	Mild ↓	Variable	↓	↓
Plasma glucose	↑/↑↑	↑↑↑	↓/Normal	Normal	↓/Normal	Normal	Normal
Plasma ketones	+++	+/−	Mild +	−	+	−	−
Anion gap	↑/↑↑	Normal	Mild ↑	Mild ↑	↑	↑	↑
Osmolality	↑	↑↑	Normal	↑↑	Normal	Normal	↑↑

DKA, diabetic ketoacidosis; HHS, hyperglycemic hyperosmolar state.

initiating dipeptidyl peptidase 4 (DPP4).[26] These rates are approximately 10-fold higher than the rates of DKA found in the large phase 4 trials demonstrating cardiovascular and kidney protection.[27] Of note, half of the patients with DKA in the CANVAS trial appeared to actually be type 1 diabetics who had been misdiagnosed as type 2.[28] SGLT2i cause DKA when the drug-induced glucosuria suppresses insulin while stimulating glucagon; however, these patients have less hepatic gluconeogenesis along with continued urinary loss of glucose resulting in mild or absent hyperglycemia. The decreased insulin and increased glucagon stimulate lipolysis, leading to ketoacidosis as in standard DKA pathophysiology.[29] Treatment requires both insulin to reverse the ketosis and glucose to prevent insulin-induced hypoglycemia.[30] The low blood sugars minimize osmotic diuresis and much of the metabolic findings of DKA. Patients tend to have very high anion gaps, often above 30, and require prolonged insulin infusions to correct the acidosis.[31,32]

Continuous Kidney Replacement Therapy

Patients undergoing continuous kidney replacement therapy (CKRT) can sometimes develop euglycemic ketosis. Two groups have reported cases, both involving glucose-free replacement fluids.[33,34] Patients were not eating because of multiorgan failure and glucose-free dialysate can remove 30 to 60 g of glucose a day, quickly depleting glycogen stores, suppressing insulin, and stimulating counterregulatory hormones, putting the patient into ketosis.[35] Patients quickly responded to glucose and insulin infusions.

End-stage Kidney Disease

Hyperglycemic crises in anuric end-stage kidney disease (ESKD) are quite different than in patients with preserved kidney function because of the lack of osmotic diuresis. This means they do not have the profound volume deficiency and shock that is typical of people presenting with hyperglycemic crisis. The hyperglycemia increases extracellular tonicity causing an osmotic shift of fluid from the intracellular to the extracellular compartment, making fluid overload and edema common. If patients have fluid overload, either because of normal fluid intake or because of pathologic redistribution of fluid from the intracellular to the extracellular compartment, hemodialysis may be required to restore normal volume. If anuric patients do have volume deficiency, patients should be given boluses of 250 to 500 mL followed by reevaluation rather than the more aggressive fluid resuscitation typically used in patients with DKA and intact kidney function.

The lack of osmotic diuresis also results in higher glucoses; in a case-controlled study of hyperglycemic crisis in ESKD compared to patients with normal kidney function (estimated GFR > 60 mL/min/1.73 m^2), blood sugar at presentation was 836 mg/dL with ESKD compared with 659 mg/dL with normal kidney function.[36]

ESKD patients also do not have the decreased total body potassium typical of hyperglycemic crises, so protocols that call for aggressive use of potassium supplementation need to be reconsidered.

Because sodium, potassium, and phosphate deficiency are less common in anuric ESKD, the treatment of DKA in ESKD can largely be accomplished with insulin infusions alone. Glucose should be lowered by 50 to 75 mg/dL/hr. Based on observational data, a lower rate of insulin infusion is recommended (0.05–0.07 units/kg/hr).[36,37]

References

1. Benoit SR, Zhang Y, Geiss LS, Gregg EW, Albright A. Trends in diabetic ketoacidosis hospitalizations and in-hospital mortality—United States, 2000-2014. *MMWR Morb Mortal Wkly Rep.* 2018;67(12):362-365.
2. Kitabchi AE, Umpierrez GE, Miles JM, Fisher JN. Hyperglycemic crises in adult patients with diabetes. *Diabetes Care.* 2009;32(7):1335-1343.
3. Fadini GP, de Kreutzenberg SV, Rigato M, et al. Characteristics and outcomes of the hyperglycemic hyperosmolar non-ketotic syndrome in a cohort of 51 consecutive cases at a single center. *Diabetes Res Clin Pract.* 2011;94(2):172-179.
4. Dingle HE, Evan Dingle H, Slovis C. Diabetic ketoacidosis and hyperosmolar hyperglycemic syndrome management. *Emerg Med.* 2018;50(8):161-171. doi:10.12788/emed.2018.0100
5. Umpierrez GE, Kelly JP, Navarrete JE, Casals MM, Kitabchi AE. Hyperglycemic crises in urban blacks. *Arch Intern Med.* 1997;157(6):669-675.
6. Schwab TM, Hendey GW, Soliz TC. Screening for ketonemia in patients with diabetes. *Ann Emerg Med.* 1999;34(3):342-346.
7. Ma OJ, Rush MD, Godfrey MM, Gaddis G. Arterial blood gas results rarely influence emergency physician management of patients with suspected diabetic ketoacidosis. *Acad Emerg Med.* 2003;10(8):836-841.
8. Manikkan AT. Hyperlipasemia in diabetic ketoacidosis. *Clin Diabetes.* 2013;31(1):31-32.
9. Yadav D, Nair S, Norkus EP, Pitchumoni CS. Nonspecific hyperamylasemia and hyperlipasemia in diabetic ketoacidosis: incidence and correlation with biochemical abnormalities. *Am. J. Gastroenterol.* 2000;95(11):3123-3128.
10. Adrogue HJ. Salutary effects of modest fluid replacement in the treatment of adults with diabetic ketoacidosis. Use in patients without extreme volume deficit. *JAMA.* 1989;262(15):2108-2113. doi:10.1001/jama.262.15.2108
11. Van Zyl DG, Rheeder P, Delport E. Fluid management in diabetic-acidosis—Ringer's lactate versus normal saline: a randomized controlled trial. *QJM.* 2011;105(4):337-343.
12. Williams V, Jayashree M, Nallasamy K, Dayal D, Rawat A. 0.9% saline versus Plasma-Lyte as initial fluid in children with diabetic ketoacidosis (SPinK trial): a double-blind randomized controlled trial. *Crit Care.* 2020;24(1):1.
13. Katz MA. Hyperglycemia-induced hyponatremia—calculation of expected serum sodium depression. *N Engl J Med.* 1973;289(16):843-844.
14. Goyal N, Miller JB, Sankey SS, Mossallam U. Utility of initial bolus insulin in the treatment of diabetic ketoacidosis. *J Emerg Med.* 2010;38(4):422-427.
15. Andrade-Castellanos CA, Colunga-Lozano LE, Delgado-Figueroa N, Gonzalez-Padilla DA. Subcutaneous rapid-acting insulin analogues for diabetic ketoacidosis. *Cochrane Database Syst Rev.* 2016;(1):CD011281.
16. Fayfman M, Pasquel FJ, Umpierrez GE. Management of hyperglycemic crises: diabetic ketoacidosis and hyperglycemic hyperosmolar state. *Med Clin North Am.* 2017;101(3):587-606.

17. Chua HR, Schneider A, Bellomo R. Bicarbonate in diabetic ketoacidosis—a systematic review. *Ann Intensive Care.* 2011;1(1):23.
18. Fisher JN, Kitabchi AE. A randomized study of phosphate therapy in the treatment of diabetic ketoacidosis. *J Clin Endocrinol Metab.* 1983;57(1):177-180.
19. Winter RJ, Harris CJ, Phillips LS, Green OC. Diabetic ketoacidosis. Induction of hypocalcemia and hypomagnesemia by phosphate therapy. *Am J Med.* 1979;67(5):897-900.
20. Ho J, Pacaud D, Hill MD, Ross C, Hamiwka L, Mah JK. Diabetic ketoacidosis and pediatric stroke. *CMAJ.* 2005;172(3):327-328.
21. Burzynski J. DKA and thrombosis. *CMAJ.* 2005;173(2):132; author reply 132-133.
22. Whelton MJ, Walde D, Havard CW. Hyperosmolar non-ketotic diabetic coma: with particular reference to vascular complications. *Br Med J.* 1971;1(5740):85-86.
23. Orban J-C, Maizière E-M, Ghaddab A, Van Obberghen E, Ichai C. Incidence and characteristics of acute kidney injury in severe diabetic ketoacidosis. *PLoS One.* 2014;9(10):e110925.
24. Chen J, Zeng H, Ouyang X, et al. The incidence, risk factors, and long-term outcomes of acute kidney injury in hospitalized diabetic ketoacidosis patients. *BMC Nephrol.* 2020;21(1):48.
25. Munro JF, Campbell IW, McCuish AC, Duncan LJ. Euglycaemic diabetic ketoacidosis. *Br Med J.* 1973;2(5866):578-580.
26. Fralick M, Schneeweiss S, Patorno E. Risk of diabetic ketoacidosis after initiation of an SGLT2 inhibitor. *N Engl J Med.* 2017;376(23):2300-2302.
27. Neal B, Perkovic V, Mahaffey KW, et al. Canagliflozin and cardiovascular and renal events in type 2 diabetes. *N Engl J Med.* 2017;377(7):644-657.
28. Erondu N, Desai M, Ways K, Meininger G. Diabetic ketoacidosis and related events in the Canagliflozin type 2 diabetes clinical program. *Diabetes Care.* 2015;38(9):1680-1686.
29. Rosenstock J, Ferrannini E. Euglycemic diabetic ketoacidosis: a predictable, detectable, and preventable safety concern with SGLT2 inhibitors. *Diabetes Care.* 2015;38(9):1638-1642.
30. Wang KM, Isom RT. SGLT2 inhibitor–induced euglycemic diabetic ketoacidosis: a case report. *Kidney Med.* 2020;2(2):218-221.
31. Taylor SI, Blau JE, Rother KI. SGLT2 inhibitors may predispose to ketoacidosis. *J Clin Endocrinol Metab.* 2015;100(8):2849-2852.
32. Kum-Nji JS, Gosmanov AR, Steinberg H, Dagogo-Jack S. Hyperglycemic, high anion-gap metabolic acidosis in patients receiving SGLT-2 inhibitors for diabetes management. *J Diabetes Complications.* 2017;31(3):611-614.
33. Coutrot M, Hékimian G, Moulin T, et al. Euglycemic ketoacidosis, a common and underrecognized complication of continuous renal replacement therapy using glucose-free solutions. *Intensive Care Med.* 2018;44(7):1185-1186.
34. Sriperumbuduri S, Clark E, Biyani M, Ruzicka M. High anion gap metabolic acidosis on continuous renal replacement therapy. *Kidney Int Rep.* 2020;5(10):1833-1835. doi:10.1016/j.ekir.2020.07.014
35. Stevenson JM, Heung M, Vilay AM, Eyler RF, Patel C, Mueller BA. In vitro glucose kinetics during continuous renal replacement therapy: implications for caloric balance in critically ill patients. *Int J Artif Organs.* 2013;36(12):861-868.
36. Schaapveld-Davis CM, Negrete AL, Hudson JQ, et al. End-stage renal disease increases rates of adverse glucose events when treating diabetic ketoacidosis or hyperosmolar hyperglycemic state. *Clin Diabetes.* 2017;35(4):202-208.
37. Seddik AA, Bashier A, Alhadari AK, et al. Challenges in management of diabetic ketoacidosis in hemodialysis patients, case presentation and review of literature. *Diabetes Metab Syndr.* 2019;13(4):2481-2487.

Obstetric Acute Kidney Injury

Jessica Sheehan Tangren and Michelle A. Hladunewich

INTRODUCTION

Acute kidney injury (AKI) is a rare but serious complication of pregnancy. Although any form of AKI that affects adults in the general population can also affect pregnant women, several etiologies are more common in pregnant women. The most important step in the diagnosis of AKI in pregnancy is differentiating among conditions with overlapping features, such as preeclampsia/hemolysis, elevated liver enzymes, and low platelets (HELLP); lupus nephritis; thrombotic thrombocytopenic purpura (TTP)/hemolytic uremic syndrome (HUS); and acute fatty liver of pregnancy (AFLP), as management strategies vary dramatically. In this chapter, we will review the incidence of AKI in pregnancy, the approach to diagnosis, as well as common etiologies and recommended management strategies.

EPIDEMIOLOGY OF ACUTE KIDNEY INJURY IN PREGNANCY

AKI during pregnancy is decreasing in both developing and developed countries. In India, the rates of pregnancy-associated AKI decreased from 15% in the 1980s to 1.5% in the 2010s.[1] This decline has also been associated with changes in AKI timing: most cases of AKI are now developing in the postpartum period, reflecting a decline in complications because of abortions. In a series from China, the most common causes of AKI were hypertension and postpartum hemorrhage, with 6% requiring dialysis.[2] Fortunately, the maternal mortality rate associated with AKI in pregnancy has also improved in the developing world, with current estimates around 4% to 6%, as compared with rates higher than 20% during the 1980s.

In the developed world, data on the rate of AKI are conflicting. An Italian cohort reported a decrease in pregnancy-associated AKI from 1 in 3,000 to 1 in 18,000 pregnancies from the 1960s to 1990s, whereas recent studies from Canada and the United States note an increased incidence of AKI in pregnancy.[3-5] Although the overall rates remained low, the incidence increased from 1.66 to 2.68 per 10,000 pregnancies from 2003 to 2010 in Canada and from 2.4 to 6.3 per 10,000 deliveries in 1999 to 2001 and 2010 to 2011 in the United States. Fortunately, most cases were mild and reversible (87%), suggesting at least some degree of ascertainment bias. Long-term kidney outcomes have not been well studied in women with AKI. Similar to nonpregnant patients, severe AKI demonstrates favorable kidney recovery, with only 4% to 9% of women with severe AKI remaining dialysis dependent at 4 to 6 months postpartum.[6]

REVIEW OF CHANGES IN KIDNEY FUNCTION DURING PREGNANCY AND ACUTE KIDNEY INJURY DIAGNOSIS

Pregnancy induces changes in systemic hemodynamics, leading to an increase in total circulating blood volume and cardiac output along with a decrease in systemic vascular resistance. This results in multiple changes to kidney physiology, including increased renal plasma flow, and hence glomerular hyperfiltration. As such, gestational hyperfiltration leads to decreased blood urea nitrogen and serum creatinine levels during gestation, and these adaptations are critical for favorable pregnancy outcomes.

As a result of changes in glomerular hemodynamics, serum creatinine–based formulas do not accurately to estimate glomerular filtration rate (GFR) in pregnancy, underestimating GFR measured by inulin clearance by approximately 40%.[7] Given the dynamic changes in GFR longitudinally across pregnancy, defining AKI can also be challenging. Standard definitions of AKI, including the Risk, Injury, Failure, Loss of kidney function, and End-stage kidney disease (RIFLE) and Acute Kidney Injury Network (AKIN) criteria, have not been validated in pregnant populations; however, in general, these definitions have been used to define AKI in this population in some studies. In the clinical context, however, there is reliance on serum creatinine to assess for kidney dysfunction, and it must be realized that a "normal" creatinine can reflect significant compromise in kidney function in a pregnant woman. A recent population-based study with over 300,000 measures of serum creatinine generated gestational age–specific estimates of kidney function at each stage of pregnancy and in the early postpartum.[8] They noted an approximately 0.17 mg/dL (15 μmol/L) difference between the 50th and 95th centile and suggested that values above the 95th centile at different stages of pregnancy should prompt assessment and further investigation (**Table 38.1**).

DIFFERENTIAL DIAGNOSIS OF ACUTE KIDNEY INJURY IN PREGNANCY

Like AKI in the nonpregnant population, pregnancy-associated AKI can be categorized as prerenal, intrarenal, and postrenal. The timing of AKI can be very helpful in narrowing the differential diagnosis.[9] In the first trimester, hemodynamic kidney injury (prerenal azotemia/acute tubular necrosis [ATN]) as a result of hyperemesis gravidarum or septic abortion predominates. AKI that develops in

TABLE 38.1 Range of Serum Creatinine Values During Gestation

Timing	Creatinine Range (mg/dL)
Prepregnancy	0.68-0.88
First trimester (12 wk)	0.53-0.69
Second trimester (24 wk)	0.51-0.68
Third trimester (36 wk)	0.54-0.63
Postpartum	0.71-0.95

Values above the upper limit should be considered abnormal and investigated.[8]

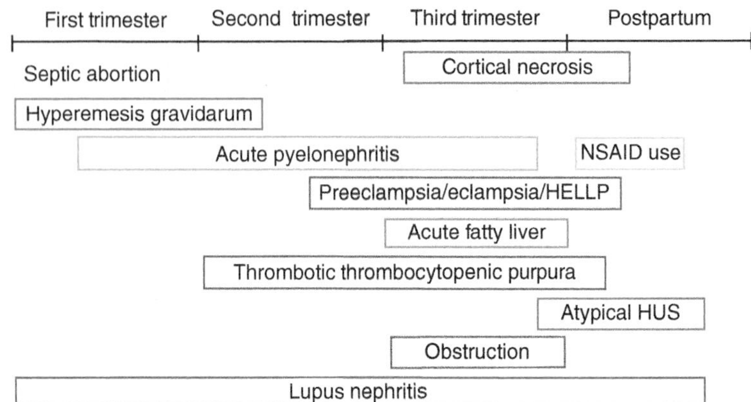

FIGURE 38.1: Etiologies of AKI at Different Stages of Gestation. HELLP, hemolysis, elevated liver enzymes, and low platelets; HUS, hemolytic uremic syndrome; NSAID, nonsteroidal anti-inflammatory drug.

the second and third trimesters can be attributed to preeclampsia/HELLP syndrome, thrombotic microangiopathies, AFLP, or obstetric hemorrhage. Atypical HUS (aHUS) and other disorders of complement regulation typically occur near term or postpartum.

Glomerulonephritis can present in any trimester of pregnancy or the postpartum period. **Figure 38.1** displays the main causes of AKI in pregnancy at different gestational ages.

Hemodynamic Kidney Injury and Bilateral Cortical Necrosis

Hemodynamic kidney injury is a common etiology of AKI in pregnancy. Injury can range from prerenal azotemia to bilateral cortical necrosis. Hypotension in pregnancy can occur from various causes including volume depletion (e.g., hyperemesis gravidarum), sepsis (e.g., septic abortion, chorioamnionitis, pyelonephritis, puerperal sepsis), or other severe obstetric complications (e.g., postpartum hemorrhage).

Bilateral renal cortical necrosis, the most extreme form of hemodynamic kidney injury, is a pathologic diagnosis characterized by diffuse cortical necrosis on kidney biopsy with evidence of intravascular thrombosis. Cortical necrosis is rare and associated with catastrophic obstetric emergencies like placental abruption with massive hemorrhage or amniotic fluid embolism, and occurs in the context of hypotensive shock often complicated by disseminated intravascular coagulation (DIC).[10] Pregnant women with severe ischemia involving the kidneys are more likely to develop cortical necrosis than the general population, presumed because of the hypercoagulable state that accompanies pregnancy in the context of endothelial dysfunction. The syndrome is characterized by sudden onset of oliguria/anuria. Computed tomography or ultrasound demonstrates hypoechoic or hypodense areas in the renal cortex. Most patients require dialysis, and long-term renal outcomes are poor.

Preeclampsia/Hemolysis, Elevated Liver Enzymes, and Low Platelets

Preeclampsia is a pregnancy-associated multisystem syndrome characterized by the development of hypertension and proteinuria after 20 weeks of gestation. It complicates approximately 5% of pregnancies in the United States. Although AKI is a rare complication of preeclampsia (1%), it is seen more frequently with HELLP syndrome (7%-15%), which is considered an extreme variant of preeclampsia. Glomerular endotheliosis or widespread glomerular endothelial swelling is the hallmark pathologic finding in the kidney in preeclampsia. Kidney failure in the setting of preeclampsia/HELLP has overlapping clinical features with other pregnancy-associated causes of AKI, including AFLP, lupus nephritis, TTP, and aHUS (**Table 38.2**). Placental antiangiogenic factors play a key role in the pathogenesis of preeclampsia. Soluble fms–like tyrosine kinase 1 (sFlt1) is a soluble vascular endothelial growth factor receptor that binds to proangiogenic factors such as placental growth factor (PlGF), neutralizing its effects.[11] Excess sFlt1 from the placenta results in widespread endothelial dysfunction. sFlt1 increases before onset of preeclampsia and correlates with disease severity.[12,13] Circulating levels of sFlt1 and PlGF have shown promise as predictive biomarkers of preeclampsia in several studies, and these biomarkers are currently being used in several countries to aid in the diagnosis of preeclampsia.[13] Women at high risk for developing preeclampsia should be given low-dose aspirin beginning before 16 weeks gestational age to help prevent the development of preeclampsia.[14]

Acute Fatty Liver of Pregnancy

AFLP is a rare condition that develops in the third trimester of pregnancy. AFLP is due to abnormal oxidation of fatty acids by fetal mitochondria. Fetal deficiency of long-chain 3-hydroxyacyl CoA dehydrogenase leads to excess fetal free fatty acids that cross the placenta and result in maternal hepatotoxicity. The clinical presentation includes fatigue, vomiting, and jaundice, with laboratory workup showing elevated serum transaminases and bilirubin levels. Thrombocytopenia, hypoglycemia, lactic acidosis, and AKI are common. Kidney biopsy findings in AFLP include ATN, fatty vacuolization of tubular cells, and occlusion of capillary lumens by fibrin-like material. Both kidney and liver failure generally resolve postpartum, but in extreme cases liver transplantation may be required.[15]

Distinguishing AFLP from HELLP syndrome can be challenging because of common lab findings. The most common clinical features of AFLP are malaise, nausea, vomiting, abdominal pain, and jaundice. HELLP syndrome more commonly presents with headache, abdominal or epigastric pain, and hypertension. Evidence of synthetic liver dysfunction, such as hypoglycemia, and abnormal coagulation parameters are characteristic of AFLP. AKI is also more common in AFLP than in HELLP.

Thrombotic Microangiopathies

TTP and HUS are important causes of AKI in pregnancy characterized by unexplained thrombocytopenia and microangiopathic hemolytic anemia. Clinically, TTP is considered when central nervous system symptoms predominate and HUS when there is profound kidney failure or when the syndrome develops in the postpartum period.

Von Willebrand factor–cleaving protease (ADAMTS-13) deficiency is the cause of TTP. In pregnancy, most cases of TTP develop during the second or third trimester. Pregnancy is associated with decreases in ADAMTS-13 levels and, thus, appears to be a trigger for new onset or a relapse of TTP. Pregnancy-related aHUS is the result of complement dysregulation most often secondary to genetic mutations in complement regulatory proteins.

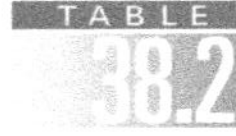

TABLE 38.2 Features of Thrombotic Microangiopathies Presenting in Pregnancy

Features	HELLP	TTP	HUS	AFLP
Clinical onset	Third trimester	Any time	Postpartum	Third trimester
Unique to pregnancy	Yes	No	No	Yes
Underlying pathophysiology	Abnormal placentation	ADAMTS-13 deficiency	Mutations in genes regulating complement function	Defective fetal mitochondrial β-oxidation of fatty acids
Hypertension	Yes	Variable	Yes	Frequently
Kidney failure	Rare	Rare	Common	Possible
Thrombocytopenia	Present	Severe	Present	Present
Liver function tests	↑↑	Normal	Normal	↑↑↑
Helpful clinical/diagnostic features	↑ sFlt:PIGF	ADAMTS-13 activity < 10%	Decreased complement levels	Abdominal pain, hypoglycemia
Management	Delivery	Plasma exchange	Eculizumab	Delivery

AFLP, acute fatty liver of pregnancy; HELLP, hemolysis, elevated liver enzymes, and low platelets; HUS, hemolytic uremic syndrome; PIGF, placental growth factor; sFlt, soluble fms–like tyrosine kinase TTP, thrombotic thrombocytopenic purpura.

Pregnancy can be a trigger for aHUS; however, more than two-thirds of cases present postpartum. Interestingly, the risk for developing aHUS is higher during a second pregnancy than during the first. Like in the nonpregnant population, genetic defects in complement regulatory proteins can be identified in more than half of patients with pregnancy-associated aHUS. Patients with detected complement gene variants are more likely to have severe disease including the need for dialysis at presentation and worse long-term outcomes, including an increased risk of relapse and progression to end-stage kidney disease (ESKD).[16] As such, a high level of suspicion for aHUS to allow for early diagnosis and treatment is critical. Misdiagnosis is common. In a Spanish cohort of pregnancy-associated aHUS cases, 17/22 met clinical criteria for preeclampsia.[17] Outcomes are better with shorter duration from diagnosis to treatment.

Distinguishing TTP/HUS from severe preeclampsia accompanied by HELLP syndrome can be challenging. Thrombocytopenia, microangiopathic hemolytic anemia, AKI, proteinuria, and hypertension occur in both TTP-HUS and HELLP, although elevated liver enzymes are more common in HELLP syndrome. As in the nonpregnant state, low levels of ADAMTS-13 are diagnostic of TTP, whereas depressed complement levels (C3) might be noted in aHUS. Antiangiogenic markers (sFlt-1/PlGF) can aid as well in the diagnosis of preeclampsia.

Lupus Nephritis and Other Glomerular Diseases

Systemic lupus erythematosus predominantly affects women of childbearing age, and clinically significant kidney disease develops in 30% of women. Pregnancy-related immunologic and hormonal changes can result in flares or de novo lupus nephritis developing in pregnancy. Preeclampsia is a frequent complication of pregnancy in women with lupus, with a higher incidence in women with lupus nephritis compared with lupus patients with no kidney involvement. Lupus nephritis flares can be difficult to distinguish from preeclampsia. The presence of low (or low-normal) circulating complement levels, anti–double-stranded DNA antibodies, active urine sediment, and extrarenal lupus manifestations can aid in diagnosis. Vasculitis is rare in women of childbearing age but should be considered in those presenting with AKI, proteinuria, and systemic disease (pulmonary-renal syndrome, joint/muscle pain, fever, poor weight gain or loss, etc.) As in the nonpregnant population, serology is diagnostic. Other glomerular diseases may require a kidney biopsy for diagnosis. When a diagnosis cannot be made on clinical grounds, expert consensus recommends kidney biopsy be performed before 32 weeks gestational age.[18] Kidney biopsy should not be performed if preeclampsia is in the differential diagnosis as hypertension and coagulopathy can develop rapidly and make this a high-risk procedure.

Pyelonephritis

Asymptomatic bacteriuria is more likely to develop into symptomatic urinary tract infections, including pyelonephritis, during pregnancy. Smooth muscle relaxation results in dilation of the urinary collecting system, which promotes bacterial translocation from the lower to the upper urinary track. Gestational pyelonephritis is associated with adverse maternal and fetal outcomes including maternal sepsis, premature labor, and fetal growth restriction. AKI develops in up to one-fourth of cases. Routine screening and treatment of asymptomatic bacteriuria has led to a reduction in the incidence of gestational pyelonephritis.[19]

Postrenal Acute Kidney Injury

Postrenal AKI is rare in pregnancy. Obstruction may be difficult to differentiate from physiologic hydronephrosis of pregnancy, which becomes more pronounced as pregnancy nears term. Cause of obstruction can include bilateral nephrolithiasis or iatrogenic injuries to the bladder and ureters during cesarean sections. Pathologic obstruction of the ureters by the uterus is unusual, but can develop in the case of multifetal pregnancies or if there are preexisting structural and anomalies involving the kidneys. Magnetic resonance imaging can help in distinguishing physiologic hydronephrosis from obstruction in pregnancy, whereas ultrasound is less reliable in such a setting.

MANAGEMENT OF ACUTE KIDNEY INJURY IN PREGNANCY

Successful management of AKI requires close collaboration between nephrologists, obstetricians, and intensivists. Identification of the underlying cause of AKI is crucial in directing management. For glomerulonephritis, steroid and immunosuppressive therapy is necessary. Pregnancy-safe immunosuppressive agents include calcineurin inhibitors prednisone, calcineurin inhibitors and azathioprine. For women with preexisting lupus, hydroxychloroquine should be continued in pregnancy, as discontinuation has been associated with lupus flares. Treatment of TTP in pregnancy is managed in the same way as in the nonpregnant patient. Plasma exchange should be initiated promptly even before the diagnosis is confirmed if TTP is suspected. Inhibition of C5 with eculizumab is the therapy of choice for aHUS and has been used safely in pregnancy for nonrenal indications.[20] For cases of severe preeclampsia/HELLP syndrome or AFLP, immediate delivery of the fetus is indicated. Intravenous (IV) magnesium is used to prevent onset of seizures in women with severe preeclampsia. Because magnesium is renally excreted, women with severe AKI are at risk for magnesium toxicity and should receive a reduced dose of magnesium and be monitored closely for toxicity (hyporeflexia, hypotension). Complications of AKI can be treated similarly to nonpregnant patients: volume overload can be treated with loop diuretics, hyperkalemia managed with cation exchange resins, metabolic acidosis with alkali therapy, and anemia with erythropoietin-stimulating agents and oral or IV iron when indicated.

For women who develop uremic symptoms, kidney replacement therapy is necessary. In almost all cases, delivery of the fetus precedes the need for kidney replacement therapy. In the rare circumstance that delivery is not indicated, kidney replacement therapy should mirror the management of dialysis in pregnant women with ESKD with longer and more frequent dialysis sessions, exercising caution not to drop maternal blood pressure.[21]

Acknowledgment

JST is supported by a research grant from the National Institutes of Health (K23DK120874).

References

1. Prakash J, Pant P, Prakash S, et al. Changing picture of acute kidney injury in pregnancy: study of 259 cases over a period of 33 years. *Indian J Nephrol.* 2016;26:262-267.
2. Huang C, Chen S. Acute kidney injury during pregnancy and puerperium: a retrospective study in a single center. *BMC Nephrol.* 2017;18:146.
3. Stratta P, Besso L, Canavese C, et al. Is pregnancy-related acute renal failure a disappearing clinical entity? *Ren Fail.* 1996;18:575-584.

4. Mehrabadi A, Dahhou M, Joseph KS, Kramer MS. Investigation of a rise in obstetric acute renal failure in the United States, 1999-2011. *Obstet Gynecol.* 2016;127:899-906.
5. Mehrabadi A, Liu S, Bartholomew S, et al. Hypertensive disorders of pregnancy and the recent increase in obstetric acute renal failure in Canada: population based retrospective cohort study. *BMJ.* 2014;349:g4731.
6. Liu Y, Ma X, Zheng J, Liu X, Yan T. Pregnancy outcomes in patients with acute kidney injury during pregnancy: a systematic review and meta-analysis. *BMC Pregnancy Childbirth.* 2017;17:235.
7. Ahmed SB, Bentley-Lewis R, Hollenberg NK, Graves SW, Seely EW. A comparison of prediction equations for estimating glomerular filtration rate in pregnancy. *Hypertens Pregnancy.* 2009;28:243-255.
8. Harel Z, McArthur E, Hladunewich M, et al. Serum creatinine levels before, during, and after pregnancy. *JAMA.* 2019;321:205-207.
9. Fakhouri F, Vercel C, Fremeaux-Bacchi V. Obstetric nephrology: AKI and thrombotic microangiopathies in pregnancy. *Clin J Am Soc Nephrol.* 2012;7:2100-2106.
10. Frimat M, Decambron M, Lebas C, et al. Renal cortical necrosis in postpartum hemorrhage: a case series. *Am J Kidney Dis.* 2016;68:50-57.
11. Maynard SE, Min J-Y, Merchan J, et al. Excess placental soluble fms-like tyrosine kinase 1 (sFlt1) may contribute to endothelial dysfunction, hypertension, and proteinuria in preeclampsia. *J Clin Invest.* 2003;111:649-658.
12. Rana S, Karumanchi SA, Levine RJ, et al. Sequential changes in antiangiogenic factors in early pregnancy and risk of developing preeclampsia. *Hypertension.* 2007;50:137-142.
13. Zeisler H, Llurba E, Chantraine F, et al. Predictive value of the sFlt-1:PlGF ratio in women with suspected preeclampsia. *N Engl J Med.* 2016;374:13-22.
14. Rolnik DL, Wright D, Poon LC, et al. Aspirin versus placebo in pregnancies at high risk for preterm preeclampsia. *N Engl J Med.* 2017;377:613-622.
15. Kushner T, Tholey D, Dodge J, Saberi B, Schiano T, Terrault N. Outcomes of liver transplantation for acute fatty liver disease of pregnancy. *Am J Transplant.* 2019;19:2101-2107.
16. Bruel A, Kavanagh D, Noris M, et al. Hemolytic uremic syndrome in pregnancy and postpartum. *Clin J Am Soc Nephrol.* 2017;12:1237-1247.
17. Huerta A, Arjona E, Portoles J, et al. A retrospective study of pregnancy-associated atypical hemolytic uremic syndrome. *Kidney Int.* 2018;93:450-459.
18. Lindheimer MD, Davison JM. Renal biopsy during pregnancy: "to b... or not to b...?". *Br J Obstet Gynaecol.* 1987;94:932-934.
19. Hill JB, Sheffield JS, McIntire DD, Wendel GD Jr. Acute pyelonephritis in pregnancy. *Obstet Gynecol.* 2005;105:18-23.
20. Kelly RJ, Hochsmann B, Szer J, et al. Eculizumab in pregnant patients with paroxysmal nocturnal hemoglobinuria. *N Engl J Med.* 2015;373:1032-1039.
21. Tangren J, Nadel M, Hladunewich MA. Pregnancy and end-stage renal disease. *Blood Purif.* 2018;45:194-200.

Postcardiac Surgery Acute Kidney Injury

Raphael Weiss and Alexander Zarbock

INTRODUCTION

Recent data suggest that the incidence of acute kidney injury (AKI) has been underestimated.[1] In this context, cardiac surgery has a special role, because it differs from other types of surgery owing to the use of cardiopulmonary bypass (CPB). Employing extracorporeal bypass during cardiac surgery may induce hemolysis, inflammation, and perfusion imbalance, which subsequently may induce organ dysfunction.[2,3] These circumstances make it necessary to monitor patients continuously far beyond the operation itself. Up to 30% to 50% of patients undergoing cardiac surgery develop AKI,[4-6] which increases intensive care unit (ICU)/hospital length of stay, morbidity, and mortality. Therefore, actions should be taken to decrease risks, avoid harmful situations and interactions, and achieve best supportive care.

PATHOPHYSIOLOGY

Perioperative circulatory depression (e.g., anesthesia, myocardial dysfunctions, circulatory instability, extracorporeal assistance), release of proinflammatory mediators (induced by surgical measures and the use of CPB), stress (increase of sympathetic activity), hormonal influence, and volume losses or redistributions reduce renal blood flow and subsequently lower oxygen delivery to the kidney. The release of hormones and the stimulation of the sympathetic nervous system lead to endothelium damage, contraction of small arterioles while vasodilation occurs triggered by the release of other hormones. Leukocytes are activated and adhere to the endothelium.[7] Hemodynamic disturbance of microcirculation[7,8] and the occlusion of small vessels by the inflammatory response lead to ischemia of the kidney which causes impaired kidney function and accumulation of fluids and waste.

Summarizing, reduced renal perfusion with concurrent ischemia and inflammation are the main risk factors for the development of AKI. Surgery and the use of CPB induce both an inflammatory reaction and an ischemia of the kidneys.

SUBCLINICAL ACUTE KIDNEY INJURY AND KIDNEY DAMAGE BIOMARKER

Recent studies have shown that various new kidney biomarkers provide information on kidney damage.[9-11] The purpose of measuring these new damage biomarkers is to identify and treat a subclinical AKI. This state describes a biomarker positive but (still) serum creatinine negative condition, which implies kidney damage without loss of function.[12] Most of the damage biomarkers are released from tubular epithelial cells. New biomarkers are superior to conventional markers in early diagnosis, prognosis, and long-term mortality.[13,14] Because biomarker-positive patients already experience a higher risk for complications (i.e., length of stay, mortality),[10,11] the "subclinical AKI" concept was proposed a couple of years ago.[15] The early release of biomarkers from stressed or damaged renal tubular epithelial cells could provide a time window to prevent further damage and a decline of kidney function.[16-18] The additional implementation of clinical risk scores (e.g., renal risk index) increases the informative value.[19] In addition, by including biomarkers in high-risk patients while considering the clinical context, the negative predictive value of biomarkers was improved.[13,14,20] For more details on biomarkers, see Chapter 16.

PREVENTIVE MEASURES

The pathophysiology of AKI is complex. Prevention of this syndrome requires a multimodal approach and high-risk patients have to be identified, because the preventive measures are especially beneficial in this patient population. As the incidence of AKI reaches 50% in these patients,[5,6,21] the number needed to treat is low. Biomarkers may help to identify patients at high risk for AKI, but also the patient, the prescribed medication, the hemodynamic situation, and other laboratory tests have to be examined to understand the underlying cause of the AKI.

Kidney Disease Improving Global Outcomes Bundle

The Kidney Disease Improving Global Outcomes (KDIGO) guidelines recommend implementing a bundle of supportive measures in patients at high risk for AKI. The KDIGO bundle consists of avoiding nephrotoxic agents, optimizing volume status and perfusion pressure, maintaining normoglycemia, monitoring of serum creatinine and urine excretion, and, if necessary, expansion of hemodynamic monitoring.[22] Two recently published randomized controlled trials demonstrated that the biomarker-guided implementation of the KDIGO bundle significantly reduced the occurrence of AKI in patients after cardiac or abdominal surgery (PrevAKI: 55.1% vs 71.1%; $p = 0.004$, BigpAK: 27.1% vs 48.0%; $p = 0.03$).[18,22,23]

Remote Ischemic Preconditioning

Remote ischemic preconditioning (RIPC) refers to the protection of a target organ (kidney) from ischemia by previously applying small periods of ischemia to a distant tissue (limb). This can be done perioperatively by using a conventional blood pressure cuff. Initially, experiments in animals showed that short ischemic episodes interrupted by reperfusion intervals have a protective effect considering ischemic organ damage on both local and remote tissues.[24-27] In most cases, RIPC is performed by a blood pressure cuff that is repeatedly pumped up beyond the patient's blood pressure (e.g., 3× for 5 minutes on one arm, 50 mm Hg above the systolic blood pressure). The effects of RIPC on kidney function have been investigated in several clinical trials with mixed results. Because of the heterogeneity of patients and different endpoints in these studies, data can only be compared to a limited extent. Some studies were able to show a protective effect of RIPC on kidney function,[28,29] whereas others did not.[30,31] One reason for the conflicting results could be the use of propofol in some studies, which is believed to attenuate the effects of RIPC.[32-35] As the preventive RIPC procedure is cheap and not harmful, it is recommended by some authors, especially in high-risk patients.[31,36]

HEMODYNAMICS

Recent literature regarding noncardiac surgery patients demonstrated that a perioperative hypotension is associated with an increased risk of developing AKI after surgery.[37,41] This affects even younger patients (<60 years).[40] Based on these data, it is likely that hypotension—especially during cardiac surgery—is associated with an increased AKI risk, because most cardiac patients already have additional AKI risk factors. Several studies including a systematic review underline this hypothesis.[42,43]

In the healthy patient, autoregulation of the kidneys maintains the glomerular filtration rate until the mean arterial pressure (MAP) falls below 80 mm Hg.[44] Comorbidities and medication might cause an impaired autoregulation, even though the MAP is in normal range.[44] In addition, during cardiac surgery, the MAP is often below the normal range and therefore often below the limits of autoregulation. Studies found that persistent hypotensive episodes result in a disruption of this process,[37] which is a common case when the kidneys get artificially perfused during times of CPB. Furthermore, during CPB, there is nonpulsatile flow. It was shown that CPB perfusion pressure and flow mode affect regional blood flow to the kidneys and other visceral organs. Studies suggest that in terms of organ perfusion and outcome, a pulsatile flow is superior to a nonpulsatile flow.[45,46] Maintaining an adequate MAP during CPB phases may have a significant effect on preventing organ dysfunctions.[47,48]

Studies have proven that regardless of the type of hemodynamic monitoring, hemodynamic surveillance significantly (i.e., stroke volume variation, cardiac output) reduced the AKI rate.[49-52] Therefore, the remaining leading question is, how high should the blood pressure be kept to prevent AKI? Some studies show that the AKI risk dramatically increases if the MAP falls below 55 mm Hg for more than 10 minutes perioperatively,[39,41] whereas other studies demonstrate that the MAP should not fall below 65 mm Hg for more than 10 minutes.[53] Another recent study found that postoperative AKI was associated with the product of hypotension duration and severity.[38] Although these studies do not include cardiac surgery patients, they underline the importance of hemodynamic management, the rationale of acuteness, and need for action. There is no reason to assume that this might be different in patients undergoing cardiac surgery, because they experience a particular risk for hemodynamic fluctuations. In the postoperative period, a reduced ejection fraction is another cause of hypotension. The heart's inability to maintain an adequate cardiac output is associated with reduced organ perfusion and might be associated with a higher risk for AKI.[54] Summarizing, hypotensive phases (only minutes—closer to seconds than to hours) during any, especially cardiac, procedure should be avoided or at least be kept as short as possible.[55] To achieve this, the underlying problem has to be identified and rectified immediately.

Right ventricular dysfunction with low cardiac output is a potential source of hypotension. If the right ventricle is compromised, venous congestion might occur, which potentially leads to reduced kidney perfusion.[54] As the kidney is encapsulated in Gerota's fascia, interstitial edema might lead to an increased pressure in the kidney. The impaired drainage increases organ resistance, which together with low cardiac output may result in a significant reduced renal blood flow and subsequently increased risk for AKI.[54] Maintaining the cardiac index seems important in this context.[56] The central venous pressure (CVP) might also provide useful information because a high CVP can point to increased venous congestion, which is, as found by different studies, associated not only with a higher risk but also with a higher severity of AKI.[57-59]

Another common reason for arterial hypotension is hypovolemia. In the past, attempts to treat a hypotension with fluids often resulted in the application of large amounts of fluid, resulting in volume overload. Nowadays, studies have shown that fluid overload is associated with organ congestion, edema formation, and increased mortality.[55] Therefore, a hypervolemia might also lead to the accumulation of fluids in the renal tissue, causing an increased pressure in the kidney that reduces renal perfusion. The choice of fluid is also important. Isotonic saline solutions contain an unphysiologically high proportion of chloride, which leads to hyperchloremic acidosis that might subsequently induce renal vasoconstriction and decrease glomerular filtration rate,[60] leading to the development of AKI.[61] Therefore, balanced crystalloid solutions are preferred.[62]

In this context, organ cross-talk should also be mentioned. The development of AKI induces increased permeability in remote organs (e.g., pulmonary edema, acute respiratory distress syndrome).[63-65] Therefore, the goal should be to maintane patients in euvolemia without tipping into either hypo- or hypervolemia.[66,67] Altogether, volume substitution has to be evaluated carefully—and so also should transfusion of blood products. Preoperative anemia (hemoglobin levels <8 mg/dL) is associated with a four-fold risk of AKI.[68,69] Unfortunately, transfusions are also an independent risk factor for AKI in both cardiac and non-cardiac surgery patients.[68-73] In cardiac surgery, some authors therefore recommend transfusions only for hemoglobin levels <8 g/dL (<5 mmol/L), unless there is hypotension.[72]

DRUGS

Another way to counter persistent hypotension in (post-)cardiac surgery patients is the addition of inotropes and vasoactive drugs. This might be necessary not only because of poor cardiac function but also because of peri-/postoperative vasoplegia. If catecholamine support is needed, most guidelines recommend norepinephrine as a first-line treatment. Although it is not yet known which vasopressor has the greatest protective effect on the development of AKI, norepinephrine increases global and medullary blood pressure. In the event of cardiac dysfunction, epinephrine may be given. However, although these agents improve cardiac output, they may also increase myocardial oxygen consumption, arrhythmias, systemic hypoperfusion, and organ ischemia.[74]

Calcium sensitizers such as levosimendan were designed to address low cardiac output but there is a growing body of evidence that these drugs do not in decrease the incidence of AKI or the need for kidney replacement therapy (KRT) and mechanical cardiac assist devices. Although they may improve cardiac indices, recent multicenter randomized trials could not demonstrate that these drugs contribute to a lower mortality or morbidity in the peri- or postoperative setting.[75-77]

Light postoperative sedation forms an essential backbone in the recovery of patients undergoing cardiac surgery. Sedation is used to reduce patient discomfort, stress, and myocardial oxygen consumption. Propofol and dexmedetomidine have become the most widely used agents in this context.[78] Dexmedetomidine is a highly selective α-2-agonist with pleiotropic effects (including sedative, analgesic, and anxiolytic effects; decreased endogenous norepinephrine release; improvement of hemodynamic stability; and balancing of myocardial oxygen demand/ supply). In the field of cardiac surgery, dexmedetomidine led to a significant reduction in AKI in patients with preoperative normal and mildly impaired (CKD Stage 2) kidney function.[79-81] The renoprotective effect caused by dexmedetomidine is believed to be due to sympatholysis and anti-inflammatory properties.[82] Furthermore, dexmedetomidine reduces the length of intubation as well as the incidence and duration of postoperative delirium.[83,84] However, larger multicenter randomized trials have to confirm the positive effects of dexmedetomidine on kidney function before it can be recommended.

It should be mentioned that there are more medications that were thought to reduce the incidence of AKI. Among the most famous are statins, sodium bicarbonate, mannitol, and *N*-acetylcysteine. However, none of the drugs has been shown to be effective in preventing or treating AKI in large multicenter trials. Therefore, it cannot be recommended to use these drugs in patients undergoing cardiac surgery.[85-98]

KIDNEY REPLACEMENT THERAPY

KRT is the only therapeutic option in patients with a severe AKI. However, the central question is when KRT should be initiated. The KDIGO guidelines currently recommend the start KRT in patients with life-threatening complications (absolute indication), including diuretic-resistant volume overload or significant metabolic/electrolyte imbalances.[22] However, the majority of patients develop severe AKI without immediate life-threatening complications, so the decision of when to start KRT is based on the assessment of the intensive care physician or nephrologist. KRT may prevent complications such as volume overload which are associated with increased mortality, whereas a premature initiation of KRT results in an invasive and expensive procedure that might have been unnecessary in the end.

The important question of when to start KRT in AKI patients without uremic symptoms, electrolyte imbalances, or volume overload remains controversial—partly because of different definitions of "early" or "late" initiation in trials.[99] However, there is only one randomized controlled trial in cardiac surgery patients. The ELAIN trial was a single-center trial that mainly recruited patients after cardiac surgery. In this trial, "early" was defined as AKI stage 2, whereas "late" was defined as AKI stage 3. The primary outcome, the all-cause 90-day mortality, was significantly lower in the "early" group compared to the "late" group.[100] Two other randomized controlled trials, mainly focusing on septic patients, showed no difference in the mortality between the "early" and "late" groups. In these studies, a large percentage of patients in the "late" group did not go on to require KRT as they spontaneously recovered from AKI. In the ELAIN trial, 90.8% of patients in the late arm received KRT.[100] Perhaps this indicates to a more appropriate selection of patients with early-stage AKI, to test the hypothesis around early versus late initiation of KRT, based on current definitions.

References

1. Li PK, Burdmann EA, Mehta RL; World Kidney Day Steering Committee 2013. Acute kidney injury: global health alert. *Kidney Int.* 2013;83(3):372-376.
2. Silvestry FE. Postoperative complications among patients undergoing cardiac surgery. UpToDate; 2015.
3. Scott Stephens R, Whitman GJR. Postoperative critical care of the adult cardiac surgical patient. Part I: routine postoperative care. *Crit Care Med.* 2015 Jul; 43(7):1477-1497.
4. Lagny MG, Jouret F, Koch JN, et al. Incidence and outcomes of acute kidney injury after cardiac surgery using either criteria of the RIFLE classification. *BMC Nephrol.* 2015 May 30;16:76.
5. Bellomo R, Kellum JA, Ronco C. Acute kidney injury. *Lancet.* 2012;380:756-766.

6. Hoste EA, Bagshaw SM, Bellomo R, et al. Epidemiology of acute kidney injury in critically ill patients: the multinational AKI-EPI study. *Intensive Care Med.* 2015;41(8):1411-1423.
7. Bonventre JV, Yang L. Cellular pathophysiology of ischemic acute kidney injury. *J Clin Invest.* 2011;121(11):4210-4221.
8. Aird WC. The role of the endothelium in severe sepsis and multiple organ dysfunction syndrome. *Blood.* 2003;101(10):3765-3777.
9. Heimbürger O, Stenvinkel P, Bárány P. The enigma of decreased creatinine generation in acute kidney injury. *Nephrol Dial Transplant.* 2012;27(11):3973-3974.
10. Nickolas TL, Schmidt-Ott KM, Canetta P, et al. Diagnostic and prognostic stratification in the emergency department using urinary biomarkers of nephron damage: a multicenter prospective cohort study. *J Am Coll Cardiol.* 2012;59(3):246-255.
11. Haase M, Devarajan P, Haase-Fielitz A, et al. The outcome of neutrophil gelatinase-associated lipocalin-positive subclinical acute kidney injury: a multicenter pooled analysis of prospective studies. *J Am Coll Cardiol.* 2011;57(17):1752-1761.
12. Haase M, Kellum JA, Ronco C. Subclinical AKI—an emerging syndrome with important consequences. *Nat Rev Nephrol.*2012;8(12):735-739.
13. Malhotra R, Siew ED. Biomarkers for the early detection and prognosis of acute kidney injury. *Clin J Am Soc Nephrol.* 2017;12(1):149-173.
14. McMahon BA, Koyner JL. Risk stratification for acute kidney injury: are biomarkers enough? *Adv Chronic Kidney Dis.* 2016; 23:167-178.
15. Chawla LS, Bellomo R, Bihorac A, et al; Acute Disease Quality Initiative Workgroup. Acute kidney disease and renal recovery: consensus report of the Acute Disease Quality Initiative (ADQI) 16 Workgroup. *Nat Rev Nephrol.* 2017;13:241-257.
16. Meersch M, Schmidt C, Hoffmeier A, et al. Prevention of cardiac surgery-associated AKI by implementing the KDIGO guidelines in high risk patients identified by biomarkers: the PrevAKI randomized controlled trial. *Intensive Care Med.* 2017;43:1551-1561.
17. Gocze I, Koch M, Renner P, et al. Urinary biomarkers TIMP-2 and IGFBP7 early predict acute kidney injury after major surgery. *PLoS One.* 2015;10(3):e0120863.
18. Meersch M, Schmidt C, Van Aken H, et al. Urinary TIMP-2 and IGFBP7 as early biomarkers of acute kidney injury and renal recovery following cardiac surgery. *PLoS One.* 2014; 9(3):e93460.
19. Basu RK, Wang Y, Wong HR, Chawla LS, Wheeler DS, Goldstein SL. Incorporation of biomarkers with the renal angina index for prediction of severe AKI in critically ill children. *Clin J Am Soc Nephrol.* 2014;9:654-662.
20. Goldstein SL, Chawla LS. Renal angina. *Clin J Am Soc Nephrol.* 2010;5:943-949.
21. Reents W, Hilker M, Börgermann J, et al. Acute kidney injury after on-pump or off-pump coronary artery bypass grafting in elderly patients. *Ann Thorac Surg.* 2014;98:9-15.
22. KDIGO. KDIGO clinical practice guideline for acute kidney injury. *Kidney Int Suppl.* 2012;2:1-138.
23. Göcze I, Jauch D, Götz M, et al. Biomarker-guided intervention to prevent acute kidney injury after major surgery: the prospective randomized BigpAK study. *Ann Surg.* 2018;267:1013-1020.
24. Murry CE, Jennings RB, Reimer KA. Preconditioning with ischemia: a delay of lethal cell injury in ischemic myocardium. *Circulation.* 1986;74:1124-1136.
25. Tapuria N, Kumar Y, Habib MM, Abu Amara M, Seifalian AM, Davidson BR. Remote ischemic preconditioning: a novel protective method from ischemia reperfusion injury—a review. *J Surg Res.* 2008;150:304-330.
26. Jensen HA, Loukogeorgakis S, Yannopoulos F. Remote ischemic preconditioning protects the brain against injury after hypothermic circulatory arrest. *Circulation.* 2011;123:714-721.
27. Er F, Nia AM, Dopp H, et al. Ischemic preconditioning for prevention of contrast medium-induced nephropathy: randomized pilot RenPro trial (renal protection trial). *Circulation.* 2012;126:296-303.
28. Zimmerman RF, Ezeanuna PU, Kane JC, et al. Ischemic preconditioning at a remote site prevents acute kidney injury in patients following cardiac surgery. *Kidney Int.* 2011;80:861-867.
29. Zarbock A, Schmidt C, Van Aken H, et al. Effect of remote ischemic preconditioning on kidney injury among high-risk patients undergoing cardiac surgery: a randomized clinical trial. *JAMA.* 2015;313:2133-2141.
30. Meybohm P, Hasenclever D, Zacharowski K. Remote ischemic preconditioning and cardiac surgery. *N Engl J Med.* 2016;374:489-492.
31. Hausenloy DJ, Candilio L, Evans R, et al. Remote ischemic preconditioning and outcomes of cardiac surgery. *N Engl J Med.* 2015;373:1408-1417.
32. Kottenberg E, Thielmann M, Bergmann L, et al. Protection by remote ischemic preconditioning during coronary artery bypass graft surgery with isoflurane but not propofol—a clinical trial. *Acta Anaesthesiol Scand.* 2012;56:30-38.

33. Ney J, Hoffmann K, Meybohm P, et al. Remote ischemic preconditioning does not affect the release of humoral factors in propofol-anesthetized cardiac surgery patients: a secondary analysis of the RIPHeart study. *Int J Mol Sci.* 2018;19(4):1094.
34. Behmenburg F, van Caster P, Bunte S, et al. Impact of anesthetic regimen on remote ischemic preconditioning in the rat heart in vivo. *Anesth Analg.* 2018;126(4):1377-1380.
35. Bunte S, Behmenburg F, Eckelskemper F, et al. Cardioprotection by humoral factors released after remote ischemic preconditioning depends on anesthetic regimen. *Crit Care Med.* 2019;47(3):e250-e255.
36. Ovize M, Bonnefoy E. Giving the ischaemic heart a shot in the arm. *Lancet.* 2010;375:699-700.
37. Gu WJ, Hou BL, Kwong JSW, et al. Association between intraoperative hypotension and 30-day mortality, major adverse cardiac events, and acute kidney injury after non-cardiac surgery: a meta-analysis of cohort studies. *Int J Cardiol.* 2018;258:68-73.
38. Maheshwari K, Turan A, Mao G, et al. The association of hypotension during non-cardiac surgery, before and after skin incision, with postoperative acute kidney injury: a retrospective cohort analysis. *Anesthesia.* 2018; 73(10):1223-1228.
39. Sun LY, Wijeysundera DN, Tait GA, Beattie WS. Association of intraoperative hypotension with acute kidney injury after elective noncardiac surgery. *Anesthesiology.* 2015;123(3):515-523.
40. Tang Y, Zhu C, Liu J, et al. Association of intraoperative hypotension with acute kidney injury after noncardiac surgery in patients younger than 60 years old. *Kidney Blood Press Res.* 2019;44(2):211-221.
41. Walsh M, Devereaux PJ, Garg AX, et al. Relationship between intraoperative mean arterial pressure and clinical outcomes after noncardiac surgery: toward an empirical definition of hypotension. *Anesthesiology.* 2013;119(3):507-515.
42. Weir MR, Aronson S, Avery EG, Pollack CV. Acute kidney injury following cardiac surgery: role of perioperative blood pressure control. *Am J Nephrol.* 2011;33(5):438-452.
43. Aronson S, Fontes ML, Miao Y, Mangano DT; Investigators of the Multicenter Study of Perioperative Ischemia Research Group; Ischemia Research and Education Foundation. Risk index for perioperative renal dysfunction/failure: critical dependence on pulse pressure hypertension. *Circulation.* 2007;115(6):733-742.
44. Abuelo JG. Normotensive ischemic acute renal failure. *N Engl J Med.* 2007;357(8):797-805.
45. Haines N, Wang S, Ündar A, Alkan T, Akcevin A. Clinical outcomes of pulsatile and non-pulsatile mode of perfusion. *J Extra Corpor Technol.* 2009;41(1):P26-P29.
46. Nakamura K, Harasaki H, Fukumura F, Fukamachi K, Whalen R. Comparison of pulsatile and non-pulsatile cardiopulmonary bypass on regional renal blood flow in sheep. *Scand Cardiovasc J.* 2004;38(1):59-63.
47. Plestis KA, Gold JP. Importance of blood pressure regulation in maintaining adequate tissue perfusion during cardiopulmonary bypass. *Semin Thorac Cardiovasc Surg.* 2001;13(2):170-175.
48. Fischer UM, Weissenberger WK, Warters RD, Geissler HJ, Allen SJ, Mehlhorn U. Impact of cardiopulmonary bypass management on postcardiac surgery renal function. *Perfusion.* 2002;17(6):401-406.
49. Pearse RM, Harrison DA, MacDonald N, et al. Effect of a perioperative, cardiac output-guided hemodynamic therapy algorithm on outcomes following major gastrointestinal surgery: a randomized clinical trial and systematic review. *JAMA.* 2014;311:2181-2190.
50. Grocott MP, Dushianthan A, Hamilton MA, et al. Perioperative increase in global blood flow to explicit defined goals and outcomes after surgery: a Cochrane systematic review. *Br J Anaesth.* 2013;111:535-548.
51. Benes J, Chytra I, Altmann P, et al. Intraoperative fluid optimization using stroke volume variation in high risk surgical patients: results of prospective randomized study. *Crit Care.* 2010;14:R118.
52. Brienza N, Giglio MT, Marucci M, Fiore T. Does perioperative hemodynamic optimization protect renal function in surgical patients? A meta-analytic study. *Crit Care Med.* 2009;37:2079-2090.
53. Wesselink EM, Kappen TH, Torn HM, Slooter AJC, van Klei WA. Intraoperative hypotension and the risk of postoperative adverse outcomes: a systematic review. *Br J Anaesth.* 2018; 121(4):706-721.
54. Mullens W, Abrahams Z, Francis GS, et al. Importance of venous congestion for worsening of renal function in advanced decompensated heart failure. *J Am Coll Cardiol.* 2009;53:589-596.
55. Haase-Fielitz A, Haase M, Bellomo R, et al. Perioperative hemodynamic instability and fluid overload are associated with increasing acute kidney injury severity and worse outcome after cardiac surgery. *Blood Purif.* 2017;43(4):298-308.
56. Westaby S, Balacumaraswami L, Sayeed R. Maximizing survival potential in very high risk cardiac surgery. *Heart Fail Clin.* 2007;3(2):159-180.

57. Tarvasmäki T, Haapio M, Mebazaa A, et al. Acute kidney injury in cardiogenic shock: definitions, incidence, haemodynamic alterations, and mortality. *Eur J Heart Fail.* 2018;20(3):572-581.
58. Chen X, Wang X, Honore PM, Spapen HD, Liu D. Renal failure in critically ill patients, beware of applying (central venous) pressure on the kidney. *Ann Intensive Care.* 2018;8(1):91.
59. Damman K, van Deursen VM, Navis G, Voors AA, van Veldhuisen DJ, Hillege HL. Increased central venous pressure is associated with impaired renal function and mortality in a broad spectrum of patients with cardiovascular disease. *J Am Coll Cardiol.* 2009;53(7):582-588.
60. Bullivant EM, Wilcox CS, Welch WJ. Intrarenal vasoconstriction during hyperchloremia: role of thromboxane. *Am J Physiol.* 1989;256:152-157.
61. McCluskey SA, Karkouti K, Wijeysundera D, Minkovich L, Tait G, Beattie WS. Hyperchloremia after noncardiac surgery is independently associated with increased morbidity and mortality: a propensity-matched cohort study. *Anesth Analg.* 2013;117:412-421.
62. Kümpers P. Volumensubstitution mit NaCl 0,9% internist. *Der Internist.* 2015;56(7):773-778.
63. Basu RK, Wheeler DS. Kidney-lung cross-talk and acute kidney injury. *Pediatr Nephrol.* 2013;28(12):2239-2248.
64. Grams ME, Rabb H. The distant organ effects of acute kidney injury. *Kidney Int.* 2012; 81(10):942-948.
65. Feltes CM, Hassoun HT, Lie ML, Cheadle C, Rabb H. Pulmonary endothelial cell activation during experimental acute kidney injury. *Shock.* 2011;36(2):170-176.
66. Shin CH, Long DR, McLean D, et al. Effects of intraoperative fluid management on postoperative outcomes: a hospital registry study. *Ann Surg.* 2018;267(6):1084-1092.
67. Chong MA, Wang Y, Berbenetz NM, McConachie I. Does goal-directed haemodynamic and fluid therapy improve peri-operative outcomes? A systematic review and meta-analysis. *Eur J Anaesthesiol.* 2018;35(7):469-483.
68. Fowler AJ, Ahmad T, Phull MK, Allard S, Gillies MA, Pearse RM. Meta-analysis of the association between preoperative anaemia and mortality after surgery. *Br J Surg.* 2015;102:1314-1324.
69. Walsh M, Garg AX, Devereaux PJ, Argalious M, Honar H, Sessler DI. The association between perioperative hemoglobin and acute kidney injury in patients having noncardiac surgery. *Anesth Analg.* 2013;117:924-931.
70. Karkouti K, Stukel TA, Beattie WS, et al. Relationship of erythrocyte transfusion with short-and long-term mortality in a population-based surgical cohort. *Anesthesiology.* 2012;117:1175-1183.
71. Karkouti K, Grocott HP, Hall R, et al. Interrelationship of preoperative anemia, intraoperative anemia, and red blood cell transfusion as potentially modifiable risk factors for acute kidney injury in cardiac surgery: a historical multicentre cohort study. *Can J Anaesth.* 2015;62:377-384.
72. Haase M, Bellomo R, Story D, et al. Effect of mean arterial pressure, haemoglobin and blood transfusion during cardiopulmonary bypass on post-operative acute kidney injury. *Nephrol Dial Transplant.* 2012;27:153-160.
73. Kindzelski BA, Corcoran P, Siegenthaler MP, Horvath KA. Postoperative acute kidney injury following intraoperative blood product transfusions during cardiac surgery. *Perfusion.* 2018;33(1):62-70.
74. Parissis JT, Rafouli-Stergiou P, Stasinos V, Psarogiannakopoulos P, Mebazaa A. Inotropes in cardiac patients: update 2011. *Curr Opin Crit Care.* 2010;16(5):432-441
75. Slawsky MT, Colucci WS, Gottlieb SS, et al. Acute hemodynamic and clinical effects of levosimendan in patients with severe heart failure. Study Investigators. *Circulation.* 2000;102(18):2222-2227.
76. Mehta RH, Leimberger JD, van Diepen S, et al. Levosimendan in patients with left ventricular dysfunction undergoing cardiac surgery. *N Engl J Med.* 2017;376(21):2032-2042.
77. Landoni G, Lomivorotov VV, Alvaro G, et al. Levosimendan for hemodynamic support after cardiac surgery. *N Engl J Med.* 2017;376(21):2021-2031.
78. Barr J, Fraser GL, Puntillo K, et al. Clinical practice guidelines for the management of pain, agitation, and delirium in adult patients in the intensive care unit. *Crit Care Med.* 2013;41:263-306.
79. Ji F, Li Z, Young JN, Yeranossian A, Liu H. Post-bypass dexmedetomidine use and postoperative acute kidney injury in patients undergoing cardiac surgery with cardiopulmonary bypass. *PLoS One.* 2013;8:e77446.
80. Xue F, Zhang W, Chu HC. Assessing perioperative dexmedetomidine reduces the incidence and severity of acute kidney injury following valvular heart surgery. *Kidney Int.* 2016;89:1164.
81. Kwiatkowski DM, Axelrod DM, Sutherland SM, Tesoro TM, Krawczeski CD. Dexmedetomidine is associated with lower incidence of acute kidney injury after congenital heart surgery. *Pediatr Crit Care Med.* 2016;17:128-134.

82. Ji F, Li Z, Young JN, Yeranossian A, Liu H. Post-bypass dexmedetomidine use and postoperative acute kidney injury in patients undergoing cardiac surgery with cardiopulmonary bypass. *PLoS One.* 2013;8:e77446.
83. Liu X, Xie G, Zhang K, et al. Dexmedetomidine vs propofol sedation reduces delirium in patients after cardiac surgery: a meta-analysis with trial sequential analysis of randomized controlled trials. *J Crit Care.* 2017;38:190-196.
84. Djaiani G, Silverton N, Fedorko L, et al. Dexmedetomidine versus propofol sedation reduces delirium after cardiac surgery: a randomized controlled trial. *Anesthesiology.* 2016;124(2):362-368.
85. Murugan R, Weissfeld L, Yende S, et al. Association of statin use with risk and outcome of acute kidney injury in community-acquired pneumonia. *Clin J Am Soc Nephrol.* 2012;7:895-905.
86. Billings FT, Hendricks PA, Schildcrout JS, et al. High-dose perioperative atorvastatin and acute kidney injury following cardiac surgery: a randomized clinical trial. *JAMA.* 2016;315:877-888.
87. Thakar CV. Perioperative acute kidney injury. *Adv Chronic Kidney Dis.* 2013;20:67-75.
88. Halliwell B, Gutteridge JM. Role of free radicals and catalytic metal ions in human disease: an overview. *Methods Enzymol.* 1990;186:1-85.
89. Haase M, Haase-Fielitz A, Plass M, et al. Prophylactic perioperative sodium bicarbonate to prevent acute kidney injury following open heart surgery: a multicenter double-blinded randomized controlled trial. *PLoS Med.* 2013;10:e1001426.
90. McGuinness SP, Parke RL, Bellomo R, Van Haren FM, Bailey M. Sodium bicarbonate infusion to reduce cardiac surgery-associated acute kidney injury: a phase II multicenter double-blind randomized controlled trial. *Crit Care Med.* 2013;41:1599-1607.
91. Bailey M, McGuinness S, Haase M, et al. Sodium bicarbonate and renal function after cardiac surgery: a prospectively planned individual patient meta-analysis. *Anesthesiology.* 2015;122(2):294-306.
92. Bragadottir G, Redfors B, Ricksten SE. Mannitol increases renal blood flow and maintains filtration fraction and oxygenation in postoperative acute kidney injury: a prospective interventional study. *Crit Care.* 2012;16(4):R159.
93. Kong YG, Park JH, Park JY, et al. Effect of intraoperative mannitol administration on acute kidney injury after robot-assisted laparoscopic radical prostatectomy: a propensity score matching analysis. *Medicine.* 2018;97(26):e11338.
94. DiMari J, Megyesi J, Udvarhelyi N, Price P, Davis R, Safirstein R. N-acetyl cysteine ameliorates ischemic renal failure. *Am J Physiol.* 1997;272:F292-F298.
95. Savluk OF, Guzelmeric F, Yavuz Y, et al. N-acetylcysteine versus dopamine to prevent acute kidney injury after cardiac surgery in patients with preexisting moderate renal insufficiency. *Braz J Cardiovasc Surg.* 2017;32(1):8-14.
96. Naughton F, Wijeysundera D, Karkouti K, Tait G, Beattie WS. N-acetylcysteine to reduce renal failure after cardiac surgery: a systematic review and meta-analysis. *Can J Anaesth.* 2008;55(12):827-835.
97. Nigwekar SU, Kandula P. N-acetylcysteine in cardiovascular-surgery associated renal failure: a meta-analysis. *Ann Thorac Surg.* 2009;87:139-147.
98. Mei M, Zhao HW, Pan QG, Pu YM, Tang MZ, Shen BB. Efficacy of N-acetylcysteine in preventing acute kidney injury after cardiac surgery: a meta-analysis study. *J Invest Surg.* 2018;31(1):14-23.
99. Wierstra BT, Kadri S, Alomar S, Burbano X, Barrisford GW, Kao RL. The impact of "early" versus "late" initiation of renal replacement therapy in critical care patients with acute kidney injury: a systematic review and evidence synthesis. *Crit Care.* 2016;20:122.
100. Zarbock A, Kellum JA, Schmidt C, et al. Effect of early vs delayed initiation of renal replacement therapy on mortality in critically ill patients with acute kidney injury: the ELAIN randomized clinical trial. *JAMA.* 2016;315(20):2190-2199.

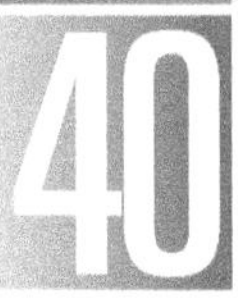

Cardiorenal Syndrome

David Mariuma and Steven Coca

INTRODUCTION, DEFINITION, AND EPIDEMIOLOGY

Recent data indicate that over 5 million emergency department (ED) visits and over 4 million hospitalizations for either primary or comorbid heart failure occur annually. Patients experiencing either acute or chronic kidney disease (CKD) in conjunction with heart failure have "cardiorenal syndrome (CRS)."[1]

CRS was formally defined in 2008 to describe the spectrum of diseases involving bidirectional dysfunction of the heart and kidney.[2] Attempts have been made to divide CRS into five classifications to distinguish between the direction of causality of heart and kidney failure and the acuity or chronicity of impairment, but in clinical practice, this directionality is difficult to ascertain and generally has no role in guiding treatment.[3] This is particularly true in the context of comorbidities such as diabetes mellitus and hypertension, which affect both organs simultaneously over time, and the prevalence of critically ill patients affected by cirrhosis or sepsis who develop CRS (classified as "CRS Type V").

Acute or chronic kidney impairment in patients admitted to the hospital with acute decompensated heart failure (ADHF) is associated with higher risk of mechanical ventilation, intensive care unit (ICU) admission, new-onset dialysis, cardiovascular mortality, and all-cause mortality compared to those with preserved kidney function.[4,5] Between 20% and 40% of patients hospitalized for ADHF will develop some degree of acute kidney injury or worsening kidney function (WRF) during admission.[6,7] It is challenging to use serum creatinine alone to define kidney dysfunction in heart failure patients, however, as decreased nutrition and muscle mass can alter serum creatinine without changing the glomerular filtration rate (GFR) and fluid overload can have a dilutional effect that falsely lowers serum creatinine and thus estimated glomerular filtration rate (eGFR). As of now, there is no easily available or routine alternative to using serum creatinine (see Chapter 16). These concerns and a paradigm shift in the theorized pathophysiology of CRS have led to significant changes in the management approach to patients with CRS over the years.

PATHOPHYSIOLOGY

Traditionally, the pathophysiology of CRS was defined by the Guyton hypothesis, which states that impaired heart function leads to reduced cardiac output, leading to underfilling of the kidney's arterioles and therefore poor kidney perfusion.[8] This results in renin release by the kidney, which increases sodium retention, vascular congestion, and afferent arteriolar vasoconstriction, which further lowers GFR.[3] However, clinical trials have failed to show a correlation between kidney dysfunction and cardiac output and that improvements in cardiac output did not result in improved kidney function in patients without cardiogenic shock.[9] Moreover, the "underfilling" theory is challenged by clinical experience, which reveals WRF in CRS patients without any episodes of overt hypotension.[6] More recently, various studies have demonstrated an important and likely leading role of increased venous congestion, right heart failure, and total body fluid overload in promoting kidney dysfunction. Increases in central venous pressure (CVP), a marker for venous congestion and volume overload, correlate with WRF in CRS patients and serve as an independent predictor of mortality.[10] Glomerular filtration depends on the difference between the mean arterial pressure (MAP) and CVP, and so, increases in CVP lead to tubular capillary distention and kidney interstitial edema. This leads to hypoxia and thus stimulation of the sympathetic nervous system (SNS), renin-angiotensin-aldosterone system (RAAS), and release of inflammatory cytokines (**Figure 40.1**). These mechanisms initially help prevent GFR decline but, over time, trigger cascading dysfunction of both the heart and kidneys.[6] Altered tubular function in the context of SNS and RAAS axis stimulation, volume overload, and immune activation further increase sodium and water retention, causing a pathologic feedback loop, which further elevates CVP.[11,12] The RAAS axis contributes to this with increased release of both angiotensin II (Ang II) and aldosterone. Ang II stimulates systemic vasoconstriction to preserve blood pressure, but also promotes increased sodium retention and extracellular volume expansion along with cardiac hypertrophy and fibrosis and kidney tubular fibrosis.[13] Aldosterone, stimulated by Ang II release, promotes further sodium and, thus, water reabsorption in the distal tubules.[14] Other mechanisms of injury in CRS include oxidative

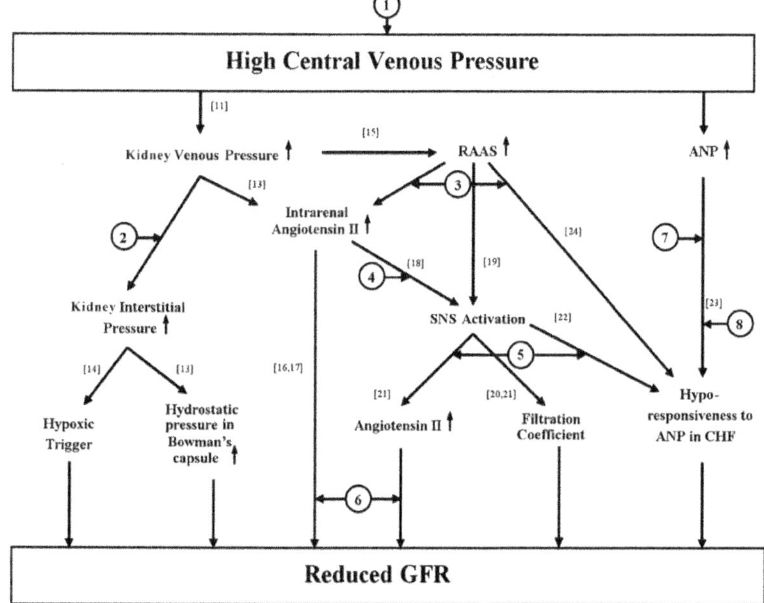

FIGURE 40.1: High central venous pressures drive hemodynamic, neurohormonal pertubations that results in reduced kidney function. From Damman K, Navis G, Smilde TD, et al. Decreased cardiac output, venous congestion and the association with renal impairment in patients with cardiac dysfunction. *Eur J Heart Fail.* 2007;9(9):872-878.

stress and mitochondrial dysfunction, the effects of protein-bound uremic toxins (PBUTs), metabolic acidosis, anemia, and electrolyte disorders.[15]

The known effects of kidney dysfunction have a harmful effect on heart function. Metabolic acidosis reduces myocardial contractility via alterations in β-receptor expression and intracellular calcium sensitivity and reduces response to vasopressors in critically hypotensive patients.[16,17] PBUTs, such as dimethylarginine, indoxyl sulfate, and p-cresyl sulfate, decrease cardiac output in humans, promote atherosclerosis, and worsen oxidative stress in both the heart and kidney.[3,18] Fibroblast growth factor 23, elevated in patients with kidney dysfunction as a mechanism to increase phosphorous excretion, has been repeatedly shown to induce left ventricular (LV) hypertrophy and is associated with increased mortality.[19] Anemia associated with erythropoietin deficiency from kidney failure can worsen oxidative stress in both the heart and kidney by decreasing delivery of antioxidants from red blood cells.[20] Perhaps most importantly, volume overload maintained by kidney dysfunction (either through anuria or increased sodium retention) propagates all the pathologic mechanisms described, such that management in CRS has shifted from raising cardiac output to prevent underfilling toward focusing on volume removal as a primary therapeutic goal.

MANAGEMENT

Goals

CRS patients should initially be categorized based on volume and perfusion status. Most patients present with a "wet and warm" state, in which venous congestion is driving end-organ damage without evidence of shock. In this case, management focuses on both pharmacologic inhibition of the downstream effects of RAAS and SNS activation as well as aggressive reduction of systemic venous congestion. Less commonly, patients present with a "wet and cold" state because of cardiogenic shock, in which case management focuses on the use of inotropes and pressors to maintain cardiac output and systemic perfusion with minimal inhibition of the RAAS and SNS axes.

In hypervolemic patients without shock, the goal is to remove fluid while minimizing the risk of frank hypotension or hypoperfusion. The clinical tension between decongestion and maintaining or maximizing kidney function is a common conundrum. However, numerous studies have repeatedly shown that WRF (defined as an increase in creatinine greater than 0.3 above baseline or a 20% decline in estimated GFR) in the context of aggressive diuresis in CRS patients is associated with a lower risk of mortality, and in critically ill patients requiring kidney replacement therapy (KRT), a negative daily fluid balance is associated with improved outcomes (**Figure 40.2**).[21-23] Moreover, post hoc analyses of the DOSE trial demonstrated that patients with improved kidney function (IKF, defined as a decrease in creatinine >0.3 below baseline) being treated for CRS had a higher composite outcome of death and rehospitalization.[24] These findings are in line with both new understandings regarding the pathophysiology of CRS and the fact that WRF may represent an unmasking of the dilutional effect of volume overload on the serum creatinine.[25] Therefore, a reasonable rise in creatinine (i.e., 20% to 30%) should not only be tolerated but seen as a positive prognostic factor in patients achieving negative daily fluid balance through diuresis in the setting of ongoing hypervolemia. An exact numerical cutoff of creatinine rise has not yet been established by studies, and further investigation is warranted to

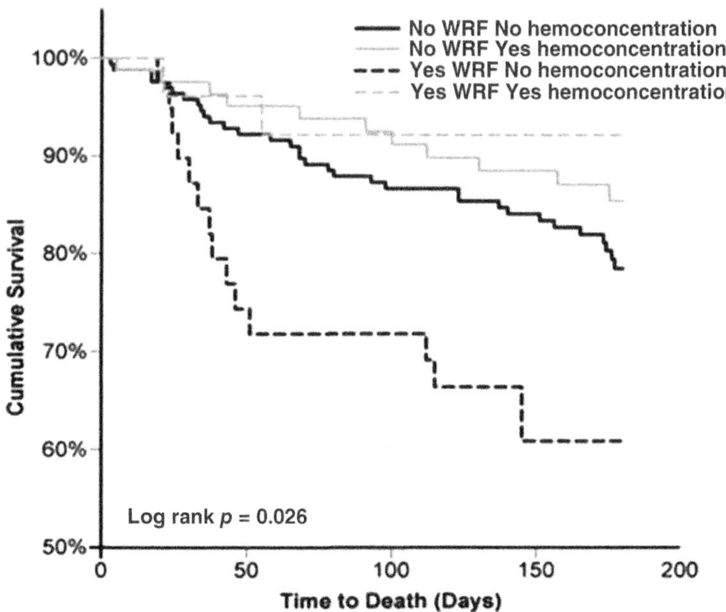

FIGURE 40.2: Patients who had WKF in the setting of achieved hemoconcentration during admission for ADHF had best 6-month survival compared to patients without hemoconcentration and no WKF. Patients who had WKF yet no hemoconcentration had the worst 6-month survival.

determine what rise in creatinine should prompt reconsideration of volume status and diuretic use.

Vasodilators and Inotropes

Consistent with the pathophysiology of CRS, which suggests that improvements in cardiac index do not improve kidney function in most CRS patients, studies have repeatedly shown no improvement in clinical or kidney outcomes in patients treated with inotropes. Notably, these studies excluded patients with cardiogenic shock, in which the standard of care is to use inotropes to maintain cardiac output. However, in patients with CRS without cardiogenic shock, inotropes such as dobutamine and dopamine have no proven benefit.[26,27] Vasodilators such as nesiritide and tezosentan, theorized to improve cardiac output and thus kidney perfusion, have shown no change in heart or kidney endpoints.[28-30] In a recent retrospective study of over 8,000 patients with ADHF, those that received acute vasodilator therapy (including nitrates) had no difference in mortality or length of ICU stay compared to those who did not receive vasodilators, except for patients with systolic blood pressures greater than 180.[31] Some data have emerged to suggest improvement in kidney function in patients with mechanical devices that increase cardiac output: one retrospective trial showed improvement in GFR in heart failure patients who received cardiac resynchronization therapy (CRT) compared to those who did not, though the follow-up period was only 6 months.[32] Ultimately, however, inotropes and vasodilators do not currently have a routine role in treating CRS patients without cardiogenic shock.

Diuretics

One of the pharmacologic mainstays to reduce venous congestion is the use of loop diuretics such as furosemide (of which intravenous [IV] dosing is equivalent to 2 times the oral dose), torsemide (20 mg of which is equivalent to 40 mg of furosemide), or bumetanide (1 mg of which is equivalent to 40 mg of furosemide). Loop diuretics can account for excretion of up to 25% of the filtered sodium load.[33] The DOSE trial was a landmark trial that randomized patients with ADHF, in a 2 × 2 factorial design, to furosemide as twice-daily IV boluses or continuous infusion, and low-dose (equal to home oral dose) or high-dose (2.5 times the home oral dose) groups. Although high-dose therapy showed modest improvement in outcomes, there were no differences in outcomes between continuous and bolus dosing.[34] Though there are no formal guidelines for diuretic dosing and up-stepping, there is an effort to establish standardized algorithms. In 2017, Ellison and Felker suggested a protocol rooted by a stepped algorithm in the CARRESS-HF trial[35] (**Table 40.1**). In this protocol, patients should be started on twice a day IV doses of furosemide to total 2.5 times the daily home dose. Daily urine output should be assessed with a goal of 3 to 5 L of urine output in 24 hours until clinical euvolemia is reached. If the goal is not achieved, the total daily furosemide dose should be calculated and used to decide the next day's bolus dose and total daily furosemide dose (given continuously or through bolus dosing), and metolazone (a thiazide diuretic) should either be added or increased in frequency.[36]

One of the challenges of using diuretics in patients with CRS is the development of diuretic resistance, in which minimal increases in urine output are achieved even with high-dose diuretics in a volume-overloaded patient. The cause of diuretic resistance is multifold. Diuretics are albumin bound, and therefore hypoalbuminemia in CRS patients leads to less delivery to the kidneys and reduced responsiveness.[6] However, there remains no evidence that administering albumin with diuresis results in improved outcomes or urine output. Bowel edema is also theorized to lead to decreased absorption of diuretics in

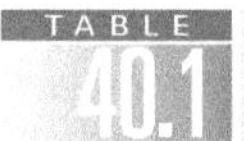

TABLE 40.1 Stepped Diuretic Regimen Depending on Current Level of Urine Output

Step[a]	Furosemide-Equivalent Dose[b]	Thiazide Dose
A	≤80 mg	N/A
B	81-160 mg	5 mg metolazone daily
C	161-240 mg	5 mg metolazone BID
D	>240 mg	5 mg metolazone BID
Urine Output	**Action**	
3-5 L	Maintain current dose	
<3 L	Advance a step	
>5 L	Reduce dose if desired[c]	

[a]Initial step: 2.5 times home PO dose.
[b]Over 24 hr. Either as BID bolus intravenous dosing or as a continuous drip with a preceding bolus.
[c]Approaching euvolemia, concern for rapid hemodynamic change, etc.

volume-overloaded patients, which is why hospitalized patients often benefit from IV diuresis instead of oral diuretic administration. Patients chronically receiving loop diuretics can develop distal convoluted tubular hypertrophy and collecting duct hypertrophy that limit therapeutic effects. This is worsened by hypokalemia through activation of the sodium chloride symporter.[37-39] One approach to this form of diuretic resistance (other than potassium repletion) is switching to continuous infusion.[36] Another approach is to target different segments of the tubule with different drugs. For example, loop diuretics, which act on the loop of Henle, can be administered concomitantly with thiazide diuretics, which act on the distal convoluted tubule, along with amiloride and mineralocorticoid receptor antagonists (MRAs), which act primarily on the collecting duct. Sodium-glucose cotransporter-2 (SGLT2) inhibitors, which have a novel role in treating diabetic nephropathy by reducing glomerular congestion and enhancing natriuresis in the proximal tubule, may also be considered. It should be noted, however, that the strategy of "sequential nephron blockade" described here has not yet been studied with high-powered randomized controlled trials (RCTs), though various observational and smaller RCTs have suggested benefit, such as when adding spironolactone to patients with diuretic resistance.[40] Though the use of multiple diuretics is often challenged by electrolyte discrepancies such as hyponatremia, hypokalemia, or hyperkalemia, these individual conditions can be treated and should not necessarily deter diuresis when it is effective in improving urine output. For example, hyperkalemia can be treated with potassium ion exchangers such as patiromer,[41] and in hypervolemic patients with diuretic-induced metabolic alkalosis, the carbonic anhydrase inhibitor acetazolamide can be used both to enhance bicarbonaturia and provide a diuretic effect. Finally, diuretic resistance can occur because of severe kidney functional impairment and reduced GFR, in which case the only feasible option is either slow continuous ultrafiltration (SCUF) or KRT.

Ultrafiltration

Another means of reducing congestion is through venovenous SCUF, an extracorporeal volume removal method that can be achieved with peripheral venous access that results in isotonic volume and sodium removal. Studies have had conflicting results when comparing SCUF to pharmacologic diuresis head-to-head, particularly in regard to efficacy of weight reduction, fluid removal, and rate of adverse effects.[35,42-44] Currently, guidelines suggest use of diuretics as a first-line treatment and initiation of SCUF only in the case of diuretic failure.[45] Generally, ultrafiltration rates should not exceed 250 mL/hr when using SCUF to avoid hemodynamic compromise.[46] Some have advocated for the use of continuous venovenous hemofiltration (CVVH), a form of dialysis, in CRS patients in place of SCUF. An observational study of 120 patients over 2 years showed improvement in mean survival time in patients on CVVH versus SCUF, but this was only seen in patients with CRS because of intrinsic cardiomyopathy (as opposed to coronary artery disease or valvular heart disease) and has not been thoroughly investigated with RCTs.[47]

Another modality for volume removal in CRS patients that has been explored is peritoneal dialysis (PD). PD is an effective means of total body sodium removal, and a standard PD prescription can be adjusted to allow for increased sodium removal. Some adjustments include the use of icodextrin as the dialysate fluid and the use of continuous ambulatory peritoneal dialysis (CAPD) instead of automated PD, as the longer cycles allow for more sodium removal through convection.[48]

Monitoring for Improvement in Volume Status

When any modality to reduce congestion is used, volume status should be routinely monitored in order to down-titrate diuretics or SCUF when euvolemia is reached. Some means of monitoring volume status include blood pressure trends, weight trends, physical examination (improvement in peripheral edema, moist or dry mucous membranes, jugular venous pressure, and skin turgor), imaging and lung auscultation to assess for pulmonary edema, inferior vena cava (IVC) diameter and collapsibility on bedside ultrasound, and, in rare cases, invasive measurement of pulmonary capillary wedge pressures and right heart venous pressures through Swan-Ganz catheterization. A post hoc study using data from the DOSE and CARRESS trials found that so long as kidney function decline was accompanied by a decline in N-terminal pro-brain natriuretic peptide (NT-proBNP) levels, the risk of mortality was lower, highlighting the importance of using congestion markers when trying to decongest patients with WRF.[49] A similar phenomenon is seen in patients that achieve hemoconcentration during treatment for ADHF, defined as an increase in hemoglobin or hematocrit above admission values. When occurring early in the course of treatment, hemoconcentration is associated with increased fluid removal and lower risk of short-term mortality and rehospitalization rates.[50]

Sympathetic Nervous System/Renin-Angiotensin-Aldosterone System Axis Inhibition

Inhibition of the effects of the SNS and RAAS axes constitutes another arm of the management of CRS, though this should be avoided in cases of cardiogenic shock. Although formal guidelines[51] focus on using these medications primarily for congestive heart failure irrespective of concomitant kidney dysfunction or WRF, various trials have shown a reduction in hospitalization, cardiovascular events, mortality, and symptoms when using these drugs compared to placebo in patients with CRS.[52-54] The recommended medications include angiotensin-converting enzyme inhibitors (ACEIs) or angiotensin receptor blockers (ARBs), β-blockers, and, in some cases, MRAs. ACEIs should be uptitrated to the highest recommended dose as tolerated, typically via increases every 4 to 8 weeks. However, an increase in creatinine by more than 30% of predrug levels justifies holding the ACEI and investigating for renal artery stenosis or other causes of kidney hypoperfusion.[50] However, without evidence of hypoperfusion or hypovolemia, ACEIs should not be routinely held in the setting of WRF in patients with ADHF. Although the new sacubitril (neprilysin inhibitor)-valsartan combination pill (angiotensin receptor neprilysin inhibitor [ARNI]) has demonstrated reductions in mortality and hospitalization rates in systolic heart failure patients, many published studies excluded patients with CKD or AKI during treatment.[6] One analysis found that ARNIs, compared to ACEIs, led to a slower rate of decline in GFR, and the clinical benefit of ARNIs on cardiovascular mortality in heart failure patients was consistent among patients with CKD.[55] Although theoretically aliskiren, a direct renin inhibitor, should improve outcomes in CRS patients, studies have shown no reduction in mortality or rehospitalization with an increase in adverse effects in patients who had this added to standard therapy.[56]

References

1. Jackson SL, Tong X, King RJ, Loustalot F, Hong Y, Ritchey MD. National burden of heart failure events in the United States, 2006 to 2014. *Circulation.* 2018;11.
2. Ronco C. The cardiorenal syndrome: basis and common ground for a multidisciplinary patient-oriented therapy. *Cardiorenal Med.* 2011;1:3-4.
3. Kumar U, Wettersten N, Garimella PS. Cardiorenal syndrome: pathophysiology. *Cardiol Clin.* 2019;37:251-265.
4. Hata N, Yokoyama S, Shinada T, et al. Acute kidney injury and outcomes in acute decompensated heart failure: evaluation of the RIFLE criteria in an acutely ill heart failure population. *Eur J Heart Fail.* 2009;12:32-37.
5. Heywood JT, Fonarow GC, Costanzo MR, et al. High prevalence of renal dysfunction and its impact on outcome in 118,465 patients hospitalized with acute decompensated heart failure: a report from the ADHERE database. *J Card Fail.* 2007;13:422-430.
6. Ronco C, Bellasi A, Di Lullo L. Implication of acute kidney injury in heart failure. *Heart Fail Clin.* 2019;15:463-476.
7. Nohria A, Hasselblad V, Stebbins A, et al. Cardiorenal interactions: insights from the ESCAPE trial. *J Am Coll Cardiol.* 2008;51:1268-1274.
8. Ronco C, Cicoira M, McCullough PA. Syndrome type 1: pathophysiological crosstalk leading to combined heart and kidney dysfunction in the setting of acutely decompensated heart failure. *J Am Coll Cardiol.* 2012;60:1031-1042.
9. Binanay C, Califf RM, Hasselblad V, et al. Evaluation study of congestive heart failure and pulmonary artery catheterization effectiveness: the ESCAPE trial. *JAMA.* 2005;294:1625-1633.
10. Damman K, van Deursen VM, Navis G, et al. Increased central venous pressure is associated with impaired renal function and mortality in a broad spectrum of patients with cardiovascular disease. *J Am Coll Cardiol.* 2009;53:582-588.
11. Mullens W, Abrahams Z, Francis GS, et al. Importance of venous congestion for worsening of renal function in advanced decompensated heart failure. *J Am Coll Cardiol.* 2009;53:589-596.
12. Colombo PC, Jorde UP. The active role of venous congestion in the pathophysiology of acute decompensated heart failure. *Rev Esp Cardiol.* 2010;63:5-8.
13. Brilla CG, Rupp H. Myocardial collagen matrix remodeling and congestive heart failure. *Cardiologia.* 1994;39:389-393.
14. Harrison-Bernard LM. The renal renin-angiotensin system. *Adv Physiol Educ.* 2009;33:270-274.
15. Di Lullo L, Reeves PB, Bellasi A, Ronco C. Cardiorenal syndrome in acute kidney injury. *Semin Nephrol.* 2019;39:31-40.
16. Saegusa N, Garg V, Spitzer KW. Modulation of ventricular transient outward K^+ current by acidosis and its effects on excitation-contraction coupling. *Am J Physiol Heart Circ Physiol.* 2013;304:H1680-H1696.
17. Nimmo AJ, Than N, Orchard CH, Whitaker EM. The effect of acidosis on beta-adrenergic receptors in ferret cardiac muscle. *Exp Physiol.* 1993;78:95-103.
18. Kielstein JT, Impraim B, Simmel S, et al. Cardiovascular effects of systemic nitric oxide synthase inhibition with asymmetrical dimethylarginine in humans. *Circulation.* 2004;109:172-177.
19. Faul C, Amaral AP, Oskouei B, et al. FGF23 induces left ventricular hypertrophy. *J Clin Invest.* 2011;121:4393-4408.
20. Grune T, Sommerburg O, Siems WG. Oxidative stress in anemia. *Clin Nephrol.* 2000;53:S18-S22.
21. Grams ME, Estrella MM, Coresh J, Brower RG, Liu KD. Fluid balance, diuretic use, and mortality in acute kidney injury. *Clin J Am Soc Nephrol.* 2011;6:966-973.
22. Bellomo R, Cass A, Cole L, et al. RENAL replacement therapy study investigators: an observational study fluid balance and patient outcomes in the randomized evaluation of normal vs. augmented level of replacement therapy trial. *Crit Care Med.* 2012;40:1753-1760.
23. Testani JM, Chen J, McCauley BD, et al. Potential effects of aggressive decongestion during the treatment of decompensated heart failure on renal function and survival. *Circulation.* 2010;122:265-272.
24. Brisco MA, Zile MR, Hanberg JS, et al. Relevance of changes in serum creatinine during a heart failure trial of decongestive strategies: insights from the DOSE trial. *J Card Fail.* 2016;22:753-760.
25. Testani JM, McCauley BD, Chen J, Shumski M, Shannon RP. Worsening renal function defined as an absolute increase in serum creatinine is a biased metric for the study of cardio-renal interactions. *Cardiology.* 2010;116:206-212.
26. Bellomo R, Chapman M, Finfer S, Hickling K, Myburgh J. Low-dose dopamine in patients with early renal dysfunction: a placebo-controlled randomised trial. Australian and New Zealand Intensive Care Society (ANZICS) Clinical Trials Group. *Lancet.* 2000;356:2139-2143.

27. Lauschke A, Teichgräber UKM, Frei U, EcKardt KU. "Low-dose" dopamine worsens renal perfusion in patients with acute renal failure. *Kidney Int.* 2006;69:1669-1674.
28. O'Connor CM, Starling RC, Hernandez AF, et al. Effect of Nesiritide in patients with acute decompensated heart failure. *N Engl J Med.* 2011;365:32-43.
29. Witteles RM, Kao D, Christophers D, et al. Impact of Nesiritide on renal function in patients with acute decompensated heart failure and pre-existing renal dysfunction. *J Am Coll Cardiol.* 2007;50:1835-1840.
30. McMurray JJ, Teerlink RJ, Cotter G, et al. Effects of Tezosentan on symptoms and clinical outcomes in patients with acute heart failure. *JAMA.* 2007;298:2009-2019.
31. Shiraishi Y, Kohsaka S, Katsuki T. Benefit and harm of intravenous vasodilators across the clinical profile spectrum in acute cardiogenic pulmonary oedema patients. *Eur Heart J Acute Cardiovasc Care.* 2020. doi:10.1177/2048872619891075
32. Boerrigter G, Costello-Boerrigter LC, Abraham WT. Cardiac resynchronization therapy improves renal function in human heart failure with reduced glomerular filtration rate. *J Card Fail.* 2008;14:539-546.
33. Puschett JB. Pharmacological classification and renal actions of diuretics. *Cardiology.* 1994;84:4-13.
34. Felker GM, Lee KL, Bull DA, et al. Diuretic strategies in patients with acute decompensated heart failure. *N Engl J Med.* 2011;364:797-805.
35. Bart BA, Goldsmith SR, Lee KL, et al. Ultrafiltration in decompensated heart failure with cardiorenal syndrome. *N Engl J Med.* 2012;367:2296-2304.
36. Ellison DH, Felker GM. Diuretic treatment in heart failure—from physiology to clinical trials. *N Engl J Med.* 2017;377:1964-1975.
37. Terker AS, Zhang C, McCormick JA, et al. Potassium modulates electrolyte balance and blood pressure through effects on distal cell voltage and chloride. *Cell Metab.* 2015;21:39-50.
38. Wade JB, Liu J, Coleman RA, Grimm PR, Delpire E, Welling PA. SPAK mediated NCC regulation in response to low K+ Diet. *Am J Physiol Renal Physiol.* 2015;308:F923-F931.
39. Vitzthum H, Seniuk A, Schulte LH, Muller ML, Hetz H, Ehmke H. Functional coupling of renal K+ and Na+ handling causes high blood pressure in Na+ replete mice. *J Physiol.* 2014;592:1139-1157.
40. Bansal S, Munoz K, Brune S, Bailey S, Prasad A, Velagapudi C. High-dose spironolactone when patients with acute decompensated heart failure are resistant to loop diuretics: a pilot study. *Ann Intern Med.* 2019;171:443.
41. Di Lullo L, Ronco C, Granata A, et al. Chronic hyperkalemia in cardiorenal patients: risk factors, diagnosis, and new treatment options. *Cardiorenal Med.* 2019;9:8-21.
42. Costanzo MR, Saltzberg MT, Jessup M, et al. Ultrafiltration is associated with fewer rehospitalizations than continuous diuretic infusion in patients with decompensated heart failure: results from UNLOAD. *J Card Fail.* 2010;16:277-284.
43. Costanzo MR, Ronco C. Isolated ultrafiltration in heart failure patients. *Curr Cardiol Rep.* 2012;14:254-264.
44. Bart BA, Boyle A, Bank AJ, et al. Ultrafiltration versus usual care for hospitalized patients with heart failure: the relief for acutely fluid-overloaded patients with decompensated congestive heart failure (RAPID-CHF) trial. *J Am Coll Cardiol.* 2005;46:2043-2046.
45. Yancy CW, Jessup M, Bozkurt B, et al. 2013 ACCF/AHA guideline for the management of heart failure: executive summary: a report of the American College of Cardiology Foundation/American Heart Association Task Force on practice guidelines. *Circulation.* 2013;128:1810.
46. Gheorghiade M, Follath F, Ponikowski P, et al. Assessing and grading congestion in acute heart failure: a scientific statement from the acute heart failure committee of the heart failure association of the European Society of Cardiology and endorsed by the European Society of Intensive Care Medicine. *Eur J Heart Fail.* 2010;12:423-433.
47. Premuzic V, Basic-Jukic N, Jelakovic B, Kes P. Continuous veno-venous hemofiltration improves survival of patients with congestive heart failure and cardiorenal syndrome compared to slow continuous ultrafiltration. *Ther Apher Dial.* 2017;21:279-286.
48. Kazory A, Koratala A, Ronco C. Customization of peritoneal dialysis in cardiorenal syndrome by optimization of sodium extraction. *Cardiorenal Med.* 2019;9:117-124.
49. McCallum W, McCallum W, Tighiouart H, Kiernan MS, Huggins GS, Sarnak MJ. Relation of kidney function decline and NT-proBNP with risk of mortality and readmission in acute decompensated heart failure. *Am J Med.* 2020;133(1):115-122.e2.
50. Rubinstein J, Sanford D. Treatment of cardiorenal syndrome. *Cardiol Clin.* 2019;37:267-273.
51. Ponikowski P, Voors AA, Anker SD, et al. 2016 ESC guidelines for the diagnosis and treatment of acute and chronic heart failure. *Eur Heart J.* 2016;27:2129-2200.
52. Bowling CB, Sanders PW, Allman RM, et al. Effects of enalapril in systolic heart failure patients with and without chronic kidney disease: insights from the SOLVD treatment trial. *Int J Cardiol.* 2013;167:151-156.

53. Anand IS, Bishu K, Rector TS, et al. Proteinuria, chronic kidney disease, and the effect of an angiotensin receptor blocker in addition to an angiotensin-converting enzyme inhibitor in patients with moderate to severe heart failure. *Circulation.* 2009;120:1577-1584.
54. Florea VG, Rector TS, Anand IS, Cohn JN. Heart failure with improved ejection fraction: clinical characteristics, correlates of recovery, and survival: results from the Valsartan Heart Failure Trial. *Circ Heart Fail.* 2016;9(7).
55. Damman K, Gori M, Claggett B, et al. Renal effects and associated outcomes during angiotensin-neprilysin inhibition in heart failure. *JACC Heart Fail.* 2018;6:489-498.
56. Gheorghiade M, Bohm M, Greene SJ, et al. Effect of aliskiren on post-discharge mortality and heart failure readmissions among patients hospitalized for heart failure. *JAMA.* 2013;309:1125-1135.

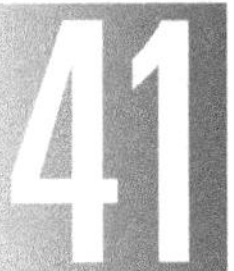

Left Ventricular Assist Devices in the Intensive Care Unit

Bethany Roehm, Gaurav Gulati, and
Daniel E. Weiner

INTRODUCTION

There are an estimated 6.5 million people in the United States with heart failure, often coincident with chronic kidney disease (CKD).[1] Those with advanced heart failure with or without CKD have a 1-year survival of 25%; this may improve more than 3-fold with left ventricular assist device (LVAD) implantation (**Visual Abstracts 41.1** and **41.2**).[2] Since 2006, over 25,000 adults have received LVADs in the United States.[3]

BASIC LEFT VENTRICULAR ASSIST DEVICES PRINCIPLES

Left Ventricular Assist Device Indications and Types

An LVAD is a mechanical pump that is surgically attached to a patient's left ventricular apex via an inflow cannula and to their aorta via an outflow cannula, moving blood from the heart to the rest of the body as a means of augmenting cardiac output.[4] LVADs may be a "bridge to transplant" to support patients while awaiting heart transplantation, a permanent "destination" therapy if a patient is not a heart transplant candidate, or a "bridge to decision" if heart transplant eligibility is unclear. Indications and contraindications for LVAD are listed in **Table 41.1**.[4-6]

Current LVADs include the HeartMate II, which utilizes an axial flow pump and lies extrapericardial; the HeartWare ventricular assist device, an intrapericardial centrifugal flow pump whose impeller is partially magnetically levitated; and

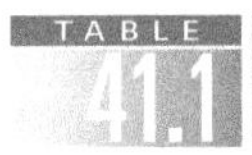

TABLE 41.1 Indications and Contraindications for Left Ventricular Assist Device

Indications	Contraindications
Stage D heart failure	Severe right heart failure
≥3 Hospitalizations/yr for heart failure	Anatomic issues
Inotrope dependence	Inability to take warfarin
Kidney dysfunction from heart failure	Active infection
Liver dysfunction from heart failure	Significant medical comorbidities

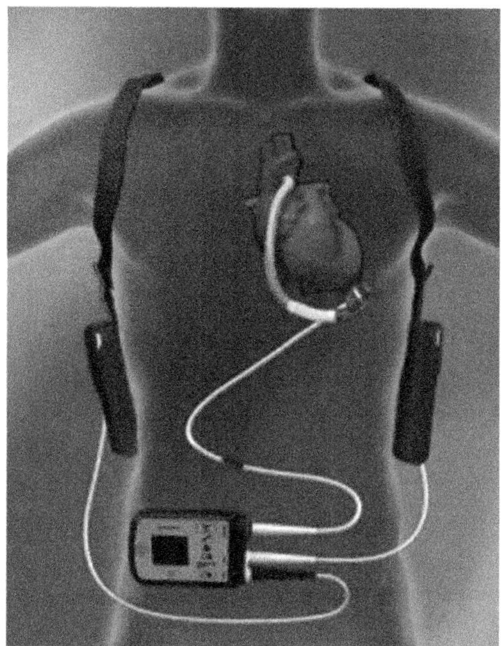

FIGURE 41.1: HeartMate 3 left ventricular assist device.

the HeartMate 3 (**Figure 41.1**), an intrapericardial centrifugal flow pump with a fully magnetically levitated impeller. The HeartMate 3 is currently favored over the two older devices because of lower risk of pump thrombosis, with fewer than 2% of HeartMate 3 LVADs complicated by pump thrombosis as compared to 14% of axial flow LVADs in a recent seminal trial.[7]

General Mechanics

Current LVADs are continuous rather than pulsatile flow devices. LVAD flow depends on preload, afterload, and pump speed; pump speed is programmed by the cardiologist and is individualized based on patient factors. A pressure differential exists between the inflow cannula in the left ventricle and the outflow cannula in the aorta that the LVAD must pump against. Higher flow is generated during ventricular systole, when the difference between left ventricular and aortic pressure is smallest.[8] Flow is estimated by the device from the set pump speed and measured power usage. The pulsatility index measures the difference between maximum and minimum flows over time and is affected by several factors, including pump speed, volume status, left ventricular afterload, and right ventricular function.

Common Left Ventricular Assist Device Alarms

Many LVAD alarms relate to issues with flow. High-power alarms may occur if there is obstruction in the pump, as seen in pump thrombosis where power increases in an attempt to maintain pump speed. Low-flow alarms may be seen in states of low circulating volume or with obstructive events such as cannula obstruction and cannula tamponade. Suction event alarms occur when the inflow cannula pulls against the intraventricular septum, such as when left ventricular preload is insufficient to meet the demands of pump speed. Both these events often are initially treated with a volume infusion; suction events may also respond to decreasing the pump speed.

LEFT VENTRICULAR ASSIST DEVICE PATIENT CARE IN THE INTENSIVE CARE UNIT SETTING

Blood Pressure and Left Ventricular Assist Devices

Many LVAD patients do not have a palpable pulse, making traditional blood pressure measurement using an automated cuff or auscultation not possible. Accordingly, blood pressure is typically assessed using a Doppler probe; this "opening pressure" approximates the mean arterial pressure (MAP) in patients with low pulsatility.[9] In the rare patient with significant residual heart contractility, a palpable pulse may be felt and measured with an automated cuff. In these patients, if a Doppler probe is used, the "opening pressure" more closely approximates the systolic blood pressure than the MAP. An arterial line may also be used in critical care settings. Goal MAP is 70 to 90 mm Hg, with hypotension defined as MAP less than 60 mm Hg.[10] Both hyper- and hypotension should be avoided. Higher afterload from poorly controlled hypertension leads to decreased flow through the LVAD and is associated with an increased risk of stroke, thromboembolic events, and aortic insufficiency.[11] In cases of hypotension, vasopressors and inotropes may be used in consultation with a heart failure cardiologist, but ultimately the cause of hypotension should be addressed.

Anticoagulation

All LVAD patients are anticoagulated with antithrombotic and antiplatelet agents. Aspirin and warfarin are used in the outpatient setting, with typical target international normalized ratio (INR) of 2 to 3. Intravenous unfractionated heparin and enoxaparin are used as bridge therapies for procedures or subtherapeutic INR. In cases of heparin-induced thrombocytopenia, direct thrombin inhibitors replace heparin.[6] Direct oral anticoagulants such as apixaban have not been formally studied in LVAD patients.

Cardiopulmonary Resuscitation

There is a theoretical concern that standard chest compressions could dislodge the LVAD cannula, though two small studies showed no cannula dislodgement after cardiopulmonary resuscitation (CPR).[12,13] Because LVAD patients are often pulseless, assessing cardiac arrest can be challenging, and blood pressure should be measured using a Doppler probe. Indications for chest compressions include hypotension with unresponsiveness or no flow through the LVAD, and CPR follows usual advanced cardiac life support (ACLS) guidelines. Similarly, there are no contraindications to external defibrillation or cardioversion.

LEFT VENTRICULAR ASSIST DEVICE COMPLICATIONS

Right-Sided Heart Failure

Right ventricular failure usually occurs in the first few weeks following LVAD implantation, though late right ventricular failure can occur. There are two major mechanisms for right ventricular failure. First, when the LVAD offloads the left ventricle, the interventricular septum shifts to the left, changing the shape of the right ventricle and reducing its contractility. Second, when cardiac output from the left ventricle improves with LVAD, the right ventricle must be able to match that cardiac output. This may be difficult because many patients have concomitant right ventricular dysfunction and also because long-standing left ventricular failure can lead to pulmonary hypertension with resultant increased afterload on an already compromised right ventricle.[14] Management of right ventricular failure in an LVAD recipient is beyond the scope of this chapter.

Pump Thrombosis

LVAD pump thrombosis is the formation of thrombus on the impeller. LVAD power spikes and laboratory signs of hemolysis suggest pump thrombosis, with lactate dehydrogenase more than 2.5 times the upper limit of normal considered diagnostic.[15] Other laboratory markers include hemoglobinuria and elevated plasma-free hemoglobin. Pump thrombosis can also be diagnosed with an echocardiogram by demonstrating failure to decompress the left ventricle with increasing pump speeds or, in rare cases, by directly visualizing a thrombus with contrast-enhanced computed tomography (CT) imaging. Medical management includes intravenous anticoagulation with unfractionated heparin or direct thrombin inhibitors, or even thrombolysis. Surgery to exchange the LVAD may be indicated. Stenting can be done if the thrombus is in the outflow cannula.[11]

Gastrointestinal Bleeding

LVAD patients are prone to gastrointestinal (GI) bleeding because of systemic anticoagulation and a propensity to develop arteriovenous (AV) malformations, thought to be due to acquired von Willebrand syndrome because of increased clearance of von Willebrand factor related to higher shear stress in the LVAD,[16] similar to the pathophysiology of aortic stenosis–related GI bleeding. This may be particularly common with coincident CKD. Management is similar to the general population, with careful risk assessment of anticoagulation utilization.[11,16] Octreotide and thalidomide are emerging as potential therapies for refractory cases.

Stroke

LVAD patients are at high risk for both ischemic and hemorrhagic stroke. Observational data suggest lower ischemic stroke risk with MAP less than 85 mm Hg as well as with use of antiplatelet agents and warfarin.[11,17] The most recent 2019 European Association for Cardio-Thoracic Surgery (EACTS) guidelines recommend against systemic thrombolytics in LVAD patients with acute ischemic stroke because of an unacceptably high bleeding risk.[11] Hemorrhagic stroke results in a 1-month survival of 45% and 1-year survival of 30%.[18] Management is challenging, but typically involves reversal of anticoagulation.[11]

Device Infections

Pump-related infections are the most common device-related complication after the initial implantation period.[2,3] Device infections can involve any part of the LVAD and may result from infection elsewhere seeding the device or may enter via the driveline. Skin flora, such as *Staphylococcus aureus* and *Staphylococcus epidermidis*, accounts for over half of all infections.[19,20] Treatment can be challenging, with prolonged treatment and sometimes lifelong suppressive therapy required.[19]

LEFT VENTRICULAR ASSIST DEVICES AND THE KIDNEY

The interaction between the mechanical circulatory support provided by an LVAD and kidney function is complex. While the majority of patients have improved kidney function following LVAD implantation, over time this improvement is not sustained (**Visual Abstract 41.3**).

Acute Kidney Injury and Acute Dialysis

LVAD patients are at high risk for acute kidney injury (AKI) and may require kidney replacement therapy. AKI most often occurs in the perioperative and immediate postoperative period following LVAD implantation because of hemodynamic insults. Other AKI etiologies include any cause of shock, right heart failure, and pump thrombosis. Mortality is high among patients who develop AKI, reaching 75% in those requiring dialysis.[21,22] It is unclear if kidney failure itself causes increased mortality risk or if kidney failure is a marker of multiorgan failure.[23] If hemodynamically unstable, continuous kidney replacement therapy may be the initial modality, prior to transitioning to intermittent hemodialysis (IHD) or peritoneal dialysis.

Maintenance Dialysis

Although many LVAD recipients who require acute kidney replacement therapy will die, some will have recovery of kidney function, whereas others will require maintenance dialysis. IHD is the most frequently used maintenance modality, but peritoneal dialysis and daily home hemodialysis are also options.[23-25] The latter two modalities may be preferable given lower ultrafiltration rates with resultant lower cardiac demand, particularly for those with right ventricular failure.

Catheters are most frequently used for hemodialysis access in LVAD patients receiving dialysis despite the high risk for infection and complexity of bloodstream infections should they occur. Frequent catheter use reflects the often acute nature of kidney injury as well as potentially limited vein options because of procedures such as implantable cardiac devices with transvenous leads and peripherally inserted central catheter (PICC) placement for home inotropes. These procedures can damage vessels, limiting AV fistula and graft options.[26] If there are adequate vessels, an AV fistula or graft should be considered; several reports describe successful AV fistula creation in LVAD patients, even those without pulsatile flow,[27-29] underscoring the importance of vein-sparing strategies in LVAD patients at risk for kidney failure.

Erythropoiesis-stimulating agents (ESAs) are often avoided in LVAD patients because of concern for increased risk of pump thrombosis, based on an observational report of a dose-dependent increased risk of LVAD thrombosis in ESA recipients with mean estimated glomerular filtration rate (eGFR) >60 mL/min/1.73 m^2 and without severe anemia.[30] Given the limitations of this report, it appears reasonable to consider ESA use in LVAD patients with advanced kidney disease per current guidelines for kidney failure populations, avoiding high-dose ESA administration. Care should be individualized to each patient, weighing the potential risks and benefits.

Although many critically ill LVAD patients requiring kidney replacement therapy will initially be started on continuous kidney replacement therapy once hemodynamically stable, LVAD patients often will transition to IHD. Particularly among those patients who remain critically ill in the intensive care unit (ICU) setting, establishing and achieving a "dry weight" may be a challenge.

This is particularly notable given the cachexia that often occurs with prolonged hospitalization.

Volume assessment incorporates not only physical examination findings but also data that may be available from existing right heart catheters and data derived from the LVAD itself. As discussed earlier, blood pressure can be monitored through an arterial line if present or via the Doppler pressure. Pulsatility index can be used in conjunction with these methods to help determine volume status but should not be used as the sole means of assessing volume status. Recall that pulsatility index reflects the magnitude of difference between the maximum and minimum LVAD flows over time.[8] Higher preload can cause left ventricular distension leading to a higher pulsatility index, thus suggesting hypervolemia; conversely, hypovolemia can cause a lower pulsatility index.[31] However, other factor such as high afterload can cause high pulsatility index. Right ventricular failure, tamponade, or pump thrombosis can cause low pulsatility index irrespective of volume status.[31,32] Recognizing these clinical factors that may impact the pulsatility index and incorporating this with other existing data may help optimize volume status.

CONCLUSIONS

Critically ill LVAD patients are complex, often have multiple organ involvement, including acute kidney disease or CKD, and require a multidisciplinary approach. A heart failure cardiologist with expertise in LVAD patients should always be involved. LVAD patients with concurrent kidney disease, particularly those on dialysis, have poor outcomes.

Acknowledgments

Bethany Roehm is funded by NIH T32 DK007777. Gaurav Gulati is funded by NIH F32HL149251 and TL1TR002546.

References

1. Benjamin EJ, Virani SS, Callaway CW, et al. Heart disease and stroke statistics—2018 update: a report from the American Heart Association. *Circulation.* 2018;137:e67-e492.
2. Kirklin JK, Pagani FD, Kormos RL, et al. Eighth annual INTERMACS report: special focus on framing the impact of adverse events. *J Heart Lung Transplant.* 2017;36:1080-1086.
3. Kormos RL, Cowger J, Pagani FD, et al. The Society of Thoracic Surgeons Intermacs database annual report: evolving indications, outcomes, and scientific partnerships. *J Heart Lung Transplant.* 2019;38:114-126.
4. Englert JAR 3rd, Davis JA, Krim SR. Mechanical circulatory support for the failing heart: continuous-flow left ventricular assist devices. *Ochsner J.* 2016;16:263-269.
5. Ammirati E, Oliva F, Cannata A, et al. Current indications for heart transplantation and left ventricular assist device: a practical point of view. *Eur J Intern Med.* 2014;25:422-429.
6. Miller LW, Guglin M. Patient selection for ventricular assist devices: a moving target. *J Am Coll Cardiol.* 2013;61:1209-1221.
7. Mehra MR, Uriel N, Naka Y, et al. A fully magnetically levitated left ventricular assist device—final report. *N Engl J Med.* 2019;380:1618-1627.
8. Tchoukina I, Smallfield MC, Shah KB. Device management and flow optimization on left ventricular assist device support. *Crit Care Clin.* 2018;34:453-463.
9. Bennett MK, Roberts CA, Dordunoo D, et al. Ideal methodology to assess systemic blood pressure in patients with continuous-flow left ventricular assist devices. *J Heart Lung Transplant.* 2010;29:593-594.
10. Feldman D, Pamboukian SV, Teuteberg JJ, et al. The 2013 International Society for Heart and Lung Transplantation Guidelines for mechanical circulatory support: executive summary. *J Heart Lung Transplant.* 2013;32:157-187.
11. Potapov EV, Antonides C, Crespo-Leiro MG, et al. 2019 EACTS Expert Consensus on long-term mechanical circulatory support. *Eur J Cardiothorac Surg.* 2019;56:230-270.

12. Shinar Z, Bellezzo J, Stahovich M, et al. Chest compressions may be safe in arresting patients with left ventricular assist devices (LVADs). *Resuscitation.* 2014;85:702-704.
13. Garg S, Ayers CR, Fitzsimmons C, et al. In-hospital cardiopulmonary arrests in patients with left ventricular assist devices. *J Card Fail.* 2014;20:899-904.
14. Bellavia D, Iacovoni A, Scardulla C, et al. Prediction of right ventricular failure after ventricular assist device implant: systematic review and meta-analysis of observational studies. *Eur J Heart Fail.* 2017;19:926-946.
15. Scandroglio AM, Kaufmann F, Pieri M, et al. Diagnosis and treatment algorithm for blood flow obstructions in patients with left ventricular assist device. *J Am Coll Cardiol.* 2016;67:2758-2768.
16. Kim JH, Brophy DF, Shah KB. Continuous-flow left ventricular assist device-related gastrointestinal bleeding. *Cardiol Clin.* 2018;36:519-529.
17. Teuteberg JJ, Slaughter MS, Rogers JG, et al. The HVAD left ventricular assist device: risk factors for neurological events and risk mitigation strategies. *JACC Heart Fail.* 2015;3:818-828.
18. Acharya D, Loyaga-Rendon R, Morgan CJ, et al. INTERMACS analysis of stroke during support with continuous-flow left ventricular assist devices: risk factors and outcomes. *JACC Heart Fail.* 2017;5:703-711.
19. Kusne S, Mooney M, Danziger-Isakov L, et al. An ISHLT consensus document for prevention and management strategies for mechanical circulatory support infection. *J Heart Lung Transplant.* 2017;36:1137-1153.
20. Gordon RJ, Weinberg AD, Pagani FD, et al. Prospective, multicenter study of ventricular assist device infections. *Circulation.* 2013;127:691-702.
21. Topkara VK, Coromilas EJ, Garan AR, et al. Preoperative proteinuria and reduced glomerular filtration rate predicts renal replacement therapy in patients supported with continuous-flow left ventricular assist devices. *Circ Heart Fail.* 2016;9(12):e002897.
22. Walther CP, Winkelmayer WC, Niu J, et al. Acute kidney injury with ventricular assist device placement: national estimates of trends and outcomes. *Am J Kidney Dis.* 2019;74(5):650-658.
23. Roehm B, Vest AR, Weiner DE. Left ventricular assist devices, kidney disease, and dialysis. *Am J Kidney Dis.* 2018;71:257-266.
24. Guglielmi AA, Guglielmi KE, Bhat G, et al. Peritoneal dialysis after left ventricular assist device placement. *ASAIO J.* 2014;60:127-128.
25. Hanna RM, Cruz D, Selamet U, et al. Left ventricular assist device patient maintained on home hemodialysis: a novel class of patients to the home dialysis population. *Hemodial Int.* 2018;22:E36-E38.
26. Drew DA, Meyer KB, Weiner DE. Transvenous cardiac device wires and vascular access in hemodialysis patients. *Am J Kidney Dis.* 2011;58:494-496.
27. Schaefers JF, Ertmer C. Native arteriovenous fistula placement in three patients after implantation of a left ventricular assist device with non-pulsatile blood flow. *Hemodial Int.* 2017;21:E54-E57.
28. Chin AI, Tong K, McVicar JP. Successful hemodialysis arteriovenous fistula creation in a patient with continuous-flow left ventricular assist device support. *Am J Kidney Dis.* 2017;69:314-316.
29. Sasson T, Wing RE, Foster TH, et al. Assisted maturation of native fistula in two patients with a continuous flow left ventricular assist device. *J Vasc Interv Radiol.* 2014;25:781-783.
30. Nassif ME, Patel JS, Shuster JE, et al. Clinical outcomes with use of erythropoiesis stimulating agents in patients with the HeartMate II left ventricular assist device. *JACC Heart Fail.* 2015;3:146-153.
31. Schaefer JJ, Sajgalik P, Kushwaha SS, et al. Left ventricular assist device pulsatility index at the time of implantation is associated with follow-up pulmonary hemodynamics. *Int J Artif Organs.* 2020;43(7):452-460.
32. Uriel N, Morrison KA, Garan AR, et al. Development of a novel echocardiography ramp test for speed optimization and diagnosis of device thrombosis in continuous-flow left ventricular assist devices: the Columbia ramp study. *J Am Coll Cardiol.* 2012;60:1764-1775.

What was the initial experience of using LVADs in patients as a bridge to transplantation?

Case Control Study

			 Median age	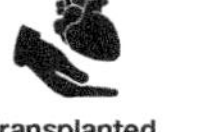 Cause of cardiomyopathy	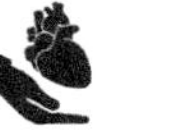 Median implant duration	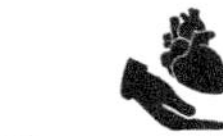 Transplanted	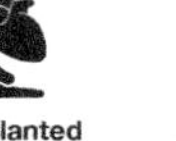 60 day mortality
August 1985 to February 1991	 HeartMate 1000 IP LVAD Candidate for heart transplant Meets hemodynamic criteria for LVAD + PCWP 20 mmHg + cardiac index 2L/min/m^2 OR systolic BP 80 mmHg Does not meet exclusion criteria	Met study criteria + Received an LVAD n = 26	46 IQR 39 - 49	Idopathic	37 IQR 10 - 114	74%	35%
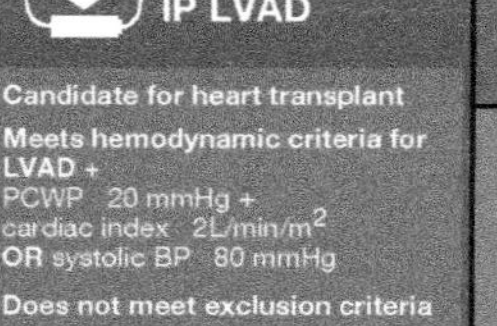		Did not meet study criteria + Received an LVAD n = 8	52.5 IQR 41 - 55	Idopathic + Ischemic	3 IQR 1 - 24	38%	88%
7 Medical Centers in USA	No LVAD	Met study criteria + Did not receive an LVAD n = 6	51 IQR 29 - 53	Ischemic	N/A	50%	83%

Conclusion: The HeartMate 1000 IP LVAD was shown to provide an effective means of supporting end-stage cardiomyopathy patients to transplantation.

Frazier OH, Rose EA, Macmanus Q, et al. ***Multicenter clinical evaluation of the HeartMate 1000 IP left ventricular assist device.*** Ann Thorac Surg. 1992;53(6):1080-90.

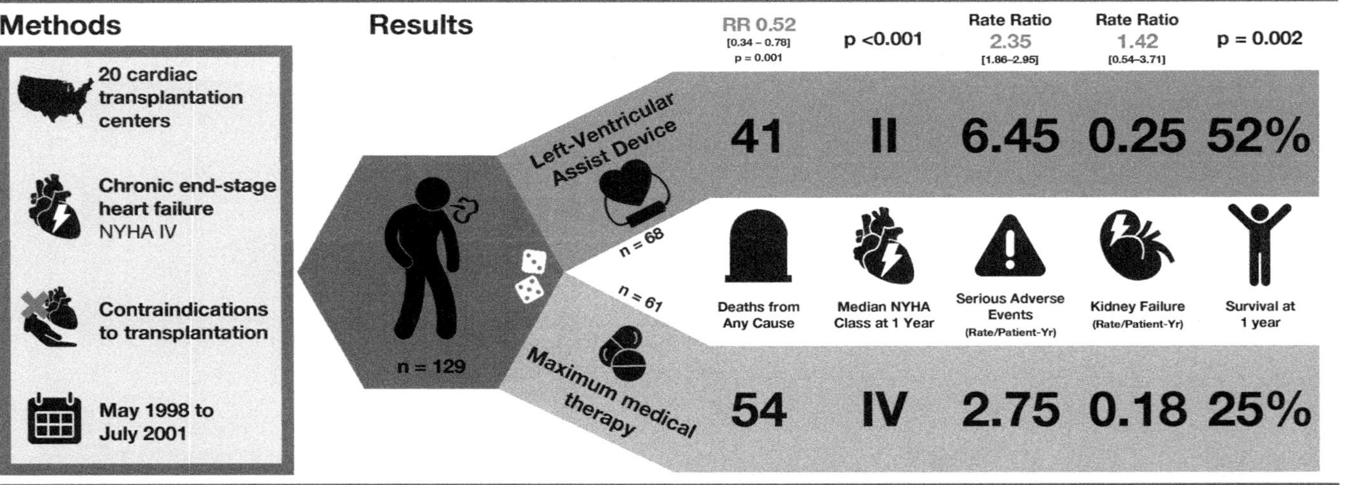

Conclusion: The use of a LVAD in patients with advanced heart failure resulted in a clinically meaningful survival benefit and an improved quality of life. A LVAD could be an alternative therapy in selected patients who are not candidates for cardiac transplantation.

Rose EA, Gelijns AC, Moskowitz AJ, et al. ***Long-term use of a left ventricular assist device for end-stage heart failure.*** N Engl J Med. 2001;345(20):1435-43.

VISUAL ABSTRACT 41.2

How does kidney function change after mechanical circulatory support device implantation?

Methods

INTERMACS Registry
Medicare and Medicaid Services –approved mechanical circulatory support implantation centers

Device implantation
Excluded total artificial heart or right ventricular support only

Creatinine measurements
at baseline and 1 month

June 2006 to March 2011

Results

n = 3363

Changes in eGFR post device insertion

	1 Month	3 Months	6 Months	1 Year
↑ ≥50%	39%	28%	21%	19%
↓ ≥25%	10%	28%	39%	41%
↓ ≥50%	3%	4%	7%	9%

Median improvement in eGFR at 1 year: **2.6** [IQR 10.1–17.2] mL/min/1.73 m^2

Late decline in eGFR: predominantly restricted to patients with early improvement in kidney function

Conclusion: Post mechanical circulatory support device implantation, most patients experience a substantial early improvement in kidney function, which is not sustained.

Brisco MA, Kimmel SE, Coca SG, et al. ***Prevalence and prognostic importance of changes in kidney function after mechanical circulatory support.*** Circ Heart Fail. 2014;7(1):68-75.

VISUAL ABSTRACT 41.3

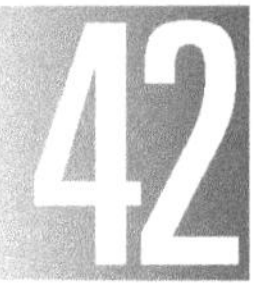

Acute Kidney Injury in Liver Disease

Yan Zhong, Claire Francoz, Francois Durand, and Mitra K. Nadim

INTRODUCTION

Acute kidney injury (AKI) is a common complication seen in cirrhotic patients, occurring in approximately 50% of hospitalized cirrhotic patients. In the setting of cirrhosis, vasoconstriction within the kidney along with changes in systemic circulation (hypotension) result in decreased blood flow to the kidneys and are central to the development of AKI. Early recognition and diagnosis of AKI etiology are crucial in identifying appropriate therapeutic measures.

PATHOPHYSIOLOGY

Current advances in our understanding of the pathophysiology of hepatorenal syndrome (HRS) suggest the involvement of systemic inflammation and intrarenal circulatory changes in parallel with systemic and splanchnic circulatory changes (**Figure 42.1**).[1,2] In decompensated cirrhosis, the increased cardiac output no longer meets the demand of systemic vasodilation effect, resulting in low effective volume and subsequent activation of renin-angiotensin-aldosterone system (RAAS), sympathetic nervous system (SNS), and vasopressin. As liver failure proceeds with unchecked systemic vasodilation, the potent vasoconstriction effect from RAAS, SNS, and vasopressin overrides the vasodilation effect of prostaglandins, causing circulatory failure within the kidney.

Alterations of gut permeability, a characteristic feature of portal hypertension, facilitate translocation of bacteria and bacterial products, which result in increased levels of circulating proinflammatory cytokines as well as increased levels of vasoactive factors. These inflammatory mediators may lead to further impairment of circulatory dysfunction, aggravating the development of HRS.[2]

ASSESSMENT OF KIDNEY FUNCTION

Serum creatinine (sCr) remains the basis of existing clinical definitions of AKI and is a key component in the Model for End-Stage Liver Disease (MELD) score. However, in patients with cirrhosis, sCr overestimates glomerular filtration rate (GFR) because of a combination of decreased creatine production by the liver, protein calorie malnutrition, muscle wasting, and large volume of distribution in the setting of fluid overload. Thus, sCr within the normal

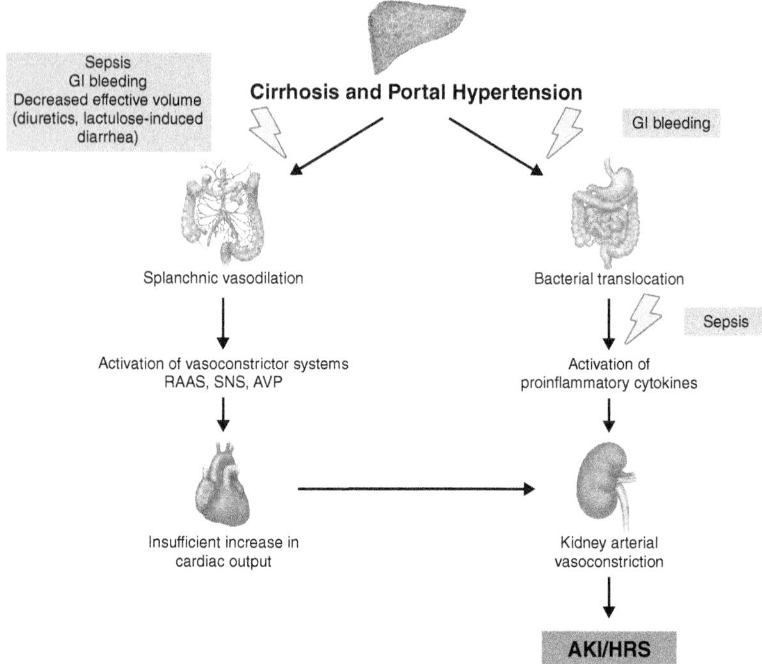

FIGURE 42.1: Mechanisms contributing to acute kidney injury (AKI) in decompensated cirrhosis. In decompensated cirrhosis several factors such as sepsis, gastrointestinal (GI) bleeding, hypovolemia from diuretics, and diarrhea result in decreased effective volume and profound splanchnic/systemic vasodilation, resulting in subsequent activation of renin-angiotensin-aldosterone system (RAAS), sympathetic nervous system (SNS), and arginine vasopressin (AVP). Together with insufficient increase in cardiac output, the potent vasoconstrictor systems cause circulatory failure within the kidneys leading to the development of hepatorenal syndrome (HRS). In addition, systemic inflammation induced by gut bacterial translocation results in activation of circulating proinflammatory cytokines as well as increased levels of vasoactive factors. These inflammatory mediators may lead to further impairment of circulatory dysfunction, aggravating the development of HRS.

range does not exclude kidney impairment. Cystatin C is less affected by age, gender, and muscle mass compared with sCr and appears to detect AKI earlier than sCr. However, it remains costly and not widely available. The clearance of inulin or radioisotopes is considered the gold standard for GFR assessment. Nevertheless, they are not routinely used in clinical practice and have not been rigorously studied in patients with advanced cirrhosis and ascites. When properly performed, timed urinary collection of creatinine and urea overcomes some of these limitations. However, these are subject to inaccurate or incomplete collection, primarily because of increased tubular secretion of creatinine as GFR declines.

In patients with cirrhosis, the precision of all estimated GFR (eGFR) equations is poor and tends to overestimate true GFR, especially in patients with GFR less than 40 mL/min. Modified Diet in Renal Disease 6 (MDRD-6) equation has been shown to be the most accurate creatinine-based equation in cirrhosis.[3]

More recently, however, in a single-center study of over 10,000 iothalamate samples, GRAIL equation (glomerular filtration rate assessment in liver disease; www.bswh.md/grail) demonstrated more precision and less bias compared with MDRD-6 equation in patients with low GFR and correctly classified 75% of the cohort as having a measured GFR less than 30 mL/min/1.73 m^2 versus 52.8% in MDRD-6 ($p < 0.01$).[4]

DEFINITION OF ACUTE KIDNEY INJURY AND HEPATORENAL SYNDROME

In 2010, the Acute Disease Quality Initiative (ADQI) proposed a new definition for AKI in patients with cirrhosis, which was based on the Acute Kidney Injury Network (AKIN) criteria.[5] In 2015, the International Club of Ascites (ICA) revised the definition of AKI on the basis of the Kidney Disease Improving Global Outcomes (KDIGO) sCr criteria alone and included changes to the definition of baseline sCr and HRS.[6] According to the ICA criteria, the most recent sCr value within the past 3 months should be considered as baseline sCr. As a result of the change in definition of AKI, the definition of HRS was also modified and, instead of the traditional definition of using a fixed sCr cutoff value greater than 1.5 mg/dL, it is defined on the basis of KDIGO definition of AKI for sCr. Other criteria for HRS, which is unchanged from previous criteria, include (a) no response after 2 consecutive days of diuretic withdrawal and plasma volume expansion with albumin, (b) absence of shock, (c) no current or recent use of nephrotoxic drugs, (d) no signs of structural kidney injury as indicated by proteinuria (>500 mg/d), microhematuria (>50 red blood cells per high-power field), and/or abnormal kidney ultrasonography. In addition, the acute form of HRS, previously HRS-1, has been renamed AKI-HRS and the more chronic form, previously HRS-2, has been renamed chronic kidney disease (CKD)-HRS. Although oliguria was not included in the current definition of AKI in patients with liver disease, urine output has been found to be a sensitive and early marker for AKI and to be associated with adverse outcomes in critically ill patients.[7] A recent international consensus meeting on the management of critically ill cirrhotic patients has recommended that regardless of any rise in sCr, oliguria (urine output <400 mL/24 hr) should be considered as AKI in patients with cirrhosis until proven otherwise.[8]

ETIOLOGY OF KIDNEY DYSFUNCTION

The most common causes of AKI in hospitalized patients are prerenal azotemia (majority because of hypovolemia-induced AKI and only one-third because of HRS), followed by acute tubular necrosis (ATN). The cause of AKI is generally distinguished by the preceding history as well as urinalysis and response to diuretic withdrawal and volume challenge. A trial of volume expansion should be initiated, both as a potential therapeutic measure and as a diagnostic tool (in differentiating HRS-AKI from other forms of prerenal azotemia). Fluid choices include blood (in cases of GIB), isotonic crystalloid (in cases of diarrhea or overdiuresis), and albumin (in cases of HRS, SBP, or unknown precipitant) (**Figure 42.2**). However, these criteria may be misleading in certain circumstances such as presence of CKD or recent diuretic use. Recent studies have suggested the use of urine biomarkers, in addition to urine microalbuminuria or fractional excretion of sodium, to enable differentiation

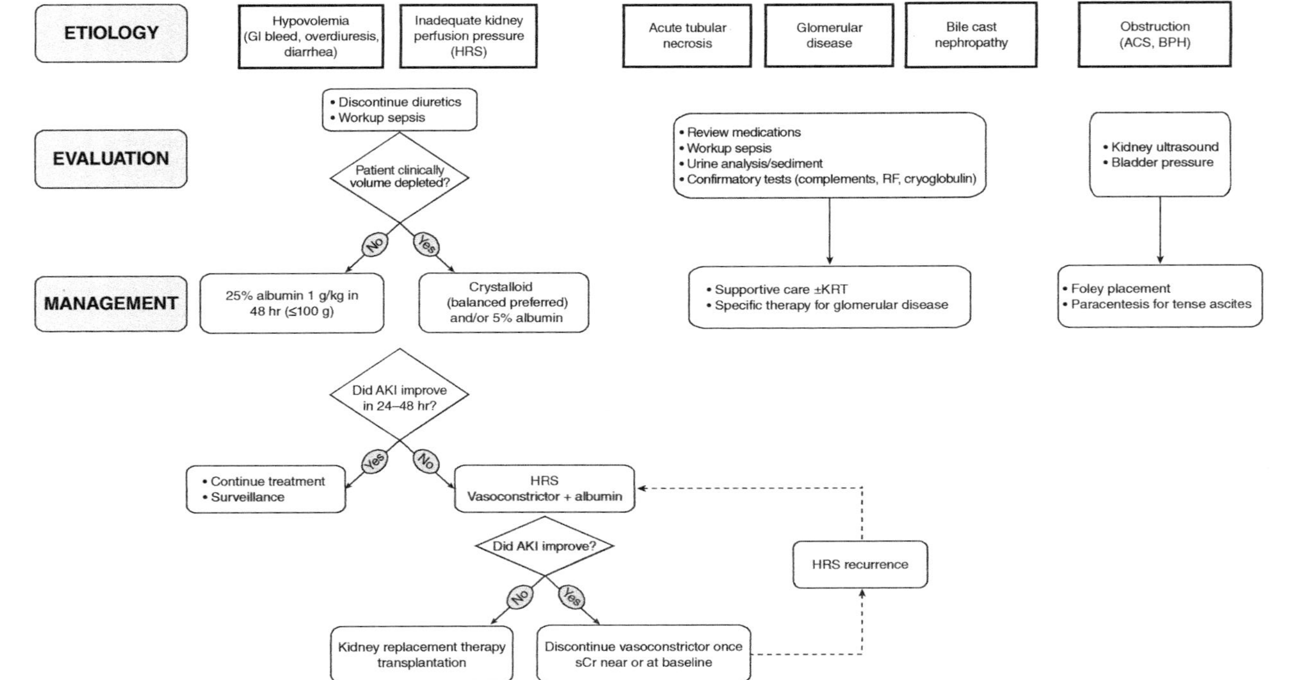

FIGURE 42.2: Algorithm for evaluation and management of acute kidney injury (AKI). ACS, acute coronary syndrome; BPH, benign prostatic hyperplasia; GI, gastrointestinal; HRS, hepatorenal syndrome; RF, kidney failure; KRT, kidney replacement therapy; sCr, serum creatinine.

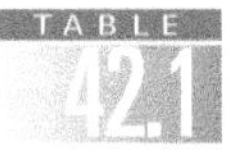

Renal Conditions Associated With Liver Disease

Liver Disease	Renal Condition
Hepatitis C	MPGN; membranous nephropathy; cryoglobulinemia; tubulointerstitial nephritis; fibrillary GN; IgA nephropathy
Hepatitis B	Membranous nephropathy; FSGS; MPGN; polyarteritis nodosa; IgA nephropathy
Alcoholic cirrhosis	IgA nephropathy
Primary biliary cirrhosis	Distal RTA; tubulointerstitial nephritis; ANCA positive vasculitis; anti-GBM disease; membranous nephropathy; microscopic polyangiitis
Primary sclerosing cholangitis	Membranous nephropathy; MPGN; ANCA positive vasculitis
Nonalcoholic steatohepatitis (NASH)	Diabetic nephropathy
Autoimmune hepatitis	Immune complex GN; RTA
Hyperbilirubinemia	Bile cast nephropathy

ANCA, antineutrophil cytoplasmic antibody; FSGS, focal-segmental glomerulosclerosis; GBM, glomerular basement membrane; GN, glomerulonephritis; IgA, immunoglobulin A; MPGN, membranoproliferative glomerulonephritis; PCKD, polycystic kidney disease; RTA, renal tubular acidosis.

between HRS versus ATN.[9,10] However, in all these studies, the diagnosis of ATN was based on nonspecific criteria without a gold standard (biopsy) and therefore should be interpreted with caution. In addition to the above-mentioned causes of AKI, patients with liver disease may present with a variety of specific conditions affecting the kidneys that should be considered when evaluating patients with AKI (**Table 42.1**).

PREVENTION OF ACUTE KIDNEY INJURY

It is important to identify and remove potential precipitating agents in the development of AKI/HRS and to prevent factors that further impair circulatory status and reduce kidney perfusion. Cautious use of diuretics, albumin infusion during large-volume paracentesis (6-8 g/L of ascitic fluid removed over 5 L), antibiotic prophylaxis following GI bleeding, early administration of broad-spectrum antibiotics have all been shown to reduce the incidence of HRS. Long-term administration of albumin in patients with decompensated cirrhosis has been shown in a large randomized controlled trial to be associated with reduced rates of spontaneous bacterial peritonitis (SBP), bacterial infections other than SBP, HRS-1, kidney dysfunction as defined by sCr greater than 1.5 mg/dL, and improved survival.[11]

TREATMENT OF ACUTE KIDNEY INJURY

Volume expansion is crucial not only in the treatment but also in the differential diagnosis of etiology of AKI. The type of fluid needed for resuscitation should be tailored on the basis of the cause of AKI and volume status of the patient (Figure 42.2). It is imperative to exercise caution when administrating fluids in cirrhotic patients with AKI to avoid development of fluid overload and pulmonary edema.

Pharmacologic Therapy

Once a diagnosis of HRS is made, the goal of medical therapy is to improve systemic hemodynamics with vasoconstrictors and restore effective circulatory volume with albumin (**Table 42.2**). It is recommended to use concentrated albumin 1 g/kg with a maximum of 100 g initially followed by doses of 20 to 40 g/d. Choice of vasoconstrictors is guided by location of hospitalized patients (ICU vs general ward) and availability because terlipressin is currently not available in many countries, including the United States. Several randomized controlled trials have shown that the combination of terlipressin and albumin (given at an initial dose of 1 g/kg of 20%-25% albumin, followed by daily doses of 20-50 g) was more effective than albumin alone in HRS reversal (**Visual Abstract 42.1** and **42.2**). For critically ill patients and those in the ICU, combination treatment with norepinephrine (goal 10-15 mm Hg increase in mean arterial pressure) and albumin may be used. However, no significant difference has been noted comparing terlipressin with noradrenaline.[12] For patients on the ward, especially in countries where terlipressin is not available, a combination of midodrine 7.5 to 12.5 mg orally thrice daily (an orally administered alpha-adrenergic agonist) and octreotide 100 to 200 μg subcutaneously thrice daily (a long-acting somatostatin analog) may be used to reduce portal hypertension and splanchnic vasoconstriction. Predictors of response include increase in mean arterial pressure of greater than 5 mm Hg, initiation of vasoconstrictors when sCr is less than 5 mg/dL, and serum bilirubin less than 10 mg/dL. Treatment with vasoconstrictors should be discontinued if there is no improvement in sCr after 5 to 7 days, in patients initiated on kidney replacement therapy (KRT), or in those who exhibit side effects.

Time-Limited Trial of Kidney Replacement Therapy

Initiation of KRT in patients who are not transplant candidates, especially those with HRS, has been controversial. However, the severity of illness and number of organ failure in patients with acute on chronic liver failure have been shown to be more predictive of mortality than etiology of AKI.[13,14] As such, the authors believe that a trial of KRT in selected patients should be considered regardless of transplant candidacy or etiology of AKI. The initiation of KRT should be made on clinical grounds (**Table 42.3**) and should be considered in the broader clinical context, for therapeutic and/or supportive treatment of "non-kidney" indications, before overt complications from AKI have developed, and the threshold for initiation should be lowered when AKI occurs as part of multiorgan failure.[8,15] Continuous KRT should be preferred to other modalities in patients with severe hemodynamic instability.

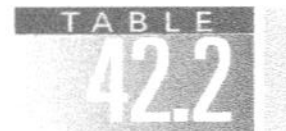

TABLE 42.2 Vasoconstrictors for the Treatment of Hepatorenal Syndrome

Drug	Mechanism of Action	Dose	Comments
Terlipressin	Vasopressin analog	1 mg every 4-6 hr either as IV bolus or through continuous IV infusion. Dose can be increased to 2 mg IV every 4-6 hr after 48 hr if sCr has not decreased by >25% from baseline up to a maximum of 12 mg/d as long as there are no side effects. Maximal treatment 14 d	Not available in the United States In countries where terlipressin is not available, the combination of octreotide/midodrine can be initiated, and if there is no decline in sCr within a maximum of 3 d then the patient should be transferred to the ICU for a trial of noradrenaline. Contraindicated in patients with preexisting ischemic heart disease, cerebrovascular disease, peripheral arterial disease, hypertension, or asthma
Noradrenaline	Alpha-adrenergic agonist	0.5-3.0 mg/hr (continuous infusion). Titrate to achieve a 15 mm Hg increase in MAP.	Requires ICU
Midodrine + octreotide	Alpha-adrenergic agonist (midodrine) Somatostatin analog (octreotide)	7.5 mg orally TID with an increase to 12.5-15 mg TID as needed to increase MAP by 15 mm Hg Octreotide SQ 100 μg TID, titrated to 200 μg TID on day 2, if kidney function has not improved	

ICU, intensive care unit; IV, intravenous; MAP, mean arterial pressure; sCr, serum creatinine; SQ, subcutaneous; TID, three times daily.

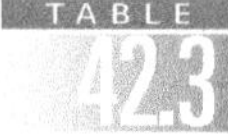

TABLE 42.3 Considerations for Initiation of Kidney Replacement Therapy in Patients With Liver Disease

- Acute kidney injury
- Fluid overload with or without pulmonary edema with failure to achieve negative fluid balance
- Patients at risk of developing fluid overload (e.g., need for massive blood products, TPN, high-volume antibiotics)
- Severe/life-threatening electrolyte and acid-base abnormalities
- Diuretic resistant/intolerant
- Uremic complications—pericarditis, bleeding, pericardial effusion, encephalopathy
- Hyperammonemia (>100-120 mmol/L) with or without hepatic encephalopathy in setting of fulminant liver failure

TPN, total parenteral nutrition.

References

1. Durand F, Graupera I, Gines P, et al. Pathogenesis of hepatorenal syndrome: implications for therapy. *Am J Kidney Dis.* 2016;67:318-328.
2. Gines P, Sola E, Angeli P, et al. Hepatorenal syndrome. *Nat Rev Dis Primers.* 2018;4:23.
3. Francoz C, Nadim MK, Baron A, et al. Glomerular filtration rate equations for liver-kidney transplantation in patients with cirrhosis: validation of current recommendations. *Hepatology.* 2014;59:1514-1521.
4. Asrani SK, Jennings LW, Trotter JF, et al. A model for glomerular filtration rate assessment in liver disease (GRAIL) in the presence of renal dysfunction. *Hepatology.* 2019;69:1219-1230.
5. Nadim MK, Kellum JA, Davenport A, et al. Hepatorenal syndrome: the 8th International Consensus Conference of the Acute Dialysis Quality Initiative (ADQI) group. *Crit Care.* 2012;16:R23.
6. Angeli P, Gines P, Wong F, et al. Diagnosis and management of acute kidney injury in patients with cirrhosis: revised consensus recommendations of the International Club of Ascites. *J Hepatol.* 2015;62:968-974.
7. Amathieu R, Al-Khafaji A, Sileanu FE, et al. Significance of oliguria in critically ill patients with chronic liver disease. *Hepatology.* 2017;66:1592-1600.
8. Nadim MK, Durand F, Kellum JA, et al. Management of the critically ill patient with cirrhosis: a multidisciplinary perspective. *J Hepatol.* 2016;64:717-735.
9. Francoz C, Nadim MK, Durand F. Kidney biomarkers in cirrhosis. *J Hepatol.* 2016;65:809-824.
10. Huelin P, Sola E, Elia C, et al. Neutrophil gelatinase-associated lipocalin for assessment of acute kidney injury in cirrhosis. A prospective study. *Hepatology.* 2019;70:319-333.
11. Caraceni P, Riggio O, Angeli P, et al. Long-term albumin administration in decompensated cirrhosis (ANSWER): an open-label randomised trial. *Lancet.* 2018;391:2417-2429.
12. Best LM, Freeman SC, Sutton AJ, et al. Treatment for hepatorenal syndrome in people with decompensated liver cirrhosis: a network meta-analysis. *Cochrane Database Syst Rev.* 2019;9:CD013103.
13. Allegretti AS, Parada XV, Eneanya ND, et al. Prognosis of patients with cirrhosis and AKI who initiate RRT. *Clin J Am Soc Nephrol.* 2018;13:16-25.
14. Angeli P, Rodriguez E, Piano S, et al. Acute kidney injury and acute-on-chronic liver failure classifications in prognosis assessment of patients with acute decompensation of cirrhosis. *Gut.* 2015;64:1616-1622.
15. Rosner MH, Ostermann M, Murugan R, et al. Indications and management of mechanical fluid removal in critical illness. *Br J Anaesth.* 2014;113:764-771.

Can terlipressin with albumin REVERSE type 1 hepatorenal syndrome?

Randomized Controlled Trial

2221 Screened

North America
50 sites in USA,
2 in Canada

Adult patients
≥ 18 years

Cirrhosis and
ascites

October 2010 to
February 2013

Hepatorenal
Syndrome
Type 1
2007 International
Club of Ascites
Criteria

196

Terlipressin + Albumin

Terlipressin
1 mg every 6 hours
+ albumin
(20 – 40g/day)

97

99

Placebo
every 6 hours
+ albumin
(20 – 40g/day)

Placebo + Albumin

Results

	Confirmed Hepatorenal Syndrome reversal	Median transplant-free survival (days)	Survival rate at 90 days	Kidney replacement therapy use at day 90
	p = 0.22	NS	p = 0.60	
Terlipressin + Albumin	20%	23.8	58%	37%
Placebo + Albumin	13%	20.7	55%	42%

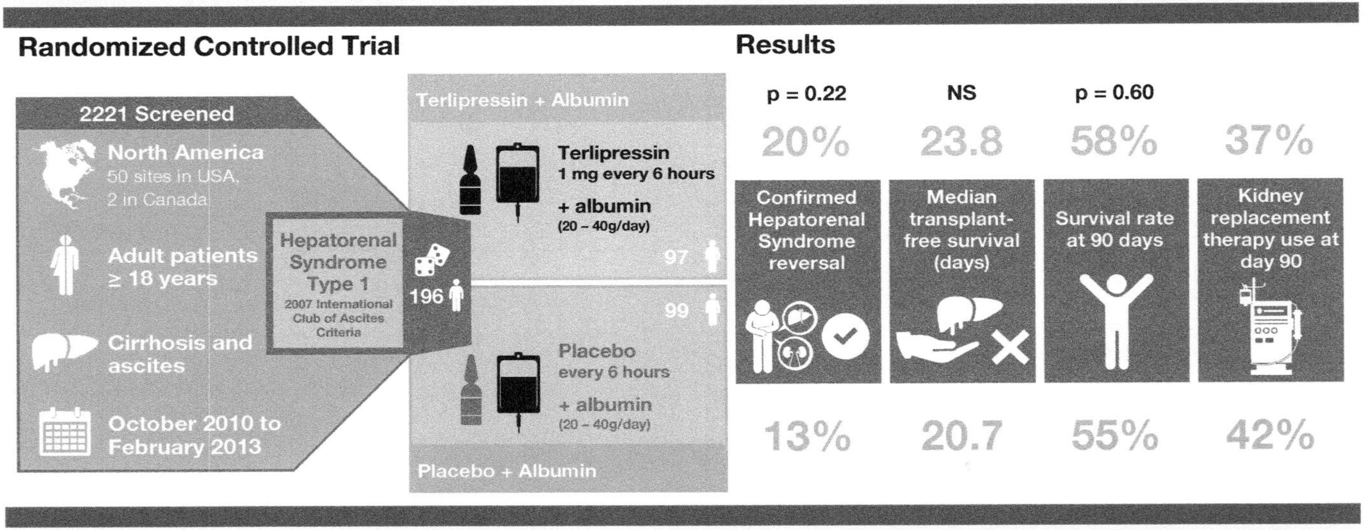

Conclusion: In this controlled trial of HRS-1 patients comparing terlipressin with placebo, there was no statistically significant difference in numbers achieving confirmed reversal of hepatorenal syndrome.

Boyer TD, Sanyal AJ, Wong F, et al. ***Terlipressin Plus Albumin Is More Effective Than Albumin Alone in Improving Kidney Function in Patients With Cirrhosis and Hepatorenal Syndrome Type 1.*** Gastroenterology. 2016;150(7):1579-1589.e2.

VISUAL ABSTRACT 42.1

Does terlipressin result in resolution of hepatorenal syndrome at day 14?

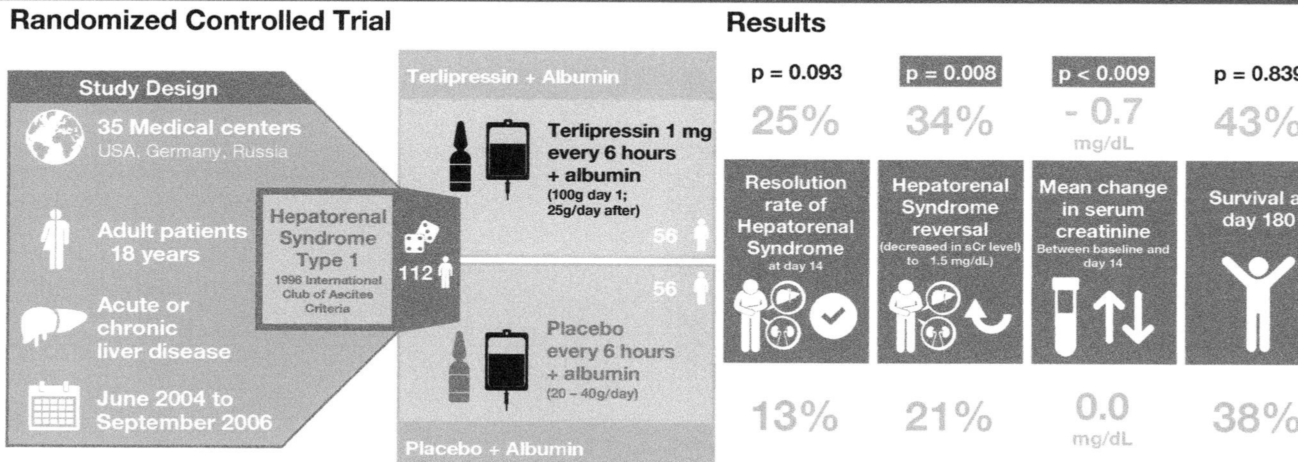

Conclusion: In a trial of terlipressin versus placebo in patients with hepatorenal syndrome, terlipressin-treated patients had significant improvements in kidney function without significant resolution rates of hepatorenal syndrome.

Sanyal AJ, Boyer T, Garcia-tsao G, et al. ***A randomized, prospective, double-blind, placebo-controlled trial of terlipressin for type 1 hepatorenal syndrome.*** Gastroenterology. 2008; 134(5):1360-8.

VISUAL ABSTRACT 42.2

43

Abdominal Compartment Syndrome

Anis Abdul Rauf, Joel M. Topf, and
Emily Temple-Woods

INTRODUCTION AND DEFINITIONS

Abdominal compartment syndrome is characterized by elevated pressure in the abdomen with consequent end-organ damage and is an important cause of morbidity and mortality in patients with intra-abdominal pathology and trauma. Kidney failure is characteristic of the syndrome along with cardiovascular collapse.[5]

The World Society of the Abdominal Compartment Syndrome (WSACS) has established consensus definitions of intra-abdominal pressure (IAP), intra-abdominal hypertension (IAH), and abdominal compartment syndrome (ACS).[1]

Measurement of IAP is performed using an intravesical pressure catheter.[1] IAP measurements are affected by patient positioning, respiratory cycle, and abdominal muscle contractions; therefore, IAP must be measured in the midaxillary line when the patient is supine, at end-expiration, without abdominal muscle contractions.[1-3]

In the normal state, IAP averages 5 to 7 mm Hg, rising to 10 mm Hg in the critically ill.[1,4] IAH is defined as sustained or repeated pressures of more than 12 mm Hg, and ACS occurs when IAP exceeds 20 mm Hg and there is a concomitant organ failure (e.g., new acute kidney injury [AKI]). The abdominal perfusion pressure (APP) is equal to the mean arterial pressure (MAP) minus the IAP; an APP less than 60 mm Hg is not necessary to diagnose ACS but is a supporting finding.[1]

In critically ill adult patients, IAH is associated with increased morbidity and mortality because of subsequent multiple organ failure, particularly cardiovascular collapse and AKI.[5] In a meta-analysis of 1,669 patients from 19 distinct centers, Malbrain and colleagues demonstrated that IAH is an independent predictor of mortality in critical illness (relative risk [RR] = 1.85; 95% confidence interval [CI]: 1.12-3.0; $p = 0.01$).[6] The earliest manifestation of IAH is AKI.[5,7]

ETIOLOGY AND PATHOPHYSIOLOGY

The causes of IAH and subsequent ACS are categorized by the underlying pathophysiology:

1. Diminished compliance of the abdominal compartment;
2. Increased intra-abdominal or intraluminal contents;
3. Third-spacing or other body water imbalances;
4. Increased thoracic pressure.[1]

The abdomen can be thought of as a simple compartment with partially compliant borders at the diaphragm and anterior abdominal wall. Any condition that decreases the compliance of the diaphragm or the anterior abdominal wall will increase IAH.[8] As volume in the abdomen begins to increase, the abdominal wall begins to compensate by stretching, ultimately changing the shape of the abdomen in the coronal section from an oval to a circle. Once the rectus abdominis and its attendant fascia are maximally stretched, further increase in the abdominal volume leads to rapid increase in IAP.[4]

The most common cause of IAH and ACS is abdominal adipose tissue and severe edema. Abdominal fat (visceral or subcutaneous) and edema cause the compartment to assume a circular coronal section even at normal IAPs, allowing a brisk progression from normal IAP to frank ACS. Eschars and adhesions decrease overall compliance by preventing the compartment from changing shape in response to increased intracompartmental volume. Similarly, diaphragmatic flattening secondary to chronic obstructive pulmonary disease (COPD) decreases the cephalad compliance of the compartment.[4]

The thoracic compartment and abdominal compartment are separated by the diaphragm, and increases in IAP will decrease the thoracic compliance and increased thoracic pressure will decrease abdominal compliance. Many critically ill patients have increased thoracic pressure because of ventilatory demands. Risk factors for the transmission of high thoracic pressure to the abdominal compartment include use of positive pressure ventilation, high positive end-expiratory pressure (PEEP), auto-PEEP, and elevation of the head of the bed by more than 30 degrees.[9,10]

At the vascular level, IAH is characterized by an initial compression of microvasculature, largely affecting the capillaries. As pressure builds up in the capillary beds, venous flow is impaired and arterial flow decreases. As IAP rises, the inferior vena cava (IVC) is compressed in the abdomen, resulting in further venous congestion. The transmission of pressure from the abdominal compartment to the thoracic compartment via the diaphragm also causes direct compression on the heart, causing tamponade-equivalent physiology (impaired filling and decreased contractility). All of these mechanisms result in visceral ischemia. Furthermore, venous congestion in both the splanchnic and portal circulation leads to edema and increases intra-abdominal volume, further increasing IAH in a positive feedback loop.[5]

Risk Factors

Table 43.1 demonstrates several established risk factors for the development of ACS.

DIAGNOSIS

The diagnosis of IAH and ACS depend on consistent and timely measurement of IAP, not physical exam or lab findings.[1,15] IAH and ACS do not have any consistent physical signs or lab abnormalities beyond those derangements that typically indicate end-organ damage. Furthermore, WSACS recommends serial measurement of IAP (every 4 hours) in patients at risk and in those who have an elevated IAP.[1] Measurement of femoral venous pressure (FVP) is not an adequate substitute for intravesical measurement of IAP, but FVP or intragastric manometry can be used as an estimate when intravesical measurement is contraindicated.[8,16]

Signs of IAH and ACS are manifestations of end-organ failure. In critically ill patients, with multiple etiologies of organ damage, other pathophysiologic processes may obscure signs of ACS.

TABLE 43.1 Risk Factors for the Development of ACS

History	Comorbidities	Treatment	Surgical	Ventilator
Age[7]	Obesity[11]	Early or high-volume crystalloid administration[8]	Eschar[8]	Prone positioning[12,a]
Intra-abdominal adhesions[8]	ARDS[5]	Shock[8]	Laparotomy on day of admission[10,11]	PEEP >10 cm H_2O[10]
Cirrhosis, ascites[11]	Acute pancreatitis[13,b]	Ileus[8]	ECMO or bypass[14,c]	PaO_2/FiO_2 <300[11]
	Abdominal trauma[8]	Need for pressors or inotropes		
	Severe burns[8]			
	GI bleed[8]			
	Ruptured AAA[8]			

AAA, abdominal aortic aneurysm; ACS, abdominal compartment syndrome; ARDS, acute respiratory distress syndrome; ECMO, extracorporeal membrane oxygenation; GI, gastrointestinal; IAP, intra-abdominal pressure; PEEP, positive end-expiratory pressure.

[a]Proning causes increased IAP, but there is no evidence for clinical significance in the setting of ACS.

[b]Independent risk factors for the development of ACS in the setting of acute pancreatitis include positive fluid balance in the first 24 hours of treatment, derangements in serum calcium, and multiple intra-abdominal fluid collections.[13]

[c]In cardiac surgery patients.[14]

PREVENTION

In a patient with IAH who has not yet progressed to ACS, early intervention to reduce IAP and thereby optimize perfusion to the abdominal viscera is essential. Monitoring and minimizing fluid excess can help prevent increases in IAP. WSACS recommends a goal IAP of less than 15 mm Hg.[1] APP may be a superior predictor of survival and surgical intervention than IAP.[5,17]

Fluid Balance

Avoiding excessive resuscitation and hewing to goal-directed fluid resuscitation principles can prevent fluid-based iatrogenic ACS.[1,8] Increased IAP causes IVC compression, mimicking the appearance of hypovolemia. Similarly, decreased thoracic compliance will cause an increase in pulse pressure variation (PPV), which could be mistaken for fluid-responsive hypotension. Therefore, in cases where there is known IAH, PPV and IVC diameter are not reliable indicators of hemodynamic status and can be misinterpreted, leading to fluid overload.[8]

Zero to negative fluid balance by day 3 of admission with the use of hypertonic fluids and colloids in cases where fluid resuscitation is indicated may prevent the development or worsening of IAH.[1] In service of maintaining a zero to negative fluid balance, judicious diuresis or hemodialysis with high ultrafiltrate is also recommended.[1,8]

Abdominal Wall Compliance

Increasing the compliance of the abdominal wall can lower IAH. High abdominal muscle tone, which may be due to pain and anxiety, can increased IAP. Therefore, relief of symptoms, including sedation and neuromuscular blockade, can substantially increase abdominal wall compliance.[1,8]

Body positioning can also contribute to IAH, particularly elevating the head of the bed over 30 degrees and prolonged hip flexion. Abdominal binders are associated with increased IAP and are contraindicated in IAH.[1,4,8] In the setting of postoperative IAH, an escharotomy to increase wall compliance may be indicated.[1]

Use of the Open Abdomen

Prophylactic use of the open abdomen may be indicated in trauma patients or postoperative patients with ACS. This may be needed in those with extreme intraoperative visceral or retroperitoneal swelling. In these cases, negative wound pressure systems can be used for temporary closure, but these patients require multiple repeat procedures every 48 hours.[8] The prophylactic open abdomen is contraindicated in septic patients.

Enteral and Intraperitoneal Volume

Acutely increased enteral volume is a risk factor for developing IAH and ACS. Depending on whether the increased volume is in the upper or lower gastrointestinal (GI) tract, mechanical decompressive treatment or use of prokinetic drugs may be useful.[8]

Nasogastric (NG) tubes are appropriate when other indications are present; there is no evidence for the efficacy of upper GI decompression as prophylaxis for IAH.[1,4,18] Enemas and rectal tubes can be used to decompress the lower GI tract.[1,5] Minimizing or discontinuing enteral feeding is also appropriate.[5] Colonoscopic decompression can be used in cases of Ogilvie syndrome or pseudo-obstruction; it is also useful when prokinetic agents have failed to produce substantial enteral decompression.[1,4]

Neostigmine is a potentially appropriate agent for the treatment of colonic ileus in the setting of IAH.[19] Other prokinetic agents include cisapride, metoclopramide, and erythromycin.[1,4] Paracentesis is not superior to decompressive laparotomy; however, removal of space-occupying lesions in the abdomen (e.g., hematoma over 1 L in volume) can be therapeutic.[1,4,8]

Ventilator Management

Because intrathoracic pressures are transmitted via the diaphragm to the abdominal compartment, appropriate management of airway pressures can be an important adjunct to preventing ACS. Notably, though the presence of PEEP in mechanically ventilated patients will increase IAP, it is not clear at what point this becomes clinically relevant.[8]

NATURAL HISTORY AND SEQUELAE

Left untreated, the natural history of ACS tends toward unavoidable death. Even when promptly and appropriately treated, IAH has a number of clinical sequelae, all of which can be characterized as different forms of end-organ damage.

Gastrointestinal and Hepatobiliary

Compression of the enteric lumen occurs relatively early on in the development of IAH provided that the ultimate cause of elevated IAP is not increased enteric volume. Edema of the bowel wall occurs as a sequela of ischemia because of splanchnic vascular resistance or positive fluid balance. The liver is similarly affected, with direct compression and vascular compression causing ischemia.[5,8]

Kidney

The etiology of AKI with ACS is multifactorial. Increased high pressure in the renal veins impedes glomerular blood flow and activates the renin-angiotensin-aldosterone system, causing vasoconstriction. Increased IAP is transmitted to the renal parenchyma and tubules, further damaging the kidneys.[5,8]

Respiratory

As IAP increases, the pressure is transmitted to the thoracic compartment, reducing pulmonary compliance by approximately 50% and increasing plateau, peak, and mean airway pressures, reducing tidal volume. It also causes a loss of functional residual capacity by direct compression of the lung parenchyma. The sum of these effects is a significant ventilation-perfusion mismatch.[5,8]

Cardiovascular

The increased pulmonary pressures of ACS increase right ventricular afterload and decreases pulmonary venous return, impairing cardiac output. Compression of the IVC decreases preload, further decreasing cardiac output.[8] Compression of the IVC causes high pressures in the lower extremity venous system and increased arterial resistance, reducing blood flow to the lower extremities.[8]

Neurologic

Increases in IAP are associated with increased intracranial pressure (ICP) and a concomitant decrease in cerebral perfusion pressure (CPP).[20] This is thought to be the result of caval compression causing high pressures in the jugular vein and therefore cerebral vascular congestion.[8]

TREATMENT

Cases of primary ACS—that is, those caused by a primary abdominopelvic pathology—may occur despite the clinician's best efforts at prevention. In these cases, the WSACS recommends urgent decompressive laparotomy with delayed closure and negative pressure wound care system placement rather than conservative measures.[1] The treatment of ACS is decompressive laparotomy.[8] A protocol for dealing with increased IAP and steps for medical management are described in **Figures 43.1** and **43.2**.

In cases where surgical management is not possible, medical measures of prevention may also be employed toward treatment. In these cases, APP is the most appropriate indicator of resuscitative success, superior to MAP or IAP alone, arterial pH, base deficit, lactic acid, and urinary output. Cheatham et al., performed multivariate regression analysis of APP as an endpoint in a prospective study of 149 surgical intensive care unit (SICU) and trauma patients and found it to be superior to these other resuscitative endpoints for predicting survival in patients with IAH ($p = 0.002$).[17] The importance of APP as a treatment target opens up the viability of increasing MAP through the use of pressors to temporarily manage ACS. Some experts suggest targeting an MAP of 60 mm Hg + IAP.[21]

When choosing to manage ACS with decompressive laparotomy or paracentesis, there is a possibility of hypotension and cardiovascular collapse because of the sudden decrease in abdominal pressure. This occurs because of the sudden drop in systemic vascular resistance (SVR) and the critically ill patient's inability to compensate appropriately. An element of reperfusion injury is also hypothesized to be contributory in any decompressive mode of treatment or resuscitation in these patients.[8]

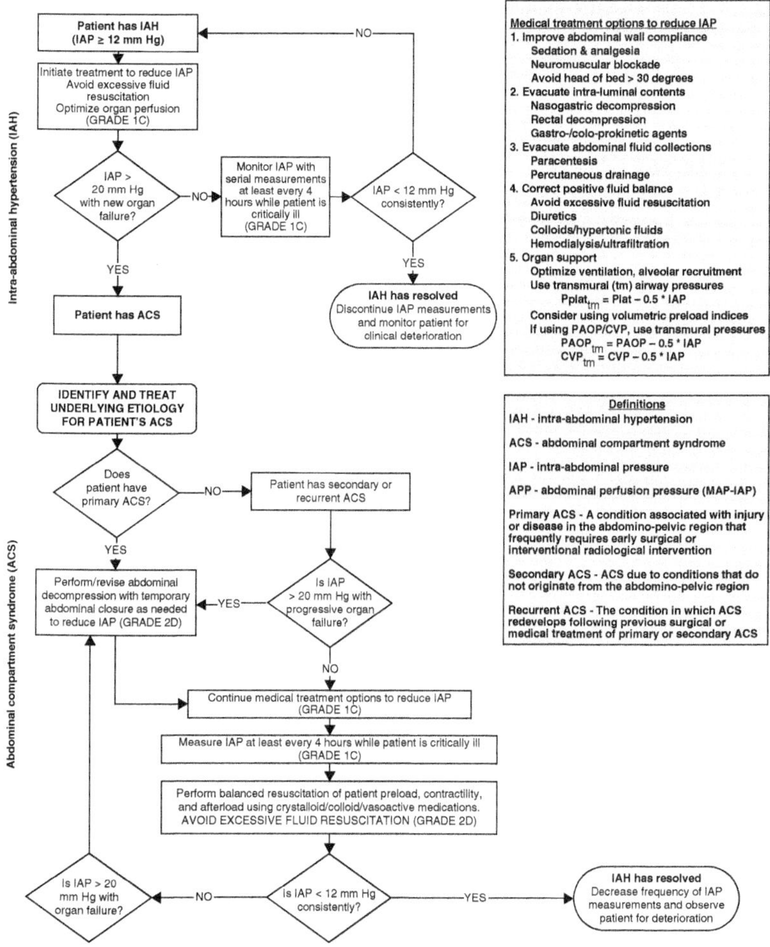

FIGURE 43.1: IAH/ACS management algorithm.

Adapted from Kirkpatrick AW, Roberts DJ, De Waele J, et al. Intra-abdominal hypertension and the abdominal compartment syndrome: updated consensus definitions and clinical practice guidelines from the World Society of the Abdominal Compartment Syndrome. *Intensive Care Med.* 2013;39(7):1190-1206. doi:10.1007/s00134-013-2906-z.

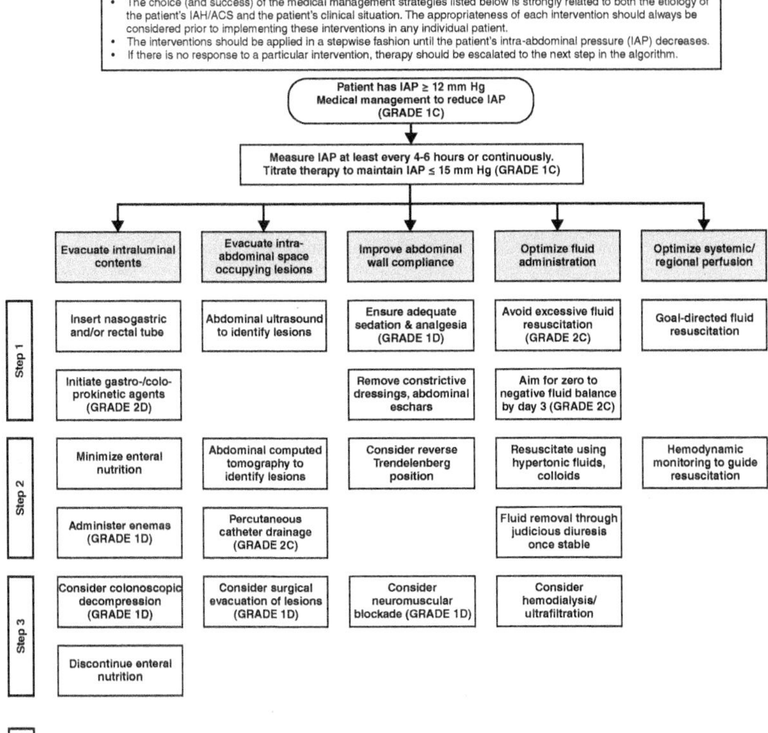

FIGURE 43.2: IAH/ACS medical management algorithm. ACS, abdominal compartment syndrome; IAH, intra-abdominal hypertension.

Adapted from Kirkpatrick AW, Roberts DJ, De Waele J, et al. Intra-abdominal hypertension and the abdominal compartment syndrome: updated consensus definitions and clinical practice guidelines from the World Society of the Abdominal Compartment Syndrome. *Intensive Care Med.* 2013;39(7):1190-1206. doi:10.1007/s00134-013-2906-z.

References

1. Kirkpatrick AW, Roberts DJ, De Waele J, et al. Intra-abdominal hypertension and the abdominal compartment syndrome: updated consensus definitions and clinical practice guidelines from the World Society of the Abdominal Compartment Syndrome. *Intensive Care Med.* 2013;39(7):1190-1206. doi:10.1007/s00134-013-2906-z
2. Cheatham ML, De Waele JJ, De Laet I, et al. The impact of body position on intra-abdominal pressure measurement: a multicenter analysis. *Crit Care Med.* 2009;37(7):2187-2190. doi:10.1097/CCM.0b013e3181a021fa

3. Yi M, Leng Y, Bai Y, Yao G, Zhu X. The evaluation of the effect of body positioning on intra-abdominal pressure measurement and the effect of intra-abdominal pressure at different body positioning on organ function and prognosis in critically ill patients. *J Crit Care.* 2012;27(2):222.e1-222.e6. doi:10.1016/j.jcrc.2011.08.010
4. Malbrain MLNG, Peeters Y, Wise R. The neglected role of abdominal compliance in organ-organ interactions. *Crit Care.* 2016;20(1):67. doi:10.1186/s13054-016-1220-x
5. Sosa G, Gandham N, Landeras V, Calimag AP, Lerma E. Abdominal compartment syndrome. *Dis Mon.* 2019;65(1):5-19. doi:10.1016/j.disamonth.2018.04.003
6. Malbrain MLNG, Chiumello D, Cesana BM, et al. A systematic review and individual patient data meta-analysis on intra-abdominal hypertension in critically ill patients: the wake-up project. World initiative on Abdominal Hypertension Epidemiology, a Unifying Project (WAKE-Up!). *Minerva Anestesiol.* 2014;80(3):293-306.
7. Dalfino L, Tullo L, Donadio I, Malcangi V, Brienza N. Intra-abdominal hypertension and acute renal failure in critically ill patients. *Intensive Care Med.* 2008;34(4):707-713. doi:10.1007/s00134-007-0969-4
8. Rogers WK, Garcia L. Intraabdominal hypertension, abdominal compartment syndrome, and the open abdomen. *Chest.* 2018;153(1):238-250. doi:10.1016/j.chest.2017.07.023
9. Kirkpatrick AW, Pelosi P, De Waele JJ, et al. Clinical review: intra-abdominal hypertension: does it influence the physiology of prone ventilation? *Crit Care.* 2010;14(4):232. doi:10.1186/cc9099
10. De Waele JJ, Malbrain ML, Kirkpatrick AW. The abdominal compartment syndrome: evolving concepts and future directions. *Crit Care.* 2015;19(1). doi:10.1186/s13054-015-0879-8
11. Blaser AR, Parm P, Kitus R, Starkopf J. Risk factors for intra-abdominal hypertension in mechanically ventilated patients. *Acta Anaesthesiol Scand.* 2011;55(5):607-614. doi:10.1111/j.1399-6576.2011.02415.x
12. Hering R, Wrigge H, Vorwerk R, et al. The effects of prone positioning on intraabdominal pressure and cardiovascular and renal function in patients with acute lung injury. *Anesth Analg.* 2001;92(5):1226-1231. doi:10.1097/00000539-200105000-00027
13. Ke L, Ni H-B, Sun J-K, et al. Risk factors and outcome of intra-abdominal hypertension in patients with severe acute pancreatitis. *World J Surg.* 2012;36(1):171-178. doi:10.1007/s00268-011-1295-0
14. Dalfino L, Sicolo A, Paparella D, Mongelli M, Rubino G, Brienza N. Intra-abdominal hypertension in cardiac surgery. *Interact Cardiovasc Thorac Surg.* 2013;17(4):644-651. doi:10.1093/icvts/ivt272
15. Kirkpatrick AW, Brenneman FD, McLean RF, Rapanos T, Boulanger BR. Is clinical examination an accurate indicator of raised intra-abdominal pressure in critically injured patients? *Can J Surg J Can Chir.* 2000;43(3):207-211.
16. De Keulenaer BL, Regli A, Dabrowski W, et al. Does femoral venous pressure measurement correlate well with intrabladder pressure measurement? A multicenter observational trial. *Intensive Care Med.* 2011;37(10):1620-1627. doi:10.1007/s00134-011-2298-x
17. Cheatham ML, White MW, Sagraves SG, Johnson JL, Block EF. Abdominal perfusion pressure: a superior parameter in the assessment of intra-abdominal hypertension. *J Trauma.* 2000;49(4):621-626; discussion 626-627. doi:10.1097/00005373-200010000-00008
18. Nelson R, Edwards S, Tse B. Prophylactic nasogastric decompression after abdominal surgery. *Cochrane Database Syst Rev.* 2007;(3):CD004929. doi:10.1002/14651858.CD004929.pub3
19. Valle RGL, Godoy FL. Neostigmine for acute colonic pseudo-obstruction: a meta-analysis. *Ann Med Surg (Lond).* 2014;3(3):60-64. doi:10.1016/j.amsu.2014.04.002
20. Deeren DH, Dits H, Malbrain MLNG. Correlation between intra-abdominal and intracranial pressure in nontraumatic brain injury. *Intensive Care Med.* 2005;31(11):1577-1581. doi:10.1007/s00134-005-2802-2
21. Farkas J. Abdominal compartment syndrome. EMCrit Project. Published March 13, 2019. Accessed November 2, 2020. https://emcrit.org/ibcc/abdominal-compartment-syndrome/

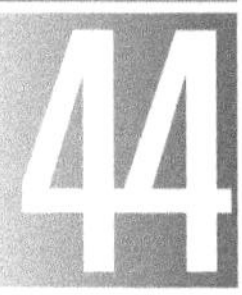

Contrast-Associated Acute Kidney Injury

Winn Cashion and Steven D. Weisbord

INTRODUCTION

Acute kidney injury (AKI) is a widely recognized complication of intravascular iodinated contrast media exposure. Contrast-associated AKI (CA-AKI) typically manifests as a small, transient decrease in kidney function that develops within 4 days of contrast administration. CA-AKI associates with serious adverse outcomes, including death and long-term loss of kidney function; however, a causal connection remains unproven. This is important considering growing evidence that clinically indicated, potentially life-saving angiographic procedures are underutilized in patients with chronic kidney disease (CKD) and acute coronary syndrome (ACS), likely because of concern by providers of precipitating CA-AKI. As patients hospitalized in the intensive care unit (ICU) frequently require contrast-enhanced imaging for diagnostic and therapeutic purposes, ICU providers should have a sound understanding of the risk factors for, outcomes associated with, and empiric evidence for the prevention of this iatrogenic complication.

PATHOPHYSIOLOGY AND INCIDENCE OF CONTRAST-ASSOCIATED ACUTE KIDNEY INJURY

Effects of intravascular contrast administration that are believed to underlie the pathophysiology of CA-AKI include mismatch of oxygen supply and demand in the renal medulla where the partial pressure of oxygen is particularly low, direct epithelial cell toxicity, and oxygen free radical generation that augments tubular epithelial injury (**Figure 44.1**). The incidence of CA-AKI varies on the basis of the patient population being studied, type of procedure performed, and the threshold increase in serum creatinine (sCr) used to define AKI. Among patients with stage 3 and 4 CKD, Weisbord et al found that CA-AKI, defined by an sCr increase of 25% or more, developed in 13.2%, 8.5%, and 6.5% following nonemergent noncoronary angiography, coronary angiography, and contrast-enhanced computed tomography (CT), respectively.[1] Among patients hospitalized in a surgical ICU, Valette et al found that CA-AKI developed in up to 19% of patients, whereas 10% of all patients required kidney replacement therapy.[2] Case and colleagues' review of epidemiologic research reported that the incidence of CA-AKI ranged from 11.5% to 19% in ICU patients.[3] Interpreting the incidence of CA-AKI requires recognition that increments in sCr may occur simultaneously yet independently of iodinated contrast administration. Bruce et al found that among CKD patients (defined as CKD stages 1 to 5, including many patients

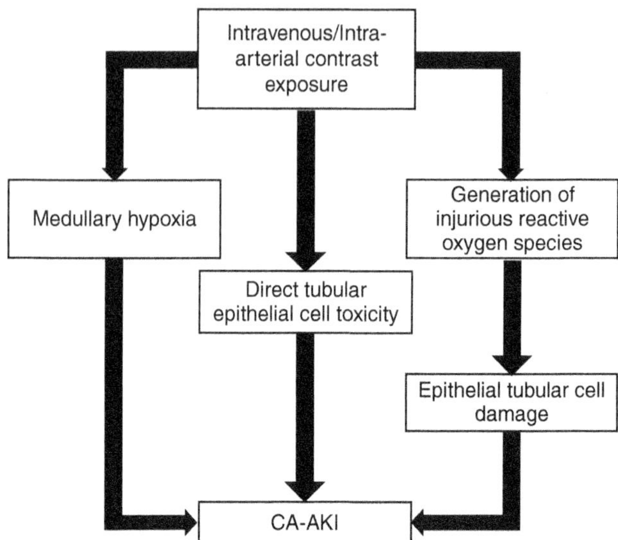

FIGURE 44.1: Pathophysiology of contrast-associated acute kidney injury (CA-AKI) involving medullary hypoxia, direct tubular toxicity, and the injurious effects of reactive oxygen species.

with estimated glomerular filtration rate [eGFR] >60 mL/min/1.73 m^2), the incidence of AKI following CT without contrast (8.8%) was comparable to that following contrast-enhanced CT (9.7% with iso-osmolar iodixanol and 9.9% with low-osmolar iohexol).[4] A series of more recent observational studies have questioned the nephrotoxicity of iodinated contrast and raised the possibility that changes in kidney function in patients undergoing contrast-enhanced procedures, including in the ICU, are often due to factors other than intravascular contrast.[5-9] A meta-analysis by McDonald et al of 13 studies found that the risk of AKI following contrast-enhanced radiographic procedures was comparable to the risk following non–contrast-enhanced radiographic procedures (relative risk = 0.79; 95% confidence interval [CI]: 0.62-1.02).[10] In an observational study of 6,877 ICU patients, this same group found no difference in AKI risk among those who received contrast (odds ratio [OR] = 0.88; 95% CI: 0.75-1.05) after propensity score adjustment.[11] Methodological limitations of this research include its observational design and likely unmeasured confounding. Nonetheless, these studies highlight the fact that baseline fluctuation in sCr and causal factors unrelated to iodinated contrast should be considered when estimating CA-AKI incidence, particularly if defined by small sCr changes.

RISK FACTORS FOR CONTRAST-ASSOCIATED ACUTE KIDNEY INJURY

Risk factors for CA-AKI are categorized as patient related and procedure related (**Table 44.1**). Underlying kidney impairment is the principal patient-related risk factor.[12] Diabetes amplifies the risk if CKD is present but does not appear to increase the risk in patients with normal kidney function. Absolute

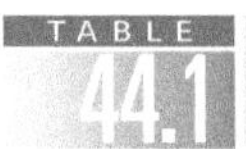

TABLE 44.1 Contrast-Associated Acute Kidney Injury Risk Factors

Patient Associated	Procedure Associated
Impairment in kidney function, acute or chronic	High-osmolal contrast
Diabetes mellitus[a]	Large volume of contrast
Reduced intravascular volume	Repeated contrast procedures
Concomitant nephrotoxic medications	

[a]Augments risk in patients with underlying impairment in kidney function.

or effective intravascular volume depletion may magnify the effect of contrast-induced renal vasoconstriction and increase CA-AKI risk.[13,14] Similarly, the use of selective and nonselective nonsteroidal anti-inflammatory medications, which inhibit the production of vasodilatory renal prostaglandins, may increase CA-AKI risk.[15] The use of large volumes of contrast increases risk, although the threshold amount beyond which at-risk patients are likely to experience kidney injury has not been definitively determined.[16-19] Repeated receipt of intravascular contrast over a short period of time also confers increased risk. Low-osmolal contrast is less nephrotoxic than high-osmolal contrast; however, at present, it is generally believed that there are no notable differences in risk of CA-AKI comparing iso-osmolal to low-osmolal contrast.[20] Finally, the risk appears to be higher following intra-arterial compared with intravenous (IV) contrast exposure.

OUTCOMES ASSOCIATED WITH CONTRAST-ASSOCIATED ACUTE KIDNEY INJURY

A multitude of studies have reported that CA-AKI is associated with increased risk for short- and long-term mortality (**Table 44.2**).[17,21-25] McCullough et al found that among patients undergoing percutaneous intervention, those who developed CA-AKI were considerably more likely to experience in-hospital death (7.1% vs 1.1%, $p < 0.0001$).[17] Solomon et al demonstrated an approximate 3-fold higher risk of death, stroke, myocardial infarction, and/or end-stage kidney disease (ESKD) at 1 year among patients who developed postangiography CA-AKI, compared with patients without CA-AKI.[26]

CA-AKI is also associated with prolonged hospitalization. Adolph et al found that patients with CA-AKI were hospitalized an average of 2 days longer than those without CA-AKI.[27] Prolonged hospitalization with CA-AKI leads to greater than $10,000 in increased costs according to a decision analysis by Subramanian et al.[28] CA-AKI is also associated with a more rapid rate of progression of underlying CKD.[29-32] Goldenberg et al demonstrated that patients who manifested transient CA-AKI experienced a larger loss of kidney function 2 years following angiography than patients without CA-AKI (ΔeGFR -20 ± 11 vs -6 ± 16 mL/min/1.73 m^2, $p = 0.02$).[30] Others have documented accelerated CKD progression in CA-AKI patients.[29,32] It is important to recognize that the causal nature of the associations of CA-AKI with serious, adverse outcomes and

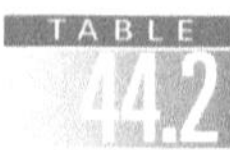

TABLE 44.2 Contrast-Associated Acute Kidney Injury (CA-AKI) and Mortality

Study Authors	(N)	CA-AKI Definition	Adjusted OR/HR	95% CI
Short-term Mortality				
Levy et al[21]	357	↑ sCr ≥ 25% to ≥2.0 mg/dL	5.5	2.9-13.2
Gruberg et al[33]	439	↑ sCr > 25%	3.9	2.0-7.6
Shema et al[34]	1,111	↑ sCr ≥ 50% or ↓ eGFR ≥ 25%	3.9	1.2-12.0
McCullough et al[17]	1,826	↑ sCr > 25%	6.6	3.3-12.9
From et al[23]	3,236	↑ sCr ≥ 25% or ≥0.5 mg/dL	3.4	2.6-4.4
Rihal et al[25]	7,586	↑ sCr > 0.5 mg/dL	10.8	6.9-17.0
Bartholomew et al[22]	20,479	↑ sCr ≥ 1.0 mg/dL	22	16-31
Weisbord et al[24]	27,608	↑ sCr 0.25-0.5 mg/dL	1.8	1.4-2.5
Long-term Mortality				
Goldenberg et al[30]	78	↑ sCr ≥ 0.5 mg/dL or ≥25%	2.7	1.7-4.5
Solomon et al[26]	294	↑ sCr ≥ 0.3 mg/dL	3.2[a]	1.1-8.7
Harjai et al[35]	985	↑ sCr ≥ 0.5 mg/dL	2.6	1.5-4.4
Roghi et al[36]	2,860	↑ sCr ≥ 0.5 mg/dL	1.8	1.0-3.4
Brown et al[37]	7,856	↑ sCr ≥ 0.5 mg/dL	3.1	2.4-4.0

[a]Denotes incident rate ratio of composite outcome of death, cerebrovascular accident, myocardial infarction, and end-stage kidney disease.

CI, confidence interval; eGFR, estimated glomerular filtration rate; HR, hazard ratio; OR, odds ratio; sCr, serum creatinine.

increased costs remains unproven. Rather than being a mediator of such outcomes, CA-AKI may simply be a marker of patients more susceptible to these outcomes through greater hemodynamic instability and diminished kidney reserve. Recognizing this possibility is important given multiple publications documenting the underutilization of clinically indicated and potentially life-saving angiographic procedures in patients with CKD and ACS, likely due to provider concern about precipitating CA-AKI. This practice, known as "renalism," was initially described by Chertow et al in a study of more than 57,000 patients with acute myocardial infarction in which those with CKD were approximately 50% less likely to undergo coronary angiography than were those without CKD.[38] These findings were recapitulated in multiple other publications.[39-42] Although presumably well intentioned, the practice of "renalism" may be iatrogenic given observational data demonstrating a survival advantage in those with CKD who undergo coronary angiography and revascularization, as well as American Heart Association/American College of Cardiology clinical practice guidelines that support the use of invasive coronary care in many CKD patients with

ACS.[38,41,43-45] In this context and with the recognition that CA-AKI has not been causally linked to adverse outcomes and, even if a causal connection indeed exists, that the net benefit of the contrast-based cardiac intervention may outweigh the renal risks, it is important that contrast-enhanced procedures are performed when clinically indicated, albeit with the implementation of evidence-based preventive care.

PREVENTION OF CONTRAST-ASSOCIATED ACUTE KIDNEY INJURY

Once determined that a procedure with intravascular iodinated contrast is required, focus should turn to implementing evidence-based preventive care. Prior research has investigated four principal preventive approaches: (a) kidney replacement therapies to remove intravascular contrast; (b) identifying less nephrotoxic contrast media; (c) use of medications that counteract the nephrotoxic effects of contrast; and (d) providing IV fluid to mitigate the adverse renal hemodynamic effects and direct tubular toxicity of contrast. Prophylactic hemodialysis has been shown to be potentially deleterious and is not a recommended preventive approach.[46] Data on the use of continuous kidney replacement therapy are conflicting with insufficient evidence to support this strategy. Over several decades, the chemical properties of iodinated contrast have evolved. Older "high-osmolal" agents were associated with a significantly elevated risk for CA-AKI compared with "low-osmolal" contrast. Conversely, trials and meta-analyses comparing low- and iso-osmolal contrast have been conflicting. As such, clinical practice guidelines from the American College of Cardiology/American Heart Association and European Society of Urogenital Radiology recommend the use of either low- or iso-osmolal contrast.[47,48]

Multiple pharmacologic agents have been evaluated for CA-AKI prevention. Some were found to be ineffective and in some cases potentially deleterious (e.g., dopamine), whereas data on other agents are mixed, with some studies demonstrating benefit and others no effect (**Table 44.3**). Conflicting findings of numerous clinical trials and meta-analyses assessing the effect of *N*-acetylcysteine (NAC) resulted in prolonged uncertainty on the benefit of this vasodilatory antioxidant. The recently published Prevention of Serious Adverse Events Following

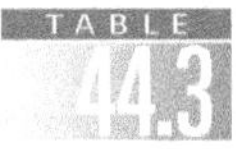
TABLE 44.3 Pharmacologic Agents Previously Tested for Contrast-Associated Acute Kidney Injury Prevention

Ineffective	Indeterminate Effectiveness
Furosemide[a]	Atrial natriuretic peptide
Dopamine[a]	Theophylline/aminophylline
Fenoldopam[a]	Atorvastatin/rosuvastatin
Calcium channel blockers	Prostaglandin analogs
N-acetylcysteine	Allopurinol
	Acetazolamide

[a]Potentially deleterious.

Angiography (PRESERVE) trial, which enrolled 4,993 patients undergoing nonemergent angiography, demonstrated that compared with oral placebo, 5 days of oral NAC (600 mg twice daily) was not associated with a reduction in 90-day death, need for dialysis, or persistent impairment in kidney function (OR = 1.02; 95% CI: 0.78-1.33) or CA-AKI, defined as an increase in sCr of greater than or equal to 25% or 0.5 mg/dL at 4 days following angiography (OR = 1.06; 95% CI: 0.87-1.28). Hence, there is presently no role for NAC or other pharmaceutical interventions for the prevention of CA-AKI (**Visual Abstract 44.1**).

Recent research on IV fluid composition and the prevention of CA-AKI has focused on the comparative effects of isotonic sodium bicarbonate and isotonic sodium chloride. The initial trial by Merten et al enrolled 119 patients and showed a lower incidence of CA-AKI with IV isotonic bicarbonate compared with IV isotonic saline (1.6% vs 13.6%, $p = 0.02$).[49] This finding resulted in a proliferation of clinical trials and meta-analyses, some reporting a lower incidence of CA-AKI with IV sodium bicarbonate and others demonstrating no difference.[27,31,50-64] To definitively address the persistent clinical equipoise on the role of IV sodium bicarbonate, the PRESERVE trial randomized high-risk patients to receive IV isotonic sodium bicarbonate ($N = 2{,}511$) or IV isotonic sodium chloride ($N = 2{,}482$) before, during, and following angiography.[65] Compared with IV sodium chloride, sodium bicarbonate did not result in a decrease in 90-day death, need for dialysis, or persistent impairment in kidney function (OR = 0.93; 95% CI: 0.72-1.22) or in the incidence of CA-AKI (OR=1.16; 95% CI: 0.96-1.41).[65] Thus, given present data, IV isotonic crystalloid should be considered the standard of care IV fluid intervention for the prevention of CA-AKI and associated adverse outcomes.

Current Recommendations for the Prevention of Contrast-Associated Acute Kidney Injury

For patients deemed at risk for CA-AKI, options for alternative imaging techniques that do not require iodinated contrast but that provide comparable diagnostic yield should be considered. Among those requiring intravascular contrast, nonsteroidal anti-inflammatories should be discontinued before contrast administration and held until CA-AKI has been ruled out. The lowest required volume of either low- or iso-osmolal contrast should be used. Isotonic IV sodium chloride should be administered before, during, and after the procedure provided there is low risk for physiologically detrimental volume overload (e.g., patient already in decompensated heart failure before IV fluid load).[65] For those who are hospitalized undergoing nonemergent procedures, regimens that are appropriate include 1 mL/kg/hr for 12 hours preceding, during, and following the procedure or 3 mL/kg/hr for 1 hour before, 1 to 1.5 mL/kg/hr during, and 4 to 6 hours following contrast exposure. The Prevention of Contrast Renal Injury with Different Hydration Strategies (POSEIDON) trial demonstrated that administering IV fluid to patients undergoing coronary angiography with elevated left ventricular end-diastolic pressure is both effective and safe.[66] Therefore, isotonic IV sodium chloride should be administered to patients with nondecompensated heart failure, albeit with careful monitoring for the development of pulmonary congestion. Available data do not support the discontinuation of diuretics or renin-angiotensin-aldosterone axis inhibitors before contrast administration. Furthermore, there are insufficient data at present to support the routine use of statins to mitigate the risk of CA-AKI. In patients at risk for CA-AKI, including those receiving appropriate preventive care, it is essential to assess sCr 48 to 96 hours following contrast administration to determine whether CA-AKI has developed, thus alerting the physician to provide supportive kidney care.

NEPHROGENIC SYSTEMIC FIBROSIS

Phenotype of Nephrogenic Systemic Fibrosis and Gadolinium Toxicology

Nephrogenic systemic fibrosis (NSF, previously known as nephrogenic fibrosing dermatopathy) is characterized by fibrosis of the skin and connective tissues and can involve internal organs. The condition is associated with the administration of gadolinium-based contrast media in patients with severe impairment in kidney function in the setting of magnetic resonance imaging (MRI).[67,68] Gadolinium interferes with calcium metabolic and signaling pathways, and NSF is characterized histologically by fibroblast and macrophage infiltrates.[69,70] Gold standard diagnosis requires skin and soft tissue biopsy and clinical/histologic correlation.[71]

Free gadolinium itself is highly toxic. In gadolinium-based contrast agents (GBCA), the gadolinium is complexed to a linear (group I) or macrocyclic (group II) ligand, which very avidly binds gadolinium.[70] Before the recognition of NSF, gadolinium-enhanced MRIs were a preferred imaging modality in patients with kidney disease owing to concern about precipitating AKI with the administration of iodinated contrast media in this population.[70]

Epidemiology of Nephrogenic Systemic Fibrosis

To date, a small number of NSF cases have been reported in the literature, with few cases documented since 2009 when the association with GBCA was established.[72] The vast majority of NSF cases have occurred in patients with ESRD, stage 5 CKD, or severe AKI, although rare cases in CKD stage 4 have been documented.[68,73] Conversely, partial or complete NSF resolution has been reported following AKI recovery or kidney transplantation.[74,75]

Despite gadolinium having been used since 1988, NSF was not recognized until 2000 in a Lancet publication of 15 cases traced as far back as 1997.[76,77] The association with gadolinium was first suggested in 2006.[78] Onset of NSF symptoms typically occurs within weeks to months of gadolinium exposure, although cases as soon as the day of MRI and as late as years later have been reported.[70]

The Food and Drug Administration (FDA) issued a boxed warning of gadolinium risk in 2007, with a subsequent drop in the number of new NSF cases being reported.[79] For example, a 2019 systematic review of 173 publications and 639 patients with biopsy-confirmed NSF found that only 7 of the 639 cases occurred with gadolinium administered after 2008.[72] There is evidence that the risk for NSF is strongly dependent on the type of gadolinium exposure; macrocyclic (group II) formulations have been empirically shown to be at much lower risk. A 2020 meta-analysis of nearly 5,000 patients with CKD stage 4 to 5 and group II GCA exposure observed no subsequent NSF cases.[80]

Hemodialysis to Potentially Prevent Nephrogenic Systemic Fibrosis

Among critically ill patients, the decision to use GBCA in the setting of advanced CKD or AKI needs to be individualized on the basis of the need for the imaging procedure and the assessed risk for NSF. When alternative imaging that does not require GBCA is available and considered to be equivalent in diagnostic capacity, it should be strongly considered. Among patients in whom contrast-enhanced MRI is required, judicious gadolinium volumes and gadolinium formulations associated with lower rates of NSF should be used. In the past, there were recommendations to provide three daily hemodialysis (HD) sessions to patient who were administered a GBCA in order to reduce the risk of NSF;[72] however more recent guidance from the National Kidney Foundation and the American College of Radiology no longer support this practice.[81] Further there are no sound data on the use of hemodialysis among patients who are not on this therapy before GBCA administration or among those receiving chronic peritoneal dialysis.

CONCLUSION

The risks and benefits of iodinated and gadolinium contrast must be balanced in individual patients. The administration of intravascular iodinated contrast media is associated with AKI, an observation that has likely contributed to the underutilization of indicated, contrast-requiring diagnostic and therapeutic procedures in CKD patients. However, the causal nature of these associations remains unproven and foregoing these procedures may have harmful clinical implications. Therefore, patients with clinical indications for procedures that require intravascular iodinated contrast who are at increased risk for CA-AKI should undergo these procedures, albeit with the implementation of evidence-based preventive care. The cornerstone of prevention is periprocedural isotonic IV crystalloid. Additional well-designed research is needed to determine if (and the extent to which) CA-AKI mediates serious, adverse outcomes and, if so, to identify other effective preventive care for this iatrogenic condition. The indication for gadolinium-enhanced MRI, the specific gadolinium formulation, and the contrast volume should be chosen to maximize MRI diagnostic yield while minimizing NSF risk.

References

1. Weisbord SD, Mor MK, Resnick AL, et al. Prevention, incidence, and outcomes of contrast-induced acute kidney injury. *Arch Intern Med.* 2008;168:1325-1332.
2. Valette X, Parienti JJ, Plaud B, et al. Incidence, morbidity, and mortality of contrast-induced acute kidney injury in a surgical intensive care unit: a prospective cohort study. *J Crit Care.* 2012;27:322.e1-322.e5.
3. Case J, Khan S, Khalid R, et al. Epidemiology of acute kidney injury in the intensive care unit. *Crit Care Res Pract.* 2013;2013:479730.
4. Bruce RJ, Djamali A, Shinki K, et al. Background fluctuation of kidney function versus contrast-induced nephrotoxicity. *AJR Am J Roentgenol.* 2009;192:711-718.
5. McDonald JS, McDonald RJ, Carter RE, et al. Risk of intravenous contrast material-mediated acute kidney injury: a propensity score-matched study stratified by baseline-estimated glomerular filtration rate. *Radiology.* 2014;271:65-73.
6. McDonald JS, McDonald RJ, Lieske JC, et al. Risk of acute kidney injury, dialysis, and mortality in patients with chronic kidney disease after intravenous contrast material exposure. *Mayo Clin Proc.* 2015;90:1046-1053.
7. McDonald RJ, McDonald JS, Bida JP, et al. Intravenous contrast material-induced nephropathy: causal or coincident phenomenon? *Radiology.* 2013;267:106-118.
8. McDonald RJ, McDonald JS, Newhouse JH, et al. Controversies in contrast material-induced acute kidney injury: closing in on the truth? *Radiology.* 2015;277:627-632.
9. Wilhelm-Leen E, Montez-Rath ME, Chertow G. Estimating the risk of radiocontrast-associated nephropathy. *J Am Soc Nephrol.* 2017;28:653-659.

10. McDonald JS, McDonald RJ, Comin J, et al. Frequency of acute kidney injury following intravenous contrast medium administration: a systematic review and meta-analysis. *Radiology.* 2013;267:119-128.
11. McDonald JS, McDonald RJ, Williamson EE, et al. Post-contrast acute kidney injury in intensive care unit patients: a propensity score-adjusted study. *Intensive Care Med.* 2017;43:774-784.
12. McCullough PA, Adam A, Becker CR, et al. Risk prediction of contrast-induced nephropathy. *Am J Cardiol.* 2006;98:27K-36K.
13. Taliercio CP, Vlietstra RE, Fisher LD, et al. Risks for renal dysfunction with cardiac angiography. *Ann Intern Med.* 1986;104:501-504.
14. Gomes AS, Baker JD, Martin-Paredero V, et al. Acute renal dysfunction after major arteriography. *AJR Am J Roentgenol.* 1985;145:1249-1253.
15. Ahmad SR, Kortepeter C, Brinker A, et al. Renal failure associated with the use of celecoxib and rofecoxib. *Drug Saf.* 2002;25:537-544.
16. Marenzi G, Assanelli E, Campodonico J, et al. Contrast volume during primary percutaneous coronary intervention and subsequent contrast-induced nephropathy and mortality. *Ann Intern Med.* 2009;150:170-177.
17. McCullough PA, Wolyn R, Rocher LL, et al. Acute renal failure after coronary intervention: incidence, risk factors, and relationship to mortality. *Am J Med.* 1997;103:368-375.
18. Nyman U, Almen T, Aspelin P, et al. Contrast-medium-Induced nephropathy correlated to the ratio between dose in gram iodine and estimated GFR in ml/min. *Acta Radiol.* 2005;46:830-842.
19. Worasuwannarak S, Pornratanarangsi S. Prediction of contrast-induced nephropathy in diabetic patients undergoing elective cardiac catheterization or PCI: role of volume-to-creatinine clearance ratio and iodine dose-to-creatinine clearance ratio. *J Med Assoc Thai.* 2010;93(suppl 1):S29-S34.
20. Laskey W, Aspelin P, Davidson C, et al. Nephrotoxicity of iodixanol versus iopamidol in patients with chronic kidney disease and diabetes mellitus undergoing coronary angiographic procedures. *Am Heart J.* 2009;158:822-828.e3.
21. Levy EM, Viscoli CM, Horwitz RI. The effect of acute renal failure on mortality. A cohort analysis. *JAMA.* 1996;275:1489-1494.
22. Bartholomew BA, Harjai KJ, Dukkipati S, et al. Impact of nephropathy after percutaneous coronary intervention and a method for risk stratification. *Am J Cardiol.* 2004;93:1515-1519.
23. From AM, Bartholmai BJ, Williams AW, et al. Mortality associated with nephropathy after radiographic contrast exposure. *Mayo Clin Proc.* 2008;83:1095-1100.
24. Weisbord SD, Chen H, Stone RA, et al. Associations of increases in serum creatinine with mortality and length of hospital stay after coronary angiography. *J Am Soc Nephrol.* 2006;17:2871-2877.
25. Rihal CS, Textor SC, Grill DE, et al. Incidence and prognostic importance of acute renal failure after percutaneous coronary intervention. *Circulation.* 2002;105:2259-2264.
26. Solomon RJ, Mehran R, Natarajan MK, et al. Contrast-induced nephropathy and long-term adverse events: cause and effect? *Clin J Am Soc Nephrol.* 2009;4:1162-1169.
27. Adolph E, Holdt-Lehmann B, Chatterjee T, et al. Renal Insufficiency Following Radiocontrast Exposure Trial (REINFORCE): a randomized comparison of sodium bicarbonate versus sodium chloride hydration for the prevention of contrast-induced nephropathy. *Coron Artery Dis.* 2008;19:413-419.
28. Subramanian S, Tumlin J, Bapat B, et al. Economic burden of contrast-induced nephropathy: implications for prevention strategies. *J Med Econ.* 2007;10:119-134.
29. James MT, Ghali WA, Tonelli M, et al. Acute kidney injury following coronary angiography is associated with a long-term decline in kidney function. *Kidney Int.* 2010;78:803-809.
30. Goldenberg I, Chonchol M, Guetta V. Reversible acute kidney injury following contrast exposure and the risk of long-term mortality. *Am J Nephrol.* 2009;29:136-144.
31. Maioli M, Toso A, Leoncini M, et al. Sodium bicarbonate versus saline for the prevention of contrast-induced nephropathy in patients with renal dysfunction undergoing coronary angiography or intervention. *J Am Coll Cardiol.* 2008;52:599-604.
32. James MT, Ghali WA, Knudtson ML, et al. Associations between acute kidney injury and cardiovascular and renal outcomes after coronary angiography. *Circulation.* 2011;123:409-416.
33. Gruberg L, Mintz GS, Mehran R, et al. The prognostic implications of further renal function deterioration within 48 h of interventional coronary procedures in patients with pre-existent chronic renal insufficiency. *J Am Coll Cardiol.* 2000;36:1542-1548.
34. Shema L, Ore L, Geron R, Kristal B. Contrast-induced nephropathy among Israeli hospitalized patients: incidence, risk factors, length of stay and mortality. *Isr Med Assoc J.* 2009;11:460-464.

35. Harjai KJ, Raizada A, Shenoy C, et al. A comparison of contemporary definitions of contrast nephropathy in patients undergoing percutaneous coronary intervention and a proposal for a novel nephropathy grading system. *Am J Cardiol.* 2008;101:812-819.
36. Roghi A, Savonitto S, Cavallini C, et al. Impact of acute renal failure following percutaneous coronary intervention on long-term mortality. *J Cardiovasc Med (Hagerstown).* 2008;9:375-381.
37. Brown JR, Block CA, Malenka DJ, et al. Sodium bicarbonate plus N-acetylcysteine prophylaxis: a meta-analysis. *JACC Cardiovasc Interv.* 2009;2:1116-1124.
38. Chertow GM, Normand SL, McNeil BJ. "Renalism": inappropriately low rates of coronary angiography in elderly individuals with renal insufficiency. *J Am Soc Nephrol.* 2004;15:2462-2468.
39. Han JH, Chandra A, Mulgund J, et al. Chronic kidney disease in patients with non-ST-segment elevation acute coronary syndromes. *Am J Med.* 2006;119:248-254.
40. Szummer K, Lundman P, Jacobson SH, et al. Relation between renal function, presentation, use of therapies and in-hospital complications in acute coronary syndrome: data from the SWEDEHEART register. *J Intern Med.* 2010;268:40-49.
41. Goldenberg I, Subirana I, Boyko V, et al. Relation between renal function and outcomes in patients with non-ST-segment elevation acute coronary syndrome: real-world data from the European Public Health Outcome Research and Indicators Collection Project. *Arch Intern Med.* 2010;170:888-895.
42. Nauta ST, van Domburg RT, Nuis RJ, et al. Decline in 20-year mortality after myocardial infarction in patients with chronic kidney disease: evolution from the prethrombolysis to the percutaneous coronary intervention era. *Kidney Int.* 2013;84:353-358.
43. Amsterdam EA, Wenger NK, Brindis RG, et al. 2014 AHA/ACC guideline for the management of patients with non-ST-elevation acute coronary syndromes: a report of the American College of Cardiology/American Heart Association Task Force on Practice Guidelines. *Circulation.* 2014;130:e344-e426.
44. Amsterdam EA, Wenger NK. The 2014 American College of Cardiology ACC/American Heart Association guideline for the management of patients with non-ST-elevation acute coronary syndromes: ten contemporary recommendations to aid clinicians in optimizing patient outcomes. *Clin Cardiol.* 2015;38:121-123.
45. Fox CS, Muntner P, Chen AY, et al. Use of evidence-based therapies in short-term outcomes of ST-segment elevation myocardial infarction and non-ST-segment elevation myocardial infarction in patients with chronic kidney disease: a report from the National Cardiovascular Data Acute Coronary Treatment and Intervention Outcomes Network registry. *Circulation.* 2010;121:357-365.
46. Reinecke H, Fobker M, Wellmann J, et al. A randomized controlled trial comparing hydration therapy to additional hemodialysis or N-acetylcysteine for the prevention of contrast medium-induced nephropathy: the Dialysis-versus-Diuresis (DVD) Trial. *Clin Res Cardiol.* 2007;96:130-139.
47. Anderson JL, Adams CD, Antman EM, et al. 2012 ACCF/AHA focused update incorporated into the ACCF/AHA 2007 guidelines for the management of patients with unstable angina/non-ST-elevation myocardial infarction: a report of the American College of Cardiology Foundation/American Heart Association Task Force on Practice Guidelines. *Circulation.* 2013;127:e663-e828.
48. European Society of Urogenital Radiology. ESUR guidelines on contrast media. 2008. www.esur.org
49. Merten GJ, Burgess WP, Gray LV, et al. Prevention of contrast-induced nephropathy with sodium bicarbonate: a randomized controlled trial. *JAMA.* 2004;291:2328-2334.
50. Brar SS, Shen AY, Jorgensen MB, et al. Sodium bicarbonate vs. sodium chloride for the prevention of contrast medium-induced nephropathy in patients undergoing coronary angiography: a randomized trial. *JAMA.* 2008;300:1038-1046.
51. Kanbay M, Covic A, Coca SG, et al. Sodium bicarbonate for the prevention of contrast-induced nephropathy: a meta-analysis of 17 randomized trials. *Int Urol Nephrol.* 2009;41:617-627.
52. Masuda M, Yamada T, Mine T, et al. Comparison of usefulness of sodium bicarbonate versus sodium chloride to prevent contrast-induced nephropathy in patients undergoing an emergent coronary procedure. *Am J Cardiol.* 2007;100:781-786.
53. Ozcan EE, Guneri S, Akdeniz B, et al. Sodium bicarbonate, N-acetylcysteine, and saline for prevention of radiocontrast-induced nephropathy. A comparison of 3 regimens for protecting contrast-induced nephropathy in patients undergoing coronary procedures. A single-center prospective controlled trial. *Am Heart J.* 2007;154:539-544.
54. Pakfetrat M, Nikoo MH, Malekmakan L, et al. A comparison of sodium bicarbonate infusion versus normal saline infusion and its combination with oral acetazolamide for prevention of contrast-induced nephropathy: a randomized, double-blind trial. *Int Urol Nephrol.* 2009;41:629-634.

55. Recio-Mayoral A, Chaparro M, Prado B, et al. The reno-protective effect of hydration with sodium bicarbonate plus N-acetylcysteine in patients undergoing emergency percutaneous coronary intervention: the RENO Study. *J Am Coll Cardiol.* 2007;49:1283-1288.
56. Vasheghani-Farahani A, Sadigh G, Kassaian SE, et al. Sodium bicarbonate plus isotonic saline versus saline for prevention of contrast-induced nephropathy in patients undergoing coronary angiography: a randomized controlled trial. *Am J Kidney Dis.* 2009;54:610-618.
57. Zoungas S, Ninomiya T, Huxley R, et al. Systematic review: sodium bicarbonate treatment regimens for the prevention of contrast-induced nephropathy. *Ann Intern Med.* 2009;151:631-638.
58. Navaneethan SD, Singh S, Appasamy S, et al. Sodium bicarbonate therapy for prevention of contrast-induced nephropathy: a systematic review and meta-analysis. *Am J Kidney Dis.* 2009;53:617-627.
59. Meier P, Ko DT, Tamura A, et al. Sodium bicarbonate-based hydration prevents contrast-induced nephropathy: a meta-analysis. *BMC Med.* 2009;7:23.
60. Hoste EA, De Waele JJ, Gevaert SA, et al. Sodium bicarbonate for prevention of contrast-induced acute kidney injury: a systematic review and meta-analysis. *Nephrol Dial Transplant.* 2010;25(3):747-758.
61. Joannidis M, Schmid M, Wiedermann CJ. Prevention of contrast media-induced nephropathy by isotonic sodium bicarbonate: a meta-analysis. *Wien Klin Wochensch.* 2008;120:742-748.
62. Hogan SE, L'Allier P, Chetcuti S, et al. Current role of sodium bicarbonate-based preprocedural hydration for the prevention of contrast-induced acute kidney injury: a meta-analysis. *Am Heart J.* 2008;156:414-421.
63. Ho KM, Morgan DJ. Use of isotonic sodium bicarbonate to prevent radiocontrast nephropathy in patients with mild pre-existing renal impairment: a meta-analysis. *Anaesth Intensive Care.* 2008;36:646-653.
64. Kunadian V, Zaman A, Spyridopoulos I, et al. Sodium bicarbonate for the prevention of contrast induced nephropathy: a meta-analysis of published clinical trials. *Eur J Radiol.* 2011;79(1):48-55.
65. Weisbord SD, Gallagher M, Jneid H, et al. Outcomes after angiography with sodium bicarbonate and acetylcysteine. *N Engl J Med.* 2018;378(7):603-614.
66. Brar SS, Aharonian V, Mansukhani P, et al. Haemodynamic-guided fluid administration for the prevention of contrast-induced acute kidney injury: the POSEIDON randomised controlled trial. *Lancet.* 2014;383:1814-1823.
67. Galan A, Cowper SE, Bucala R. Nephrogenic systemic fibrosis (nephrogenic fibrosing dermopathy). *Curr Opin Rheumatol.* 2006;18(6):614-617.
68. Rudnick M, Wahba I, Miskulin D. Nephrogenic systemic fibrosis/nephrogenic fibrosing dermopathy in advanced kidney disease. *UpToDate.* Retrieved June 22, 2020. https://www.uptodate.com/contents/nephrogenic-systemic-fibrosis-nephrogenic-fibrosing-dermopathy-in-advanced-kidney-disease?search=NSF&source=search_result&selectedTitle=1~41&usage_type=default&display_rank=1
69. Idée JM, Port M, Raynal I, et al. Clinical and biological consequences of transmetallation induced by contrast agents for magnetic resonance imaging: a review. *Fundam Clin Pharmacol.* 2006;20(6):563-576.
70. Wagner B, Drel V, Gorin Y. Pathophysiology of gadolinium-associated systemic fibrosis. *Am J Physiol Renal Physiol.* 2016;311(1):F1-F11.
71. Girardi M, Kay J, Elston DM, et al. Nephrogenic systemic fibrosis: clinicopathological definition and workup recommendations. *J Am Acad Dermatol.* 2011;65(6):1095-1106.e7.
72. Attari H, Cao Y, Elmholdt TR, et al. A systematic review of 639 patients with biopsy-confirmed nephrogenic systemic fibrosis. *Radiology.* 2019;292(2):376-386.
73. Shibui K, Kataoka H, Sato N, et al. A case of NSF attributable to contrast MRI repeated in a patient with Stage 3 CKD at a renal function of eGFR >30 mL/min/1.73 m^2. *Jpn J Nephrol.* 2009;51:676.
74. Leung N, Shaikh A, Cosio FG, et al. The outcome of patients with nephrogenic systemic fibrosis after successful kidney transplantation. *Am J Transplant.* 2010;10(3):558-562.
75. Wilson J, Gleghorn K, Seigel Q, et al. Nephrogenic systemic fibrosis: a 15-year retrospective study at a single tertiary care center. *J Am Acad Dermatol.* 2017;77(2):235-240.
76. Lohrke J, Frenzel T, Endrikat J, et al. 25 years of contrast-enhanced MRI: developments, current challenges and future perspectives. *Adv Ther.* 2016;33(1):1-28.
77. Cowper SE, Robin HS, Steinberg SM, et al. Scleromyxoedema-like cutaneous diseases in renal-dialysis patients. *Lancet.* 2000;356(9234):1000-1001.
78. Grobner T. Gadolinium—a specific trigger for the development of nephrogenic fibrosing dermopathy and nephrogenic systemic fibrosis? *Nephrol Dial Transplant.* 2006;21(4):1104-1108.
79. U.S. Food & Drug Administration. FDA Drug Safety Communication: new warnings for using gadolinium-based contrast agents in patients with kidney dysfunction. 2018. https://www

.fda.gov/drugs/drug-safety-and-availability/fda-drug-safety-communication-new-warnings-using-gadolinium-based-contrast-agents-patients-kidney

80. Woolen SA, Shankar PR, Gagnier JJ, et al. Risk of nephrogenic systemic fibrosis in patients with stage 4 or 5 chronic kidney disease receiving a group II gadolinium-based contrast agent: a systematic review and meta-analysis. *JAMA Intern Med.* 2019;180(2):223-230.
81. Weinreb JC, Rodby RA, Yee J, et al. Use of intravenous gadolinium-based contrast media in patients with kidney disease: consensus statements from the American College of Radiology and the National Kidney Foundation. *Radiology.* 2021;298(1):28-35. doi:10.1148/radiol.2020202903

Does intravenous sodium bicarbonate or acetylcysteine prevent contrast-associated acute kidney injury?

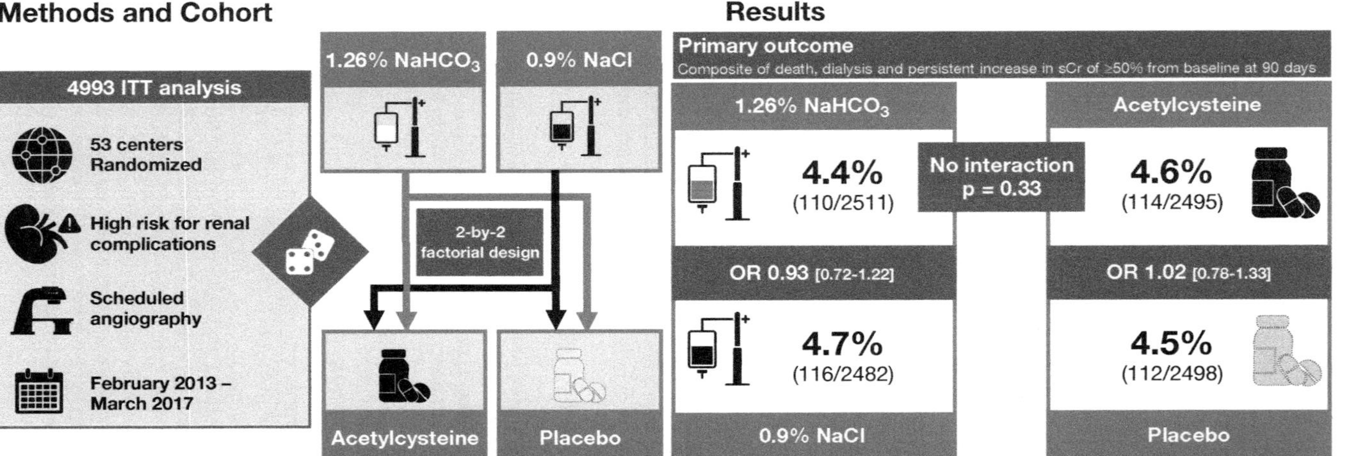

Conclusion: There was no benefit of intravenous sodium bicarbonate over intravenous sodium chloride or of oral acetylcysteine over placebo for the prevention of death, need for dialysis, or persistent decline in kidney function at 90 days or for the prevention of contrast-associated acute kidney injury in this cohort.

Weisbord SD, Gallagher M, Jneid H et al; PRESERVE Trial Group. ***Outcomes after angiography with Sodium Bicarbonate and Acetylcysteine***. N Engl J Med. 2018 Feb 15;378(7):603-614.

VISUAL ABSTRACT 44.1

Hypertensive Emergency

Waleed E. Ali and George L. Bakris

INTRODUCTION

Severe and major blood pressure (BP) elevations in adults are characterized and defined based on the evidence of acute target organ damage. Hypertensive emergencies, defined as a systolic BP greater than 180 mm Hg and/or diastolic BP greater than 120 mm Hg with signs or symptoms of acute end-organ damage.

By contrast, hypertensive urgencies are relatively or completely asymptomatic despite BP elevation being in the same range. The treatment approach is different where hypertensive emergencies require immediate medical attention and treatment with intravenous (IV) antihypertensive agents under close monitoring to ensure fast but controlled BP reduction in order to protect target organ function. Hypertensive urgencies need gradual BP reduction over longer time and ensuring adequate follow-up to improve long-term hypertension control. This chapter discusses the pathogenesis, epidemiology, and diagnostic approach of hypertensive emergencies and urgencies and presents current pharmacologic options for the treatment of these conditions.

A *hypertensive emergency* is defined as an acute increase in BP associated with severe potentially life-threatening target organ damage, such as coronary ischemia, dissecting aortic aneurysm, pulmonary edema, hypertensive encephalopathy, cerebral hemorrhage, and eclampsia. In this condition, hospitalization and admission to an intensive care unit (ICU) are often required for prompt BP control within minutes to 1 hour using parenteral drug therapy to limit end-organ damage.[1]

Hypertensive *urgency* is present in a clinical setting of significant BP elevation without acute target organ dysfunction. Such patients require neither hospitalization nor acute lowering of BP and can safely be managed in the outpatient setting to gradually lower BP within hours with oral antihypertensive drug therapy.[2-4]

ETIOLOGY AND PATHOGENESIS

Hypertensive emergencies and urgencies, that is, hypertensive crises, are associated with adverse outcomes and higher rate of rehospitalizations and utilization of the health care system. In this context, understanding the etiology and risk factors is a first step in reducing health care burden.[5] **Box 45.1** illustrates the most common etiologies of hypertensive crises. Several studies have evaluated characteristics of both the health care system and patients' behavior to address risk factors associated with hypertensive crisis. It was reported that male sex, older age, and history of cardiovascular comorbidities increase the likelihood of hypertensive crisis.[6] Poor access to health care and lack of insurance were also found to be strong predictors in inner-city minority populations where financial challenges contribute to poor BP control and subsequently hypertensive crisis.[6,7]

Box 45.1 Common Triggers of Hypertensive Crisis

Acceleration of chronic hypertension

- Cardiovascular Conditions
  - Acute myocardial ischemia/infarction caused by coronary artery disease
  - Acute aortic dissection
  - Severe hypertension after coronary bypass or other vascular surgery
- Kidney Conditions
  - Acute or rapidly progressive glomerulonephritis
  - Kidney-vascular hypertension
  - Kidney crises from scleroderma or collagen vascular disease
- Neurologic Conditions
  - Hypertensive encephalopathy
  - Intracerebral hemorrhage
  - Subarachnoid hemorrhage
  - Acute head trauma
- Excess Circulating Catecholamine Conditions
  - Pheochromocytoma crisis
  - Interactions of tyramine-containing foods with monoamine oxidase inhibitors
  - Rebound hypertension after sudden withdrawal of centrally acting α_2-agonists (clonidine, methyldopa, or other)
  - Use of sympathomimetic drugs (phencyclidine, phenylpropanolamine, cocaine, or other)
  - Automatic hyperreflexia after spinal cord injury
- Pregnancy-Related Condition
  - Preeclampsia and eclampsia

In some hypertensive crisis, a triggering factor or an underlying condition is the clear cause of acute BP elevation (Box 45.1). However, in some cases, it may be difficult to differentiate whether BP elevation is the cause or the result of a hypertensive crisis. For example, in a patient with intracerebral hemorrhage, an acute marked BP increase may be the primary cause; alternatively, a hemorrhage of other etiology (i.e., coagulation deficit) may have occurred, followed by BP elevation to preserve cerebral tissue blood supply. Thus, a careful diagnostic evaluation of hypertensive emergencies and urgencies is essential to guide proper treatment.

The precise pathogenesis of the hypertensive crisis is complex and incompletely understood. However, at least two integrated mechanisms are proposed to play a major role in the pathophysiology of the hypertensive crisis. The first mechanism, believed to play a central role, is the failure of the intrinsic capacity of blood vessels to dilate or to constrict in response to changes in perfusion pressure, so-called autoregulation. Thus, arteries from normotensive individuals can maintain flow over a wide range of mean arterial pressures, 70 to 150 mm Hg, associated with systolic BP of around 90 to 180 mm Hg. Chronic BP elevations, however, cause compensatory changes in the arteriolar circulation and allow hypertensive patients to maintain normal perfusion at higher BP levels.[8,9] Over time, these compensatory mechanisms may lead to a progressive inability of the arterioles to autoregulate properly.[4,10,11]

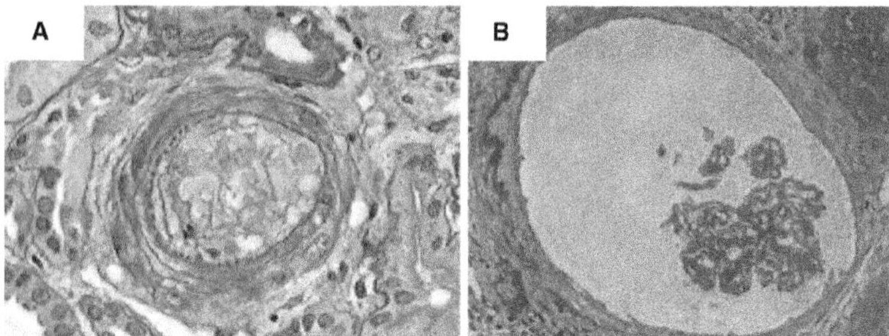

FIGURE 45.1: Hypertensive nephrosclerosis with fibrinoid changes—consequences of years of poorly controlled hypertension. **A:** Effects of long standing very high blood pressures. **B:** Fibrinoid necrosis.

The second mechanism involves the activation of the renin-angiotensin system (RAS) following kidney dysfunction and small arteriolar nephrosclerosis as a result of chronically elevated BP. This, in turn, promotes further vasoconstriction and thus generates a vicious cycle of endothelial vascular injury and sustained elevation in BP. Consequently, these harmful events increase tissue ischemia and ultimately lead to fibrinoid necrosis (**Figure 45.1**).[4,9]

Studies that examined the histologic and pathologic changes of patients with hypertensive emergency–related nephropathy demonstrated characteristic structural kidney changes described as concentric subendothelial edematous thickening (onion skin appearance) of small arteries. Fibrinoid necrosis and thrombotic microangiopathy of small arteries, albeit prevalent in many pathologic processes, are less common in hypertensive emergencies.[10]

EPIDEMIOLOGY

Despite the importance and clinical implications of hypertensive crisis, the exact incidence and burden of the disease remains controversial and varies with the population under study. Previous reports estimated 1% to 2% of individuals with hypertension develop hypertensive emergencies at some point in their lives.[12,13] A recent study investigated the incidence of hypertensive emergency in the emergency department (ED) nationwide in the period from 2006 through 2013.[14] The authors reported an increase in the total number of hypertensive emergencies by 16.2% per year from 2006 to 2013. In this study, among the diagnosis of acute organ damage, heart failure was the most common presentation followed by stroke and cerebrovascular complications.

Conversely, hypertensive urgencies are much more common and accounted for 5% of patients presenting to the ED, either because of uncontrolled BP or for some other reasons. One study found that hypertensive urgencies were prevalent in 5% of patients in the outpatient setting.[15] In contrast to hypertensive emergencies, no study has concluded that hypertensive urgencies pose a similar acute risk over short-term follow-up. However, severely uncontrolled BP over extended period portends adverse cardiovascular and kidney outcomes.[16] In a study of 120 patients with malignant hypertension and a median follow-up of 67 months, 24% of the patients developed end-stage kidney disease (ESKD) and started dialysis and another 7% had an estimated glomerular filtration rate (eGFR) decline of 50% or more.[17]

DIAGNOSTIC EVALUATION

The primary goal of the diagnostic process is differentiation of a true hypertensive emergency from a hypertensive urgency, because of the different therapeutic approaches. To that goal, the diagnostic evaluation should focus on targeted clinical history, attentive physical exam, and some laboratory examinations to differentiate the two disorders and to identify and rapidly assess the type and severity of ongoing target organ damage (**Box 45.2**). In some hypertensive emergencies, the history (e.g., acute head trauma, preeclampsia, scleroderma) or overt symptoms and signs (e.g., chest/back pain, dyspnea, throbbing abdominal mass) may guide the diagnosis, whereas in other cases (e.g., severe hypertension with altered mental status), the evaluation is more comprehensive.

Signs of secondary hypertension should not be missed in this initial examination. For example, an abdominal bruit may indicate renovascular hypertension; a palpable abdominal mass suggests abdominal aneurysm or polycystic kidneys; a radial-femoral pulse delay suggests aortic coarctation; abdominal striae and central obesity are observed with Cushing syndrome; and exophthalmos may indicate hyperthyroidism. Patients with features of hemolytic anemia and thrombocytopenia should be evaluated for causes of thrombotic microangiopathy.

The initial laboratory studies are important valuable methods to investigate and document acute organ damage. The laboratory examinations should include: (1) a complete blood count with peripheral smear, to look for a fragmented red blood cell, suggesting microangiopathic hemolytic anemia, (2) a complete

Box 45.2 Diagnostic Evaluation for Hypertensive Emergencies and Urgencies

History

- Symptoms, previous diagnoses, and treatment of cardiac, cerebral, kidney, and visual damage
- Intake of pressor agents: sympathomimetics, illicit substances

Physical Examination

- Repeated blood pressure measurements (first measurement in both arms)
- Cardiac
- Pulmonary
- Neurologic
- Optic fundi

Laboratory and Imaging Studies

- Complete blood count (red cells, platelets, white cells), urinalysis, creatinine, urea, electrolytes
- Plasma renin activity, aldosterone, and catecholamines if secondary hypertension is suspected
- Electrocardiography
- Chest radiograph
- Kidney ultrasound
- Brain CT scan or MRI
- Echocardiography (transthoracic, transesophageal)
- Thoracoabdominal CT scan or MRI

CT, computed tomography; MRI, magnetic resonance imaging.

metabolic panel (creatinine and urea concentration, and electrolyte values), and (3) urinalysis with focus on red blood cell products and casts, an important finding in acute glomerular and tubular injury.[4,18] If a secondary form of hypertension is suspected, samples for plasma renin activity, aldosterone concentration, and plasma free catecholamines and metanephrines should also be drawn *before* initiation of treatment. Electrocardiography to rule out myocardial ischemia and left ventricular strain or hypertrophy, as well as chest radiography, should be performed in symptomatic patients.[18] Kidney ultrasound is also useful to rule out abnormalities such as differences in size or perfusion, especially in patients with altered kidney function or with abnormalities on urinalysis.

Head imaging in emergency settings is best performed with computed tomography (CT) as it provides a definite diagnosis in the setting of acute neurologic symptoms related to hypertensive emergencies. Echocardiography, thoracoabdominal CT or MRI, or abdominal ultrasound may be needed in patients with suspected aortic dissection or pheochromocytoma.

TREATMENT

General Principles for Managing Hypertensive Emergencies

There is no evidence from randomized controlled trials (RCTs) to support that treatment of hypertensive emergency reduces morbidity or mortality; however, left untreated it carries a 1-year mortality rate of 79% and a median survival of 10.4 months.[19] Moreover, clinical experience demonstrates that the treatment of hypertensive emergency could limit or prevent further target organ damage. Although therapy with parenteral antihypertensive agents may be initiated in the ED, patients with a hypertensive emergency should be admitted to an ICU for continuous BP monitoring, clinical surveillance, and continued parenteral administration of an appropriate agent (**Tables 45.1** and **45.2**). The need for gradual and tightly controlled BP reduction requires the use of short-acting IV drugs (Table 45.1), the effects of which can be promptly reversed if the response is excessive. Previous systematic reviews and meta-analyses showed minor differences in the degree of BP lowering and no differences in morbidity or mortality among these agents, because of the relative paucity of large RCTs with appropriate follow-up.[20,21] Table 45.1 provides pharmacologic characteristics and adverse effects of agents that have been used in the treatment of hypertensive emergencies. Table 45.2 includes a general guide for the use of these drugs according to the type of hypertensive emergency.[1]

Understanding of autoregulation is crucial for therapeutic decisions. In most patients with a hypertensive emergency, the BP-blood flow curve is shifted to the right, maintaining reasonable tissue perfusion at higher BP levels.[9] A sudden lowering of BP into a "normal" range could, therefore, lead to inadequate tissue perfusion and ischemic events.[22] Clinical data document that lowering BP in hypertensive emergencies is beneficial: papilledema and exudates regress, hypertensive encephalopathy vanishes, pulmonary edema resolves, and kidney function improves. However, there is also evidence that abrupt lowering of BP can be harmful. For example, the use of sublingual nifedipine with potent but unpredictable BP lowering may shunt blood away from the penumbra of the brain (ischemic penumbra), resulting in a vascular infarct.[23,24] Thus, the goal of antihypertensive therapy is not to normalize BP rapidly but to prevent target organ damage by gradually reducing BP while minimizing the risk of hypoperfusion.

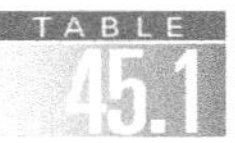

TABLE 45.1 Pharmacologic Agents for Treatment of Hypertensive Emergencies

Drug	Mechanism of Action	Dose	Onset of Action	Duration of Action	Adverse Effects[a]	Special Indications
Vasodilators						
Nicardipine hydrochloride	Calcium channel blocker	5-15 mg IV every hour	5-15 min	15-30 min, may exceed 4 hr	Tachycardia, headache, flushing, nausea, vomiting, local phlebitis	Most hypertensive emergencies except acute heart failure
Fenoldopam mesylate	Dopamine-1 receptor agonist	0.1-0.3 μg/kg/min IV infusion	>5 min	30 min	Tachycardia, headache, nausea, flushing	Most hypertensive emergencies; caution with glaucoma
Clevidipine butyrate	Calcium channel blocker	1-2 mg/hr IV infusion; increase every 5-10 min up to 16 mg/hr	2-4 min	5-15 min	Tachycardia, headache, flushing, heart failure deterioration	Most hypertensive emergencies; caution with severe aortic stenosis
Sodium nitroprusside	↑ Cyclic GMP, blocks intracellular Ca^{2+} increase	0.25-10 μg/kg/min IV infusion[b]	Immediate	1-2 min	Nausea, vomiting, muscle twitching, thiocyanate and cyanide intoxication, impaired cerebral autoregulation, coronary steal syndrome	Caution in situations associated with CNS manifestations, hepatic or kidney failure; probably should be avoided if given other agents, especially fenoldopam
Nitroglycerin	↑ Nitrate receptors	5-100 μg/min IV infusion	2-5 min	5-10 min	Headache, vomiting, methemoglobinemia, tachyphylaxis	Coronary ischemia, pulmonary edema

(*continued*)

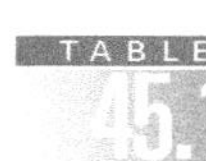

TABLE 45.1 Pharmacologic Agents for Treatment of Hypertensive Emergencies (*continued*)

Drug	Mechanism of Action	Dose	Onset of Action	Duration of Action	Adverse Effects[a]	Special Indications
Enalaprilat	ACE inhibitor	1.25-5 mg every 6 hr IV	15-30 min	6-12 hr	Precipitous fall in BP in high-renin states, variable response, acute kidney failure	Acute left ventricular failure; avoid in acute myocardial infarction
Isradipine	Calcium channel blocker	0.15 μg/kg/min IV, increase by 0.0025 μg/kg/min every 15 min. Maintenance infusion 0.15 μg/kg/min	1-10 min	1-2 hr	Headache, flushing, peripheral edema, dizziness, tachycardia	Perioperative, pregnancy
Hydralazine hydrochloride	Opens K^+ channels	10-20 mg IV	10-20 min	1-4 hr	Tachycardia, flushing, headache, vomiting, aggravation of angina	Must be given with concomitant IV β-blockers to avoid precipitation of angina. *Not* a preferred initial choice of treatment
Adrenergic Inhibitors						
Labetalol hydrochloride	α_1-, β-Blocker	20-80 mg IV bolus every 10 min *or* 0.5-2 mg/min IV infusion	5-10 min	3-6 hr	Nausea, vomiting, scalp tingling, bronchoconstriction, dizziness, heart block, heart failure	Most hypertensive emergencies except acute heart failure

Esmolol hydrochloride	β_1-Blocker	0.5-2.0 mg/min IV infusion *or* 250-500 μg/kg/min IV bolus, then 50-100 μg/kg/min by infusion; may repeat bolus after 5 min or increase infusion to 300 μg/min	1-2 min	10-30 min	Nausea, bronchoconstriction, first-degree heart block, heart failure, thrombophlebitis, COPD	Aortic dissection, perioperative, increased cardiac output or heart rate
Urapidil	α_1-Blocker, serotonin (5-HT1A) receptor agonist	12.5-25 mg IV bolus followed by 5-40 mg/hr IV infusion	3-5 min	4-6 hr	Headache, dizziness	Perioperative
Phentolamine	α-Blocker	5-15 mg IV bolus	1-2 min	10-30 min	Tachycardia, flushing, headache	Catecholamine excess

ACE, angiotensin-converting enzyme; BP, blood pressure; CNS, central nervous system; COPD, chronic obstructive pulmonary disease; GMP, guanosine monophosphate; IV, intravenous(ly).

[a]Hypotension may occur with all agents.

[b]Requires light-resistant delivery system.

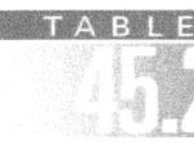

TABLE 45.2 Management of Specific Types of Hypertensive Emergencies

Type of Emergency	First-Choice Drug(s)	Second-Choice or Additional Drug(s)	Drugs to Avoid	Aim of BP Reduction
Cardiac				
Coronary ischemia/infarction	Nitroglycerin, nicardipine, clevidipine, labetalol	Sodium nitroprusside, esmolol if heart failure absent	Diazoxide, hydralazine	Improvement in cardiac perfusion
Heart failure, pulmonary edema	Nitroglycerin, fenoldopam, clevidipine	Sodium nitroprusside, enalaprilat; loop diuretics	Diazoxide, hydralazine; β-blockers	Decrease in afterload
Aortic dissection	Labetalol or combination of esmolol with sodium nitroprusside, fenoldopam, or nicardipine		Diazoxide, hydralazine	Decrease of aortic wall stress with systolic BP reduction <100-120 mm Hg in 20 min (if possible)
Renal				
Acute glomerulonephritis, collagen vascular renal disease, or renal artery stenosis	Fenoldopam	Nicardipine, labetalol, clevidipine; diuretics for volume overload	Sodium nitroprusside; ACE inhibitors and ARBs	Reduction in vascular resistance and volume overload without compromise of renal blood flow or glomerular filtration rate
Scleroderma crisis	Enalaprilat or another ACE inhibitor	ARB, fenoldopam	Corticosteroids,[a] diuretics	Decrease in BP to <140/90 mm Hg with long-term goal of <130/85 mm Hg

Neurologic			
Hypertensive encephalopathy	Nicardipine, fenoldopam, labetalol, clevidipine	Nitroprusside, esmolol, urapidil	20%-25% reduction in mean BP over 1-2 hr
Ischemic stroke	Nicardipine, labetalol, clevidipine	Nitroprusside, nimodipine, esmolol, urapidil	Reduction of BP if above 220/120 mm Hg (mean BP >130) by no more than 10%-15% within first 24 hr to avoid impairing cerebral blood flow in penumbra
Intracerebral hemorrhage	Nicardipine, labetalol, clevidipine	Fenoldopam, nitroprusside, esmolol, urapidil, nimodipine for subarachnoid hemorrhage	For patients presenting with SBP 150-220 mm Hg and without contraindication to acute BP treatment, decrease SBP to 140 mm Hg, as it is safe and can improve functional outcome. For patients presenting with SBP >220 mm Hg, it may be reasonable to consider aggressive reduction of BP with a continuous intravenous infusion and frequent BP monitoring for subarachnoid hemorrhage in normotensive patients, reduction to systolic BP of 130-160 mm Hg

(*continued*)

TABLE 45.2 Management of Specific Types of Hypertensive Emergencies (*continued*)

Type of Emergency	First-Choice Drug(s)	Second-Choice or Additional Drug(s)	Drugs to Avoid	Aim of BP Reduction
Catecholamine Excess States				
Pheochromocytoma	Phentolamine or labetalol	β-Blocker in the presence of phentolamine, sodium nitroprusside	Diuretics, β-blockers alone	Control of paroxysmal BP from sympathetic stimulation
Ingestion of cocaine or other sympathomimetic	Phentolamine or labetalol	β-Blocker in the presence of phentolamine, sodium nitroprusside	Diuretics	Control of paroxysmal BP from sympathetic stimulation
Perioperative/Postoperative Hypertension				
Coronary artery surgery	Nitroglycerin, nicardipine, clevidipine	Esmolol, labetalol, fenoldopam, isradipine, urapidil		Protection against target organ damage and surgical complications (keep BP <140/90 or mean BP <105 mm Hg)
Noncardiac surgery	Esmolol, labetalol, fenoldopam, nicardipine, clevidipine, urapidil, nitroglycerin			Protection against target organ damage and surgical complications
Pregnancy Related				
Eclampsia	Labetalol, urapidil	Nifedipine, isradipine, nicardipine, $MgSO_4$, methyldopa	Nitroprusside, ACE inhibitors, ARBs	Control BP (typically <90 mm Hg diastolic but often lower) and protect placental blood flow

ACE, angiotensin-converting enzyme; ARB, angiotensin receptor blocker; BP, blood pressure; SBP, systolic blood pressure.

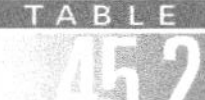

With the exception of situations requiring rapid BP reduction, the mean BP in most patients with a hypertensive emergency should be reduced gradually by no more than 20% to 25% within the first hour, then to 160/100 to 110 mm Hg over the next 2 to 6 hours.[7,12,25] Reduction of diastolic pressure to less than 90 mm Hg or by 35% of the initial mean BP has been associated with major organ dysfunction, coma, and death. If the degree of BP reduction is well tolerated, and the patient is clinically stable, further gradual reductions toward levels below 140/90 mm Hg should be implemented within the next 24 to 48 hours.

An important consideration before initiation of IV therapy is an assessment of the patient's volume status. With the exception of patients presenting with volume overload and pulmonary edema, several patients with hypertensive emergency may be volume depleted because of pressure natriuresis, and diuretics are not typically recommended; rather, fluid administration may help restore organ perfusion and prevent a precipitous fall in BP.[4] However, cautious use of diuretics could be considered after prolonged use of IV vasodilating agents (except fenoldopam) that typically cause water retention and resistance to further reduction in BP levels.

Major exceptions to these treatment recommendations include (a) patients with acute stroke. In ischemic stroke, there is no clear evidence to support immediate BP lowering, except for patients who are eligible for treatment with thrombolytic therapy or presented with extreme hypertension. In these scenarios, early initiation of treatment is recommended to avoid hemorrhagic transformations[26]; (b) patients with hemorrhagic stroke require a different approach and more intensive BP lowering. The Intensive Blood Pressure Reduction in Acute Cerebral Hemorrhage Trial (INTERACT2) in patients with recent hemorrhagic stroke showed that lowering systolic BP to less than 140 mm Hg within an hour is safe and may improve functional outcome,[27] leading to change in relevant guidelines[7]; and (c) patients with acute aortic dissection should have their systolic BP lowered to levels between 100 and 120 mm Hg.[12,18]

After the BP is reduced to safe levels over a sufficient period, typically 12 to 24 hours, allowing reestablishment of autoregulation, oral therapy can be started with continuous tapering of parenteral BP medications to avoid rebound hypertension. Typically, a calcium channel blocker (CCB), α- and β-blocker, or RAS blocker can be used, depending on the suspected cause and possible ongoing investigations for secondary hypertension.[11]

Treatment of Hypertensive Urgencies

Although hypertensive urgencies are particularly common, quality studies on the value of extensive diagnostic testing for target organ damage, the need of hospitalization, the type of treatment, and the optimal follow-up in asymptomatic patients with BP elevation are clearly missing.[28] All patients with hypertensive urgency should be provided a quiet room in which to rest because this maneuver was associated with BP fall of greater than or equal to 20/10 mm Hg in one-third of such patients.[29]

As there is no proven benefit from rapid BP reduction in asymptomatic patients without evidence of acute target organ damage, there is evidence of harm including the development of stroke and even death. Thus, most agree that BP lowering should occur over a period of hours to days. BP reduction to levels below

160/100 mm Hg may be accomplished within 2 to 4 hours in the ED with the oral drugs described later. The most important aspect of treatment of hypertensive urgency is not achieving a BP goal but rather ensuring adequate follow-up, generally within 1 week, to an appropriate site of care for chronic hypertension in order to optimize care and improve BP control of uncontrolled hypertensive patients.[4,18,22] There are data, however, suggesting that most of these patients do not receive medications or instructions in the emergency room as traditionally described in the literature and providers overestimate how often they refer patients for follow-up, resulting in questionable improvement in long-term outpatient BP control.[28]

Another major factor to consider before prescribing medication is the assessment of pain. Patients with severe pain not secondary to cardiac or cerebral origin should be given analgesics first to improve pain. If such patients present with hypertensive urgency and are given acute acting medications such as clonidine or labetalol, they could become hypotensive once pain is alleviated with nonsteroidal agents, opioids, or steroids.

The choice of drugs for the treatment of hypertensive urgencies is much broader than for emergencies because almost all antihypertensives lower BP effectively over a reasonable time (**Table 45.3**). Keep in mind that the drugs used should be ones associated with good adherence, affordable, and most likely the patient will take. Hence, clonidine, captopril, and labetalol, which must be taken three times a day, are not ideal agents. Use of once-daily calcium antagonists with a once-daily angiotensin receptor blocker and diuretic in combination in low to moderate doses is reasonable for discharge with a follow-up appointment within 2 to 3 weeks by a primary care physician.

Angiotensin-converting enzyme (ACE) inhibitors must be used with caution because they can cause or exacerbate kidney impairment in the occasional patient with critical renal artery stenosis.[9,18] Furosemide can also effectively lower BP if elevated pressure is related to volume overload, especially if kidney dysfunction is present. However, a common physiologic response of the kidney to elevated BP is natriuresis, so many patients, especially those with normal kidney function, are volume depleted rather than volume expanded.[4,18] Further, furosemide is not considered a drug of choice for primary hypertension because of its short duration of action.

As noted earlier, sublingual or oral short-acting nifedipine, although once frequently used, is now contraindicated secondary to a higher incidence of stroke, myocardial infarction, and death related to precipitous hypotensive episodes after ED release.[23,24] An exception to this rule is possibly pregnant patients with acute BP elevations, where oral nifedipine was shown to reduce BP faster than IV labetalol and without safety concerns in randomized studies.[30] Longer-acting CCBs, such as once-daily nifedipine or nifedipine XL, amlodipine, and sustained-release isradipine, do not have a role in reducing BP in the ED. However, these and long-acting agents from other major antihypertensive classes are valuable tools for long-term BP control. The most important aspects of management in these patients have already been discussed.

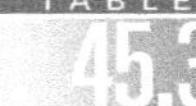

TABLE 45.3 Pharmacologic Agents for Treatment of Hypertensive Urgencies

Drug[a]	Mechanism of Action	Dose	Onset of Action	Duration of Action	Adverse Effects	Special Indications
Captopril	ACE inhibitor	12.5-25 mg PO every 1-2 hr	15-30 min	4-6 hr	Angioedema, cough, acute kidney failure	Known or suspected renal artery stenosis
Clonidine	Central α_2-agonist	0.1-0.2 mg PO every 1-2 hr	30-60 min	6-8 hr	Sedation, dry mouth, bradycardia, rebound hypertension after withdrawal	None
Labetalol	α_1-, β-Blocker	200-400 mg PO every 2-3 hr	30-120 min	6-8 hr	Bronchoconstriction, heart block, congestive heart failure	Ruptured aneurysm, arrhythmia
Furosemide	Loop diuretic	20-40 mg PO every 2-3 hr	30-60 min	8-12 hr	Volume depletion, hyponatremia, hypokalemia	Volume overload from kidney or heart failure
Isradipine	Calcium channel blocker	5-10 mg PO every 4-6 hr	30-90 min	8-16 hr	Headache, tachycardia, flushing, peripheral edema	Arterial vasospasm

ACE, angiotensin-converting enzyme; PO, taken orally.

[a]Short-acting agents that are commonly used in the emergency room setting. However, as noted in the text, sometimes longer-acting drugs can also be used.

References

1. Muiesan ML, Salvetti M, Amadoro V, et al. For the working Group on Hypertension, Prevention, Rehabilitation of the Italian Society of Cardiology, the Societa' Italiana dell'Ipertensione Arteriosa: an update on hypertensive emergencies and urgencies. *J Cardiovasc Med (Hagerstown)*. 2015;16(5):372-382.
2. Elliott WJ. Clinical features and management of selected hypertensive emergencies. *J Clin Hypertens (Greenwich)*. 2004;6:587-592.
3. Rosei EA, Salvetti M, Farsang C. European Society of Hypertension Scientific Newsletter: treatment of hypertensive urgencies and emergencies. *J Hypertens*. 2006;24(12):2482-2485.
4. Sarafidis PA, Georgianos PI, Malindretos P, Liakopoulos V. Pharmacological management of hypertensive emergencies and urgencies: focus on newer agents. *Expert Opin Investig Drugs*. 2012;21:1089-1106.
5. Benenson I, Waldron FA, Jadotte YT, et al. Risk factors for hypertensive crisis in adult patients: a systematic review protocol. *JBI Database System Rev Implement Rep*. 2019;17(11):2343-2349.
6. Hyman DJ, Pavlik VN. Characteristics of patients with uncontrolled hypertension in the United States. *N Engl J Med*. 2001;345(7):479-486.
7. Shea S, Misra D, Ehrlich MH, et al. Predisposing factors for severe, uncontrolled hypertension in an inner-city minority population. *N Engl J Med*. 1992;327(11):776-781.
8. Palmer BF. Renal dysfunction complicating the treatment of hypertension. *N Engl J Med*. 2002;347:1256-1261.
9. Kaplan NM, Victor RG. Hypertensive crises. In: Kaplan NM, Victor RG, eds. *Kaplan's Clinical Hypertension*. Wolters Kluwer; 2014.
10. Nonaka K, Ubara Y, Sumida K, et al. Clinical and pathological evaluation of hypertensive emergency-related nephropathy. *Intern Med*. 2013;52:45-53.
11. Ruland S, Aiyagari V. Cerebral autoregulation and blood pressure lowering. *Hypertension*. 2007;49(5):977-978.
12. Marik PE, Rivera R. Hypertensive emergencies: an update. *Curr Opin Crit Care*. 2011;17:569-580.
13. Chobanian AV, Bakris GL, Black HR, et al; National Heart, Lung, and Blood Institute Joint National Committee on Prevention, Detection, Evaluation, and Treatment of High Blood Pressure; National High Blood Pressure Education Program Coordinating Committee. The Seventh Report of the Joint National Committee on Prevention, Detection, Evaluation, and Treatment of High Blood Pressure: the JNC 7 report [published correction appears in *JAMA*. 2003;290(2):197]. *JAMA*. 2003;289:2560-2572.
14. Janke A, McNaughton C, Body A, et al. Trends in the incidence of hypertensive emergencies in US Emergency Departments from 2006 to 2013. *J Am Heart Assoc*. 2016;5(12) e004511.
15. Patel KK, Young L, Howell EH, et al. Characteristics and outcomes of patients presenting with hypertensive urgency in the office setting. *JAMA Intern Med*. 2016;176(7):981-988.
16. Lewington S, Clarke R, Qizilbash N, et al; Prospective Studies Collaboration. Age-specific relevance of usual blood pressure to vascular mortality: a meta-analysis of individual data for one million adults in 61 prospective studies. *Lancet*. 2002;360(9349):1903-1913.
17. Amraoui F, Bos S, Vogt L, van den Born BJ. Long-term renal outcome in patients with malignant hypertension: a retrospective cohort study. *BMC Nephrol*. 2012;13:71.
18. Agabiti-Rosei E, Salvetti M, Farsang C. European Society of Hypertension Scientific Newsletter: treatment of hypertensive urgencies and emergencies. *J Hypertens*. 2006;24:2482-2485.
19. Keith NM, Wagener HP, Barker NW. Some different types of essential hypertension: their course and prognosis. *Am J Med Sci*. 1974;268(6):336-345.
20. Cherney D, Straus S. Management of patients with hypertensive urgencies and emergencies: a systematic review of the literature. *J Gen Intern Med*. 2002;17:937-945.
21. Perez MI, Musini VM. Pharmacological interventions for hypertensive emergencies: a Cochrane systematic review. *J Hum Hypertens*. 2008;22:596-607.
22. Elliott WJ. Clinical features in the management of selected hypertensive emergencies. *Prog Cardiovasc Dis*. 2006;48:316-325.
23. Messerli FH, Grossman E. The use of sublingual nifedipine: a continuing concern. *Arch Intern Med*. 1999;159:2259-2260.
24. Chobanian AV, Bakris GL, Black HR, et al. Seventh Report of the Joint National Committee on Prevention, Detection, Evaluation, and Treatment of High Blood Pressure. *Hypertension*. 2003;42:1206-1252.
25. Mancia G, Fagard R, Narkiewicz K, et al. 2013 ESH/ESC guidelines for the management of arterial hypertension: the Task Force for the management of arterial hypertension of the European Society of Hypertension (ESH) and of the European Society of Cardiology (ESC). *J Hypertens*. 2013;31:1281-1357.

26. Wajngarten M, Silva GS. Hypertension and stroke: update on treatment. *Eur Cardiol.* 2019;14(2):111-115.
27. Anderson CS, Heeley E, Huang Y, et al. Rapid blood-pressure lowering in patients with acute intracerebral hemorrhage. *N Engl J Med.* 2013;368:2355-2365.
28. Wolf SJ, Lo B, Shih RD, Smith MD, Fesmire FM. Clinical policy: critical issues in the evaluation and management of adult patients in the emergency department with asymptomatic elevated blood pressure. *Ann Emerg Med.* 2013;62:59-68.
29. Grassi D, O'Flaherty M, Pellizzari M, et al. Hypertensive urgencies in the emergency department: evaluating blood pressure response to rest and to antihypertensive drugs with different profiles. *J Clin Hypertens (Greenwich).* 2008;10:662-667.
30. Shekhar S, Sharma C, Thakur S, Verma S. Oral nifedipine or intravenous labetalol for hypertensive emergency in pregnancy: a randomized controlled trial. *Obstet Gynecol.* 2013;122:1057-1063.

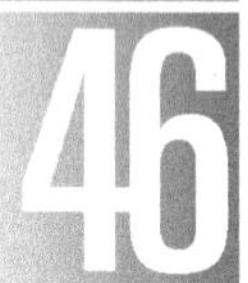

Acute Kidney Injury in Burns Patients

Anthony P. Basel, Garrett W. Britton, and Kevin K. Chung

INTRODUCTION

The care of critically ill burn patients is both complex and challenging. The severely burned are a particularly vulnerable population owing to the nature of burn injury. Burn intensive care unit (ICU) patients are at risk for developing recurrent shock throughout their course, each episode increasing the risk for organ failure and mortality. The successful management of burn injury comprises largely of multiorgan support while protecting the patient from further insult until the burn wounds are healed. Because of the complex pathophysiology and constant threat, burn injury is associated with staggering morbidity and mortality, particularly in patients who developed acute kidney injury (AKI). In the past, AKI associated with burn trauma portended an estimated mortality of 50% to 100%, with the highest mortality experienced by those who required kidney replacement therapy (KRT).[1,2]

This chapter provides insight into the occurrence of AKI in the burn population, highlights the concept of functional injury versus cellular damage, provides an overview in the resuscitation of burn trauma, and discusses the application of KRT and other extracorporeal modalities specific to severely burn patients.

PREVALENCE, STAGING, AND IMPACT

Over the last decade, validated and standardized definitions of AKI have been applied within the burn population, revealing 20% to 40% of burn patients admitted to the ICU develop some degree of AKI compared to 1% to 2% of burn patients not requiring ICU-level care.[3-5] When the Risk, Injury, Failure, Loss, and End-Stage Renal Disease (RIFLE) system and the Acute Kidney Injury Network (AKIN) criteria have been applied in head-to-head studies, it was found that some degree of AKI was present in 24% and 33% of ICU burn patients, respectively.[4,6] Interestingly, the application of the AKIN criteria identified a cohort of patients that were otherwise missed by application of the RIFLE system owing to small changes in serum creatinine. The importance of detecting early-stage AKI is delineated by the associated increased length of stays, increases in mortality, and to guide specific therapies. The Kidney Disease: Improving Global Outcomes (KDIGO) definition of AKI is even more specific than the AKIN criteria, again owing to smaller changes in serum creatinine over a larger period of time. KDIGO has yet to be validated in the burn population but research is ongoing.[7,8]

In the burn population, AKIN stage I has been shown to be associated with 8% to 12% mortality, whereas AKIN stages II and III are associated with 15% to 19% and 53% to 57% mortality, respectively.[6] Burn patients requiring some form of KRT experienced the highest mortality (62% to 100%).[4,9]

EARLY DETECTION OF ACUTE KIDNEY INJURY (FUNCTIONAL VS CELLULAR DAMAGE)

The limitations of serum creatinine and urine output for the assessment of AKI are well known, and the introduction of novel biomarkers for the detection of renal cellular injury has changed the paradigm of AKI detection. The utility of many novel serum and urine biomarkers has been assessed with respect to their ability to predict development of AKI by formal criteria as discussed in Chapter 16. Plasma and urine neutrophil gelatinase–associated lipocalin (NGAL) have been shown to outperform serum cystatin C and serum creatinine alone for the prediction of developing AKI in the burn population.[10,11] Many other biomarkers have been assessed for the detection of AKI in the burn population with mixed results, and research is ongoing.

MANAGEMENT

The largest contributor to mortality among burn patients is the extent of injured and unhealed wound burden.[12] The goal of early resuscitation for the severely burned patient is optimizing perfusion to preserve end organ function and microcirculation to the wound beds. Aggressive goal-directed resuscitation and reversal of shock allow patients to receive surgical intervention earlier when the wound beds are largest and capable of accepting grafted tissue.[13]

Many formulae have been utilized to predict the adequate volume of resuscitation needed during the first 24 to 48 hours after burn injury. At the US Army Institute of Surgical Research (USAISR), the "Rule of 10s" was developed from the principle that all of the other calculations used to estimate fluid resuscitation are applied as starting rates and that ongoing titrations should be made based on patients' response. The Rule of 10s estimates starting fluid rate in milliliters per hour by multiplying the affected total body surface area (TBSA %), to the nearest 10%, by 10 and adding 100 mL/hr for every 10 kg for those patients above 80 kg.[14] Following the initial rate, additional fluid administration is individualized based on the clinical scenario and guided by various endpoints of resuscitation such as urine output and serum lactate. The treating clinician, however, must remain vigilant to avoid over-resuscitation. A resuscitation volume larger than 250 mL/kg applied over a 24-hour period (the Ivy Index) is often cited as a runaway resuscitation and increases the risk of abdominal compartment syndrome.[15] Adjunctive therapies used to prevent a runaway resuscitation and decrease morbidity and mortality include colloid resuscitation by which 5% albumin dosed at one-third the hourly rate of the crystalloid infusion is initiated.[16,17] Another adjunct that is coming back in favor and currently being studied is the use of plasma resuscitation to limit fluid creep in burn resuscitation.[18] Lastly, high-dose vitamin C is thought to restore endothelial glycocalyx and limit edema formation and intravascular fluid loss.[19] Of note, oxalate nephropathy has been reported with use of high-dose vitamin C.[20]

AKI prevention in burn trauma centers on early and aggressive resuscitation and avoidance of kidney insult. Early detection of AKI is paramount to the management of burn victims. We believe a theragnostic approach utilizing novel biomarkers would allow clinicians to tailor therapies in a more patient-specific manner. Identifying high-risk patients could prevent unnecessary exposure to nephrotoxins such as intravenous contrast and certain antimicrobial agents and perhaps ultimately provide early identification of those who would benefit from KRT.

Kidney Replacement Therapy

Historically, the need for KRT in patients with severe burns portended a reported mortality rate as high as 100%.[5] Intermittent hemodialysis (IHD) is challenging to implement, because of the often tenuous hemodynamic status of these patients.[21] As technology has advanced and different methods of KRT have been implemented, improvement in patient outcomes has been observed.

Continuous Kidney Replacement Therapy

Continuous kidney replacement therapy (CKRT) has been adopted widely over the last decade in the burn community. It is well known and documented that continuous therapies are much better tolerated and thus more desirable for patients who are hemodynamically unstable. This makes CKRT an ideal modality for the burn patient particularly in the post-autografting period as to maintain adequate perfusion to the vulnerable newly grafted tissue.[1,21,22] The USAISR group revealed a significant reduction in 28-day mortality when comparing continuous venovenous hemofiltration (CVVH) versus historical controls, who largely did not receive any KRT (38% vs 71%, $p = 0.011$).[23] The largest multicenter observational trial that included eight different burn centers and 170 patients treated mostly with CKRT demonstrated the lowest in-hospital mortality reported to date at 50%, with a less than 10% need for long-term KRT among survivors.[22] Based on the aforementioned data, CKRT seems safe, effective, and should be considered standard care in critically ill burn patients with AKI who are hemodynamically unstable.

Initiation of Continuous Kidney Replacement Therapy

The traditional indications for KRT have been known to manifest quickly and sometimes unexpectedly to the novice burn clinician. Early initiation of CKRT remains controversial as studies in medical and surgical ICUs have been mixed in regards to its benefit.[24-26] Though readers are referred to chapter 30 on the timing of KRT, they should keep in mind that it is likely inappropriate to extrapolate these findings to the care of burn patients with AKI. An early and aggressive approach to the initiation of CVVH appeared to improve outcomes compared to those in the historical control who died prior to meeting any traditional criteria.[23] In the recent multicenter observational study, half of the patients were initiated on KRT with AKIN stage II or less. In fact, 6% of patients did not meet any criteria for AKI.[22] The synthesis of these aforementioned data suggests early and aggressive application of KRT may be beneficial in burn patients with AKI.

Continuous Kidney Replacement Therapy Dosing

A dose of 20 to 30 mL/kg/hr is considered standard in the general ICU population with AKI requiring CKRT.[27,28] High-volume hemofiltration (HVHF) as a therapy for both renal and extrarenal manifestations of AKI in septic shock remains controversial in the general ICU population. Where small single-center studies have touted the potential benefits of modulating hemodynamics, immune system responses to sepsis, removal of toxins, and other inflammatory mediators contributing to organ failure in septic shock, larger trials have failed to show benefit.[29-32]

HVHF has shown promise in critical care burn patients with AKI (**Visual Abstracts 46.1** and **46.2**). This is likely due to the profound metabolic disturbances seen in this special population. Most of the earlier reports of the use of CKRT in the burn population used higher than normal replacement doses (ranging from 30 to 120 mL/kg/hr).[21,23] A recent multicenter randomized controlled trial examined the impact of HVHF (70 mL/kg/hr vs standard doses) in critically ill burn patients. Although it was terminated because of slow enrollment, in the patients studied, vasopressor dependency at 48 hours decreased in the HVHF group, whereas it did not in the control, validating prior observations. No difference in inflammatory markers or mortality was found.[12,21,23] When considering HVHF, it is important to consider its impact on drug pharmacokinetics and electrolyte abnormalities. Also, it can be rather labor intensive for nursing and support staff given the need for frequent replacement fluid bag changes. It is important to incorporate a team dynamic to include pharmacy, extra support staff, and protocols for drug and electrolyte monitoring and replacement.[12]

We cannot stress enough that using HVHF in the burn population is very different than its controversial use in the general ICU population. HVHF appears effective in expediting the reversal of shock and severe metabolic derangements in the burn population. Further clinical trials are needed to solidify its effects on outcomes like mortality. Either way, dosing of CKRT should be individualized to each patient and their clinical circumstance. CKRT doses higher than the typical 20 to 30 mL/kg/hr may be required for burn patients with severe metabolic derangements secondary to AKI. Consider using HVHF with doses of 70 mL/kg/hr for up to 48 hours in patients suffering from burn shock and/or severe metabolic derangements.

EXTRACORPOREAL THERAPIES: A FUTURE OUTLOOK

Extracorporeal membrane oxygenation (ECMO) allows for both oxygenation and carbon dioxide removal through blood flow across a membrane and can provide partial or total pulmonary and/or cardiac support. Our experience with ECMO in the burn population has been increasing. Multiple groups have reported a favorable survival rate among critically ill burn patients with severe acute respiratory distress syndrome (ARDS) treated with ECMO.[33,34] Small polymer gas-exchange filters known as membrane lungs can attach to standard CKRT platforms, and although they cannot provide oxygenation, they can provide greater than 50% carbon dioxide removal at blood flows of 250 mL/min. This "partial lung support" may be ideal for augmenting lung-protective strategies, allowing for maximal reduction in tidal volumes in burn patients with severe inhalational injury and ARDS.[35] Blood purification has been shown to improve outcomes in some forms of septic shock.[36] Peng et al were able to show significant decreases in levels of endotoxins in burn patients using blood purification. Further studies are needed.[37] As this field grows, it is rapidly expanding the capabilities of the critical care team. Severely burn injured patients have some of the severest multiorgan dysfunctions requiring multiple extracorporeal therapies, yet survive to discharge and have functional and fulfilling lives. As technologies advance, perhaps one day we will see a multiorgan support therapy (MOST) that incorporates multiple extracorporeal therapies onto a single circuit and system that can be deployed in even remote or resource-limited areas.

Acknowledgment

The authors would like to thank Dr. John Fletcher for his assistance with formatting, editing, and reference management.

References

1. Chung KK, Wolf SE, Cancio LC, et al. Resuscitation of severely burned military casualties: fluid begets more fluid. *J Trauma.* 2009;67(2):231-237.
2. Mustonen K, Vuola J. Acute renal failure in intensive care burn patients. *J Burn Care Res.* 2008;29(1):227-237.
3. Clemens MS, Stewart IJ, Sosnov JA, et al. Reciprocal risk of acute kidney injury and acute respiratory distress syndrome in critically ill burn patients. *Crit Care Med.* 2016;44(10):e915-e922.
4. Stewart IJ, Tilley MA, Cotant CL, et al. Association of AKI with adverse outcomes in burned military casualties. *Clin J Am Soc Nephrol.* 2011;7(2):199-206.
5. Brusselaers N, Monstrey S, Colpaert K, et al. Outcome of acute kidney injury in severe burns: a systematic review and meta-analysis. *Intensive Care Med.* 2010;36(6):915-925.
6. Chung KK, Stewart IJ, Gisler C, et al. The Acute Kidney Injury Network (AKIN) criteria applied in burns. *J Burn Care Res.* 2012;33(4):483-490.
7. Clark A, Neyra JA, Madni T, et al. Acute kidney injury after burn. *Burns.* 2017;43(5):898-908.
8. Coca SG, Bauling P, Schifftner T, et al. Contribution of acute kidney injury toward morbidity and mortality in burns: a contemporary analysis. *Am J Kidney Dis.* 2007;49(4):517-523.
9. Mosier MJ, Pham TN, Klein MB, et al. Early acute kidney injury predicts progressive renal dysfunction and higher mortality in severely burned adults. *J Burn Care Res.* 2010;31(1):83-92.
10. Kashani K, Al-Khafaji A, Ardiles T, et al. Discovery and validation of cell cycle arrest biomarkers in human acute kidney injury. *Crit Care.* 2013;17(1):R25.
11. Sen S, Godwin ZR, Palmieri T, et al. Whole blood neutrophil gelatinase–associated lipocalin predicts acute kidney injury in burn patients. *J Surg Res.* 2015;196(2):382-387.
12. Chung KK, Coates EC, Smith DJ, et al. High-volume hemofiltration in adult burn patients with septic shock and acute kidney injury: a multicenter randomized controlled trial. *Crit Care.* 2017;21(1):289.
13. Rowan MP, Cancio LC, Elster EA, et al. Burn wound healing and treatment: review and advancements. *Crit Care.* 2015;19(1):243.
14. Parrillo JE, Dellinger RP, eds. *Critical Care Medicine: Principles of Diagnosis and Management in the Adult.* 5th ed. Elsevier; 2019.
15. Ivy ME, Atweh NA, Palmer J, et al. Intra-abdominal hypertension and abdominal compartment syndrome in burn patients. *J Trauma.* 2000;49(3):387-391.
16. Navickis RJ, Greenhalgh DG, Wilkes MM. Albumin in burn shock resuscitation. *J Burn Care Res.* 2016;37(3):e268-e278.
17. Joint Trauma System. Published March 15, 2019. Retrieved April 19, 2019. https://jts.amedd.army.mil/assets/docs/cpgs/JTS_Clinical_Practice_Guidelines_(CPGs)/Burn_Care_11_May_2016_ID12.pdf
18. O'Mara MS, Slater H, Goldfarb IW, et al. A prospective, randomized evaluation of intra-abdominal pressures with crystalloid and colloid resuscitation in burn patients. *J Trauma.* 2005;58(5):1011-1018.
19. Tanaka, H., Matsuda, T., Miyagantani, Y., et al. Reduction of resuscitation fluid volumes in severely burned patients using ascorbic acid administration: a randomized, prospective study. *Archives of Surgery.* 2000;135(3):326-331.
20. Buehner M, Pamplin J, Studer L, et al. Oxalate nephropathy after continuous infusion of high-dose vitamin C as an adjunct to burn resuscitation. *J Burn Care Res.* 2016;37(4):e374-e379.
21. Chung K, Juncos L, Wolf S, et al. Continuous renal replacement therapy improves survival in severely burned military casualties with acute kidney injury. *J Trauma.* 2008;64(suppl):S179-S187.
22. Chung KK, Coates EC, Hickerson WL, et al. Renal replacement therapy in severe burns: a multicenter observational study. *J Burn Care Res.* 2018;39(6):1017-1021.
23. Chung KK, Lundy JB, Matson JR, et al. Continuous venovenous hemofiltration in severely burned patients with acute kidney injury: a cohort study. *Crit Care.* 2009;13(3):R62.
24. Zarbock A, Kellum JA, Schmidt C, et al. Effect of early vs delayed initiation of renal replacement therapy on mortality in critically ill patients with acute kidney injury. *JAMA.* 2016;315(20):2190.
25. Gaudry S, Hajage D, Schortgen F, et al. Initiation strategies for renal replacement therapy in the intensive care unit. *N Engl J Med.* 2016;375(2):122-133.
26. Bhatt GC, Das RR. Early versus late initiation of renal replacement therapy in patients with acute kidney injury—a systematic review & meta-analysis of randomized controlled trials. *BMC Nephrol.* 2017;18(1):78.

27. Palevski PM, Zhang JH, O'Conner T, et al. Intensity of renal support in critically ill patients with acute kidney injury. *N Engl J Med.* 2008;359(1):7-20.
28. Bellomo R, Cass A, Cole L, et al. Intensity of renal-replacement therapy in critically ill patients. *N Engl J Med.* 2009;361(17):1627-1638.
29. Joannes-Boyau O, Honore PM, Perez P, et al. High-volume versus standard volume haemofiltration for septic shock patients with acute kidney injury (IVOIRE study): a multicenter randomized controlled trial. *Intensive Care Med.* 2013;39:1535-1546.
30. Boussekey N, Chiche A, Faure K, et al. A pilot randomized study comparing high and low volume hemofiltration on vasopressor use in septic shock. *Intensive Care Med.* 2008;34(9):1646-1653.
31. Bellomo R, Lipcsey M, Calzavacca P, et al. Early acid-base and blood pressure effects of continuous renal replacement therapy intensity in patients with metabolic acidosis. *Intensive Care Med.* 2013;39:429-436.
32. Borthwick EM, Hill CJ, Rabindranath KS, et al. High-volume haemofiltration for sepsis in adults. *Cochrane Database Syst Rev.* 2017;1:1-39.
33. Ainsworth CR, Dellavolpe J, Chung KK, et al. Revisiting extracorporeal membrane oxygenation for ARDS in burns: a case series and review of the literature. *Burns.* 2018;44(6):1433-1438.
34. Chiu Y, Ma H, Liao W, et al. Extracorporeal membrane oxygenation support may be a lifesaving modality in patients with burn and severe acute respiratory distress syndrome: experience of Formosa Water Park dust explosion disaster in Taiwan. *Burns.* 2018;44(1):118-123.
35. Neff LP, Cannon JW, Stewart IJ, et al. Extracorporeal organ support following trauma: the dawn of a new era in combat casualty critical care. *J Trauma Acute Care Surg.* 2013;75(2 suppl 2):S121-S129.
36. Cruz DN, Antonelli M, Fumagalli R, et al. Early use of polymyxin B hemoperfusion in abdominal septic shock: the EUPHAS randomized controlled trial. *JAMA.* 2009;301:2445-2452.
37. Peng Y, Yuan Z, Li H. Removal of inflammatory cytokines and endotoxin by veno-venous continuous renal replacement therapy for burned patients with sepsis. *Burns.* 2005;31:623-628.

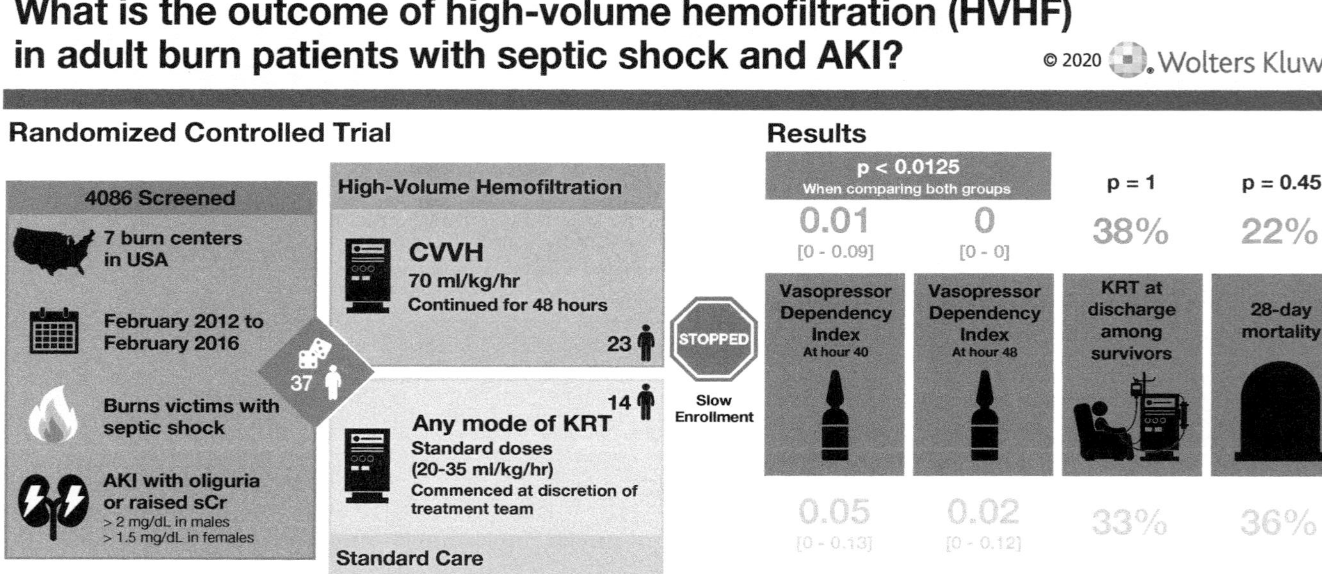

Conclusion: HVHF was effective in reversing shock and improving organ function in burn patients with septic shock and AKI and appears safe. Whether reversal of shock in these patients can improve survival is yet to be determined.

Chung KK, Coates EC, Smith DJ, et al. ***High-volume hemofiltration in adult burn patients with septic shock and acute kidney injury: a multicenter randomized controlled trial. Crit Care.*** 2017;21(1):289.

Does high-dose CVVH confer any benefit in patients with AKI and severe burns?

 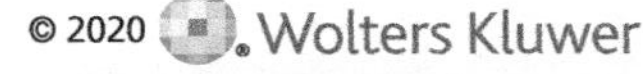

Retrospective Cohort Study

US Army Burn Center, Texas

CVVH Group		
Burns 40% total body surface area	Age	27 ± 8
AKI treated with CVVH	Total Body Surface Area	64 ± 18%
November 2005 to August 2007	AKIN 3	70%
n = 29	ALI/ARDS	55%

Control Group		
Burns 40% total body surface area	Age	38 ± 18
CVVH not available	Total Body Surface Area	58 ± 18%
March 2003 to November 2005	AKIN 3	71%
n = 28	ALI/ARDS	71%

Results

	28-day mortality	In-hospital mortality	Vasopressors at 24 hours	Vasopressors at 48 hours	Received IHD
	p = 0.011	p = 0.04	p < 0.0001	p< 0.001	
CVVH Group	38%	62%	43%	24%	N/A
Control Group	71%	86%	100%	94%	7% (2/28)

Conclusion: The application of CVVH in adult patients with severe burns and AKI was associated with a decrease in 28-day and hospital mortality when compared with a historical control group, which largely did not receive any form of kidney replacement.

Chung KK, Lundy JB, Matson JR, et al. ***Continuous venovenous hemofiltration in severely burned patients with acute kidney injury: a cohort study.*** Crit Care. 2009;13(3):R62.

VISUAL ABSTRACT 46.2

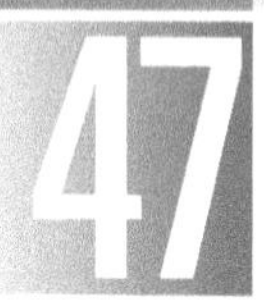

Trauma-Associated Acute Kidney Injury

Zane Perkins, Ryan W. Haines, and John R. Prowle

OUTLINE

Acute kidney injury (AKI) complicates around one in five critical illness cases following major trauma. Major trauma often impacts younger patients with less comorbidity and represents an abrupt transition from health to critical illness. Consequently, AKI in these settings may have injury-specific causes. As AKI is a marker of the severity of acute physiologic derangement caused by injuries, it is strongly associated with the risk of death. The care of trauma patients with or at risk of AKI requires consideration with regard to cause and mechanism of AKI in this setting.

BACKGROUND

Trauma is a global public health problem. The World Health Organization estimates that trauma causes 5.1 million deaths per year worldwide and is responsible for over 80 million lost disability-adjusted life years (DALYs).[1-3] Although the majority of trauma deaths occur rapidly after injury, because of exsanguination or traumatic brain injury, an important group of potentially preventable late deaths occurs, which are associated with prolonged critical illness and multiorgan failure.[4,5] In critically ill patients that survive their initial injuries after trauma, AKI is common. In this setting, AKI, which causes an abrupt decrease in kidney function, represents a heterogeneous collection of underlying syndromes.[6] Each case of AKI has a specific etiology, pathogenesis, and treatment, which may result in renal dysfunction that ranges from mild impairment to need for kidney replacement therapy (KRT). Overall, trauma patients that develop AKI suffer higher mortality rates and longer hospital admissions than those without AKI.[7,8] In addition, it remains unclear to what degree kidney function recovers after AKI, and survivors may be prone to develop chronic kidney disease (CKD) and late morbidity and mortality, something that may be of particular significance in a younger population.[9] As advances in trauma systems and care improve immediate survival, the management of organ failure, including AKI, will likely present a growing challenge to clinicians and place an increasing demand on resources.

EPIDEMIOLOGY

The development and standardization of diagnosis and staging of AKI[10] have allowed more rigorous study of its epidemiology in trauma populations, most thoroughly studied in populations of injured patients admitted to critical care units. Two recent systematic reviews demonstrate a pooled incidence of trauma-associated AKI in critically ill patients of approximately 20% to 24%.[7,8] The majority (56% to 59%) of these AKI episodes are mild (Stage 1), whereas 23% to 30% are moderate (Stage 2) and 14% to 18% are severe (Stage 3). Overall, around 1 in 10 trauma patients who develop AKI will require KRT.[7,11]

The reported incidence of AKI in the general trauma populations is more difficult to determine. Issues include greater clinical (e.g., differences in exposures and the distribution of risk factors in study populations) and methodological (differences in diagnostic criteria and how baseline serum creatinine is estimated) variability between studies. Two recent large observational studies of injured patients in London[11] and Paris[12] demonstrated an overall AKI incidence of 13%. The majority (>95%) of patients that developed AKI were admitted to a critical care unit, with approximately 58% of AKI episodes mild (Stage 1), 23% moderate (Stage 2), and 19% severe (Stage 3). In addition, a recent analysis of almost 1 million trauma cases in the United States demonstrated a 0.68% incidence of severe (Stage 3) AKI.[13]

The majority of cases (75% to 95%) of trauma-associated AKI develop within 5 days of injury, with a median time from injury to meeting AKI diagnostic criteria of 2 to 3 days.[7,11,12]

ETIOLOGY AND RISK FACTORS

Several pathophysiologic mechanisms may contribute to the development of AKI in trauma patients. Because, in the vast majority of patients, AKI develops within the first few days following trauma, this suggests that AKI generally occurs as a direct sequelae of the traumatic injury rather than as a result of other complications.[7,11,12] These early causes of AKI include hemorrhagic shock, rhabdomyolysis, direct kidney injury, a complication of massive blood transfusion, and the systemic inflammatory response following massive release of damage-associated molecular patterns. Although less common, delayed causes of AKI are also important, as many cases are potentially preventable. Late causes of AKI include exposure to nephrotoxins and complications such as sepsis or abdominal compartment syndrome.

Several clinical measures of these causal mechanisms demonstrate a strong association with the development of AKI (**Table 47.1**). For example, clinical markers of shock that are strongly associated with AKI include prehospital and admission hypotension,[7,11,12,14-16] tachycardia,[12] raised admission lactate,[11,12,17] coagulopathy,[14] hypothermia,[17] acidosis,[15] volume of resuscitation fluid administered,[18] volume of blood products transfused,[7,11,12,17,19-21] and vasopressor requirements.[12,18] Furthermore, many clinical variables associated with AKI may be markers of more than one mechanism of AKI. For example, the presence of a significant abdominal injury[7,21] may indicate an increased risk of hypovolemic shock, direct kidney injury, or abdominal compartment syndrome; and treatment with antibiotics may indicate sepsis[7] or, with certain antibiotics, exposure to nephrotoxins.[11] Similarly, a high injury severity score (ISS)[7,11,12,14,16,19] may act as a marker of the degree of tissue injury or an increased risk of hemorrhage and hypovolemic shock as well as exposure to massive transfusion. Blood transfusion has been consistently demonstrated as one of the most important risk factors for AKI in the trauma setting.[7,11,12,20] The risk increases with each unit of blood transfused in the first 24 hours following injury (adjusted odds ratio 1.08),[11,17,20] and transfusions of all components

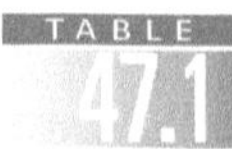

Etiologic Factors and Pathogenesis of Acute Kidney Injury After Major Trauma

Finding	Etiology	Pathophysiology	Timing
Hypovolemic shock	Hemorrhage Extravasation of plasma water	Low cardiac output Tissue hypoperfusion Secondary reperfusion injury after resuscitation	Immediate
Direct kidney injury	Abdominopelvic trauma	May be directly to the kidney, to the lower urinary tract, or the vascular supply to the kidneys	Immediate
Rhabdomyolysis	Crush injury Therapeutic embolization or vascular occlusion devices for bleeding	Hypovolemia Heme pigment nephropathy Calcium phosphate Uric acid	Early
Massive transfusion	Massive hemorrhage and consumptive coagulopathy	Heme pigment nephropathy Systemic inflammation Immunosuppression	Early
Coagulopathy	Consumptive coagulopathy	Systemic inflammation Microvascular thrombosis	Early
Intra-abdominal hypertension	Primary abdominal injuries requiring major surgery	Renal venous congestion, compression, and hypoperfusion	Early
Systemic inflammation	Direct and reperfusion tissue injury with release of *damage-associated molecular patterns*	Vasoplegia and systemic hypotension Endothelial activation and microvascular injury	Early-late
Nephrotoxins	Need for emergent radiocontrast investigations and procedures Medications including antibiotics and nonsteroidal anti-inflammatories	Direct nephrotoxic injury particular in combination with shock and systemic inflammation	Early-late
Secondary sepsis	Trauma and transfusion-induced immunosuppression	Sepsis-associated AKI	Late
Preexisting comorbidities	CKD, diabetes, chronic liver disease, heart failure	Preexisting AKI risk factors	Any

AKI, acute kidney injury; CKD, chronic kidney disease.

(red blood cells, plasma, and platelets) are associated with an increased risk of developing AKI.[12,21] Although the volume of blood transfusion is a surrogate marker of hemorrhagic shock, studies have reported that the strong association of blood transfusion with AKI over other measures of injury severity suggests additional transfusion-specific risk factors. These include exposure to products of hemolysis, plasma-free heme and iron,[22,23] and transfusion-related immunosuppression.[24] Overall, AKI is generally associated with the presence of multiple potential causal insults, and it is often not possible to differentiate the individual contribution of each factor.

Finally, exposure to iodinated contrast material is believed to be an important cause of avoidable AKI and is something most polytrauma patients are exposed to early in admission. However, there is only weak evidence to support a clinically significant causal relationship between contemporary low- or iso-osmolality contrast agents.[25,26] Meta-analyses of large mixed hospital populations demonstrate no significant difference in rates of AKI, need for KRT, or survival between patients who underwent procedures with intravenous (IV) contrast administration and those who underwent procedures without.[27,28] A recent meta-analysis in trauma demonstrated similar results, with, in fact, a lower risk of AKI in trauma patients who received contrast compared to those who did not.[7] Certainly, there is no current evidence to justify limiting the use of radiologic contrast in necessary diagnostic and therapeutic procedures in trauma patients because of concerns of contrast-associated AKI.

Baseline Risk Factors for Acute Kidney Injury

Although many trauma patients are young with few comorbidities, some injured patients may have preexisting risk factors that increase AKI susceptibility to a variety of causative insults. In the context of major trauma, older age, diabetes mellitus, chronic hypertension, CKD, obesity, and African race have all been described as risk factors for the development of AKI.[7,13,29] There is conflicting evidence on the effect of gender in the trauma literature, with reports of greater risk in females,[30] males,[7,16] or no effect.[11,20] Importantly, confounding variables such as mechanism of injury are unevenly distributed between male and female patient groups.

PATHOPHYSIOLOGY

As trauma-associated AKI is a complex heterogeneous condition with multiple etiologic factors, a number of distinct pathophysiologic mechanisms may be involved in its development (Table 47.1). Broadly, these may be divided into alterations in systemic and glomerular hemodynamics resulting in decreased filtration and/or ischemic kidney injury and local and systemic release of damage-associated molecular patterns, nephrotoxins and inflammatory mediators resulting in a local inflammatory response to endothelial injury, microcirculatory dysfunction, and tubular cell injury. Interaction between these various mechanisms is complex and occurs at the level of the microcirculation, on the whole organ, the nephron unit, and in the microcirculation. An overview of these processes is given in **Figure 47.1**; in any individual patient, differing mechanisms may apply to differing degrees and at varying stages in the evolution of AKI.[6] Understandably, given this complexity, intervention at any given downstream pathway in isolation may not significantly affect the overall course of illness.

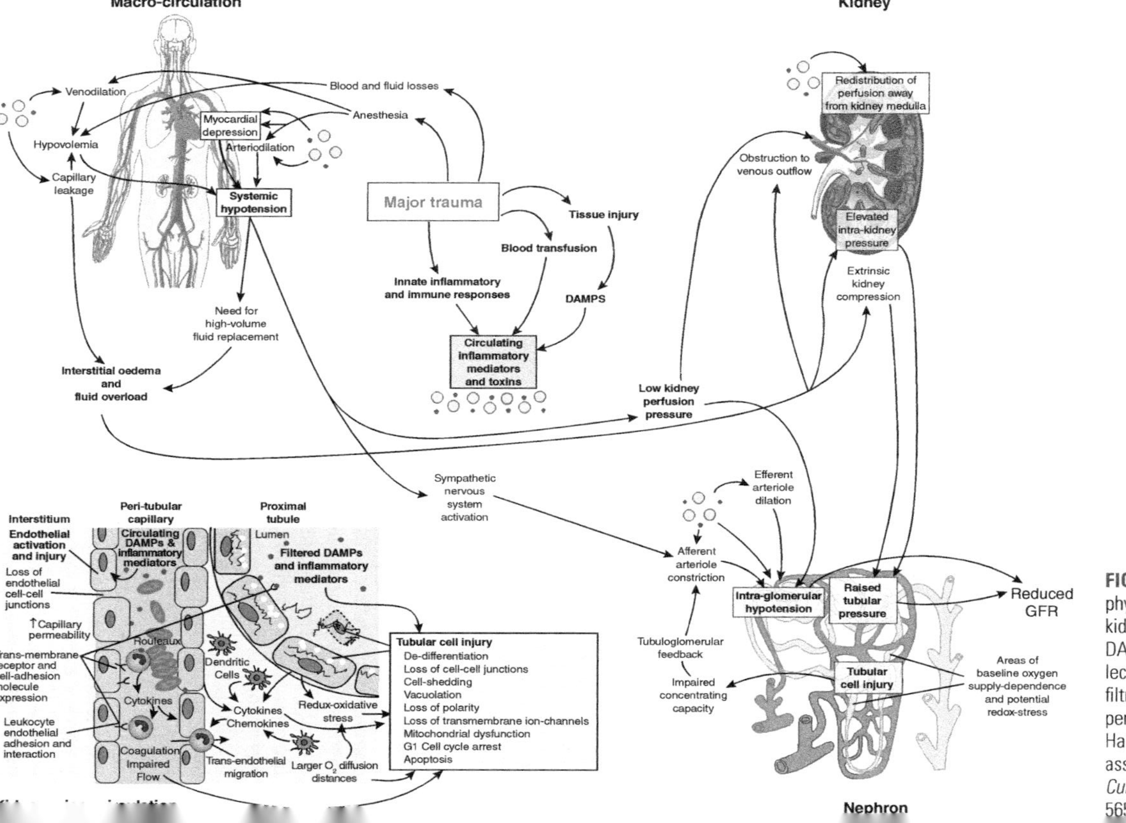

FIGURE 47.1: Principal pathophysiologic mechanisms of acute kidney injury following trauma. DAMP, damage-associated molecular pattern; GFR, glomerular filtration rate. Reproduced with permission from Perkins ZB, Haines RW, Prowle JR. Trauma-associated acute kidney injury. *Curr Opin Crit Care*. 2019;25(6):565-572.

MANAGEMENT

There are a few studies that provide prospective evidence regarding the management of trauma-associated AKI. Inferences can be made from studies examining AKI settings, including postoperative AKI; however, trauma-associated AKI has unique aspects and often involves a more heterogeneous group of critically ill patients.[31] There is, however, a well-established evidence base regarding the initial management of major polytrauma that has evolved over the last 20 years. In the time course of a trauma patient's journey from prehospital management to immediate life-saving surgery, modern trauma management including permissive hypotension, early use of blood products, and damage control surgery have been consistently demonstrated to improve prehospital and in-hospital mortality.[32,33] Thus, these necessary management steps take precedence over any AKI-specific approaches, at least initially. In developed trauma systems, hypotensive resuscitation has been shown to be associated with improved survival, and a recent meta-analysis reported no increase in the incidence of AKI when this strategy was applied,[34] suggesting this approach is generally safe for the kidney. There are little data examining blood pressure targets beyond 24 hours of traumatic injury; therefore, clinicians caring for patients after major trauma adhere to general, recommended perfusion parameters, often a mean arterial pressure (MAP) of more than or equal to 65. Vasopressors are regularly used in this phase of illness, and ongoing research is awaited to help guide the choice of vasopressors both after major trauma and in other intensive care unit (ICU) settings.

Importantly, although current AKI guidelines such as those from the Kidney Disease: Improving Global Outcomes group provide guidance on best supportive care for the prevention and management of AKI, their constituent elements are generally only suggestions with, on the whole, low-quality evidence in support.[35] This requires clinicians to adapt these measures appropriately to individual patients and clinical scenarios, which is generally after the initial 24 hours of trauma management, often when patients are managed in critical care.

Volume and choice of fluid therapy are important factors in the management of trauma patients both in early resuscitation and in later stages of management. Commonly, blood products are the preferred resuscitation choice and crystalloids are avoided.[36] As discussed previously, high-volume transfusion requirement is consistently associated with AKI after trauma. Restrictive versus liberal transfusion targets, when patients are hemodynamically stable, have been shown to be safe in other critically ill cohorts such as cardiac surgery,[37] and such strategies could be examined in trauma; however, in general, the volume of transfusion is driven by severity of the hemorrhage and ongoing bleeding rather than the level of transfusion target.

Modern trauma management restricts the use of crystalloid therapy in the prehospital and acute resuscitation setting because of the adverse effect of hemodilution on coagulation, continued hemorrhage, and oxygen delivery.[36] Recent observations have shown increased mortality in patients with more liberal use of crystalloids during the first 24 to 48 hours of admission in adult[38] and pediatric trauma patients.[39] Furthermore, there is growing evidence that more restrictive use of fluid throughout the time course of critical illness might be beneficial,[40,41] with more liberal fluid administration over the first 7 days of trauma admission being associated with longer duration of mechanical ventilation and ICU stay.[42] The adoption of more restrictive use of fluid and impact on morality and AKI is being tested in multicenter randomized controlled trials (RCTs) in patients with septic shock. If ongoing studies confirm observational associations, the application of fluid restriction to trauma patients will need appropriate investigation. Finally, when fluid is required, the use of balanced crystalloid solutions compared to normal saline, especially when larger volumes are required, is seen as a safer option in general critical care patients,[43,44] and this is likely to extend to the trauma population.

Rhabdomyolysis is a specific AKI etiology that is common in trauma patients. Current renal management follows general rhabdomyolysis protocols (see Chapter 47). Importantly, prevention and/or mitigation of AKI associated with rhabdomyolysis first involves recognition and treatment of the underlying cause (such as relief of compartment syndrome), whereas maintenance of urine output to dilute nephrotoxic exposure to myoglobin should be regarded only as an adjunct to removal of the source if possible.

Kidney Replacement Therapy

Optimal timing of KRT initiation in critical illness in general remains controversial, with continued uncertainty despite recent RCTs,[45,46] and little evidence exists to guide us in the management of trauma-associated AKI. Not infrequently, very early KRT to combat the metabolic impact of massive transfusion is required, potentially at higher than standard protocol clearance rates to achieve electrolyte homeostasis. Later in the clinical course, when AKI is overt, optimal timing of KRT is uncertain, and this is discussed in more detail in Chapter 30.

CONCLUSION

Trauma-associated AKI is common, predictable, and associated with poor patient outcomes. Overall, it is generally multifactorial in nature, with specific risks for immediate, early, or late AKI occurring in combination. These risk factors may interact in a complex fashion. Given this interplay of causative factors, the management of AKI risk in the trauma patient should focus on both optimal management of the primary source of injury and avoidance of secondary injury—particularly through minimizing avoidable nephrotoxin exposure and prevention of important complications such as sepsis.

References

1. Lozano R, Naghavi M, Foreman K, et al. Global and regional mortality from 235 causes of death for 20 age groups in 1990 and 2010: a systematic analysis for the Global Burden of Disease Study 2010. *Lancet.* 2012;380(9859):2095-2128.
2. Murray CJ, Vos T, Lozano R, et al. Disability-adjusted life years (DALYs) for 291 diseases and injuries in 21 regions, 1990-2010: a systematic analysis for the Global Burden of Disease Study 2010. *Lancet.* 2012;380(9859):2197-2223.
3. Haagsma JA, Graetz N, Bolliger I, et al. The global burden of injury: incidence, mortality, disability-adjusted life years and time trends from the Global Burden of Disease study 2013. *Inj Prev.* 2016;22(1):3-18.
4. Sauaia A, Moore FA, Moore EE, et al. Epidemiology of trauma deaths: a reassessment. *J Trauma Acute Care Surg.* 1995;38(2):185-193.
5. Sobrino J, Shafi S, eds. *Timing and Causes of Death After Injuries.* Taylor & Francis; 2013.
6. Kellum JA, Prowle JR. Paradigms of acute kidney injury in the intensive care setting. *Nat Rev Nephrol.* 2018;14(4):217-230.
7. Søvik S, Isachsen MS, Nordhuus KM, et al. Acute kidney injury in trauma patients admitted to the ICU: a systematic review and meta-analysis. *Intensive Care Med.* 2019;45(4):407-419.
8. Haines RW, Fowler AJ, Kirwan CJ, et al. The incidence and associations of acute kidney injury in trauma patients admitted to critical care: a systematic review and meta-analysis. *J Trauma Acute Care Surg.* 2019;86(1):141-147.

9. Gallagher M, Cass A, Bellomo R, et al. Long-term survival and dialysis dependency following acute kidney injury in intensive care: extended follow-up of a randomized controlled trial. *PLoS Med.* 2014;11(2):e1001601.
10. Kellum JA, Lameire N. Diagnosis, evaluation, and management of acute kidney injury: a KDIGO summary (Part 1). *Crit Care.* 2013;17(1):204.
11. Perkins ZB, Captur G, Bird R, et al. Trauma induced acute kidney injury. *PLoS One.* 2019;14(1):e0211001.
12. Harrois A, Soyer B, Gauss T, et al. Prevalence and risk factors for acute kidney injury among trauma patients: a multicenter cohort study. *Crit Care.* 2018;22(1):344.
13. Farhat A, Grigorian A, Nguyen NT, et al. Obese trauma patients have increased need for dialysis. *Eur J Trauma Emerg Surg.* 2019:1-8.
14. Ferencz S-AE, Davidson AJ, Howard JT, et al. Coagulopathy and mortality in combat casualties: do the kidneys play a role? *Mil Med.* 2018;183(suppl_1):34-39.
15. Skinner DL, Hardcastle TC, Rodseth RN, et al. The incidence and outcomes of acute kidney injury amongst patients admitted to a level I trauma unit. *Injury.* 2014;45(1):259-264.
16. Harbrecht BG, Broughton-Miller K, Frisbie M, et al. Risk factors and outcome of acute kidney injury in elderly trauma patients. *Am J Surg.* 2019;218(3):480-483.
17. Bihorac A, Delano MJ, Schold JD, et al. Incidence, clinical predictors, genomics, and outcome of acute kidney injury among trauma patients. *Ann Surg.* 2010;252(1):158-165.
18. Yuan F, Hou FF, Wu Q, et al. Natural history and impact on outcomes of acute kidney injury in patients with road traffic injury. *Clin Nephrol.* 2009;71(6):669-679.
19. Eriksson M, Brattström O, Mårtensson J, et al. Acute kidney injury following severe trauma: risk factors and long-term outcome. *J Trauma Acute Care Surg.* 2015;79(3):407-412.
20. Haines RW, Lin S-P, Hewson R, et al. Acute kidney injury in trauma patients admitted to critical care: development and validation of a diagnostic prediction model. *Sci Rep.* 2018;8(1):3665.
21. Shashaty MGS, Meyer NJ, Localio AR, et al. African American race, obesity, and blood product transfusion are risk factors for acute kidney injury in critically ill trauma patients. *J Crit Care.* 2012;27(5):496-504.
22. Rother RP, Bell L, Hillmen P, et al. The clinical sequelae of intravascular hemolysis and extracellular plasma hemoglobin: a novel mechanism of human disease. *JAMA.* 2005;293(13):1653-1662.
23. Jones AR, Bush HM, Frazier SK. Injury severity, sex, and transfusion volume, but not transfusion ratio, predict inflammatory complications after traumatic injury. *Heart Lung.* 2017;46(2):114-119.
24. Torrance HD, Brohi K, Pearse RM, et al. Association between gene expression biomarkers of immunosuppression and blood transfusion in severely injured polytrauma patients. *Ann Surg.* 2015;261(4):751-759.
25. Wilhelm-Leen E, Montez-Rath ME, Chertow G. Estimating the risk of radiocontrast-associated nephropathy. *J Am Soc Nephrol.* 2017;28(2):653-659.
26. Mehran R, Dangas GD, Weisbord SD. Contrast-associated acute kidney injury. *N Engl J Med.* 2019;380(22):2146-2155.
27. Aycock RD, Westafer LM, Boxen JL, et al. Acute kidney injury after computed tomography: a meta-analysis. *Ann Emerg Med.* 2018;71(1):44-53.
28. McDonald JS, McDonald RJ, Comin J, et al. Frequency of acute kidney injury following intravenous contrast medium administration: a systematic review and meta-analysis. *Radiology.* 2013;267(1):119-128.
29. Fujinaga J, Kuriyama A, Shimada N. Incidence and risk factors of acute kidney injury in the Japanese trauma population: a prospective cohort study. *Injury.* 2017;48(10):2145-2149.
30. Bagshaw SM, George C, Gibney RTN, et al. A multi-center evaluation of early acute kidney injury in critically ill trauma patients. *Ren Fail.* 2008;30(6):581-589.
31. Lyons RA, Kendrick D, Towner EM, et al. Measuring the population burden of injuries—implications for global and national estimates: a multi-centre prospective UK longitudinal study. *PLoS Med.* 2011;8(12):e1001140.
32. Rehn M, Weaver A, Brohi K, et al. Effect of prehospital red blood cell transfusion on mortality and time of death in civilian trauma patients. *Shock.* 2019;51(3):284-288.
33. Glen J, Constanti M, Brohi K, et al. Assessment and initial management of major trauma: summary of NICE guidance. *BMJ.* 2016;353:i3051.
34. Owattanapanich N, Chittawatanarat K, Benyakorn T, et al. Risks and benefits of hypotensive resuscitation in patients with traumatic hemorrhagic shock: a meta-analysis. *Scand J Trauma Resusc Emerg Med.* 2018;26(1):107.
35. Pickkers P, Ostermann M, Joannidis M, et al. The intensive care medicine agenda on acute kidney injury. *Intensive Care Med.* 2017;43(9):1198-1209.
36. Harris T, Davenport R, Mak M, et al. The evolving science of trauma resuscitation. *Emerg Med Clin North Am.* 2018;36(1):85-106.

37. Mazer CD, Whitlock RP, Fergusson DA, et al. Restrictive or liberal red-cell transfusion for cardiac surgery. *N Engl J Med.* 2017;377(22):2133-2144.
38. Jones DG, Nantais J, Rezende-Neto JB, et al. Crystalloid resuscitation in trauma patients: deleterious effect of 5L or more in the first 24h. *BMC Surg.* 2018;18(1):93.
39. Coons BE, Tam S, Rubsam J, et al. High volume crystalloid resuscitation adversely affects pediatric trauma patients. *J Pediatr Surg.* 2018;53(11):2202-2208.
40. Hjortrup PB, Haase N, Bundgaard H, et al. Restricting volumes of resuscitation fluid in adults with septic shock after initial management: the CLASSIC randomised, parallel-group, multicentre feasibility trial. *Intensive Care Med.* 2016;42(11):1695-1705.
41. Silversides JA, Fitzgerald E, Manickavasagam US, et al. Deresuscitation of patients with iatrogenic fluid overload is associated with reduced mortality in critical illness. *Crit Care Med.* 2018;46(10):1600-1607.
42. Mezidi M, Ould-Chikh M, Deras P, et al. Influence of late fluid management on the outcomes of severe trauma patients: a retrospective analysis of 294 severely-injured patients. *Injury.* 2017;48(9):1964-1971.
43. Semler MW, Kellum JA. Balanced crystalloid solutions. *Am J Respir Crit Care Med.* 2019; 199(8):952-960.
44. Semler MW, Self WH, Rice TW. Balanced crystalloids versus saline in critically ill adults. *N Engl J Med.* 2018;378(20):1951.
45. Zarbock A, Kellum JA, Schmidt C, et al. Effect of early vs delayed initiation of renal replacement therapy on mortality in critically ill patients with acute kidney injury: the ELAIN randomized clinical trial. *JAMA.* 2016;315(20):2190-2199.
46. Gaudry S, Hajage D, Schortgen F, et al. Initiation strategies for renal-replacement therapy in the intensive care unit. *N Engl J Med.* 2016;375(2):122-133.

48 Neurologic Emergencies in the Intensive Care Unit

Fernando D. Goldenberg, Christopher Kramer, Christos Lazaridis, and Hussain Aboud

INTRODUCTION

Acute kidney injury (AKI) and chronic kidney disease (CKD) have the potential to directly or indirectly adversely impact the function of the entire neuroaxis, from the brain down to the peripheral nerves. Moreover, the various treatments of both AKI and CKD, including dialysis and kidney transplantation, have the potential to independently induce or exacerbate neurologic injury.[1,2] Some of these associated conditions are emergencies and require prompt recognition and timely management to potentially avoid permanent neurologic damage and resultant disability (see **Table 48.1**).[3,4]

Conversely, AKI is one of the most commonly encountered pathologies in neurocritical care, with an incidence of 5.3% to 15%. The common co-occurrence of acute brain and kidney injury is associated with staggering consequences, including a higher rate of other in-hospital complications, hemorrhagic conversion of ischemic stroke, poorer neurologic outcome, and increased mortality relative to patients who sustained an acute brain injury without AKI. Although sepsis is the most common cause of AKI in the neurointensive care unit, CKD is a prominent independent risk factor for the development of AKI as well.[2,4-7]

In this chapter, we will explore the most common ways kidney dysfunction and its treatment may acutely and adversely affect the nervous system.

UREMIC ENCEPHALOPATHY

Encephalopathy is commonly encountered in patients with kidney dysfunction and can be precipitated by a variety of causes. These causes include the accumulation of toxins in kidney failure, imbalance of excitatory and inhibitory neurotransmitters, significant disruption in the metabolism of certain endogenous compounds as well as decreased transport functions, and increased permeability of the central nervous system leading to neuronal dysfunction. Furthermore, metabolites of certain drugs may be increased in uremia because of the inhibition of the organic anion transporter (OAT) importantly, plasma levels of opiates may increase because of decreased excretion.[8] Other causes of encephalopathy in kidney failure may include thiamine deficiency, osmolar shifts in the setting of dialysis, cerebral ischemia related to hypotension from dialysis, cerebral vasogenic edema (posterior reversible encephalopathy syndrome or PRES) secondary to hypertension, or electrolyte and acid-base abnormalities.[9-12] The precipitation of encephalopathy is more common in patients with AKI than CKD

TABLE 48.1 Neurologic Emergencies Associated With Kidney Disease and Dialysis

Localization	Disease	Symptoms	Mechanism	Prevention/Treatment
Intracranial, extra-axial compartment	Subdural hematoma	Alteration in mental status, focal neurologic deficits, seizures	Coagulopathy due to use of anticoagulant or uremic effect	Consider treatment with DDAVP, consider utilizing continuous dialysis, slowing or shortening intermittent dialysis, neurology/neurosurgery consultation
Predominantly cerebral cortical involvement (although subcortical tissue can be involved as well)	Encephalopathy	Confusion, depressed level of consciousness, agitation, myoclonus, asterixis	• Accumulation of endogenous toxic metabolites, hormonal disturbances, neurotransmitter imbalances • Electrolyte disorders (sodium, calcium, phosphorus), acid-base derangements • Impaired clearance of medications • Severe hypertension	Dialysis, electrolyte supplementation/elimination, avoid medications that are excreted by the kidneys, careful and gradual reduction in blood pressure
	Ischemic stroke	Focal neurologic deficits	• Comorbid vascular risk factors • Hypercoagulable state including elevated homocysteine • Accelerated atherosclerosis • Paradoxical embolus from line-associated thrombus • Septic emboli • Hypotension during dialysis with preexisting cerebrovascular stenosis	Neurology consultation, aggressive management of vascular risk factors, evaluation and treatment of line-associated complications, avoid hypotension during dialysis Consider use of systemic thrombolysis and/or mechanical thrombectomy in the appropriate patient

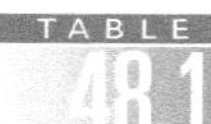

	Dialysis disequilibrium syndrome (DDS)	Nausea/emesis, cramps, encephalopathy, seizures, coma	• Reverse urea hypothesis • Idiogenic osmole hypothesis	• Identify patients at high risk of DDS (see text) and employ measures to reduce the risk of DDS (see Table 48.3) • Consider neurology consultation and osmotherapy in severe cases
	Posterior reversible encephalopathy syndrome	Headache, confusion/agitation, depressed level of consciousness, nausea/emesis, focal neurologic deficits, seizures	• Blood pressure fluctuations • Hypertension • Immunosuppression after renal transplant	Minimize blood pressure fluctuations, careful reduction in blood pressure, hold and consider changing immunosuppressive medication, neurology consultation, consider need for antiepileptic medication

DDAVP, desmopressin.

because of the rapidity of onset and relative lack of time for neural compensatory mechanisms to buffer the insult.

Symptoms and signs common to all patients with encephalopathy include changes in attention and level of alertness ranging from agitation to obtundation, alteration in cognition (including disorientation, perseveration, decreased executive functioning, and impaired memory), psychomotor disturbances (e.g., asterixis, myoclonus, paratonia), emotional dysregulation, and circadian rhythm disturbance. Uremic encephalopathy, hypertensive encephalopathy/PRES, and various electrolyte disturbances can also be associated with a lowering of the seizure threshold. In this chapter, we will focus on uremic encephalopathy, one of the most common forms of encephalopathy encountered in the acute setting.[7,8]

Uremic encephalopathy is not usually encountered until the glomerular filtration rate (GFR) drops to less than 15 mL/min, though more rapid declines in GFR may result in more severe symptoms or clinical manifestations at higher baseline GFRs. The precipitation of uremic encephalopathy is thought to result from the accumulation of hundreds of endogenous toxic metabolites in addition to hormonal disturbances and neurotransmitter imbalances. Urea, guanidine compounds, myo-inositol, uric acid, and other molecules are examples of some of the implicated toxic molecules that have been found to be highly increased in serum, cerebrospinal fluid (CSF), and brain in patients with uremic encephalopathy. Activation of the excitatory *N*-methyl D-aspartate (NMDA) neurotransmitter receptor and concomitant inhibition of the inhibitory gamma-aminobutyric acid type A (GABA(A)) neurotransmitter receptors have also been encountered in patients with uremic encephalopathy and may also explain the higher frequency of seizures in these patients.[11,12] Additionally, inhibition of transketolase, a thiamine-dependent enzyme of the pentose pathway that is important for the maintenance of myelin, is more common in uremic patients. Finally, hormonal disturbances, including increased insulin resistance and significant reduction of insulin clearance when GFR is less than 20 mL/min, increased parathyroid hormone, increased prolactin levels, and decreased luteinizing hormone production, may also contribute to uremic encephalopathy.[12,13]

Psychomotor symptoms, including tremor, myoclonus, and asterixis, are a very common feature of uremic encephalopathy, but are not specific for the disease.[7-9] Asymmetry in the motor examination, gaze deviation, or other focal neurologic findings can be rarely encountered, though they often fluctuate in severity and side. These symptoms may improve with dialysis though mandatory workup should exclude other causes for focal neurologic deficits, including stroke. Electroencephalogram (EEG) usually demonstrates background slowing, theta and delta wave bursts, and many times triphasic waves, all of which are nonspecific and may not immediately recover after hemodialysis. Brain magnetic resonance imaging (MRI) can be normal but may show increased T2 signal in the basal ganglia (see **Figure 48.1**), though diffusion restriction and T2 hyperintensities can also be sometimes seen in the cortex and subcortex. Many of these imaging findings resolve after resolution of AKI.[14]

When consistent with the goals of care, solute removal is the treatment for uremic encephalopathy and should result in normalization of clinical findings with the exception of patients with CKD who may have subtle residual long-term cognitive deficits. However, a lag of 1 to 2 days is common from the initiation of dialysis to clinical improvement. The failure of a patient with suspected uremic encephalopathy to improve several days after dialysis should prompt consideration of an alternative mechanism of encephalopathy.

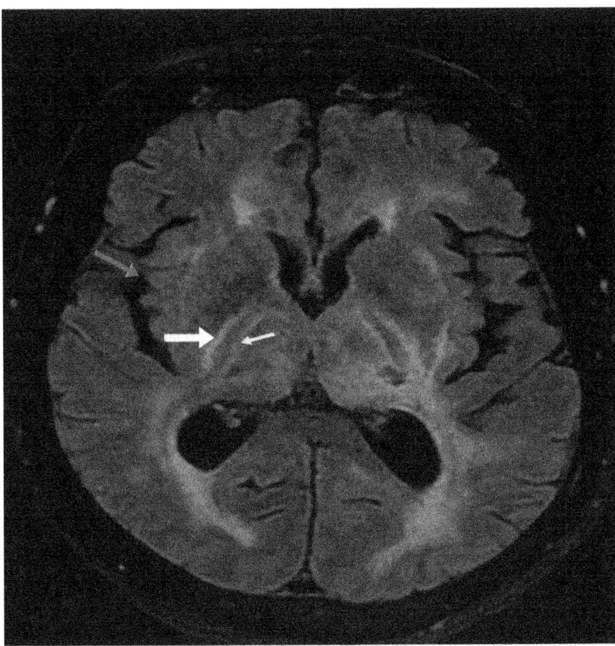

FIGURE 48.1: Axial MRI of the brain, FLAIR sequence demonstrating the "lentiform fork sign," T2 hyperintensity in the external capsule (red arrow), the external medullary lamina (white arrow), and the internal medullary lamina (yellow arrow) that outline several nuclei (putamen and globus pallidum) within the basal ganglia. FLAIR, fluid-attenuated inversion recovery; MRI, magnetic resonance imaging.

DIALYSIS DISEQUILIBRIUM SYNDROME

Dialysis disequilibrium syndrome (DDS) most commonly manifests as acute encephalopathy following (or during) conventional hemodialysis where sudden and marked osmotic shifts result.[15-17] The symptoms of DDS range from nausea and cramps to encephalopathy, seizures, coma, cerebral edema, brain herniation, and potentially death (**Figure 48.2**). The signs and symptoms associated with DDS present a temporal relationship to the development of cerebral edema and to the dialysis procedure.

Symptoms are most likely to appear toward the end of the dialysis session, as they reflect the changes in urea that occur earlier in the treatment. There is no threshold urea reduction ratio below which DDS is less likely as reductions as low as 17% have been associated with DDS.[15]

The main precipitating factors of DDS are described in **Table 48.2.**[15,18,19]

Although the pathophysiology of DDS is likely multifactorial, the most popular pathophysiologic explanation is the *reverse urea hypothesis.* According to this hypothesis, urea is unable to move freely between the extra- and intracellular spaces in neuronal tissue because of the presence of tight junctions and other components of the blood-brain barrier (BBB).

When urea is rapidly removed from the plasma water during intermittent dialysis, urea molecules are slow to move out of the cells (including neurons), and CSF which results in a temporary increase in intracellular urea concentration

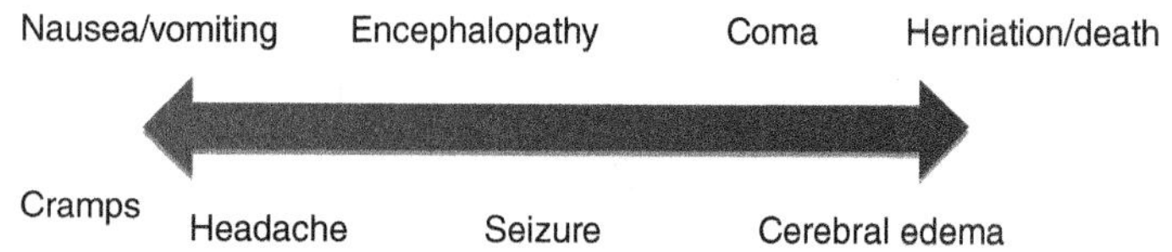

FIGURE 48.2: Clinical spectrum of dialysis disequilibrium syndrome (DDS).

relative to plasma (it can take up to 12-24 hours for the urea in the brain to equilibrate with blood). Given that the water movement through aquaporins is about 20 times faster than urea transport, water will move along the concentration gradient generated by the difference in urea concentration, passing into the brain and leading to the development of brain swelling and eventual increase in the intracranial pressure (ICP) (**Figure 48.3**).[20-23] In an elegant study, Walters et al imaged the brain of kidney patients before and immediately after dialysis and control subjects and demonstrated that those with kidney disease had an increase in cerebral volume following dialysis that averaged 32.8 mL (corresponding to 3% of the brain volume). Patients with the highest predialysis urea and greatest absolute reductions in urea typically developed more cerebral edema.[24]

Another pathophysiologic explanation for DDS is the *idiogenic osmole hypothesis*. Idiogenic osmoles are osmotically active particles created by brain cells in the context of hypernatremia and hyperglycemia (e.g., taurine, glycine, inositol).[25] In 1973, Arieff et al proposed that they would also develop during rapid hemodialysis in dogs, leading to the development of cerebral edema,[26] although it seems unlikely that the generation of idiogenic osmoles plays a significant role in the development of DDS associated with CKD.[27]

Another potential contributor to cerebral edema formation is the high dialysate bicarbonate concentration. The rapid increase in blood pH during dialysis generates a disequilibrium. As bicarbonate is charged, it can only slowly cross lipid-rich cell membranes, although in plasma bicarbonate reacts with hydrogen ions to form water and carbon dioxide, which can then rapidly cross cell membranes. Once the water and carbon dioxide are inside brain cells, they generate hydrogen ions, creating a paradoxical intracellular acidosis, increasing intracellular osmolarity further and promoting water entry and cerebral edema.[28,29]

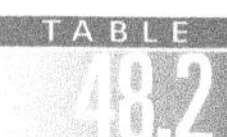

Risk Factors for Developing DDS

- First dialysis treatment
- Children
- Elderly
- High BUN (e.g., >175 mg/dL or 60 mmol/L)
- Hypernatremia
- Hyperglycemia
- Metabolic acidosis
- Preexisting neurologic disorders
- Preexisting cerebral edema and/or increased BBB permeability

BBB, blood-brain barrier; BUN, blood urea nitrogen; DDS, dialysis disequilibrium syndrome.

Modified from Mistry K. Dialysis disequilibrium syndrome prevention and management. *Int J Nephrol Renovasc Dis*. 2019;12:69-77 and Agarwal R. Dialysis disequilibrium syndrome. *UpToDate*. https://www.uptodate.com/contents/dialysis-disequilibrium-syndrome

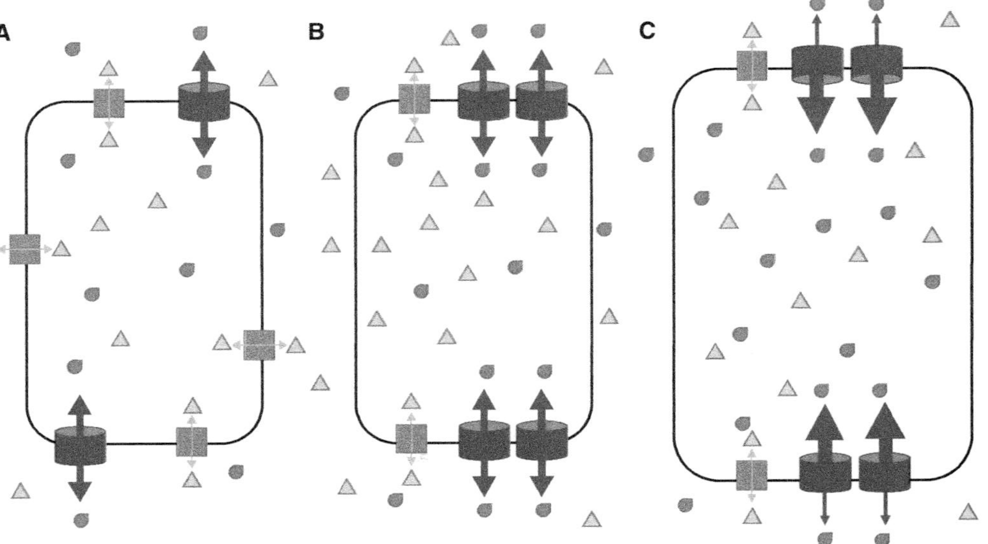

FIGURE 48.3: The reverse urea hypothesis. Under normal conditions **(A)**, the extracellular and intracellular concentrations of water (blue teardrop) and urea (orange triangles) are maintained in a state of equilibrium across the cell membrane by urea transporters (green squares) and aquaporin channels (purple cylinders). As urea accumulates in kidney failure **(B)**, the cell adapts by decreasing the number of urea transporters and increasing the number of aquaporin channels. As a result of dialysis, urea is rapidly cleared from the extracellular space. However, the downregulation of urea transporters slows the diffusion of urea out of the intracellular space and water, facilitated by the upregulated aquaporin channels, rushes into the relatively hypertonic intracellular space, and results in cell swelling **(C)**.

Adapted from Patel N, Dalal P, Panesar M. Dialysis disequilibrium syndrome: a narrative review. *Semin Dial.* 2008;21(5):493-498. doi:10.1111/j.1525-139X.2008.00474.x

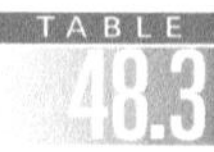

Table 48.3 Methods Used to Reduce Risk of DDS During Dialysis

- Using dialyzer membrane with smaller surface area
- Using slower blood flow rates (50-200 mL/min) or CKRT
- Reducing dialysis session time (2 hr); increasing frequency of dialysis, if necessary
- Increasing osmotically active material in the serum through sodium modeling and giving mannitol infusion during the second hour of dialysis
- Increasing sodium concentration in dialysate (143-146 mEq/L)
- Reducing bicarbonate concentration in the dialysate
- Maintaining hemodynamic stability during dialysis
- Providing solute clearance as needed and use isolated ultrafiltrate for fluid removal when feasible
- Cooling dialysate to 35°C

CKRT, continuous kidney replacement therapy; DDS, dialysis disequilibrium syndrome; HD, hemodialysis.

Recognition of patients at high risk for DDS is essential as alterations in the dialysis prescription can reduce the incidence of DDS (see **Table 48.3**).[18,19] The development of acute encephalopathy during dialysis, especially in high-risk patients, should be followed by immediate cessation of dialysis. After assuring patency of the airway and cardiopulmonary stability, administration of osmotherapy with hypertonic saline and/or mannitol should be emergently considered especially in patients that demonstrate acute clinical signs of increased ICP or brain herniation such as stupor or coma, acute pupillary abnormalities, and motor posturing response (either flexor/decorticate or extensor/decerebrate motor posturing). Brain imaging (usually noncontrast computed tomography [CT] scan of the brain is sufficient as a first step) should be rapidly obtained to assess for the presence of cerebral edema and to rule out other possible acute neurologic injuries. Invasive monitoring of ICP is very rarely required but could be considered in addition to more aggressive ICP-reducing therapies in exceptional cases without contraindications. Notation of the dialysis settings and pre- and postdialysis labs, in addition to clinical response to therapy and overall clinical trajectory, should guide the next treatment. Patients with severe DDS may need continuous kidney replacement therapy (CKRT) initially as part of their management to further minimize osmolar shifts while providing the needed clearance and ultrafiltration.[18, 19, 30-33] See **Figure 48.4** for a case example of DDS.

KIDNEY REPLACEMENT THERAPY IN THE SETTING OF REDUCED CEREBRAL COMPLIANCE OR INCREASED INTRACRANIAL PRESSURE

The cranial vault is a fixed space inside which normally resides brain tissue, CSF, and blood. The sum of volumes of these three noncompressible intracranial components is constant and is known as the Monro-Kellie hypothesis. An increase in one of the components should cause a decrease in one or both of the remaining two. Compensatory mechanisms allow for some displacement of CSF and/or blood outside of the intracranial space, creating space to accommodate an increased volume of some of the other components. Those compensatory mechanisms are limited and allow accommodation for just small-volume

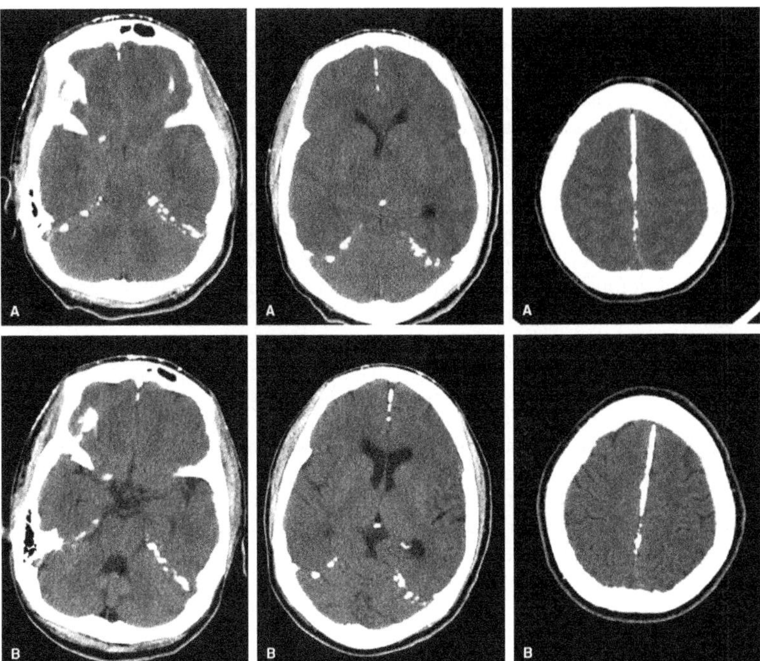

FIGURE 48.4: **A** and **B:** Axial noncontrast computerized tomography (CT) of the head in a patient with dialysis disequilibrium syndrome (DDS). A 56-year-old man with history of hypertension (HTN), diabetes mellitus (DM), end-stage kidney disease (ESKD) on dialysis presents w/encephalopathy after missing the last three doses of dialysis. Blood urea nitrogen (BUN) on admission: 212 mg/dL, Cr: 10.2 mg/dL, K^+: 6.6 mEq/L, Na^+: 138 mEq/L, HCO_3: 14 mEq/L. He undergoes dialysis and becomes acutely comatose with fixed and dilated pupils. Emergently intubated for airway protection; head CT demonstrates diffuse cerebral edema with obliteration of all the cerebral sulcus and basilar cisterns as well as bilateral uncal/downward transtentorial herniation **(A)**. He receives aggressive osmotherapy with rapid return of pupillary reactivity. Postdialysis pertinent labs: BUN: 94 mg/dL, Na: 136 mEq/L, HCO_3: 20 mEq/L. Repeat CT of the head performed 20 hours after the first one demonstrates complete resolution of the cerebral edema **(B)**. Over the course of 2 days the patient returned to his neurologic baseline function.

additions. Therefore, the addition of a significant acute space-occupying lesion, whether it is a hematoma, vasogenic or cytotoxic edema, or excess CSF because of obstructed drainage, has the potential of increasing the pressure inside of the rigid cranium (ICP).[34] The relationship between the volume of the space-occupying lesion and the degree to which it increases the ICP is not linear and becomes logarithmic after the compensatory mechanisms have been exhausted—initially, CSF and some blood can be diverted outside of the skull to accommodate the presence of a new lesion without increasing the ICP. However, as CSF and the intracranial blood volume only comprise approximately 20% of the total intracranial content, there becomes a point where the compensatory mechanisms become overwhelmed as the lesion continues to expand. When this happens, even small increases in the volume of an intracranial lesion will result in a relatively large increase in ICP. A sudden and sustained spike in ICP can potentially result in global brain ischemia by opposing the pressure driving blood flow into the brain, the mean arterial pressure (MAP), thereby reducing the cerebral perfusion pressure (CPP), which is the net blood pressure perfusing the brain (CPP = MAP − ICP).[35] Additionally, ICP gradients generated by a space-occupying mass can lead to brain herniations around rigid openings and fibrous bands that divide it into its various compartments, causing further compression and potentially local ischemia.

As all forms of KRT have the potential to precipitate brain edema, as discussed in the DDS section, so too can it cause or worsen elevated ICP. It is relatively uncommon for patients with DDS to have severely elevated ICP because of diffuse brain edema from large osmotic shifts; however, patients with acute brain injury and compromised cerebral compliance who require dialysis commonly develop intracranial hypertension during dialysis,[36-38] as only a relatively small increase in brain edema will translate to a large ICP spike.

Other dialysis-related issues can also potentially result in secondary brain injury in these patients—patients with acute brain injury are often managed with high serum sodium targets as a result of osmotherapy, which can be acutely reduced with dialysis. A relatively rapid drop in the serum sodium can precipitate an ICP crisis, compromise brain perfusion, and eventually induce brain herniation. Given that many patients that suffer intracranial hypertension have been receiving hypertonic saline solutions and are already hypernatremic, special emphasis should be placed on maintaining those serum sodium levels during and after KRT and avoiding significant fluctuations. Standard commercially available premixed replacement fluid used for CKRT contains a sodium concentration of 140 mEq/L, which is usually lower than the serum sodium in this group of patients. Therefore, continuous postfilter infusion of 3% hypertonic saline solution (Na^+ concentration of 513 mEq/L) is suggested to maintain or induce hypernatremia. There is a formula that allows for determining the 3% NaCl infusion rate = (target serum Na^+ − 140 mEq/L)/(513 mEq/L − 140 mEq/L) × desired clearance (L/hr - replacement fluid / dialysate flow rate). This formula applies when aiming at inducing hypernatremia and not necessarily when the same degree of an already established hypernatremia needs to be maintained. Also, this formula considers only the flow rate of either replacement or hemodialysis fluid and the one of hypertonic saline. The separate effect of all other intravenous fluids that contribute to the final electrolyte and water delivery must also be considered. We recommend that serum Na^+ concentration in these circumstances should be checked every 4 to 6 hours and corrected accordingly.[39,40]

Additionally, thrombocytopenia and inhibition of platelet aggregation are common complications of AKI, dialysis, and kidney disease, which can be problematic in patients with intracranial hemorrhage. Although platelet dysfunction has been described in these patients, the roles of quantification of the defect and corrective measures in patients with intracranial bleeding have not been investigated exhaustively. In patients who require a surgical intracranial procedure and present evidence of platelet dysfunction, attempts at correction can be done using desmopressin. The effect of desmopressin usually lasts 4 to 8 hours and tachyphylaxis typically develops after the second dose.

Furthermore, hospitalized patients with acute brain injury have high rates of deep venous thrombosis and thromboembolism, which can be further exacerbated by the need for large-bore central venous access for KRT. As the venous drainage of the brain occurs predominantly through the internal jugular (IJ) veins, any impediment to this drainage can result in increased ICP from the ensuing backup of blood inside the skull. For this reason, IJ lines, which are commonly used in other settings, are typically avoided if a temporary dialysis catheter is needed.

Finally, a sudden drop in the MAP associated with dialysis can result in a decrease in CPP and potential cerebral ischemia, even if the ICP is in the normal range. In patients in whom cerebral autoregulation is preserved, drops in the MAP will promote cerebral vasodilatation in order to maintain a normal cerebral blood flow (CBF). That vasodilatation leads to an increase in the intracranial blood volume (one of the three intracranial components) that can promote or exacerbate intracranial hypertension, compromising the CPP even further.

In a small retrospective study comparing intermittent hemodialysis (IHD) with CKRT in patients with acute brain injury, ICP was elevated with both modalities; however, the ICP peak was reached earlier with IHD in comparison with CKRT (75 vs 375 minutes after initiation of the treatment, respectively).[41] However, in the majority of the literature and our own experience, the use of CKRT has been associated with less frequent and less severe elevations of the ICP in patients with acute brain injury and ICP monitoring. We suggest using CKRT in those patients with suspected low cerebral compliance or elevated ICP. The latest guidelines for the management of severe traumatic brain injury use a threshold of 22 mm Hg of ICP to indicate treatment of intracranial hypertension.[42]

Additionally, dialysate with the highest sodium concentration should be utilized and the administration of hypertonic saline should be initiated or increased if there is a desire to maintain the serum sodium level higher than the dialysis bath.

There are no clear guidelines on when to transition from CKRT to IKRT in patients with acute brain injury. Under ideal circumstances, that transition can be tried while an ICP monitor is still in place and once the intracranial hypertension has resolved and the cerebral compliance is permissive. Transitioning under those conditions will allow the clinician to observe the clinical and ICP behavior as well as the patient's tolerance to that change and also act immediately if ICP elevations are detected. We suggest a careful and conservative approach whenever possible.

References

1. Ali T, Khan I, Simpson W, et al. Incidence and outcomes in acute kidney injury: a comprehensive population-based study. *J Am Soc Nephrol.* 2007;18:1292-1298.
2. Covic A, Schiller A, Mardare NG, et al. The impact of acute kidney injury on short-term survival in an eastern European population with stroke. *Nephrol Dial Transplant.* 2008;23:2228-2234.
3. Khatri M, Himmelfarb J, Adams D, Becker K, Longstreth WT, Tirschwell DL. Acute kidney injury is associated with increased hospital mortality after stroke. *J Stroke Cerebrovasc Dis.* 2014;23(1):25-30.
4. Tsagalis G, Akrivos T, Alevizaki M, et al. Long-term prognosis of acute kidney injury after first acute stroke. *Clin J Am Soc Nephrol.* 2009;4:616-622.
5. Bagshaw SM, George C, Bellomo R. Early acute kidney injury and sepsis: a multicentre evaluation. *Crit Care.* 2008;12:R47.
6. Büttner S, Stadler A, Mayer C, et al. Incidence, risk factors, and outcome of acute kidney injury in neurocritical care. *J Intensive Care Med.* 2020;35(4):338-346.
7. Mahoney CA, Arieff AI. Uremic encephalopathies: clinical, biochemical, and experimental features. *Am J Kidney Dis.* 1982;2(3):324-336.
8. Seifter JL, Samuels MA. Uremic encephalopathy and other brain disorders associated with renal failure. *Semin Neurol.* 2011;31:139-143.
9. Kunze K. Metabolic encephalopathies. *J Neurol.* 2002;249(9):1150-1159.

10. Hou SH, Bushinsky DA, Wish JB, Cohen JJ, Harrington JT. Hospital-acquired renal insufficiency: a prospective study. *Am J Med.* 1983;74(2):243-248.
11. Guisado R, Arieff AI, Massry SG, Lazarowitz V, Kerian A. Changes in the electroencephalogram in acute uremia. Effects of parathyroid hormone and brain electrolytes. *J Clin Invest.* 1975;55(4):738-745.
12. Vanholder R, De Smet R, Glorieux G, et al; European Uremic Toxin Work Group. Review on uremic toxins: classification, concentration, and interindividual variability. *Kidney Int.* 2003;63(5):1934-1943.
13. De Deyn PP, D'Hooge R, Van Bogaert PP, Marescau B. Endogenous guanidino compounds as uremic neurotoxins. *Kidney Int Suppl.* 2001;78:S77-S83.
14. Kim DM, Lee IH, Song CJ. Uremic encephalopathy: MR imaging findings and clinical correlation. *Am J Neuroradiol.* 2016;37:1604-1609.
15. Lopez-Almaraz E, Correa-Rotter R. Dialysis disequilibrium syndrome and other treatment complications of extreme uremia: a rare occurrence yet not vanished. *Hemodial Int.* 2008;12:301-306.
16. United States Renal Data System. *2018 USRDS Annual Data Report. Epidemiology of Kidney Disease in the United States.* National Institutes of Health, National Institute of Diabetes and Digestive and Kidney Diseases; 2018.
17. Dalia T, Tuffaha AM. Dialysis disequilibrium syndrome leading to sudden brain death in a chronic hemodialysis patient. *Hemodial Int.* 2018;22(3):E39-E44.
18. Mistry K. Dialysis disequilibrium syndrome prevention and management. *Int J Nephrol Renovasc Dis.* 2019;12:69-77.
19. Meyer TW, Hostetter TH. Approaches to uremia. *JASN.* 2014:25(10):2151-2158.
20. Schoolar JC, Barlow CF, Roth LJ. The penetration of carbon-14 urea into cerebrospinal fluid and various areas of the cat brain. *J Neuropathol Exp Neurol.* 1960;19:216-227.
21. Kleeman CR, Davson H, Levin E. Urea transport in the central nervous system. *Am J Physiol.* 1962;203:739-747.
22. Rosen SM, O'Connor K, Shaldon S. Haemodialysis disequilibrium. *Br Med J.* 1964;2(5410):672-675.
23. Arieff AI, Kleeman CR. Studies on mechanisms of cerebral edema in diabetic comas. Effects of hyperglycemia and rapid lowering of plasma glucose in normal rabbits. *J Clin Invest.* 1973;52(3):571-583.
24. Walters RJL, Fox NC, Crum WR, Taube D, Thomas DJ. Haemodialysis and cerebral oedema. *Nephron.* 2001;87:143-147.
25. Lien YH, Shapiro JI, Chan L. Effects of hypernatremia on organic brain osmoles. *J Clin Invest.* 1990;85(5):1427-1435.
26. Arieff AI, Massry SG, Barrientos A, Kleeman CR. Brain water and electrolyte metabolism in uremia: effects of slow and rapid hemodialysis. *Kidney Int.* 1973;4(3):177-187.
27. Silver SM. Cerebral edema after rapid dialysis is not caused by an increase in brain organic osmolytes. *J Am Soc Nephrol.* 1995;6(6):1600-1606.
28. Tratchtman H, Futterweit S, Tonidandel W, Gullans SR. The role of organic osmolytes in the cerebral cell volume regulatory response to acute and chronic renal failure. *J Am Soc Nephrol.* 1993;3(12):1913-1919.
29. Posner JB, Plum F. Spinal-fluid pH and neurologic symptoms in systemic acidosis. *N Engl J Med.* 1967;277(12):605-613.
30. Davenport A. Practical guidance for dialyzing a hemodialysis patient following acute brain injury. *Hemodial Int.* 2008;12:307-312.
31. Davenport A. Renal replacement therapy for the patient with acute traumatic brain injury and severe acute kidney injury. *Contrib Nephrol.* 2007;156:333-339.
32. Port FK, Johnson WJ, Klass DW. Prevention of dialysis disequilibrium syndrome by use of high sodium concentration in the dialysate. *Kidney Int.* 1973;3(5):327-333.
33. Bagshaw SM, Peets AD, Hameed M, Boiteau PJ, Laupland KB, Doig CJ. Dialysis disequilibrium syndrome: brain death following hemodialysis for metabolic acidosis and acute renal failure—a case report. *BMC Nephrol.* 2004;5:9.
34. Macintyre I. A hotbed of medical innovation: George Kellie (1770-1829), his colleagues at Leith and the Monro-Kellie doctrine. *J Med Biogr.* 2014;22(2):93-100.
35. Rosner MJ, Rosner SD, Johnson AH. Cerebral perfusion pressure: management protocol and clinical results. *J Neurosurg.* 1995;83:949-962.
36. Kumar A, Cage A, Dhar R. Dialysis induced worsening of cerebral edema in intracranial hemorrhage: a case series and clinical perspective. *Neurocrit Care.* 2015;22(2):283-287.
37. Kennedy AC, Linton AL, Luke RG, Renfrew S, Dinwoodie A. The pathogenesis and prevention of cerebral dysfunction during dialysis. *Lancet.* 1964;1(733):790-793.

38. Davenport A. Changing the hemodialysis prescription for hemodialysis patients with subdural and intracranial hemorrhage. *Hemodial Int.* 2013;17:S22-S27.
39. Yessayan L, Frinak S, Szamosfalvi B. Continuous renal replacement therapy for the management of acid-base and electrolyte imbalances in acute kidney injury. *Adv Chronic Kidney Dis.* 2016;23(3):203-210
40. Fulop T, Zsom L, Rodriguez RD, Chabrier-Rosello JO, Hamrahian M, Koch CA. Therapeutic hypernatremia management during continuous renal replacement therapy with elevated intracranial pressures and respiratory failure. *Rev Endocr Metab Disord.* 2019;20:65-75.
41. Lund A, Damholt MB, Wiis J, Kelsen J, Strange DG, Møller K. Intracranial pressure during hemodialysis in patients with acute brain injury. *Acta Anaesthesiol Scan.* 2019;63:493-499.
42. Carney N, Totten AM, O'Reilly C, et al. Guidelines for the management of severe traumatic brain injury, fourth edition. *Neurosurgery.* 2017;80(1):6-15.

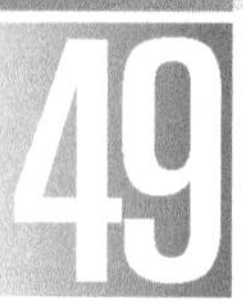

Rhabdomyolysis

Maria Clarissa Tio and Gearoid M. McMahon

INTRODUCTION

Rhabdomyolysis is a syndrome due to skeletal muscle necrosis and the subsequent release of intracellular contents into the circulation. Patients present with altered electrolytes, increased creatine kinase (CK), lactate dehydrogenase (LDH), alanine aminotransferase (ALT), aspartate aminotransferase (AST), and myoglobin. Myoglobin is a 17-kDa oxygen carrier[1] that is implicated in the pathogenesis of rhabdomyolysis-associated acute kidney injury (AKI).[2-4] Rhabdomyolysis was first reported in 1940 by Bywaters and Beall, who detailed the clinical course of four patients crushed by collapsed buildings during World War II.[5] These four victims, rescued at various time points, presented with significant limb trauma, volume depletion, shock, nausea, vomiting, fevers, serum chemistry abnormalities, and swollen limbs, with impairments in sensation, temperature, and pulsation. Notably, all four of them developed oligoanuria, three were reported to have electrocardiogram changes (such as widened QRS, Q waves, T-wave changes, and bundle branch block), and all died with "nitrogen retention." Autopsies showed pigmented casts obstructing the renal tubules. Moreover, the authors noted the similarity between this pathology and with those who had received mismatched blood transfusions or who had eclampsia. In the 1970s, nontraumatic causes of rhabdomyolysis were also recognized.[6,7]

PATHOPHYSIOLOGY OF ACUTE KIDNEY INJURY IN RHABDOMYOLYSIS

The mechanism by which rhabdomyolysis leads to AKI is not certain; therefore, several processes have been implicated, including vasoconstriction within the kidney and ischemic tubular injury, cast formation, and myoglobin-induced direct tubular toxicity (**Table 49.1**).[2,3,8,9] Renal vasoconstriction is universal in patients with rhabdomyolysis and results from a combination of systemic and local factors. Volume depletion as a result of edema and third spacing in necrotic muscles leads to the activation of the renin-angiotensin system and sympathetic nervous system. Muscle necrosis releases endogenous toxins and cytokines into the circulation, contributing to renal vasoconstriction, whereas locally, myoglobin appears to scavenge nitric oxide, an endogenous vasodilator.[8,10,11]

Brown pigmented casts were noted in autopsy specimens from the first identified patients with rhabdomyolysis. These acellular casts result from the precipitation of myoglobin with Tamm-Horsfall proteins. For this to occur, there needs to be an increase in myoglobin concentration in the renal tubules (usually as a result of volume depletion with consequent reduced renal blood flow and increased production by damaged skeletal muscle cells) and an acidic urinary environment that favors precipitation.[3,4,9] These casts cause kidney injury by two mechanisms: tubular obstruction leading to a reduction in glomerular filtration rate (GFR) and

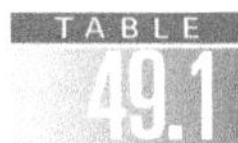

Potential Mechanisms of Rhabdomyolysis-Induced Acute Kidney Injury

Vasoconstriction within the Kidney and Ischemic Tubular Injury	Cast Formation	Myoglobin-Induced Direct Tubular Toxicity
Muscle necrosis leads to third spacing, release of endotoxins and cytokines, and volume depletion.	Results from the interaction of Tamm-Horsfall proteins with myoglobin. Formation of casts is enhanced by renal vasoconstriction and low tubular pH.	Heme component of myoglobin is implicated in ischemic tubular injury, ATP depletion, oxidative stress, and lipid peroxidation.
Hypovolemia results in the activation of RAAS, leading to renal vasoconstriction.	Cast formation leads to tubular obstruction, thus increasing intraluminal pressure and decreasing glomerular filtration.	Myoglobin-induced tubular toxicity is exacerbated by hypovolemia and aciduria.
Hastens cast formation and worsens the myoglobin-induced tubular toxicity		

ATP, adenosine triphosphate; RAAS, renin-angiotensin-aldosterone system.

direct tubular toxicity contributing to the development of acute tubular necrosis.[8,12,13] It is unclear if myoglobin itself is directly nephrotoxic, but some studies have suggested that there may be some direct myoglobin-induced tubular toxicity through lipid peroxidation, inflammation, and oxidative injury.[8,14,15]

ETIOLOGIES OF RHABDOMYOLYSIS

Table 49.2 lists the eight major categories of injury that lead to rhabdomyolysis.[2-4,9] The outcome of rhabdomyolysis is highly dependent on the underlying cause, and thus establishing the etiology at the time of presentation is key to help

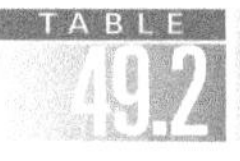

Common Causes of Rhabdomyolysis

Physical causes	Endocrinopathies and rheumatologic causes	Infections
Crush syndrome	Adrenal insufficiency	Influenza A and B viruses
Trauma	Hypothyroidism	Coxsackievirus
Strenuous/prolonged exercise	Hyperaldosteronism	Epstein-Barr virus
Alcohol withdrawal syndrome	Diabetic ketoacidosis	Herpes virus
Overuse of involuntary muscles—seizures and status asthmaticus	Hyperosmolarity	Human immunodeficiency virus
Severe agitation	Dermatomyositis	*Legionella*
Electrocution	Polymyositis	*Streptococcus pyogenes*
		Staphylococcus aureus
		Clostridium
		Salmonella
		Falciparum malaria

(*continued*)

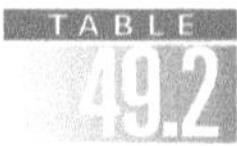

Common Causes of Rhabdomyolysis (*continued*)

Muscle ischemia/ hypoxia	Changes in body temperature	Electrolyte abnormalities
Limb occlusion from prolonged immobilization Pressure-related muscle injury in obese patients or nonobese patients undergoing prolonged surgeries Arterial or venous thrombosis Diffuse vascular occlusion (e.g., sickle cell, vasculitis) Compartment syndrome Carbon monoxide exposure Cyanide exposure	Hypothermia Heat stroke Malignant hyperthermia Neuroleptic malignant syndrome (quetiapine, aripiprazole)	Hypophosphatemia Hypokalemia Hypocalcemia Hyponatremia
Genetic defects and disorders of metabolism	**Drugs and toxins**	
Disorders of glycolysis or glycogenolysis Disorders of lipid metabolism Mitochondrial disorders G6PD deficiency Myoadenylate deaminase deficiency McArdle disease	Statins and fibrates, especially when taken with cytochrome P450 inhibitors such as cyclosporine, warfarin, amiodarone, azole antifungals, and calcium channel blockers Propofol Daptomycin Alcohol (immobilization, malnutrition, electrolyte abnormalities) Heavy metals Heroin Cocaine Amphetamine/ methamphetamine Bath salts (mephedrone, methylenedioxypyrovalerone) Organic toxins from bees, wasps, hornets, ants, centipedes, scorpions, brown recluse spiders	

G6PD, glucose-6-phosphate dehydrogenase.

determine the need for aggressive fluid management. New causes of rhabdomyolysis are being identified regularly with the development of synthetic recreational drugs and new tools in diagnosing genetic and metabolic diseases.

CLINICAL FEATURES

Although rhabdomyolysis is classically characterized by the triad of muscle pain, weakness, and dark urine, less than 50% of cases present with muscle pain. Moreover, objective physical examination findings, such as muscle tenderness and swelling, are seen in less than 10% of cases. When swelling of the muscles does occur, it is usually seen after fluid administration.[16]

Rhabdomyolysis is diagnosed by an increase in the serum CK, myoglobin, and other muscle enzymes. Owing to its slow clearance and degradation, CK is a more reliable marker of the presence and extent of muscle injury compared to myoglobin.[2] A specific CK cutoff value has not been established; however, an arbitrary value used in the diagnosis of rhabdomyolysis is a CK level 5 times the upper limit of normal.[4,16-18] It should be noted that CK is a poor predictor of AKI in rhabdomyolysis. Levels greater than 40,000 U/L are associated with an increased risk of AKI[19]; although AKI can be seen at lower levels, this is often in the context of other systemic disorders, such as sepsis or recent surgery, and is not necessarily primarily due to myoglobin-induced kidney injury.

The metabolic derangements seen in rhabdomyolysis are a consequence of the release of intracellular contents of necrotic muscle and their accumulation in the setting of reduced clearance secondary to kidney failure. These include hyperkalemia, hyperphosphatemia, hyperuricemia from nucleoside release, hypermagnesemia, elevated LDH, and high anion gap metabolic acidosis (lactic acid, phosphates, and other organic anions).[2-4] Interestingly, the development of hypocalcemia in these patients is independent of kidney function, but rather a consequence of calcium binding to damaged muscle. This has important clinical implications because as the injury resolves, calcium is released from the muscle, which can lead to significant hypercalcemia and even metastatic calcification. This is exacerbated by an increase in 1,25-dihydroxyvitamin D production.[20,21] Thus, overly aggressive calcium supplementation during the hypocalcemic phase should be avoided.[2]

A urine dipstick test (UDT) is a useful screening test for rhabdomyolysis. Over 80% of cases have been reported to be positive for blood in the UDT.[7,22] The peroxidase agent reacts with heme, a compound contained in both hemoglobin and myoglobin, leading to a false-positive test for the presence of blood.[23] In a retrospective study of 1,796 patients with rhabdomyolysis, 85% had a blood-positive UDT, whereas only half had red blood cells (RBCs) identified on urine sediment analysis.[22] Thus, it is an excellent screening test for rhabdomyolysis, and a blood-positive UDT in the absence of RBCs should prompt further investigation. From a diagnostic perspective, UDT can be a reliable predictor of the absence of myoglobinuria.[23]

Although myoglobin in the urine can be detected and quantified, its clinical utility is unclear, especially in its role in AKI prediction, and so routine testing is not recommended.[24] Pigmented casts are classically seen in the urine sediment, particularly in patients with significant AKI, but are not specific for the diagnosis of rhabdomyolysis. They may have a role in predicting prognosis in patients with AKI.[25]

PROGNOSIS

The outcomes of rhabdomyolysis vary widely from being benign and asymptomatic to life-threatening electrolyte abnormalities, such as AKI, including the need for kidney replacement therapy (KRT), and death. Among hospitalized patients with rhabdomyolysis, 13% to 50% develop AKI, 4% to 13% require KRT, and 1.7% to 46% die during the hospitalization.[4,9,17,19,26-28] In-hospital mortality rates are significantly higher in rhabdomyolysis patients who develop AKI compared to those who remain AKI free (22%-62% vs 7%-18%).[19,28] Although an elevated CK suggests the presence of rhabdomyolysis, the degree of its elevation alone is a weak predictor of the development of AKI and the need for KRT[16,17,28] and may also be dependent on the clinical context. In a study of exercise-induced rhabdomyolysis among 203 healthy volunteers tasked to perform 50 maximal eccentric contractions of the elbow flexor muscle, the mean CK 4 days following exercise was 6,400 U/L, and no kidney impairment was found even among participants with CK levels above 10,000 U/L.[29]

The Rhabdomyolysis Risk Score is a risk prediction score for the composite outcome of KRT and in-hospital mortality (**Table 49.3**). Important clinical variables that predict these outcomes include age, female sex, etiology of rhabdomyolysis, initial creatine, initial CK within 72 hours of admission, and serum

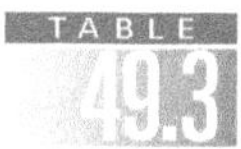

TABLE 49.3 The Rhabdomyolysis Risk Score

Variable	Score
Age, in years	
>50 to <70	1.5
>70 to <80	2.5
>80	3
Female sex	1
Initial creatinine	
1.4-2.2 mg/dL (124-195 μmol/L)	1.5
>2.2 mg/dL (>195 μmol/L)	3
Initial calcium <7.5 mg/dL (<1.88 mmol/L)	2
Initial CPK >40,000 U/L	2
Origin not seizures, syncope, exercise, statins, or myositis	3
Initial phosphate	
4.0-5.4 mg/dL (1.0-1.4 mmol/L)	1.5
>5.4 mg/dL (>1.4 mmol/L)	3
Initial bicarbonate <19 mEq/L (19 mmol/L)	2

A score of <5 confers a 2.3% risk of death or KRT requirement, whereas a score>10 confers a 61.2% risk of death or KRT.

CPK, creatine phosphokinase; KRT, kidney replacement therapy.

Source: McMahon GM, Zeng X, Waikar SS. A risk prediction score for kidney failure or mortality in rhabdomyolysis. *JAMA Intern Med.* 2013;173(19):1821-1828. doi:10.1001/jamainternmed.2013.9774

concentrations of phosphate, calcium, and bicarbonate. With a score of 5 as the cutoff, the McMahon score has a 97% negative predictive value and 29.6% positive predictive value for the composite outcome of KRT and death. Every 1 point increase in the score is associated with almost 1.5 times the increase in odds of developing these outcomes.[19] This score was validated in a retrospective study of patients with rhabdomyolysis in the intensive care unit (ICU) setting and found that a score of 6 on admission was 83% sensitive and 55% specific for the prediction of need for KRT.[28]

MANAGEMENT

Medical Management

The cornerstones of medical management include cessation or reversal of the cause of rhabdomyolysis to prevent further skeletal muscle injury, prevention of kidney injury, and treatment of life-threatening metabolic complications. Aggressive resuscitation with intravenous fluids is vital because patients with rhabdomyolysis are usually significantly volume depleted from water sequestration into injured muscles.[3] At present, there is no clear evidence of which resuscitation fluid is more superior in rhabdomyolysis. A 0.9% saline (normal saline or NS) is generally administered to aim for a urine output greater than 200 mL/hr, in order to prevent AKI by preventing cast formation.

A small randomized controlled trial (RCT) of 28 patients with rhabdomyolysis who ingest doxylamine compared the use of lactated Ringer (LR) versus NS for resuscitation and found that the NS group required more sodium bicarbonate supplementation for acidosis and diuretic augmentation. No participant required KRT.[30] There are theoretic benefits from urinary alkalization in patients with rhabdomyolysis. Data from animal models suggest that the nephrotoxic effects of myoglobin are enhanced when the urine is acidic, leading to increased cast formation,[14] increased oxidative stress and lipid peroxidation,[31] and myoglobin-induced vasoconstriction.[32] In humans, however, an RCT of 98 patients with doxylamine-induced rhabdomyolysis, given either NS or bicarbonate, did not find a difference in AKI incidence between the two groups.[33] Alkalization also has significant potential adverse consequences, the most important of which is worsening of hypocalcemia by increasing protein binding.[9] There is also a risk of increased calcium phosphate deposition in the kidney.[3,34,35] Taken together, we do not feel that alkalization should be used as a first-line treatment in severe rhabdomyolysis, because it likely has little effect in less severe cases where the potential for adverse effects is lower. The combined use of sodium bicarbonate and mannitol has also been studied in rhabdomyolysis because mannitol is a known osmotic diuretic with antioxidant properties[2,3]; however, whether this combination prevents AKI is uncertain.[36-40] Moreover, mannitol is known to be nephrotoxic at high levels through vasoconstriction and tubular toxicity.[3,41,42]

A 2013 review by Sever and Vanholder[43] on the management of crush victims in mass disasters recommended NS as the fluid of choice, given its efficacy in volume expansion and wide availability. Fluid administration should be initiated during the period of extrication if possible, with recommended infusion rates of 1,000 mL/hr for the first 2 hours. If the extrication procedure takes longer than 2 hours, the volume of fluids should be reduced to at least 50% thereafter. Exact infusion rates may vary depending on the clinical situation and degree of urine output, but total fluid resuscitation of 3 to 6 L/d is reasonable if close monitoring cannot be done.[43,44] Although the authors recommended against the use of LR and other potassium-containing fluids in crush injuries, given the victims' higher risk of developing fatal hyperkalemia, it has not been shown that LR is a cause of increased potassium levels in these patients.[43,45]

Loop diuretics have also been used to augment urinary flow to prevent myoglobin precipitation; however, there is no clear evidence that they specifically reduce the risk of AKI.[3] Indications for their use in rhabdomyolysis are no different than its role in managing volume overload in other causes of AKI.[3]

KIDNEY REPLACEMENT THERAPY

Initiation of KRT is indicated when refractory hyperkalemia, metabolic acidemia, or volume overload has occurred. Most studies of KRT in rhabdomyolysis have focused on myoglobin clearance.

Conventional hemodialysis is ineffective and inefficient in removing myoglobin owing to the following reasons: (a) myoglobin is a charged molecule with a nonspherical shape; (b) it has a large molecular weight of 17 kDa, and thus, convection is the preferred method for its removal; and (c) it is distributed in two pools in humans—the intravascular compartment and muscle tissues. In the past, older cellulose membranes were relatively impermeable to myoglobin, however modern high-flux dialyzers do not have this issue.[46,47] Micro-crimping, a technique that results in a more wavy hollow fiber, increases myoglobin clearance by 30% to 60% in in vitro studies.[48]

Continuous kidney replacement therapy (CKRT) addresses the limitations of intermittent hemodialysis in myoglobin clearance. An early study of CKRT demonstrated a myoglobin clearance of 4.6 mL/min, with myoglobin removal rate of 0.08 g/treatment hour.[49,50] Since then, various filters have been developed and studied. Naka and colleagues used a novel super high-flux (SHF) membrane with a molecular cutoff point of 100 kDa for a patient with an initial serum myoglobin concentration of 100,000 μg/L, which resulted in a myoglobin clearance of up to 30.5 to 39.2 mL/min (with replacement fluid rates of up to 3-4 L/hr) and myoglobin removal rates of 0.18 to 0.21 g/treatment hour. A problem with SHF filters is the loss of serum albumin (69 kDa), which necessitates albumin replacement (100 g over 24 hours for this patient). The possible loss of protein-bound drugs and clotting factors is also a concern.[51] Premru and colleagues used a high cutoff (HCO) hemofilter (45 kDa cutoff) for hemodiafiltration lasting 6 to 12 hours per treatment in a case series of six patients with AKI from rhabdomyolysis. Their results showed efficient myoglobin clearance of 81 mL/min, with as high as 5 g of myoglobin removed in a day. Aggressive albumin replacement was necessary, and the authors noticed a significant rebound in serum myoglobin, as high as 244% of the post-hemodiafiltration myoglobin level.[52]

At present, there are no established RCTs that compare immediate- and long-term outcomes between early and late KRT initiation in rhabdomyolysis. Data on head-to-head comparisons among KRT modalities have also been sparse. A meta-analysis of RCTs and quasi-RCTs for CKRT in rhabdomyolysis included only three small studies from China, with a total of 101 participants. In this report, although CKRT was associated with a significant decrease in serum myoglobin, improvement in metabolic parameters (creatinine, blood urea nitrogen, and potassium), shortened time in the oliguric phase, and reduced in-hospital stay, no differences in mortality rates were seen. Moreover, the authors noted the overall poor methodological quality in these studies and the inadequate assessment of important clinical outcomes.[53]

Overall, based on current data on the management of rhabdomyolysis and recognizing the absence of good clinical trials, our recommendations are summarized in **Table 49.4. Table 49.5** summarizes several of the key points from the chapter.

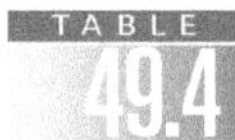

The Authors' Recommendations on the Management of Rhabdomyolysis

Suggested Guidelines for the Management of Rhabdomyolysis

1. Assess likelihood of developing AKI based on the etiology of rhabdomyolysis and laboratory abnormalities on admission.
2. If the patient is at high risk for AKI, administer IV fluids to target a urine output of >200 mL/hr.
3. NS or LR is the fluid of choice. Bicarbonate should be reserved for patients with acidemia.
4. If bicarbonate is used, target a urine pH >6.5 and closely monitor for hypocalcemia.
5. Diuretics may be used for augmentation if the urine output is lower than the desired range despite adequate volume resuscitation.
6. There is no clear current role for prophylactic dialysis for the prevention of rhabdomyolysis-associated AKI, but in the event that KRT is needed, high-flux dialyzers are more efficient at reducing myoglobin levels.

AKI, acute kidney injury; IV, intravenous; LR, lactated Ringer; KRT, kidney replacement therapy; NS, normal saline.

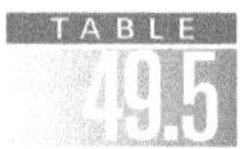

Rhabdomyolysis Key Points

Rhabdomyolysis is due to the breakdown of striated skeletal muscles that results in the release of intracellular components, leading to complications, including clinically significant electrolyte abnormalities and AKI secondary to myoglobinuria.

Etiologies of rhabdomyolysis include trauma, exercise-induced, ischemia/hypoxia, electrical injuries, genetic and metabolism disorders, infections, electrolyte abnormalities, and drugs and toxins.

Myoglobin causes AKI through three mechanisms: (1) renal vasoconstriction exacerbated by volume depletion, (2) heme-pigment cast formation resulting from the interaction of myoglobin and Tamm-Horsfall proteins, and (3) direct heme toxicity through oxidative stress and lipid peroxidation.

Rhabdomyolysis is both a clinical and biochemical diagnosis. An increase in the biomarker creatinine kinase is used in its diagnosis, with the usual accepted cutoff value of >5 times the upper limit of normal. Typical biochemical abnormalities in rhabdomyolysis include hyperkalemia, hyperphosphatemia, hypocalcemia, elevated creatinine and blood urea nitrogen, and a blood-positive UDT.

The Rhabdomyolysis Risk Score is a clinical calculator that predicts the need for KRT and in-hospital mortality among hospitalized patients with rhabdomyolysis. A score of 5 or below confers a low risk for a patient to need KRT or die. Every 1 point increase in the score is associated with almost 1.5 times the increase in odds of developing these outcomes.

Rhabdomyolysis is managed medically until a need for KRT arises, when medical management has failed. Medical management consists of aggressive fluid repletion. At present, no studies have shown a clear superiority of one fluid composition over the other. The use of mannitol has been controversial as well.

(*continued*)

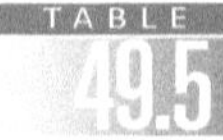

Rhabdomyolysis Key Points (*continued*)

At present, there are no large randomized controlled trials that compare KRT modalities for rhabdomyolysis. Myoglobin can only be removed via hemofiltration owing to its charge, shape, and size. High-flux dialyzers presently used for intermittent hemodialysis are compatible with myoglobin removal. Continuous KRT modalities have the advantage of better myoglobin clearance. SHF and high cutoff membranes have been studied and shown to be more efficient in the removal of myoglobin, though a trade-off exists, given that these membranes result in a significant loss in albumin and, possibly, other protein-bound drugs and clotting factors.

AKI, acute kidney injury; KRT, kidney replacement therapy; SHF, super high flux; UDT, urine dipstick test.

References

1. Zaia J, Annan RS, Biemann K. The correct molecular weight of myoglobin, a common calibrant for mass spectrometry. *Rapid Commun Mass Spectrom.* 1992;6(1):32-36. doi:10.1002/rcm.1290060108
2. Vanholder R, Sever MS, Erek E, Lameire N. Rhabdomyolysis. *J Am Soc Nephrol.* 2000;11(8):1553-1561.
3. Bosch X, Poch E, Grau JM. Rhabdomyolysis and acute kidney injury. *N Engl J Med.* 2009;361(1):62-72. doi:10.1056/NEJMra0801327
4. Zimmerman JL, Shen MC. Rhabdomyolysis. *Chest.* 2013;144(3):1058-1065. doi:10.1378/chest.12-2016
5. Bywaters EG, Beall D. Crush injuries with impairment of renal function. *Br Med J.* 1941;1(4185):427-432. doi:10.1136/bmj.1.4185.427
6. Grossman RA, Hamilton RW, Morse BM, Penn AS, Goldberg M. Nontraumatic rhabdomyolysis and acute renal failure. *N Engl J Med.* 1974;291(1):807-811. doi:10.1056/NEJM197410172911601
7. Koffler A, Friedler RM, Massry SG. Acute renal failure due to nontraumatic rhabdomyolysis. *Ann Intern Med.* 1976;85(1):23-28. doi:10.7326/0003-4819-85-1-23
8. Zager RA. Rhabdomyolysis and myohemoglobinuric acute renal failure. *Kidney Int.* 1996;49(2):314-326. doi:10.1038/ki.1996.48
9. Huerta-Alardín AL, Varon J, Marik PE. Bench-to-bedside review: rhabdomyolysis—an overview for clinicians. *Crit Care.* 2005;9:158-169. doi:10.1186/cc2978
10. Better OS. The crush syndrome revisited (1940–1990). *Nephron.* 1990;55(2):97-103. doi:10.1159/000185934
11. Vetterlein F, Hoffmann F, Pedina J, Neckel M, Schmidt G. Disturbances in renal microcirculation induced by myoglobin and hemorrhagic hypotension in anesthetized rat. *Am J Physiol.* 1995;268:F839-F846. doi:10.1152/ajprenal.1995.268.5.f839
12. Zager RA, Burkhart KM, Conrad DS, Gmur DJ. Iron, heme oxygenase, and glutathione: effects on myohemoglobinuric proximal tubular injury. *Kidney Int.* 1995;48:1624-1634. doi:10.1038/ki.1995.457
13. Zager RA. Myoglobin depletes renal adenine nucleotide pools in the presence and absence of shock. *Kidney Int.* 1991;39:111-119. doi:10.1038/ki.1991.14
14. Zager RA. Studies of mechanisms and protective maneuvers in myoglobinuric acute renal injury. *Lab Invest.* 1989;60:619-629.
15. Nara A, Yajima D, Nagasawa S, Abe H, Hoshioka Y, Iwase H. Evaluations of lipid peroxidation and inflammation in short-term glycerol-induced acute kidney injury in rats. *Clin Exp Pharmacol Physiol.* 2016;43:1080-1086. doi:10.1111/1440-1681.12633
16. Gabow PA, Kaehny WD, Kelleher SP. The spectrum of rhabdomyolysis. *Medicine (Baltimore).* 1982;61(3):141-152. doi:10.1097/00005792-198205000-00002
17. Melli G, Chaudhry V, Cornblath DR. Rhabdomyolysis: an evaluation of 475 hospitalized patients. *Medicine (Baltimore).* 2005;84(6):377-385. doi:10.1097/01.md.0000188565.48918.41
18. Chavez LO, Leon M, Einav S, Varon J. Beyond muscle destruction: a systematic review of rhabdomyolysis for clinical practice. *Crit Care.* 2016;20(1):135. doi:10.1186/s13054-016-1314-5
19. McMahon GM, Zeng X, Waikar SS. A risk prediction score for kidney failure or mortality in rhabdomyolysis. *JAMA Intern Med.* 2013;173(19):1821-1828. doi:10.1001/jamainternmed.2013.9774
20. Akmal M, Goldstein DA, Telfer N, Wilkinson E, Massry SG. Resolution of muscle calcification in rhabdomyolysis and acute renal failure. *Ann Intern Med.* 1978;89(6):928-930. doi:10.7326/0003-4819-89-6-928

21. Akmal M, Bishop JE, Telfer N, Norman AW, Massry SG. Hypocalcemia and hypercalcemia in patients with rhabdomyolysis with and without acute renal failure. *J Clin Endocrinol Metab.* 1986;63(1):137-142. doi:10.1210/jcem-63-1-137
22. Alhadi SA, Ruegner R, Snowden B, Hendey GW. Urinalysis is an inadequate screen for rhabdomyolysis. *Am J Emerg Med.* 2014;32(3):260-262. doi:10.1016/j.ajem.2013.10.045
23. Schifman RB, Luevano DR. Value and use of urinalysis for myoglobinuria. *Arch Pathol Lab Med.* 2019;143(11):1378-1381. doi:10.5858/arpa.2018-0475-OA
24. Rodríguez-Capote K, Balion CM, Hill SA, Cleve R, Yang L, El Sharif A. Utility of urine myoglobin for the prediction of acute renal failure in patients with suspected rhabdomyolysis: a systematic review. *Clin Chem.* 2009;55(12):2190-2197. doi:10.1373/clinchem.2009.128546
25. Perazella MA, Coca SG, Hall IE, Iyanam U, Koraishy M, Parikh CR. Urine microscopy is associated with severity and worsening of acute kidney injury in hospitalized patients. *Clin J Am Soc Nephrol.* 2010;5(3):402-408. doi:10.2215/CJN.06960909
26. Delaney KA, Givens ML, Vohra RB. Use of RIFLE criteria to predict the severity and prognosis of acute kidney injury in emergency department patients with rhabdomyolysis. *J Emerg Med.* 2012;42(5):521-528. doi:10.1016/j.jemermed.2011.03.008
27. Sever MS, Erek E, Vanholder R, et al. The Marmara earthquake: epidemiological analysis of the victims with nephrological problems. *Kidney Int.* 2001;60(3):1114-1123. doi:10.1046/j.1523-1755.2001.0600031114.x
28. Simpson JP, Taylor A, Sudhan N, Menon DK, Lavinio A. Rhabdomyolysis and acute kidney injury: creatine kinase as a prognostic marker and validation of the McMahon Score in a 10-year cohort: a retrospective observational evaluation. *Eur J Anaesthesiol.* 2016;33(12):906-912. doi:10.1097/EJA.0000000000000490
29. Clarkson PM, Kearns AK, Rouzier P, Rubin R, Thompson PD. Serum creatine kinase levels and renal function measures in exertional muscle damage. *Med Sci Sports Exerc.* 2006;38(4):623-627. doi:10.1249/01.mss.0000210192.49210.fc
30. Cho YS, Lim H, Kim SH. Comparison of lactated Ringer's solution and 0.9% saline in the treatment of rhabdomyolysis induced by doxylamine intoxication. *Emerg Med J.* 2007;24(4):276-280. doi:10.1136/emj.2006.043265
31. Moore KP, Holt SG, Patel RP, et al. A causative role for redox cycling of myoglobin and its inhibition by alkalinization in the pathogenesis and treatment of rhabdomyolysis-induced renal failure. *J Biol Chem.* 1998;273(48):31731-31737. doi:10.1074/jbc.273.48.31731
32. Heyman SN, Greenbaum R, Shina A, Rosen S, Brezis M. Myoglobinuric acute renal failure in the rat: a role for acidosis? *Exp Nephrol.* 1997;5(3):210-216.
33. Kim E, Choi YH, Lim JY, Lee J, Lee DH. The effect of early urine alkalinization on occurrence rhabdomyolysis and hospital stay in high dose doxylamine ingestion. *Am J Emerg Med.* 2018;36(7):1170-1173. doi:10.1016/j.ajem.2017.11.058
34. Better OS, Abassi ZA. Early fluid resuscitation in patients with rhabdomyolysis. *Nat Rev Nephrol.* 2011;7(7):416-422. doi:10.1038/nrneph.2011.56
35. Holt SG, Moore KP. Pathogenesis and treatment of renal dysfunction in rhabdomyolysis. *Intensive Care Med.* 2001;27(5):803-811. doi:10.1007/s001340100878
36. Gunal AI, Celiker H, Dogukan A, et al. Early and vigorous fluid resuscitation prevents acute renal failure in the crush victims of catastrophic earthquakes. *J Am Soc Nephrol.* 2004;15(7):1862-1867. doi:10.1097/01.ASN.0000129336.09976.73
37. Altintepe L, Guney I, Tonbul Z, et al. Early and intensive fluid replacement prevents acute renal failure in the crush cases associated with spontaneous collapse of an apartment in Konya. *Ren Fail.* 2007;29(6):737-741. doi:10.1080/08860220701460095
38. Brown CV, Rhee P, Chan L, Evans K, Demetriades D, Velmahos GC. Preventing renal failure in patients with rhabdomyolysis: do bicarbonate and mannitol make a difference? *J Trauma.* 2004;56(6):1191-1196. doi:10.1097/01.ta.0000130761.78627.10
39. Homsi E, Leme Barreiro MFF, Orlando JMC, Higa EM. Prophylaxis of acute renal failure in patients with rhabdomyolysis. *Ren Fail.* 1997;19(2):283-288. doi:10.3109/08860229709026290
40. Scharman EJ, Troutman WG. Prevention of kidney injury following rhabdomyolysis: a systematic review. *Ann Pharmacother.* 2013;47(1):90-105. doi:10.1345/aph.1r215
41. Better OS, Rubinstein I, Winaver JM, Knochel JP. Mannitol therapy revisited (1940–1997). *Kidney Int.* 1997;52(4):886-894. doi:10.1038/ki.1997.409
42. Visweswaran P, Massin EK, DuBose TD. Mannitol-induced acute renal failure. *J Am Soc Nephrol.* 1997;8(6):1028-1033.
43. Sever MS, Vanholder R. Management of crush victims in mass disasters: highlights from recently published recommendations. *Clin J Am Soc Nephrol.* 2013;8(2):328-335. doi:10.2215/CJN.07340712
44. Sever MS, Vanholder R, Ashkenazi I, et al. Recommendations for the management of crush victims in mass disasters. *Nephrol Dial Transplant.* 2012;27:i1-i67. doi:10.1093/ndt/gfs156

45. Sever MS, Erek E, Vanholder R, et al. Serum potassium in the crush syndrome victims of the Marmara disaster. *Clin Nephrol.* 2003;59(5):326-333. doi:10.5414/CNP59326
46. Ronco C. Extracorporeal therapies in acute rhabdomyolysis and myoglobin clearance. *Crit Care.* 2005;9(2):141-142. doi:10.1186/cc3055
47. Cruz DN, Bagshaw SM. Does continuous renal replacement therapy have a role in the treatment of rhabdomyolysis complicated by acute kidney injury? *Semin Dial.* 2011;24(4):417-420. doi:10.1111/j.1525-139X.2011.00892.x
48. Leypoldt JK, Cheung AK, Chirananthavat T, et al. Hollow fiber shape alters solute clearances in high flux hemodialyzers. *ASAIO J.* 2003;49(1):81-87. doi:10.1097/00002480-200301000-00013
49. Sorrentino SA, Kielstein JT, Lukasz A, et al. High permeability dialysis membrane allows effective removal of myoglobin in acute kidney injury resulting from rhabdomyolysis. *Crit Care Med.* 2011;39(1):184-186. doi:10.1097/CCM.0b013e3181feb7f0
50. Bellomo R, Daskalakis M, Parkin G, Boyce N. Myoglobin clearance during acute continuous hemodiafiltration. *Intensive Care Med.* 1991;17(8):509.
51. Naka T, Jones D, Baldwin I, et al. Myoglobin clearance by super high-flux hemofiltration in a case of severe rhabdomyolysis: a case report. *Crit Care.* 2005;9(2):R90-R95. doi:10.1186/cc3034
52. Premru V, Kovač J, Buturovič-Ponikvar J, Ponikvar R. High cut-off membrane hemodiafiltration in myoglobinuric acute renal failure: a case series. *Ther Apher Dial.* 2011;15(3):287-291. doi:10.1111/j.1744-9987.2011.00953.x
53. Zeng X, Zhang L, Wu T, Fu P. Continuous renal replacement therapy (CRRT) for rhabdomyolysis. *Cochrane Database Syst Rev.* 2014;(6):CD008566. doi:10.1002/14651858.CD008566.pub2

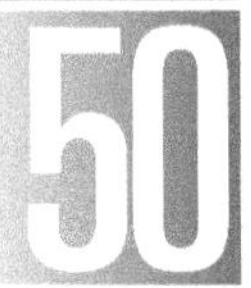

Onconephrology Emergencies

Krishna Sury and Mark A. Perazella

Patients with cancer commonly develop acute kidney injury (AKI), which portends a higher morbidity and mortality.[1-4] There are a variety of mechanisms by which cancer or its treatment may lead to kidney injury. The malignancy may directly induce AKI through infiltration or external compression of the kidney, or indirectly by paraneoplastic effects and metabolic complications. Cancer therapies may directly injure kidney tissue or may trigger systemic inflammation that leads to AKI. The severity of kidney injury varies depending on the etiology. Those etiologies of cancer-related AKI that lead to critical illness requiring intensive medical care are discussed in this chapter.

CANCER AND KIDNEY INJURY

Kidney Infiltration of the Kidney

One mechanism of cancer-related AKI is direct infiltration of cancer cells into kidney parenchyma, a relatively common finding in B-cell lymphoproliferative disorders. AKI is seen in up to 85% of cases, most often because of lymphomatous or leukemic infiltration of the kidney interstitium.[5,6] Infiltration can only be definitively diagnosed by kidney biopsy, because urine studies and advanced imaging techniques have inherent limitations in spatial resolution, leaving small foci of tissue infiltration undetected. Massive nephromegaly seen on imaging may be a tip-off to malignant infiltration. Early identification of cancer spread to the kidney is paramount; although most reported cases of infiltration-related kidney failure have achieved only partial recovery following cancer therapy,[6,7] there are some cases of complete kidney recovery following prompt and successful treatment of the malignancy.[8]

Obstructive Nephropathy

With certain malignancies, obstructive AKI because of involvement of the collecting system, ureters, bladder, and urethra may occur. Examples include prostate cancer causing bladder outlet obstruction, bladder cancer obstructing ureteral orifices, and cancer of the kidney, particularly in cases of renal cell carcinoma following nephrectomy where unilateral ureteral obstruction can cause fulminant AKI in the remaining kidney. In addition, bulky lymphomas and solid-organ cancers in the abdomen or pelvis cause extrinsic compression of the urinary outflow tract. Percutaneous nephrostomy tubes, ureteral stents, or bladder catheter placement often partially or completely restores kidney function. Hydronephrosis should prompt immediate intervention to relieve obstruction, although the absence of hydronephrosis does not rule out malignant obstruction in all cases, because cancer can encase the collecting system and prevent its dilatation.

Myeloma Light-Chain Cast Nephropathy

Multiple myeloma (MM) is a common cause of AKI and can be life-threatening.[9] MM is associated with kidney injury through various mechanisms, including common paraneoplastic effects occurring from monoclonal immunoglobulin and light-chain (LC) production, metabolic disturbances (hypercalcemia, tumor lysis syndrome [TLS]), and drug-induced nephrotoxicity.[10] Paraprotein production can induce injury in the vascular, glomerular, and tubulointerstitial compartments of the kidney.[10] As LC cast nephropathy is the most common kidney lesion, it is the focus of this section.

LC cast nephropathy occurs because of aggregation of LCs and uromodulin, which is due to a binding site on LCs that interacts with a carbohydrate moiety on uromodulin and leads to precipitation of insoluble casts within the tubular lumens.[11] Cast formation stimulates a monocytic reaction in the interstitium, causing further injury to the tubulointerstitium.[10] This may result in tubular obstruction, tubular rupture with resulting atrophy, and tubulointerstitial inflammation. In this setting, AKI develops. In the absence of effective therapy, dialysis requirement and chronic kidney disease (CKD) may result. Thus, early, effective therapy is crucial to salvaging kidney function.

Therapy for AKI from cast nephropathy hinges primarily on effective eradication of the malignant clone. A number of drugs (proteasome inhibitors, steroids, cyclophosphamide, others) are effective and can reverse or stabilize kidney function.[9,10] Extracorporeal removal of LCs with plasmapheresis to treat cast nephropathy is fraught with mixed data, and the modality is considered second line. In view of this, high cutoff hemodialysis (HCO-HD), which more efficiently removes LCs, was studied in two randomized controlled trials.[12,13] Patients with dialysis-requiring AKI from cast nephropathy were randomized to either standard myeloma therapy alone or standard therapy plus HCO-HD. The EuLITE (**Visual Abstract 50.1**) and MYRE (**Visual Abstract 50.2**) trials showed no benefit for the primary end point (freedom from dialysis) or mortality, although there was a signal for AKI recovery at 6 and 12 months in the MYRE trial. Thus, the utility of this modality remains unproven.

METABOLIC COMPLICATIONS OF CANCER AND KIDNEY INJURY

Hypercalcemia

Hypercalcemia is a common complication of cancer, occurring in up to 30% of all malignancies.[1,14] Symptoms of hypercalcemia are nonspecific and often go unnoticed until they become severe (see Chapter 22).[14,15]

Malignancy-related hypercalcemia may arise because of tumor invasion of bone causing osteolysis and calcium release, malignancy-generated active vitamin D (lymphomas) causing excess gut absorption of calcium, and malignancy-secreted parathyroid hormone–related protein (PTHrP), which acts to increase calcium release from bone and increase gut absorption.[14]

Hypercalcemia exerts deleterious effects on the kidney by reducing glomerular filtration rate (GFR) through direct renal vasoconstriction,[16,17] while also activating the calcium-sensing receptor on the thick ascending limb of the loop of Henle (inactivates NA-K-2Cl cotransporter), which leads to significant natriuresis and AKI from volume depletion.[18] Hypercalcemia also impairs water reabsorption in the distal nephron (disturbs antidiuretic hormone [ADH] effect), contributing to more fluid loss and hypernatremia.[14] These effects reduce GFR and further impair urinary calcium excretion, exacerbating hypercalcemia.

The mainstay of acute hypercalcemia treatment is aggressive volume expansion with intravenous saline, with the goal of restoring a euvolemic state and improving the GFR. Loop diuretics were previously recommended as an adjunct to saline; however, they are now recognized as retarding efforts at volume expansion and, therefore, should not be used unless the patient is hypervolemic.[19] If saline cannot be safely administered because of anuric AKI and/or significant hypervolemia, HD with a low calcium bath may be required. When bone calcium release is the culprit, therapy must be directed at inhibiting osteoclastic bone resorption (**Table 50.1**; **Figure 50.1**). Calcitonin, the bisphosphonates, and denosumab (reviewed in Chapter 22) may be employed to reduce calcium release from bone. Severe AKI contraindicates zoledronate therapy, whereas pamidronate can be used at a lower dose (60 mg) with a longer infusion time (4-6 hours). The anti–receptor activator of nuclear factor kappa-B ligand (RANKL) antibody denosumab is an excellent alternative when AKI is present, in that it is highly effective and safe in those with impaired kidney function. When hypercalcemia is due to malignancy-related excess active vitamin D, corticosteroids are often effective.[14]

Tumor Lysis Syndrome (TLS)

TLS is a constellation of specific metabolic derangements that arise when tumor cells die and intracellular contents are released into the systemic circulation. Characteristic findings include hyperkalemia, hyperphosphatemia, hypocalcemia, and hyperuricemia, which range from mild to severe and life-threatening. TLS is subcategorized as either laboratory TLS (specified degrees of deviation of each metabolic derangement, as well as criteria defining onset and duration) or clinical TLS (laboratory TLS along with evidence of organ dysfunction).

The TLS definition initially put forth by Cairo and Bishop has been modified over the years, but all versions distinguish laboratory from clinical TLS, highlighting the fact that laboratory derangements may occur without causing organ dysfunction, as summarized in **Table 50.2**.[20-23] This is possible because when hyperkalemia or hyperphosphatemia occurs with normal kidney function, renal excretion of potassium and phosphorus restores serum levels to the normal range and minimizes the risk of hypocalcemia. Similarly, uric acid is excreted by the kidneys; however, with severe hyperuricemia, volume depletion, and urine pH less than 7.0, uric acid precipitates within tubular lumens, thus causing AKI from acute uric acid nephropathy.

In the setting of oliguric or anuric AKI, electrolyte derangements such as hyperkalemia and hyperphosphatemia may be difficult to manage, leading to life-threatening cardiac arrhythmias and hypocalcemic seizure. Intravenous saline is employed to maintain high urine flow rates and prevent volume depletion. Urinary alkalinization is no longer recommended because of the risk of calcium

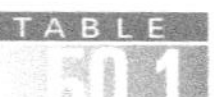

TABLE 50.1 Treatment of Acute Hypercalcemia

Therapy	Mechanism of Action	Reasons for Use	Limitations of Use
Calcitonin	Blocks kidney tubules from reabsorbing calcium Interferes with osteoclast activity	Rapid onset, works within hours to lower serum calcium	Tachyphylaxis occurs within 2 d
Bisphosphonates Pamidronate Zoledronate Ibandronate	Structural analogs of pyrophosphate; incorporated into osteoclast ATP that renders it nonfunctional Disrupts the osteoclast cytoskeleton, so it cannot maintain contact with the bone surface	Sustained reduction in serum calcium levels	Slow onset of action, takes 48-72 hr to see full effect Zoledronate is more effective than pamidronate but is contraindicated in AKI or advanced CKD with serum Cr of 4.5 mg/dL or greater or CrCl <30 mL/min. Pamidronate can be used in AKI but requires dose reduction to 60 mg and prolonged infusion time of 4-6 hr.
Denosumab	Antibody against RANKL; RANKL is secreted by osteoblasts to bind to the RANK receptor on osteoclasts and drives bone breakdown. Denosumab blocks the binding of RANKL to RANK, inhibiting the maturation, activation, and function of osteoclasts.	Sustained reduction in serum calcium levels with no limitations of use in patients with impaired kidney function	Serum calcium levels must be closely monitored after denosumab administration, as there is a risk for hypocalcemia. Small risk of atypical femur fractures
Corticosteroids	Malignant cells recruit macrophages to express 1-alpha-hydroxylase to convert calcidiol into calcitriol (active vitamin D). Steroids inhibit 1-alpha-hydroxylase and activate 24-hydroxylase, thus limiting the formation of activated vitamin D and reducing hypercalcemia.	Malignancy-related hypercalcemia characterized by elevated vitamin D production	Blood sugar levels must be monitored.

AKI, acute kidney injury; ATP, adenosine triphosphate; CKD, chronic kidney disease; Cr, creatinine; CrCl, creatinine clearance; RANKL, receptor activator of nuclear factor kappa-B ligand.

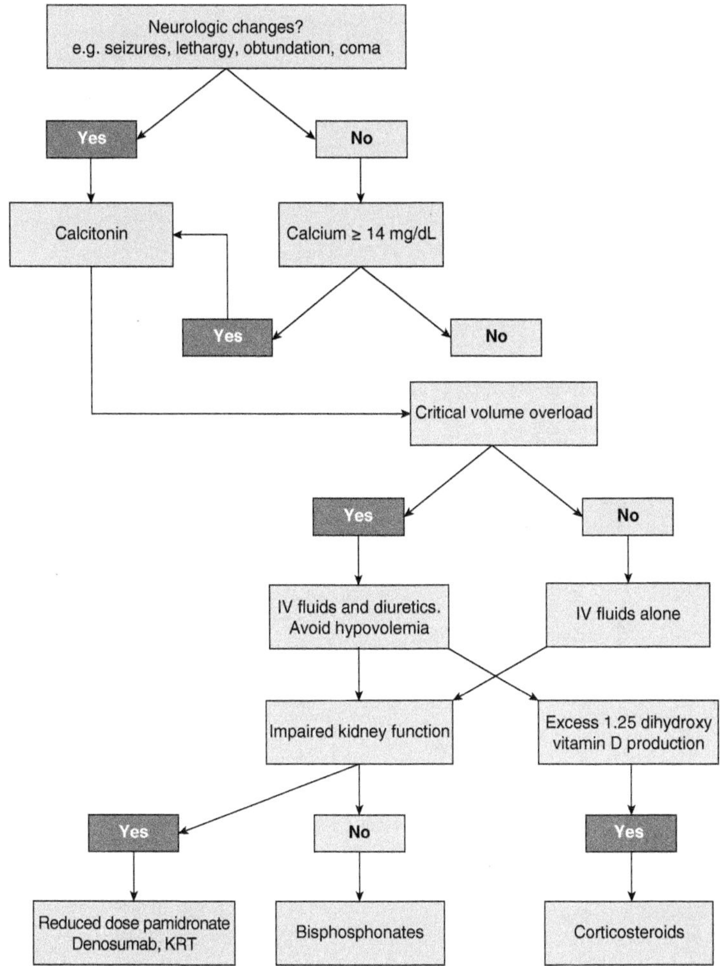

FIGURE 50.1: Algorithm for the management of acute hypercalcemia. Initial assessment and management of patients with acute hypercalcemia focus on neurologic status. In cases where neurologic function is preserved or pharmacologically restored, further management centers on volume expansion with saline (limited only in cases where the patient is at risk for critical volume overload) and disruption of osteoclast activity. IVF, intravenous fluids; KRT, kidney replacement therapy.

phosphate and xanthine crystal precipitation within tubules. Management of each specific electrolyte derangement is well described,[24] with kidney replacement therapy (KRT) required in some cases (**Figure 50.2**). Allopurinol is used to prevent hyperuricemia, but rasburicase is often required to rapidly and effectively correct hyperuricemia with TLS.[24]

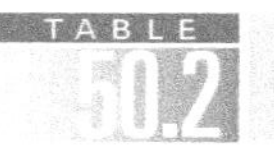

Definition of Tumor Lysis Syndrome

Laboratory Tumor Lysis Syndrome (LTLS)[a]	Clinical Tumor Lysis Syndrome (CTLS)[b]
Serum uric acid ≥ 8 mg/dL (≥476 μmol/L) or 25% increase from baseline	Creatinine ≥1.5 times greater than the institutional ULN if below the age/gender-defined ULN, for patients >12 yr of age
Serum potassium ≥ 6 meq/L (≥6 mmol/L) or 25% increase from baseline	Cardiac arrhythmia/sudden death not directly or probably attributable to a therapeutic agent
Serum phosphorus ≥ 6.5 mg/dL (≥ 2.1 mmol/L) in children, ≥ 4.5 mg/dL (≥ 1.45 mmol/L) in adults, or 25% increase from baseline	Seizure not directly or probably attributable to a therapeutic agent
Serum calcium ≤ 7.0 mg/dL (≤1.75 mmol/L or 25% decrease from baseline	

Proposed Changes

Howard et al[22]

1. Require that two or more metabolic abnormalities be present simultaneously
2. Eliminate 25% increase in criterion
3. Expand definition of CTLS to include any symptomatic hypocalcemia

Wilson and Berns[23]

1. Eliminate requirement that the patient be initiated on chemotherapy, to include spontaneous TLS
2. Change the CTLS criterion for creatinine range to an established definition inclusive of patients with chronic kidney disease, such as an absolute creatinine increase of 0.3 mg/dL or a relative increase of 50% above baseline.

ULN, upper limit of normal.

[a]The Cairo-Bishop definition of LTLS requires that two or more metabolic abnormalities are present within the 3 days preceding or 7 days following the initiation of chemotherapy. The required 25% change in metabolite serum concentration assumes the patient has received adequate hydration and a hypouricemic agent.

[b]The Cairo-Bishop definition of CTLS requires one or more clinical manifestations along with criteria for LTLS.

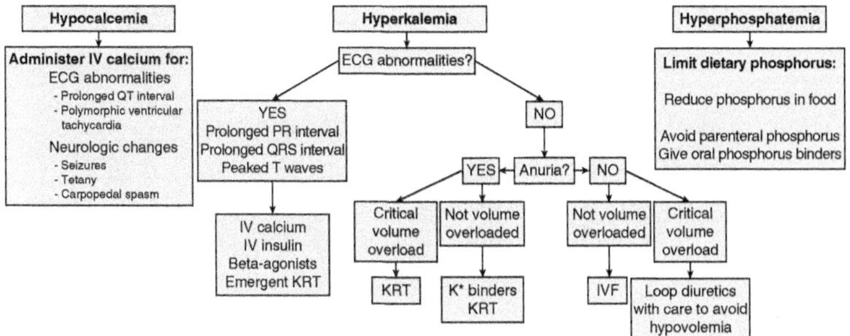

FIGURE 50.2: Algorithm for the management of TLS-related electrolyte derangements. When severe, hyperkalemia and hypocalcemia can cause life-threatening cardiac arrhythmias and must be emergently addressed. Hyperphosphatemia itself is not acutely life-threatening but can lead to hypocalcemia. ECG, electrocardiogram; IVF, intravenous fluids; KRT, kidney replacement therapy; TLS, tumor lysis syndrome.

CANCER TREATMENT AND KIDNEY INJURY

Conventional chemotherapy is the first-line treatment for most cancers, but for many advanced or chemotherapy-refractory malignancies, immunotherapy has proven effective. In contrast to conventional chemotherapy, immunotherapy utilizes the specificity of the patient's own immune system to launch a targeted attack on malignant cells. However, as with conventional chemotherapy, immunotherapy also causes kidney injury from off-target effects, which are primarily immune-related adverse events (irAEs). Although conventional chemotherapies and other targeted cancer agents cause kidney injury (**Table 50.3**), the discussion will be limited to the potentially life-threatening irAEs associated with immune-checkpoint inhibitors (ICPIs) and chimeric antigen receptor (CAR) T cells.

Immune-Checkpoint Inhibitors

The tumor microenvironment confers tumor resistance to chemotherapy, so new immunotherapies were developed by targeting specific components of the microenvironment, such as tumor-infiltrating lymphocytes (TILs), the B and T cells that surround and infiltrate tumors.[25,26] Antigen-presenting cells (APCs) use major histocompatibility complex (MHC) molecules to display an antigen to T cells, which engages with the APC through an interaction between a T-cell surface receptor and the MHC. Once the APC and T cell are connected, a B7 ligand on the APC surface interacts with either a stimulatory (CD28) or an inhibitory (cytotoxic T-lymphocyte antigen 4, CTLA-4) receptor on the T-cell surface, determining the T-cell response against that antigen. If CD28 is triggered, the T cell will be activated against that antigen, whereas CTLA-4 binding will suppress T-cell activation.[27,28] CTLA-4 acts in regional lymph nodes, whereas in peripheral tissues, T-cell activation is inhibited by binding of the T-cell surface receptor programmed death 1 (PD1) to APC surface ligand PD-L1.[28-30] Although T-cell suppression via CTLA-4 and PD1 is intended to prevent T cells from attacking healthy tissue, tumor cells upregulate the expression of CTLA-4, PD1, and PD-L1 to block the activation of T cells and stifle antitumor immune response.[31,32]

Overcoming this tumor-mediated T-cell suppression is the goal of novel immunotherapy, such as the ICPIs. These drugs are monoclonal antibodies that bind

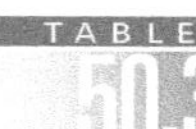

Anticancer Drug-Related Nephrotoxicity

Medications	Kidney Syndrome	Kidney Histopathology	Preventive Measures
Conventional Chemotherapy			
Gemcitabine, mitomycin C, cisplatin (rare)	AKI, HTN (new or worsened), hematuria, proteinuria	TMA	NA
Platins (cisplatin, carboplatin, oxaliplatin)	AKI, proximal tubulopathy, Fanconi syndrome, NDI, SIAD, Na^{+} and Mg^{++} wasting	ATI and ATN	Intravenous fluids, dose adjust, intravenous magnesium
Ifosfamide	AKI, proximal tubulopathy, Fanconi syndrome, NDI, SIAD	ATI and ATN, AIN	Intravenous fluids, dose adjust
Pemetrexed	AKI, proximal tubulopathy, Fanconi syndrome, NDI	ATI and ATN, interstitial fibrosis	Intravenous fluids
Methotrexate	AKI	Crystalline nephropathy and ATI	Intravenous fluids, urinary alkalinization
Antimetabolites (azacitidine, capecitabine, clofarabine, fludarabine, 5-fluorouracil, thioguanine, mercaptopurine)	AKI, Fanconi syndrome, NDI	ATI	Intravenous fluids
Cyclophosphamide, vincristine	Hyponatremia (SIAD), hemorrhagic cystitis (cyclophosphamide)	No kidney histopathologic lesion	Intravenous fluids, mesna for hemorrhagic cystitis with cyclophosphamide
Nitrosoureas	Chronic kidney disease	Chronic interstitial nephritis	Intravenous fluids

Targeted Cancer Drugs			
Anti-VEGF drugs (bevacizumab, aflibercept)	HTN, AKI, proteinuria (sometimes nephrotic)	TMA	NA
Tyrosine kinase/multikinase inhibitors (sunitinib, sorafenib, pazopanib, imatinib)	HTN, AKI, proteinuria	TMA, FSGS, AIN, ATI (imatinib)	NA
EGFR inhibitors (cetuximab, gefitinib, panitumumab, erlotinib)	Hypomagnesemia, electrolyte disorders	No kidney histopathologic lesion	NA
BRAF inhibitors (vemurafenib, dabrafenib)	AKI, electrolyte disorders	ATI and AIN	NA
ALK inhibitors (crizotinib)	AKI, electrolyte disorders, microcysts in the kidney	ATI and AIN	NA
Rituximab	AKI from tumor lysis syndrome	Uric acid nephropathy	Intravenous fluids
Other Anticancer Drugs			
Pamidronate	Nephrotic syndrome, AKI	FSGS, ATI, and ATN	Dose adjust, increase infusion time
Zoledronate	AKI, rare nephrotic syndrome	ATI and ATN	Dose adjust (contraindicated with GFR <30 mL/min)

AIN, acute interstitial nephritis; AKI, acute kidney injury; ALK, anaplastic lymphoma kinase; ATI, acute tubular injury; ATN, acute tubular necrosis; BRAF; EGFR, epidermal growth factor receptor; FSGS, focal segmental glomerulosclerosis; GN, glomerulonephritis; HTN, hypertension; MCD, minimal change disease; NA, not available; NDI, nephrogenic diabetes insipidus; SIAD, syndrome of inappropriate antidiuresis; TMA, thrombotic microangiopathy; VEGF, vascular endothelial growth factor.

CTLA-4, PD1, or PD-L1 to block tumors from suppressing TIL activity and proliferation. Preventing suppression augments the TIL-driven anticancer response, frequently resulting in irAEs that affect the kidneys. Early phase I and II trials of ICPIs estimated an incidence of AKI of 2.2%[33]; however, as ICPI use became increasingly common, many case reports and case series were published, and recent analysis suggests the true AKI incidence may be as high as 29%.[34] Making the diagnosis of ICPI-induced AKI is difficult because the available literature includes reports that vary widely with regard to the expected time lag between ICPI exposure and AKI onset, as well as the expected clinical presentation.[33-43] The most frequently described kidney pathology is acute interstitial nephritis (AIN), whereas acute tubular injury (ATI) and other kidney lesions are less common.[38,41,43] Other kidney lesions include minimal change disease, membranous nephropathy, immunoglobulin A (IgA) nephropathy, focal segmental glomerulosclerosis, lupus nephritis, thrombotic microangiopathy, immune-complex glomerulonephritis, and pauci-immune glomerulonephritis.[33-43] Proton pump inhibitor (PPI) or nonsteroidal anti-inflammatory drug (NSAID) use in patients taking ICPIs appears to increase the risk for AIN. A speculated mechanism for ICPI-associated AIN is widespread T-cell activation, leading to reduced immune tolerance to these medications.[33,35,41,42]

Development of AKI following ICPIs generally leads to ICPI cessation, but optimal management should include careful perusal of medication lists and, most importantly, a kidney biopsy. Corticosteroids are often employed for AKI, which is either proven with biopsy as AIN or clinically diagnosed as AIN.[33,35,41-43] Either complete or partial remission is observed in up to 85% of patients when drug withdrawal and corticosteroid therapy are undertaken.[41,42] In cases where ICPI-induced AKI leads to prolonged anuria or acutely life-threatening electrolyte disturbances such as hyperkalemia, HD may be necessary.

Chimeric Antigen Receptor T Cells

CAR T-cell therapy utilizes the patient's own T cells, which are removed via apheresis, whereupon a genetically engineered T-cell receptor is attached. The CAR T-cell population is then exogenously expanded with interleukin-2 (IL-2) and infused into the patient. The CAR is designed with specificity for a tumor antigen; therefore, following reinfusion, it binds the target antigen, proliferates, secretes cytokines, and launches a cytotoxic response against tumor cells.[39,44] Successful antitumor response is achieved in many cases of advanced malignancy; this is often accompanied by adverse events that impact many organs, including the kidney.

The toxicity profile of CAR T-cell therapy includes cytokine release syndrome (CRS) and hemophagocytic lymphohistiocytosis (HLH). These syndromes, caused by widespread cytokine release and immune activation, cause dysfunction of multiple organs and portend significant morbidity and mortality if not rapidly treated.[39,44] CRS is the most common irAE following CAR T-cell therapy and usually manifests within days of T-cell infusion. Severity is related to disease burden and the magnitude of CAR T-cell expansion. CRS is characterized by high fevers, hypoxia, and hypotension from vasodilatory shock, with widespread capillary leak and reduced cardiac function (which reduces organ perfusion), leading to AKI and liver dysfunction.[45] Rampant activation of the immune system may lead to HLH, which is characterized by high ferritin, low fibrinogen, cytopenias, and AKI and can be fatal unless immune dysregulation is controlled. High levels of IL-6 are a therapeutic target; the use of the anti–IL-6 antibody tocilizumab has successfully reversed life-threatening CRS.[46] Recent studies using murine models of CRS suggest that pharmacologic blockade of IL-1 may also have therapeutic potential, but this has yet to be evaluated in humans.[47]

In addition to these cytokine-mediated toxicities, CAR T-cell therapy can trigger autoimmune-mediated severe organ dysfunction known as *on-target, off-tumor toxicity*, wherein a CAR binds a tumor antigen that happens to be present in healthy tissue.[39,45,48]

CONCLUSION

AKI is commonly seen in the setting of cancer, whether secondary to the tumor or to anticancer therapies. In some cases, the kidney damage may be severe and require advanced life support, such as KRT. Identifying the etiology of cancer-related AKI is paramount in determining the optimal therapy.

References

1. Lam AQ, Humphreys BD. Onco-nephrology: AKI in the cancer patient. *Clin J Am Soc Nephrol.* 2012;7:1692.
2. Libório AB, Abreu KLS, Silva JGB, et al. Predicting hospital mortality in critically ill cancer patients according to acute kidney injury severity. *Oncology.* 2011;80:160-166
3. Darmon M, Lebert C, Perez P, et al. Acute kidney injury in critically ill patients with haematological malignancies: results of a multicentre cohort study from the Groupe de Recherche en Réanimation Respiratoire en Onco-Hématologie. *Nephrol Dial Transplant.* 2015;30:2006-2013.
4. Rosner MH, Perazella MA. Acute kidney injury in patients with cancer. *N Engl J Med.* 2017;376:1770-1781.
5. Törnroth T, Heiro M, Marcussen N, et al. Lymphomas diagnosed by percutaneous kidney biopsy. *Am J Kidney Dis.* 2003;42:960-971.
6. Corlu L, Rioux-Leclercq N, Ganard M, et al. Renal dysfunction in patients with direct infiltration by B-cell lymphoma. *Kidney Int Rep.* 2019;4:688-697.
7. Chauvet S, Bridoux F, Ecotière L, et al. Kidney diseases associated with monoclonal immunoglobulin M–secreting B-cell lymphoproliferative disorders: a case series of 35 patients. *Am J Kidney Dis.* 2015;66:756-767.
8. da Silva WF Jr, de Farias Pinho LL, de Farias CLG, et al. Renal infiltration presenting as acute kidney injury in Hodgkin lymphoma—a case report and review of the literature. *Leuk Res Rep.* 2018;10:41-43.
9. Heher EC, Rennke HG, Laubach JP, et al. Kidney disease and multiple myeloma. *Clin J Am Soc Nephrol.* 2013;8:2007-2017.
10. Shah M, Perazella MA. AKI in multiple myeloma: paraproteins, metabolic disturbances, and drug toxicity. *J Onco-Nephrol.* 2017;1:188-197.
11. Huang ZQ, Sanders PW. Localization of a single binding site for immunoglobulin light chains on human Tamm-Horsfall glycoprotein. *J Clin Invest.* 1997;99:732-736.
12. Hutchison CA, Cockwell P, Moroz V, et al. High cutoff versus high-flux haemodialysis for myeloma cast nephropathy in patients receiving bortezomib-based chemotherapy (EuLITE): a phase 2 randomised controlled trial. *Lancet Haematol.* 2019;6:e217-e228.
13. Bridoux F, Carron P-L, Pegourie B, et al. Effect of high-cutoff hemodialysis vs conventional hemodialysis on hemodialysis independence among patients with myeloma cast nephropathy: a randomized clinical trial. *JAMA.* 2017;318:2099-2110.
14. Rosner MH, Dalkin AC. Onco-nephrology: the pathophysiology and treatment of malignancy-associated hypercalcemia. *Clin J Am Soc Nephrol.* 2012;7:1722-1729.
15. Turner JJO. Hypercalcaemia—presentation and management. *Clin Med.* 2017;17:270-273.
16. Levi M, Ellis MA, Berl T. Control of renal hemodynamics and glomerular filtration rate in chronic hypercalcemia. Role of prostaglandins, renin-angiotensin system, and calcium. *J Clin Invest.* 1983;71:1624-1632.
17. Castelli I, Steiner LA, Kaufmann MA, et al. Renovascular responses to high and low perfusate calcium steady-state experiments in the isolated perfused rat kidney with baseline vascular tone. *J Surg Res.* 1996;61:51-57.
18. Moor MB, Bonny O. Ways of calcium reabsorption in the kidney. *Am J Physiol Renal Physiol.* 2016;310:F1337-F1350.

19. LeGrand SB, Leskuski D, Zama I. Narrative review: furosemide for hypercalcemia: an unproven yet common practice furosemide for hypercalcemia. *Ann Intern Med.* 2008;149:259-263.
20. Cairo MS, Bishop M. Tumour lysis syndrome: new therapeutic strategies and classification. *Br J Haematol.* 2004;127:3-11.
21. Cairo MS, Coiffier B, Reiter A, et al. Recommendations for the evaluation of risk and prophylaxis of tumour lysis syndrome (TLS) in adults and children with malignant diseases: an expert TLS panel consensus. *Br J Haematol.* 2010;149:578-586.
22. Howard SC, Jones DP, Pui C-H. The tumor lysis syndrome. *N Engl J Med.* 2011;364:1844-1854.
23. Wilson FP, Berns JS. Tumor lysis syndrome: new challenges and recent advances. *Adv Chronic Kidney Dis.* 2014;21:18-26.
24. Sury K. Update on the prevention and treatment of tumor lysis syndrome. *J Onco-Nephrol.* 2019;3:19-30.
25. Klemm F, Joyce JA. Microenvironmental regulation of therapeutic response in cancer. *Trends Cell Biol.* 2015;25:198-213.
26. Yu Y, Cui J. Present and future of cancer immunotherapy: a tumor microenvironmental perspective. *Oncol Lett.* 2018;16:4105-4113.
27. Alegre M-L, Frauwirth KA, Thompson CB. T-cell regulation by CD28 and CTLA-4. *Nat Rev Immunol.* 2001;1:220.
28. Greenwald RJ, Latchman YE, Sharpe AH. Negative co-receptors on lymphocytes. *Curr Opin Immunol.* 2002;14:391-396.
29. Iwai Y, Hamanishi J, Chamoto K, et al. Cancer immunotherapies targeting the PD-1 signaling pathway. *J Biomed Sci.* 2017;24:26.
30. Parry RV, Chemnitz JM, Frauwirth KA, et al. CTLA-4 and PD-1 receptors inhibit T-cell activation by distinct mechanisms. *Mol Cell Biol.* 2005;25:9543-9553.
31. Gatalica Z, Snyder C, Maney T, et al. Programmed cell death 1 (PD-1) and its ligand (PD-L1) in common cancers and their correlation with molecular cancer type. *Cancer Epidemiol Biomarkers Prev.* 2014;23:2965-2970.
32. Perazella MA, Shirali AC. Immune checkpoint inhibitor nephrotoxicity: what do we know and what should we do? *Kidney Int.* 2020;97(1):62-74.
33. Cortazar FB, Marrone KA, Troxell ML, et al. Clinicopathological features of acute kidney injury associated with immune checkpoint inhibitors. *Kidney Int.* 2016;90:638-647.
34. Wanchoo R, Karam S, Uppal NN, et al. Adverse renal effects of immune checkpoint inhibitors: a narrative review. *Am J Nephrol.* 2017;45:160-169.
35. Shirali AC, Perazella MA, Gettinger S. Association of acute interstitial nephritis with programmed cell death 1 inhibitor therapy in lung cancer patients. *Am J Kidney Dis.* 2016;68:287-291.
36. Mamlouk O, Selamet U, Machado S, et al. Nephrotoxicity of immune checkpoint inhibitors beyond tubulointerstitial nephritis: single-center experience. *J Immunother Cancer.* 2019;7:2.
37. Izzedine H, Mateus C, Boutros C, et al. Renal effects of immune checkpoint inhibitors. *Nephrol Dial Transplant.* 2017;32:936-942.
38. Izzedine H, Lambotte O, Goujon J-M, et al. Renal toxicities associated with pembrolizumab. *Clin Kidney J.* 2018;12:81-88.
39. Perazella MA, Shirali AC. Nephrotoxicity of cancer immunotherapies: past, present and future. *J Am Soc Nephrol.* 2018;29(8):2039-2052.
40. Sury K, Perazella MA, Shirali AC. Cardiorenal complications of immune checkpoint inhibitors. *Nat Rev Nephrol.* 2018;14:571-588.
41. Perazella MA, Shirali AC. Immune checkpoint inhibitor nephrotoxicity. What do we know and what should we do? *Kidney Int.* 2020;97(1):62-74.
42. Cortazar FB, Kibbelaar ZA, Glezerman IG, et al. Clinical features and outcomes of immune checkpoint inhibitor-associated AKI: a multicenter study. *J Am Soc Nephrol.* 2020;31(2):435-446.
43. Cassol C, Satoskar A, Lozanski G, et al. Anti-PD-1 immunotherapy may induce interstitial nephritis with increased tubular epithelial expression of PD-L1. *Kidney Int Rep.* 2019;4(8):1152-1160.
44. Jhaveri KD, Rosner MH Chimeric antigen receptor T cell therapy and the kidney: what the nephrologist needs to know. *Clin J Am Soc Nephrol.* 2018;13:796-798.
45. Neelapu SS, Tummala S, Kebriaei P, et al. Chimeric antigen receptor T-cell therapy—assessment and management of toxicities. *Nat Rev Clin Oncol.* 2018;15:47-62.
46. Teachey DT, Rheingold SR, Maude SL, et al. Cytokine release syndrome after blinatumomab treatment related to abnormal macrophage activation and ameliorated with cytokine-directed therapy. *Blood.* 2013;121:5154-5157.
47. Giavridis T, van der Stegen SJC, Eyquem J, et al. CAR T cell-induced cytokine release syndrome is mediated by macrophages and abated by IL-1 blockade. *Nat Med.* 2018;24:731-738.
48. Zhang E, Xu H. A new insight in chimeric antigen receptor-engineered T cells for cancer immunotherapy. *J Hematol Oncol* 2017;10:1.

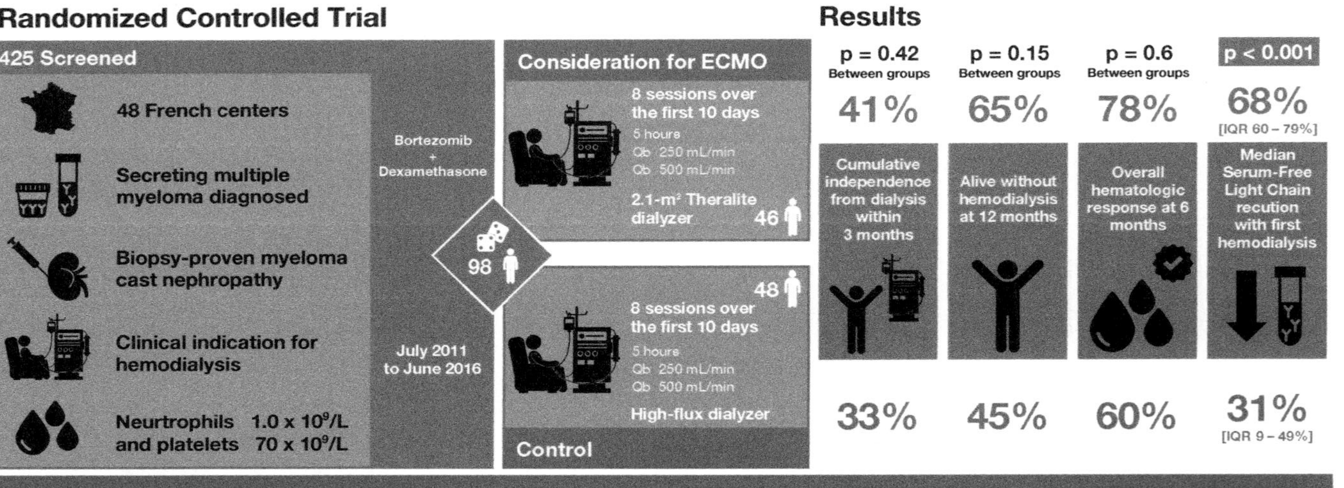

VISUAL ABSTRACT 50.1

Does high cut-off hemodialysis improve outcomes in myeloma cast nephropathy?

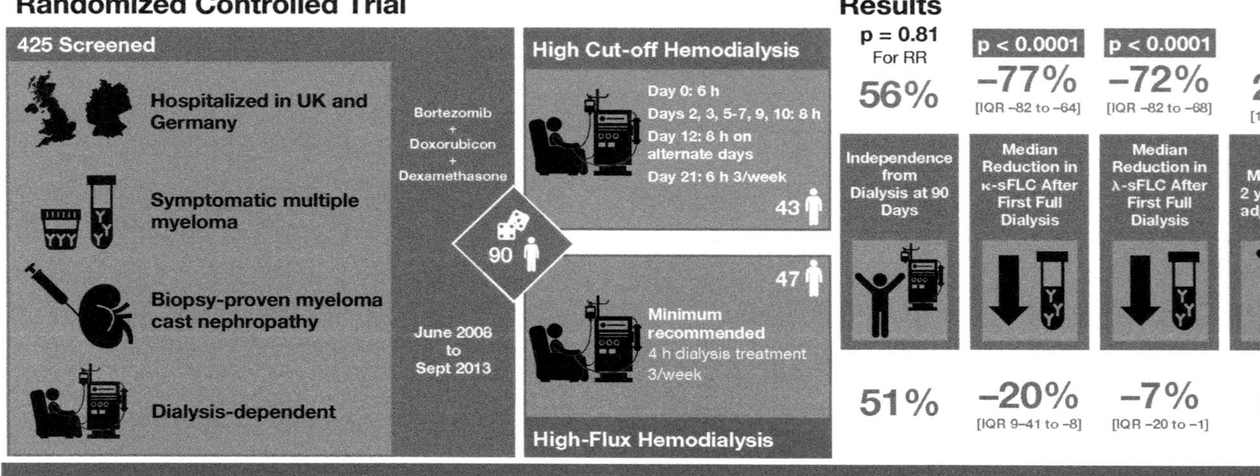

Conclusion: High cut-off hemodialysis did not improve clinical outcomes for patients with myeloma cast nephropathy requiring hemodialysis relative to those receiving high-flux hemodialysis.

Hutchison CA, Cockwell P, Moroz V, et al. ***High cutoff versus high-flux haemodialysis for myeloma cast nephropathy in patients receiving bortezomib-based chemotherapy (EuLITE): a phase 2 randomised controlled trial.*** Lancet Haematol. 2019;6(4):e217-e228.

VISUAL ABSTRACT 50.2

51 Caring for Patients After Acute Kidney Injury

Michael Heung

BACKGROUND

Acute kidney injury (AKI) is one of the most common complications in the health care setting, affecting up to one in five hospitalized patients, and is associated with significant increased risk of hospital mortality.[1] However, the impact of AKI is felt far beyond the hospitalization phase. Survivors of an AKI episode remain at higher risk for the development of chronic kidney disease (CKD) and end-stage kidney disease (ESKD),[2] recurrent AKI,[3] major adverse cardiovascular events,[4] and long-term mortality[5] (**Table 51.1**). Therefore, an important goal of post-AKI follow-up care is to reduce the risk for these complications.

FOLLOW-UP AFTER ACUTE KIDNEY INJURY

A prerequisite to appropriate management of AKI survivors is to emphasize the importance of follow-up care. Both the patients and the providers need to be properly educated on the risk for complications after an episode of AKI. The 2012 Kidney Disease Improving Global Outcomes (KDIGO) AKI guidelines recommend that patients be evaluated 3 months after an episode of AKI for resolution versus development or worsening of CKD.[6] However, rates of post-AKI nephrology follow-up appear to be poor, with less than 10% of patients referred in one study.[7] In another study from Canada, nephrologists were surveyed to determine which hypothetical AKI patient scenarios should receive follow-up nephrology care; among actual patients meeting these criteria, just 24% overall received such follow-up (**Visual abstract 51.1**).[8] Notably, in another observational study, early (within 90 days) outpatient nephrology follow-up care after an episode of severe (dialysis-requiring) AKI was associated with a reduction in mortality (**Visual abstract 51.2**).[9]

The Acute Disease Quality Initiative (ADQI) held a conference on quality of care in AKI in 2018 and recommended measuring rates of follow-up as a potential quality measure for AKI care.[10] Clearly, not all patients recovering from an episode of AKI will require nephrology specialty care, and follow-up can also be done by non-nephrologists, especially in less severe cases. Health systems and clinical practices are encouraged to develop mechanisms to monitor and ensure post-AKI follow-up care. Recently, some centers have developed specific clinics dedicated to post-AKI care,[11] and formal studies are underway to evaluate the clinical impact of such an approach.

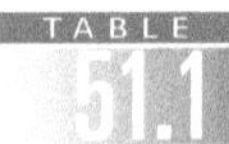

Long-Term Complications Following Acute Kidney Injury

Complication	Notes
Kidney outcomes	
CKD/ESKD	• May lead to new and/or progressive CKD • Risk progressively increases with greater severity (stage) or AKI, but is present even for mildest forms of AKI.
Proteinuria	• Strong risk factor for progressive CKD in the post-AKI period
Recurrent AKI	• Occurs in up to 30% of AKI patients • Associated with worse outcomes
Cardiovascular outcomes	
High blood pressure	• Animal models suggest possible salt-sensitive hypertension with associated ongoing kidney injury following AKI
Cardiovascular events (heart failure, myocardial infarction, stroke)	• Strongest association observed is between AKI and heart failure.
Long-term mortality	• AKI is associated with increased risk for all-cause and cardiovascular mortality. • Care remains primarily supportive and focused on modifiable risk factors.
Quality of life	• Reductions appear primarily related to limitations in physical functioning, so attention should be paid to rehabilitation needs.

AKI, acute kidney injury; CKD, chronic kidney disease; ESKD, end-stage kidney disease.

GENERAL ASPECTS OF FOLLOW-UP CARE

Several principles can be broadly applied to patients surviving an episode of AKI (**Table 51.2**). First, kidney function monitoring is required, including both an assessment of estimated glomerular filtration rate (eGFR) and evaluation for albuminuria. The exact timing of this evaluation will depend on the severity of the initial insult and the trajectory of kidney function recovery. However, even patients with recovery to baseline kidney function should have a kidney function assessment at least 2 to 3 months after the acute episode (as discussed in the Kidney Outcomes section of this chapter).[12]

Second, both the patients and the providers should be educated regarding the AKI episode and the potential downstream complications. Unfortunately, a significant proportion of patients remain unaware of their AKI diagnosis following a hospitalization—80% in a recent study.[13] This knowledge is fundamental to engaging patients in subsequent risk factor modification.

Third, the providers must carefully perform medication reconciliation, for both prescribed and over-the-counter drugs. One aspect is education around

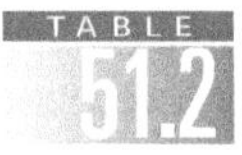

Principles of Post–Acute Kidney Injury Care

Component	Notes
Patient education	• Many patients with AKI are not aware of this diagnosis or the risk of later complications. • Quality of life assessment • Education about "sick-day protocols" for holding certain medications, such as diuretics and ACEI/ARB, during acute illness
Kidney function assessment	• Monitor for kidney recovery vs new or progressive CKD. • Both serum creatinine/eGFR and proteinuria measurement are indicated.
Medication reconciliation	• Importance of avoiding nephrotoxin exposures to the extent possible, such as NSAIDs
Medication adjustment	• For renally cleared drugs, either dose reduction (in the setting of progressive CKD) or dose increase (in the setting of kidney recovery) may be required.
Risk factor modification	• Blood pressure control • Cardiovascular risk assessment

AKI, acute kidney injury; ACEI, angiotensin-converting enzyme inhibitor; ARB, angiotensin receptor blocker; CKD, chronic kidney disease; eGFR, estimated glomerular filtration rate; NSAID, nonsteroidal anti-inflammatory drug.

potential nephrotoxin exposure, particularly in patients with delayed kidney function recovery or persistent CKD. For example, studies have shown that regular nonsteroidal anti-inflammatory drug (NSAID) use is common even among AKI survivors.[14] Another aspect is ensuring appropriate dosing of renally cleared medications. Dose reduction may be required with new-onset or worsening CKD. Conversely, posthospitalization medication dosing increases may be appropriate when further improvement in kidney function occurs, in order to avoid underdosing.

KIDNEY OUTCOMES

Chronic Kidney Disease/End-Stage Kidney Disease

In recent years, there has been increasing recognition of the bidirectional relationship between AKI and CKD.[15] The risk for later complications increases with the severity of the initial AKI insult,[16] although even relatively mild episodes of AKI are associated with significant increased risk for subsequent CKD and ESKD.[2] One study has developed a risk tool for prediction of advanced CKD after an episode of AKI,[17] providing an opportunity for a risk-stratified approach to AKI follow-up. This tool incorporates data that are readily available at the time of hospital discharge (including demographic information, severity of AKI episode [by KDIGO stage], and the degree of albuminuria) and generates a percentage estimate for the development of eGFR less than 45 within 1 year after discharge. The tool is freely available online at https://qxmd.com/calculate/calculator_451/advanced-ckd-after-aki-risk-index.

In addition to an overt decline in GFR, AKI has also been associated with subsequent development of CKD in the form of new-onset or worsening proteinuria.[18] Furthermore, post-AKI proteinuria appears to be a strong predictor for subsequent CKD progression. In the Assessment, Serial Evaluation, and Subsequent Sequelae in Acute Kidney Injury (ASSESS-AKI) study, higher post-AKI albuminuria was associated with a significant increased risk for kidney disease progression (hazard ratio [HR] 1.53, 95% confidence interval [CI]: 1.45-1.62).[12] These findings emphasize the importance of appropriate post-AKI monitoring of both kidney filtration function and urinary protein excretion.

There remains debate regarding whether the link between AKI and CKD is causal versus associative, such as simply an unmasking of underlying subclinical CKD. Animal models have demonstrated a prolonged inflammatory response after an episode of AKI, which can mediate chronic damage,[19] suggesting a pathophysiologic mechanism for the transition to CKD. In addition, interventional animal studies have found that post-AKI kidney damage can be mitigated by pharmacologic means targeting inflammatory pathways.[20,21] In one study, spironolactone was able to reduce post-AKI CKD changes in rats, postulated secondary to reducing profibrotic and inflammatory pathways mediated by transforming growth factor beta (TGF-beta).[21] Another study similarly showed that a dose of lithium, which inhibits glycogen synthase kinase 3 beta, was able to reduce post-AKI kidney tissue inflammation and promote repair.[20] Together, these studies support a causal connection between AKI and CKD and also provide a basis for future mechanistic and interventional studies. However, multiple different pathways have been implicated in the pathogenesis of AKI, and it remains unclear which pathway may predominate, or whether the pathway depends on the type of injury. Unfortunately, at present, there are no human clinical trials supporting therapies specifically for reducing the risk of CKD following AKI.

For patients who do progress to CKD, standard CKD management practices should be adopted, including focus on risk factor modification such as blood pressure control. Appropriate monitoring and recognition can provide the opportunity for early intervention, which is likely to yield the greatest benefit.

Recurrent Acute Kidney Injury

Nearly 30% of patients surviving an episode of AKI will subsequently have a recurrent hospitalization with AKI, and not surprisingly, recurrence is associated with worse outcomes.[3,22] Risk factors for recurrence include well-established AKI risk factors, such as older age, diabetes, and worse baseline kidney function. In addition, particularly high-risk groups for recurrent AKI are those with significant underlying comorbidities, including heart failure, cirrhosis, and acute coronary syndromes. Therefore, follow-up care of these patients should emphasize interspecialty communication and coordination of care because optimizing management of underlying conditions is likely to reduce the chances of AKI recurrence.
A particular area of clinical uncertainty is whether renin-angiotensin system (RAS) blockade should be used and when. In theory, RAS blockade could be nephroprotective and beneficial for progression of CKD. But in the acute setting of AKI, angiotensin receptor blockers (ARBs) and angiotensin-converting enzyme inhibitors (ACEIs) are typically held to optimize glomerular filtration. Resumption (or new initiation) of these therapies can be associated with a reduction in filtration, which may confound the clinical picture of recovering AKI, and there is concern they could contribute to recurrent AKI. As such, it seems reasonable to wait for stability in kidney function before starting or restarting RAS blockade, and this may

occur in the posthospitalization follow-up period. A retrospective cohort study suggested that new initiation of RAS blockade after AKI was relatively safe and not associated with an increased risk for recurrent AKI; patients treated with RAS blockade experienced similar rates of recurrent AKI compared to those not on RAS blockade (adjusted odds ratio [OR] 0.71, 95% CI:0.45-1.12).[23] An earlier retrospective study of post-AKI RAS blockade did show increased risk for kidney-related rehospitalization (adjusted HR 1.28, 95% CI: 1.12-1.46), but demonstrated lower risk for overall mortality (adjusted HR 0.85, 95% CI: 0.81-0.89) in patients treated with RAS blockade compared to those not treated (**Visual abstract 51.3**).[24] Taken together, these studies suggest a reasonable safety profile for RAS blockade in the post-AKI setting and potential long-term benefits. However, close monitoring is warranted, and additional studies are needed to identify which subgroups may benefit most or be at highest risk for complications.

One consideration is the employment of "sick-day protocols," whereby patients are educated to hold certain medications during periods of acute illness,[10] such as acute febrile episodes or gastrointestinal disease associated with the risk of volume depletion (e.g., vomiting and/or diarrhea). In these situations, patients are advised to temporarily discontinue diuretics and ACEI/ARB, which may exacerbate a prerenal state and lead to recurrent AKI. For patients with diabetes, metformin is also recommended to be held because of the risks associated with AKI.

CARDIOVASCULAR OUTCOMES

Hypertension

One carefully conducted observational study found that AKI was independently associated with increased risk of subsequently having an elevated blood pressure (>140/90 mm Hg) in follow-up, and this finding persisted whether or not patients had CKD.[25] Hypertension may, in turn, be a risk factor for CKD development or progression and certainly may play a role in cardiovascular disease. As such, close monitoring for blood pressure control is an important aspect of post-AKI care.

At present, there are inadequate data to recommend specific first-line agents for the management of hypertension following AKI. However, animal models of AKI have demonstrated a post-AKI predilection to salt-sensitive hypertension and worsening kidney injury.[19] Therefore, diuretic therapy may be a reasonable option. In addition, as discussed earlier, the use of ACEI or ARB may have theoretical benefits and appears to be a reasonably safe option.

Major Adverse Cardiovascular Events

Observational studies have found an association between an episode of AKI and subsequent increased risk for both cardiovascular mortality and the development of cardiac complications. The strongest association is between AKI and subsequent development of heart failure,[4] but a meta-analysis suggested overall increased risk for myocardial infarction and stroke as well.[26] The mechanisms for this increased risk remain uncertain, but appear independent of shared risk factors. Proposed factors include the post-AKI inflammatory state, neurohormonal activation (including both sympathetic and RAS), and volume expansion.

In terms of management, there are no clinical trials that have specifically examined therapeutic approaches to cardiovascular risk reduction in AKI survivors. However, recognizing that these patients are at high risk for events is a starting point, and aggressive risk factor modification (e.g., blood pressure control) would seem appropriate.

MORTALITY

AKI is associated with high in-hospital mortality. Unfortunately, beyond the initial hospitalization, AKI survivors remain at significantly increased risk of long-term cardiovascular and all-cause mortality compared to those without AKI.[5,26] Care of this population remains primarily supportive in nature. The focus of management should be on control of modifiable risk factors, such as elevated blood pressure, blood sugar, and cholesterol, or weight loss when appropriate. In patients with persistent CKD, statin therapy may be appropriate.

QUALITY OF LIFE

Another underappreciated aspect of post-AKI care is the importance of patient-reported outcomes. Early studies found a significant and prolonged reduction in health-related quality of life (HRQOL) following an episode of severe (dialysis-requiring) AKI.[27] A more recent systematic review found that severe AKI survivors do have significantly reduced HRQOL when compared to the general population, but were comparable to other survivors or critical illness.[28] Reductions in HRQOL appear to be primarily related to limitations in physical function. Therefore, physical disability should be actively screened for among AKI survivors and consideration given to rehabilitation needs.

ACUTE KIDNEY INJURY REQUIRING OUTPATIENT DIALYSIS

One particularly vulnerable population is that of AKI patients who require dialysis (AKI-D) and who remain dialysis dependent at the time of discharge. Although some of these patients will have ESKD, a significant proportion of AKI-D patients, ranging from 20% to 60%, may still recover kidney function to the point of dialysis independence after hospital discharge.[29] As such, clinicians need to optimize management of these patients to promote kidney recovery—a critical and highly patient-centered outcome.

General principles for AKI-D patients are similar to the general AKI population as outlined earlier, including education about the natural course of AKI and avoidance of nephrotoxic insults. However, AKI-D patients face an even greater adjustment following hospitalization owing to the new dialysis requirements. Such patients generally have longer hospital stays, which may have included intensive care, and, therefore, may not be as prepared for the transition to the outpatient setting. Close attention and reinforcement are needed, and the opportunity exists, given that they will be seen frequently at the dialysis center. An important aspect of care should be the regular (e.g., weekly) assessment of residual kidney function to monitor for recovery.

Specific management recommendations for AKI-D outpatients focus on dialysis prescription, with a goal of optimizing blood pressure stability. One single-center retrospective study noted that greater episodes of intradialytic hypotension were associated with lower likelihood of kidney recovery to dialysis independence among patients with AKI requiring outpatient dialysis.[30] Although additional studies are needed to confirm these results, the findings are certainly plausible. Intradialytic hemodynamic instability has been associated with a variety of adverse outcomes, such as cardiovascular events and mortality,[31] presumably secondary to impaired end-organ perfusion, and this could certainly translate to kidney ischemia, impairing kidney recovery in AKI patients. As such, it is important that AKI-D patients have a more individualized approach to dialysis prescription that contrasts with the protocol-driven approaches often employed for

ESKD patients on maintenance dialysis. Consistent with this approach, the recent ADQI recommendations emphasize lower dialysis ultrafiltration rates and even permissive mild hypervolemia in favor of optimizing intradialytic hemodynamic stability.[10]

CONCLUSIONS

In recent years, there has been increasing recognition of the significant risk for morbidity and mortality following an episode of AKI. Unfortunately, there is a paucity of specific recommendations for management, as this remains a relatively understudied area. Still, by focusing on basic principles such as ensuring appropriate follow-up and risk factor modification, there is ample opportunity to improve the survivorship of this vulnerable population.

Acknowledgment

No funding was received for this work.

References

1. Susantitaphong P, Cruz DN, Cerda J, et al. World incidence of AKI: a meta-analysis. *Clin J Am Soc Nephrol.* 2013;8(9):1482-1493.
2. Heung M, Steffick DE, Zivin K, et al. Acute kidney injury recovery pattern and subsequent risk of CKD: an analysis of veterans health administration data. *Am J Kidney Dis.* 2016;67(5):742-752.
3. Siew ED, Parr SK, Abdel-Kader K, et al. Predictors of recurrent AKI. *J Am Soc Nephrol.* 2016;27(4):1190-1200.
4. Go AS, Hsu CY, Yang J, et al. Acute kidney injury and risk of heart failure and atherosclerotic events. *Clin J Am Soc Nephrol.* 2018;13(6):833-841.
5. Lafrance JP, Miller DR. Acute kidney injury associates with increased long-term mortality. *J Am Soc Nephrol.* 2010;21(2):345-352.
6. Kidney Disease: Improving Global Outcomes (KDIGO) CKD Work Group. KDIGO 2012 clinical practice guidelines for the evaluation and management of chronic kidney disease. *Kidney Int.* 2013;3(suppl 1):1-150.
7. Siew ED, Peterson JF, Eden SK, et al. Outpatient nephrology referral rates after acute kidney injury. *J Am Soc Nephrol.* 2012;23(2):305-312.
8. Karsanji DJ, Pannu N, Manns BJ, et al. Disparity between nephrologists' opinions and contemporary practices for community follow-up after AKI hospitalization. *Clin J Am Soc Nephrol.* 2017;12(11):1753-1761.
9. Harel Z, Wald R, Bargman JM, et al. Nephrologist follow-up improves all-cause mortality of severe acute kidney injury survivors. *Kidney Int.* 2013;83(5):901-908.
10. Kashani K, Rosner MH, Haase M, et al. Quality improvement goals for acute kidney injury. *Clin J Am Soc Nephrol.* 2019;14(6):941-953.
11. Silver SA, Harel Z, Harvey A, et al. Improving care after acute kidney injury: a prospective time series study. *Nephron.* 2015;131(1):43-50.
12. Hsu C-Y, Chinchilli VM, Coca S, et al. Post-acute kidney injury proteinuria and subsequent kidney disease progression: the assessment, serial evaluation, and subsequent sequelae in acute kidney injury (ASSESS-AKI) study. *JAMA Int Med.* 2020;180(3):402-410.
13. Siew ED, Parr SK, Wild MG, et al. Kidney disease awareness and knowledge among survivors of acute kidney injury. *Am J Nephrol.* 2019;49(6):449-459.
14. Lipworth L, Abdel-Kader K, Morse J, et al. High prevalence of non-steroidal anti-inflammatory drug use among acute kidney injury survivors in the southern community cohort study. *BMC Nephrol.* 2016;17(1):189.
15. Chawla LS, Eggers PW, Star RA, et al. Acute kidney injury and chronic kidney disease as interconnected syndromes. *N Engl J Med.* 2014;371(1):58-66.
16. Coca SG, Singanamala S, Parikh CR. Chronic kidney disease after acute kidney injury: a systematic review and meta-analysis. *Kidney Int.* 2012;81(5):442-448.
17. James MT, Pannu N, Hemmelgarn BR, et al. Derivation and external validation of prediction models for advanced chronic kidney disease following acute kidney injury. *JAMA.* 2017;318(18):1787-1797.
18. Hsu CY, Hsu RK, Liu KD, et al. Impact of AKI on urinary protein excretion: analysis of two prospective cohorts. *J Am Soc Nephrol.* 2019;30(7):1271-1281.

19. Basile DP, Leonard EC, Tonade D, et al. Distinct effects on long-term function of injured and contralateral kidneys following unilateral renal ischemia-reperfusion. *Am J Physiol Renal Physiol.* 2012;302(5):F625-F635.
20. Bao H, Ge Y, Wang Z, et al. Delayed administration of a single dose of lithium promotes recovery from AKI. *J Am Soc Nephrol.* 2014;25(3):488-500.
21. Barrera-Chimal J, Perez-Villalva R, Rodriguez-Romo R, et al. Spironolactone prevents chronic kidney disease caused by ischemic acute kidney injury. *Kidney Int.* 2013;83(1):93-103.
22. Holmes J, Geen J, Williams JD, et al. Recurrent acute kidney injury: predictors and impact in a large population-based cohort. *Nephrol Dial Transplant.* 2020;35(8):1361-1369.
23. Hsu CY, Liu KD, Yang J, et al. Renin-angiotensin system blockade after acute kidney injury (AKI) and risk of recurrent AKI. *Clin J Am Soc Nephrol.* 2020;15(1):26-34.
24. Brar S, Ye F, James MT, et al. Association of angiotensin-converting enzyme inhibitor or angiotensin receptor blocker use with outcomes after acute kidney injury. *JAMA Intern Med.* 2018;178(12):1681-1690.
25. Hsu CY, Hsu RK, Yang J, et al. Elevated BP after AKI. *J Am Soc Nephrol.* 2016;27(3):914-923.
26. Odutayo A, Wong CX, Farkouh M, et al. AKI and long-term risk for cardiovascular events and mortality. *J Am Soc Nephrol.* 2017;28(1):377-387.
27. Johansen KL, Smith MW, Unruh ML, et al. Predictors of health utility among 60-day survivors of acute kidney injury in the Veterans Affairs/National Institutes of Health Acute Renal Failure Trial Network Study. *Clin J Am Soc Nephrol.* 2010;5(8):1366-1372.
28. Villeneuve PM, Clark EG, Sikora L, et al. Health-related quality-of-life among survivors of acute kidney injury in the intensive care unit: a systematic review. *Intensive Care Med.* 2016;42(2):137-146.
29. Heung M. Outpatient dialysis for acute kidney injury: progress and pitfalls. *Am J Kidney Dis.* 2019;74(4):523-528.
30. Pajewski R, Gipson P, Heung M. Predictors of post-hospitalization recovery of renal function among patients with acute kidney injury requiring dialysis. *Hemodial Int.* 2018; 22(1):66-73.
31. Stefannsson BV, Brunelli SM, Cabrera C, et al. Intradialytic hypotension and risk of cardiovascular disease. *Clin J Am Soc Nephrol.* 2014;9(12):2124-2132.

What do nephrologists think about follow-up for severe AKI? How does this compare with practice?

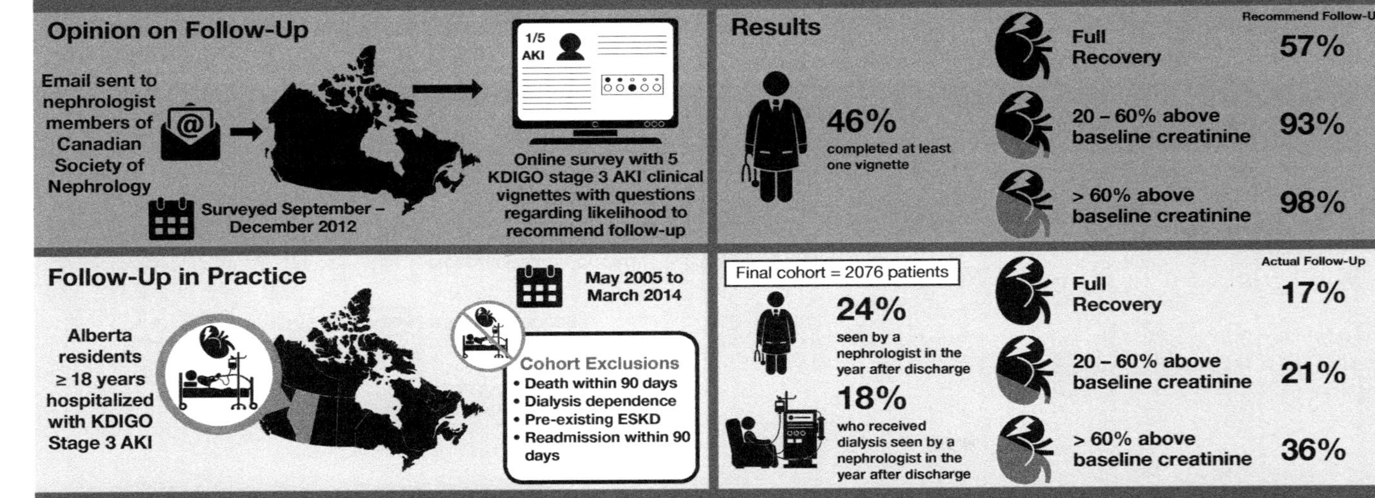

Conclusion: There is a substantial disparity between the opinions of nephrologists and actual processes of care for nephrology evaluation of patients after hospitalization with severe AKI.

Karsanji DJ, Pannu N, Manns BJ, et al. ***Disparity between Nephrologists' Opinions and Contemporary Practices for Community Follow-Up after AKI Hospitalization.*** Clin J Am Soc Nephrol. 2017;12(11):1753-1761.

VISUAL ABSTRACT 51.1

Is mortality different with versus without nephrology follow-up after dialysis-requiring AKI?

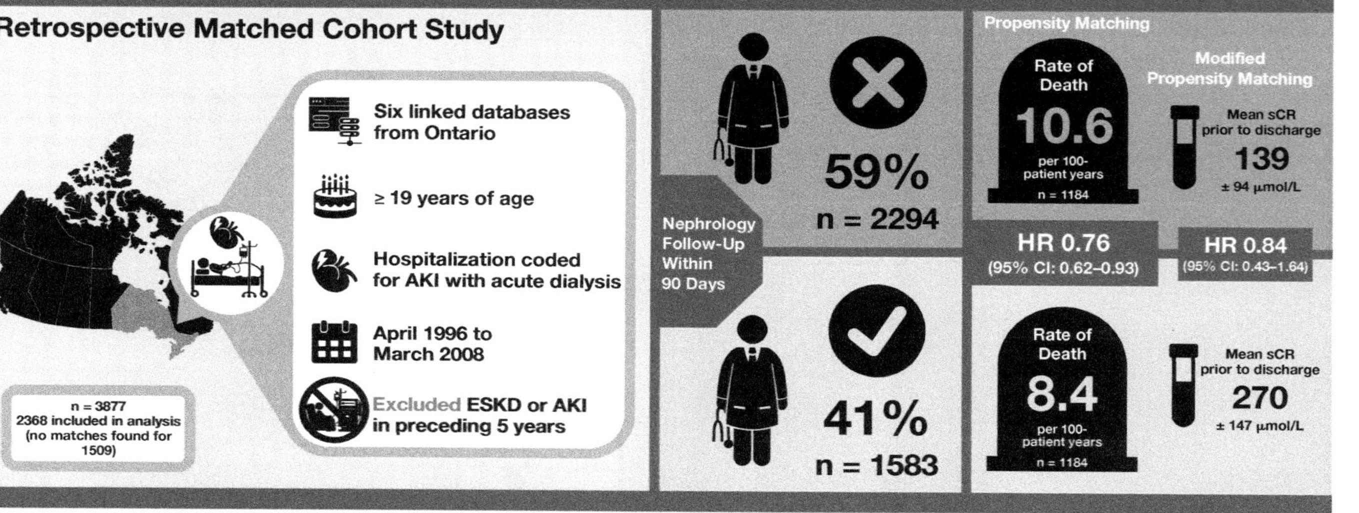

Conclusion: Using propensity matching, a visit with a nephrologist within 90 days of discharge following hospitalization with AKI-requiring dialysis was associated with a 24% lower hazard of death at 2 years.

Harel Z, Wald R, Bargman JM, et al. ***Nephrologist follow-up improves all-cause mortality of severe acute kidney injury survivors.*** Kidney Int. 2013;83(5):901-8.

VISUAL ABSTRACT 51.2

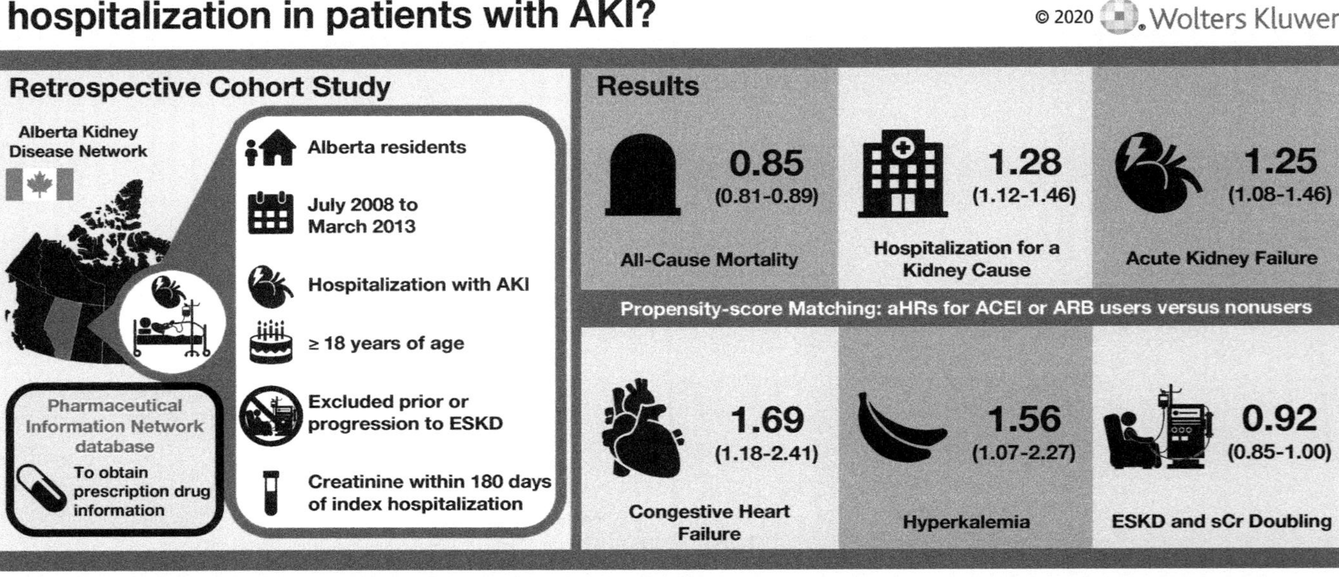

VISUAL ABSTRACT 51.3

SECTION X

Organ Transplantation

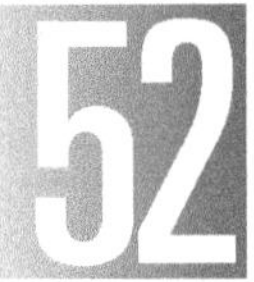

Perioperative Management of Kidney Transplant Recipients

Hunter Witt, Jaime Glorioso, Elizabeth A. King, and Jacqueline Garonzik Wang

INTRODUCTION

Kidney transplantation (KT) is the treatment of choice for suitable candidates with end-stage kidney disease (ESKD). KT not only increases patient survival but also improves quality of life and is more cost-effective in comparison to dialysis.[1-7] Despite more than 100,000 patients currently awaiting KT, only approximately 20,000 KTs are performed annually,[8] leading to organ shortage and unacceptable waitlist mortality.[9-11] Because kidney allografts represent a scare resource, it is imperative that we optimize patient selection and maximize allograft longevity through meticulous perioperative care. This chapter highlights the major principles of perioperative care of the KT recipient, including expedited preoperative evaluation at the time of organ offer and postoperative management.

PREOPERATIVE PATIENT ASSESSMENT

A successful KT begins with appropriate patient selection. Patients with ESRD frequently have other medical comorbidities that must be evaluated and optimized. A thorough history and physical examination are essential, as is an exhaustive and comprehensive medical workup.[12,13] Although the complete preoperative assessment is outside the scope of this chapter, in general, KT candidates should be evaluated for cardiopulmonary, cerebrovascular, and peripheral vascular disease (PVD). All patients should undergo a standard cardiopulmonary workup, including electrocardiogram, chest X-ray, and echocardiogram. Patients with diabetes, those older than 50 years, or with personal or a strong familial history of cardiovascular disease should have a cardiac stress test. Coronary angiography should be performed in patients with any evidence or suggestion of ischemia.[14-16] Further, candidates should be counseled on smoking cessation. Routine laboratory testing includes a complete blood count (CBC) with differential, comprehensive metabolic panel, and serologies. Cross-sectional imaging should be considered in the elderly or those with PVD, in order to assess for iliac artery calcifications that might preclude transplantation.[17] Transplant candidates should also undergo age-appropriate cancer screening.[18,19]

Often, the pretransplant workup is completed years prior to a recipient receiving an organ offer and undergoing transplantation. Therefore, it is imperative that each transplant center have an organized system for patient evaluation, routine reassessment, and an electronic record that makes this workup readily accessible when the recipient is called in for KT. Given the significant time interval between evaluation and transplantation, many aspects of the workup may have expired, or the patient's clinical status may have changed. Therefore, the following must be performed at the time of organ offer by a clinician:

1. Updated history and physical examination, focused on factors that affect peritransplant outcomes.
   a) Determine the etiology of ESKD with specific attention to recurrent diseases that may require additional perioperative therapies (i.e., focal segmental glomerulosclerosis [FSGS]).
   b) Recent/current infections (may be a contraindication to transplant)
   c) Active chest pain or shortness of breath
   d) Use of anticoagulation and last dosage
   e) If indicated, dialysis type and dialysis access, with documentation on examination of functioning access
   f) Assessment of PVD in the lower extremities, including confirmation of palpable femoral pulses for inflow of the graft (if there is any concern, an up-to-date computed tomography scan should be ordered)
   g) History of prior transplantation or prior surgeries and location of previous scars
   h) Quantification of daily urine output (if any). This information will be useful when determining perioperative allograft function.
2. Confirm the patient has an up-to-date human leukocyte antigen (HLA) sample for crossmatch (ensure no sensitizing events such as blood transfusion since the last sample was provided)
3. Standard laboratory evaluation with specific attention to the following:
   a) Potassium (to ensure they do not need dialysis prior to transplantation)
   b) Hematocrit (as many patients with ESKD are anemic at baseline and may require transfusion prior to, during, or after transplantation)
   c) Coagulation tests (especially patients on blood thinners)
   d) Active type and screen
   e) Determination of histocompatibility

The goal of this assessment should be to determine whether the patient is medically cleared for transplantation and if there is need for urgent pretransplant dialysis or additional studies. Usually, the organ has already been accepted and procured; therefore, time is of the essence to minimize cold ischemia time on the allograft.

OPERATIVE DETAILS

The KT operation remains relatively unchanged from its inception. The kidney is first prepared on the backtable. The kidney is evaluated for any trauma, surgical damage, or abnormalities. The perinephric fat is removed, and the vasculature is cleared of the surrounding tissue, taking care to ligate lymphatics. Care must be taken to preserve the periureteral tissue to maintain the blood supply to the ureter. The kidney vasculature is anastomosed to the recipient's external iliac vessels, which are most commonly accessed via a retroperitoneal approach, thus decreasing the likelihood of ileus or bowel injury. Occasionally, a transperitoneal approach is required. Depending on hospital-specific protocols, some recipients may receive intravenous heparin, Lasix, and mannitol prior to clamping of the vessels and reperfusion of the organ. The kidney is reperfused, and a ureterocystostomy is performed, frequently over a double-J stent.

IMMUNOSUPPRESSION

There are numerous intricacies to immunosuppression therapies based on center- and surgeon-specific protocols, patient sensitization, and ongoing clinical trials. The following are guidelines, based on frequently utilized therapies, and not meant to be an exhaustive resource.

Induction Immunosuppression

Induction therapy is intense immunosuppressive therapy given at the time of transplant to decrease the likelihood of rejection. Thymoglobulin (rabbit antithymocyte globulin) is a T-cell-depleting therapy.[20] This is a weight-based therapy, and the total dosage is often based on recipient sensitization and center-specific protocols. It is coadministered with steroids, which act as an additional induction agent and mitigate the cytokine release seen with thymoglobulin. A daily CBC should be closely monitored because pancytopenia is often a limiting side effect. Other induction agents that are sometimes employed include basiliximab, alemtuzumab, and OKT3.

Maintenance Immunosuppression in the Perioperative Period

Maintenance immunosuppression consists of triple therapy, including a calcineurin inhibitor, an antimetabolite, and steroid therapy.[21-24] Tacrolimus is a calcineurin inhibitor that requires drug level monitoring, given the side-effect profile, drug-drug interactions, and variability in pharmacokinetics.[24] Cyclosporine is a calcineurin inhibitor that is sometimes used as a second-line agent for patients who do not tolerate the side effects of tacrolimus. The most common antimetabolite used is one of the many formulations of mycophenolate mofetil. Azathioprine is sometimes used for patients who do not tolerate mycophenolate mofetil, those who are already on the drug for other reasons, or women of childbearing age who are considering pregnancy.[25] In addition, most recipients are placed on prednisone for maintenance immunosuppression, with some centers opting for steroid-free or steroid-minimization protocols. Finally, some centers include mammalian target of rapamycin (mTOR) inhibitors, sirolimus or everolimus, in their maintenance immunosuppression regimens.

POSTOPERATIVE MANAGEMENT

Postoperative care of the transplant recipient can be challenging because patient- and graft-related issues often have conflicting management. These patients are monitored in either an intensive care unit or a step-down unit to ensure frequent assessment of patient complaints, vitals, and fluid status. It is important to be mindful of the fact that the combination of chronic disease and intense immunosuppression can often obscure diagnosis of postoperative complications. The major tenets of postoperative care are highlighted in the subsequent section.

Perioperative Fluid Management

Management of volume status of a KT recipient can be challenging in the postoperative period. Although they are often relatively volume overloaded, KT recipients may have intravascular volume depletion from the stress associated with surgery and allograft reperfusion. Further, the transplant allograft performs better if the patient is adequately intravascularly resuscitated; however, this often conflicts with tenets of volume management in patients who are oliguric or anuric at baseline. Most centers employ the following volume administration strategy in the perioperative period to ensure adequate hydration for graft perfusion, while preventing pulmonary and cardiac complications associated with significant volume overload: the patient is placed on a small carrier fluid (e.g., 30 mL/hr of half-normal saline and mL per mL replacement of urine output with normal saline or half-normal saline).[26] This allows the amount of fluid administered to be proportional to the function of the graft. At 24 hours, fluid is dropped to an hourly rate, based on output from the previous 24 hours. The primary goal of perioperative fluid management is to ensure adequate graft perfusion, while minimizing the risks of intravenous fluid, such as volume overload and electrolyte abnormalities. Finally, serum potassium needs to be monitored frequently, even in a KT recipient with immediate graft function, as solute clearance often lags behind urine production. Although temporizing measures can be employed for hyperkalemia, the best and most appropriate treatment is often hemodialysis.[27] Patients on peritoneal dialysis who are at risk for delayed graft function should, therefore, be warned that they may need temporary hemodialysis access placed in the postoperative period.

Hemodynamic Considerations

Blood pressure management in the perioperative period is also complicated. Patients with ESKD can present with a wide span of preoperative blood pressures, ranging from patients who are severely hypertensive on multiple medications to patients with severe autonomic dysfunction or hypotension requiring midodrine.[28] Further, general anesthesia, narcotics, and thymoglobulin can potentiate hypotension, whereas pain and volume overload can potentiate hypertension. It is recommended to hold antihypertensives postoperatively to determine how the patient will respond to thymoglobulin and general anesthesia and slowly reintroduce agents as necessary, although there are limited data to support this practice. In the perioperative period, the provider will want to prevent severe hypertension (systolic blood pressure >180 mm Hg), while maintaining blood pressure for adequate allograft perfusion.[28]

Catheter and Drain Management

Patients will have a urinary bladder catheter placed at the time of surgery. This serves two purposes. First, it decompresses the bladder to allow the ureterocystostomy to heal, and second, it allows for close urine output assessment in the perioperative period. The duration of the catheter is often dictated by the integrity of the bladder, which is assessed intraoperatively. Some surgeons also perform the ureteral anastomosis over a stent to prevent leakage or stricture.[29] This is removed as an outpatient procedure approximately 1 month after the transplant. Surgical drains allow the surgeon to assess for urinary, lymphatic, or vascular leakage.

Graft Function

While the majority of recipients will have immediate graft function, given increased utilization of high kidney donor profile index (KDPI) and high terminal creatinine kidneys and many other factors, some will have slow or delayed graft function.[30,31] The crudest assessment of allograft function is based on urine output and creatinine clearance. For kidneys with immediate allograft function, the recipient will have robust urine output and a rapid drop in creatinine. Lack of urine output or a significant reduction in urine output should warrant concern and prompt recipient volume assessment and kidney ultrasound.[32] For recipients with slow or delayed graft function, a transplant duplex ultrasound confirms adequate vascular inflow and outflow and allograft perfusion. Additional studies, such as nuclear medicine kidney scintigraphy, can assess for vascular integrity and help assess for a urine leak or ureteral obstruction.[31]

Recipient Diet and Ambulation

Recipients will often start a clear liquid diet immediately after surgery and will be advanced based on return of bowel function. Patients are placed on an H2 blocker or proton pump inhibitor (PPI) for ulcer prophylaxis. Diabetic patients should be placed on a carbohydrate-controlled diet. Of note, all patients should have strict glycemic control because perioperative steroids often complicate blood glucose control.[33] Patients should be encouraged to ambulate as soon as possible, and standard deep vein thrombosis (DVT) prophylaxis should be administered including sequential compression devices (SCDs) and subcutaneous heparin, as long as there are no contraindications.

POST–KIDNEY TRANSPLANTATION COMPLICATIONS

Ureteral Complications

The incidence of urologic complications in the early posttransplant period ranges from 3% to 14%.[34] Early detection is of key importance because these complications can lead to early loss of a KT. Urine leaks generally present within the first 3 months posttransplantation. Common signs include pain and swelling in the transplant area, rising creatinine, oliguria, and/or signs of infection. Urologic complications can often be traced to technical errors or difficulties encountered during procurement, bench dissection, or implantation. The majority of leaks occur at the ureterocystostomy and are managed initially with percutaneous drainage of the collection and bladder catheterization until the leak has resolved.[35] Percutaneous nephrostomy and nephroureteral stent placement are additional adjuncts. If the leak fails to resolve with maximal decompression, then surgical exploration is required. The ureter is also at risk for stricture, often as a consequence of inadequate blood supply or injury. This frequently can be managed with stenting and ureteroplasty, but may ultimately require operative revision.[36]

Rejection

An unexpected rise in creatinine should raise concern for rejection, especially when other etiologies including infection, dehydration, or medication-induced kidney injury have been excluded.[37] When this occurs, donor-specific antibodies should be checked. Percutaneous kidney biopsy provides definitive diagnosis. Newer, noninvasive markers, including donor-derived cell-free deoxyribonucleic acid (DNA), are being explored to aid in rejection diagnosis; however, none are currently the standard of care.[38] Once rejection is suspected or diagnosed, prompt treatment based on rejection type should follow.[39]

Renal Artery Thrombosis

Recipients with a known prothrombotic state or history of venous thromboembolic events are at higher risk of renal artery thrombosis. Multiple donor arteries, donor and recipient atherosclerosis, and pediatric kidneys also increase this risk.[40] Although a rare complication (with an incidence rate of 0.1%-2%), this typically occurs within 72 hours of transplant and presents with abrupt decrease in urine output without pain over the allograft.[41] Ultrasound is the imaging study of choice to make the diagnosis. Allograft salvage with thrombectomy is rarely successful.

Renal Vein Thrombosis

Risk factors for renal vein thrombosis include prothrombotic state, kinked vessels, narrow venous anastomosis, hypotension, and acute rejection.[42] It frequently occurs soon after surgery and presents with hematuria, decrease in urine output, and significant pain. Emergent thrombectomy and anastomotic revision may result in allograft salvage.[43]

Lymphocele

A lymphocele is a collection arising from the lymphatics along the iliac vessels or the renal hilum of the donor kidney. Small lymphoceles are often asymptomatic. However, they can be large, resulting in pain, ureteral obstruction, or vascular compression.[44] Limiting the iliac vessel dissection and ensuring the lymphatics are ligated can minimize the risk of lymphocele formation. If the lymphocele results in compressive symptoms or is infected, it should be managed with a drain. Noninfected and persistent lymphoceles can be managed with internal drainage via laparoscopic marsupialization into the peritoneal cavity.[45]

Medical Complications

KT recipients are at risk for a variety of postoperative medical complications, given their comorbidity and organ failure at the time of transplant. These include, but are not limited to, myocardial infarction, pulmonary embolism, stroke, volume overload, congestive heart failure, and a variety of nosocomial and opportunistic infections.[46] Recipients are placed on prophylaxis for *Pneumocystis*, cytomegalovirus, and *Candida*. Individuals who present with glomerular disease are at risk for disease recurrence following KT. For patients with primary FSGS, the urine protein-to-creatinine ratio should be monitored, and elevation in serum creatinine should prompt early biopsy.

SUMMARY

KT has become the treatment of choice for individuals with ESKD. Owing to organ shortage, appropriate recipient selection and meticulous perioperative care to maximize the longevity of the allograft are imperative. Advancements in technique, immunosuppression, and postoperative care lead to excellent allograft and patient survival.

References

1. Wolfe RA, Ashby VB, Milford EL, et al. Comparison of mortality in all patients on dialysis, patients on dialysis awaiting transplantation, and recipients of a first cadaveric transplant. *N Engl J Med.* 1999;341(23):1725-1730.
2. Abecassis M, Bartlett ST, Collins AJ, et al. Kidney transplantation as primary therapy for end-stage renal disease: a National Kidney Foundation/Kidney Disease Outcomes Quality Initiative (NKF/KDOQITM) conference. *Clin J Am Soc Nephrol.* 2008;3(2):471-480.

3. Fisher R, Gould D, Wainwright S, et al. Quality of life after renal transplantation. *J Clin Nurs.* 1998;7(6):553-563.
4. Ichikawa Y, Fujisawa M, Hirose E, et al. Quality of life in kidney transplant patients. *Transplant Proc.* 2000;32(7):1815-1816.
5. Jofre R, Lopez-Gomez JM, Moreno F, et al. Changes in quality of life after renal transplantation. *Am J Kidney Dis.* 1998;32(1):93-100.
6. Page TF, Woodward RS. Cost-effectiveness of Medicare's coverage of immunosuppression medications for kidney transplant recipients. *Exp Rev Pharmacoecon Outcomes Res.* 2009;9(5):435-444.
7. Perovic S, Jankovic S. Renal transplantation vs hemodialysis: cost-effectiveness analysis. *Vojnosanit Pregl.* 2009;66(8):639-644.
8. Matas AJ, Smith JM, Skeans MA, et al. OPTN/SRTR 2013 Annual Data Report: kidney. *Am J Transplant.* 2015;15(suppl 2):1-34.
9. Grams ME, Massie AB, Schold JD, et al. Trends in the inactive kidney transplant waitlist and implications for candidate survival. *Am J Transplant.* 2013;13(4):1012-1018.
10. Cassuto JR, Reese PP, Sonnad S, et al. Wait list death and survival benefit of kidney transplantation among nonrenal transplant recipients. *Am J Transplant.* 2010;10(11):2502-2511.
11. Schold J, Srinivas TR, Sehgal AR, et al. Half of kidney transplant candidates who are older than 60 years now placed on the waiting list will die before receiving a deceased-donor transplant. *Clin J Am Soc Nephrol.* 2009;4(7):1239-1245.
12. Chapman JR. The KDIGO clinical practice guidelines for the care of kidney transplant recipients. *Transplantation.* 2010;89(6):644-645.
13. Bunnapradist S, Danovitch GM. Evaluation of adult kidney transplant candidates. *Am J Kidney Dis.* 2007;50(5):890-898.
14. Katta N, Balla S, Velagapudi P, et al. Preoperative cardiac evaluation in kidney transplant patients: is coronary angiography superior? A focused review. *Adv Perit Dial.* 2016;32:32-38.
15. Fossati N, Meacci L, Amorese G, et al. Cardiac evaluation for simultaneous pancreas-kidney transplantation and incidence of cardiac perioperative complications: preliminary study. *Transplant Proc.* 2004;36(3):582-585.
16. Eagle KA, Berger PB, Calkins H, et al. ACC/AHA guideline update for perioperative cardiovascular evaluation for noncardiac surgery—executive summary. A report of the American College of Cardiology/American Heart Association Task Force on Practice Guidelines (Committee to Update the 1996 Guidelines on Perioperative Cardiovascular Evaluation for Noncardiac Surgery). *Anesth Analg.* 2002;94(5):1052-1064.
17. Sarsengaliyev T, Chuvakova E, Tsoy B, et al. Computed tomography in the preoperative and postoperative evaluation of kidney transplant patients. *Exp Clin Transplant.* 2015;13(suppl 3):88-90.
18. Lambert M. Cancer screening recommendations from the ACS: a summary of the 2017 guidelines. *Am Fam Physician.* 2018;97(3):208-210.
19. Acuna SA, Huang JW, Scott AL, et al. Cancer screening recommendations for solid organ transplant recipients: a systematic review of clinical practice guidelines. *Am J Transplant.* 2017;17(1):103-114.
20. Koyawala N, Silber JH, Rosenbaum PR, et al. Comparing outcomes between antibody induction therapies in kidney transplantation. *J Am Soc Nephrol.* 2017;28(7):2188-2200.
21. Menon MC, Murphy B. Maintenance immunosuppression in renal transplantation. *Curr Opin Pharmacol.* 2013;13(4):662-671.
22. Alberu J, Urrea EM. Immunosuppression for kidney transplant recipients: current strategies. *Rev Invest Clin.* 2005;57(2):213-224.
23. Matas AJ, Kandaswamy R, Humar A, et al. Long-term immunosuppression, without maintenance prednisone, after kidney transplantation. *Ann Surg.* 2004;240(3):510-516; discussion 516-517.
24. Gaston RS. Maintenance immunosuppression in the renal transplant recipient: an overview. *Am J Kidney Dis.* 2001;38(6 suppl 6):S25-S35.
25. Wagner M, Earley AK, Webster AC, et al. Mycophenolic acid versus azathioprine as primary immunosuppression for kidney transplant recipients. *Cochrane Database Syst Rev.* 2015(12):CD007746.
26. Efune GE, Zerillo J, Zhou G, et al. Intravenous fluid management practices in kidney transplant patients: a multicenter observational cohort pilot study. *Semin Cardiothorac Vasc Anesth.* 2020;24(3):256-264.
27. Schnuelle P, Johannes van der Woude F. Perioperative fluid management in renal transplantation: a narrative review of the literature. *Transpl Int.* 2006;19(12):947-959.
28. Cheung AK, Chang TI, Cushman WC, et al. Blood pressure in chronic kidney disease: conclusions from a Kidney Disease: Improving Global Outcomes (KDIGO) controversies conference. *Kidney Int.* 2019;95(5):1027-1036.

29. Wilson CH, Rix DA, Manas DM. Routine intraoperative ureteric stenting for kidney transplant recipients. *Cochrane Database Syst Rev*. 2013;17(6):CD004925.
30. Halloran PF, Hunsicker LG. Delayed graft function: state of the art, November 10-11, 2000. Summit meeting, Scottsdale, Arizona, USA. *Am J Transplant*. 2001;1(2):115-120.
31. Siedlecki A, Irish W, Brennan DC. Delayed graft function in the kidney transplant. *Am J Transplant*. 2011;11(11):2279-2296.
32. Humar A, Matas AJ. Surgical complications after kidney transplantation. *Semin Dial*. 2005;18(6):505-510.
33. Hricik, DE, Bartucci MR, Moir EJ, et al. Effects of steroid withdrawal on posttransplant diabetes mellitus in cyclosporine-treated renal transplant recipients. *Transplantation*. 1991;51(2):374-377.
34. Pisani F, Iaria G, D'Angelo M, et al. Urologic complications in kidney transplantation. *Transplant Proc*. 2005;37(6):2521-2522.
35. Friedersdorff F, Weinberger S, Biernath N, et al. The ureter in the kidney transplant setting: ureteroneocystostomy surgical options, double-J stent considerations and management of related complications. *Curr Urol Rep*. 2020;21(1):3.
36. Buttigieg J, Agius-Anastasi A, Sharma A, et al. Early urological complications after kidney transplantation: an overview. *World J Transplant*. 2018;8(5):142-149.
37. Hanssen O, Erpicum P, Lovinfosse P, et al. Non-invasive approaches in the diagnosis of acute rejection in kidney transplant recipients. Part I. In vivo imaging methods. *Clin Kidney J*. 2017;10(1):97-105.
38. Bloom RD, Bromberg JS, Poggio ED, et al. Cell-free DNA and active rejection in kidney allografts. *J Am Soc Nephrol*. 2017;28(7):2221-2232.
39. Matas AJ, Humar A, Payne WD, et al. Decreased acute rejection in kidney transplant recipients is associated with decreased chronic rejection. *Ann Surg*. 1999;230(4):493-498.
40. Ponticelli C, Moai M, Montagnino G. Renal allograft thrombosis. *Nephrol Dial Transplant*. 2009;24(5):1388-1393.
41. McCarthy JM, Yeung CK, Keown PA. Late renal-artery thrombosis after transplantation associated with intraoperative abdominopelvic compression. *N Engl J Med*. 1990;323(26):1845.
42. El Zorkany K, Bridson JM, Halawa A. Transplant renal vein thrombosis. *Exp Clin Transplant*. 2017;12(2):123-129.
43. Kim HS, Fine DM, Atta MG. Catheter-directed thrombectomy and thrombolysis for acute renal vein thrombosis. *J Vasc Interv Radiol*. 2006;17(5):815-822.
44. Lucewicz A, Wong G, Lam VW, et al. Management of primary symptomatic lymphocele after kidney transplantation: a systematic review. *Transplantation*. 2011;92(6):663-673.
45. Joosten M, D'ancona FC, Van der Meijden WA, et al. Predictors of symptomatic lymphocele after kidney transplantation. *Int Urol Nephrol*. 2019;51(12):2161-2167.
46. Silkensen JR. Long-term complications in renal transplantation. *J Am Soc Nephrol*. 2000; 11(3):582-588.

Acute Kidney Injury in Patients with Kidney Transplants

Kalyani Chandra and Ling-Xin Chen

EPIDEMIOLOGY

Kidney transplant (KT) recipients have lower rates of hospitalization compared with dialysis-dependent patients; however, they have increased rates of acute kidney injury (AKI) when compared with the community-dwelling population.[1,2] The incidence rates of AKI and AKI-requiring dialysis in the KT population are estimated to be as much as 20- and 45-fold higher than those in the general community.[2] KT recipients are at higher risk for AKI as compared to the general population due to their solitary kidney status with lower nephron mass, higher incidence of frailty, dialysis dependency prior to transplantation, immunocompromised state, higher comorbidity burden, and calcineurin inhibitor exposure.[3,4] Lower estimated glomerular filtration rate (eGFR) was identified as the most important risk factor for AKI in a national registry-based study of AKI including 27,232 KT recipients; other risk factors include black race, diabetic status, and more recent transplantation.[2] This study found that 11.3% of Medicare-insured transplant recipients developed AKI between 6 months and 3 years post-KT, of which 14% (1.6% of the entire cohort) of patients had AKI-requiring dialysis and 12.1% lost their graft during hospitalization.[2] AKI led to a hazard ratio for transplant failure of 2.74 [95% confidence interval (CI): 2.56-2.92] when dialysis was not required and 7.35 (95% CI: 6.32-8.54) when dialysis was required (**Visual abstract 53.1**).[2]

Admission to the intensive care unit (ICU) in the KT population seems to have decreased from 41.6% in the 1990s to 4% to 7% in more recent years.[4-6] The most common indications for admission to the ICU in a single-center French study including 200 KT recipients were acute respiratory failure (27.5%) and septic shock (26.5%), followed by immediate postoperative complications (23%), cardiogenic shock (9%), neurologic complications (6%), AKI (5%), and others (3%).[5] However, 57% of KT recipients had infection at the time of ICU admission, indicating the high degree that infectious etiologies are responsible for morbidity in KT.[5] The source of infection was pulmonary (50%), urinary (22.8%), and peritonitis (24%). This cohort had a total hospital mortality of 22.5%, and 30.1% had a progression of at least one stage of CKD at 6 months posthospitalization.[5] The detrimental effects of an episode of AKI for the KT population are multiplied by the fact that lower eGFR is a predictor of cardiovascular mortality as well as long-term graft and patient survival.[6]

SPECIFIC ETIOLOGIES

The specific etiologies of AKI in KT have been summarized by time after transplantation in **Figure 53.1** and are discussed later in this chapter. Generally, as time after transplant increases, primary consideration should be given to the usual causes of AKI in native kidneys. Immediate postsurgical complications such as vascular issues (arterial or venous thrombosis and dissection), ureteral complications (ureteral leakage and obstruction), peritransplant hematomas or seromas, wound infections or dehiscence, and other postsurgical cardiovascular, respiratory, and neurologic issues are discussed in detail in Chapter 52.

Pyelonephritis

Urinary tract infection (UTI), including pyelonephritis, is the most common bacterial infection post-KT, with reported incidence rates ranging from 6% to 83% and accounting for up to 45% to 72% of all infections in solid-organ transplant recipients.[7-9] Having a shorter segment of the ureter without a native ureteral valve predisposes KT recipients to chronic mild-to-moderate vesicoureteral reflux and allows the potential for rapid progression of simple cystitis to pyelonephritis.[10] One retrospective study of UTI in 867 KT recipients followed up to 1 year posttransplant found that 21% developed a UTI at a median of 18 days posttransplantation and 15% had an episode of pyelonephritis.[11] Risk factors for pyelonephritis are variably reported in the literature, but consistent ones include early postoperative period, female gender, advanced age, and the presence of a ureteral stent (which are removed at variable times early post transplant).[11-15] The increased risk of pyelonephritis in a patient population that is often asymptomatic in the early phases of infection has led many practitioners to treat asymptomatic bacteriuria, but a multicenter prospective randomized trial demonstrated lack of benefit.[8] In 87 KT recipients without ureteral or urethral catheters within their first post transplant year who developed asymptomatic urinary bacteriuria, there was no difference between antibiotic-treated and nontreated groups in the rate of acute graft pyelonephritis, bacteremia, cystitis, need for admission, or eGFRs.[8] In fact, the treatment group had more fosfomycin-resistant, extended-spectrum beta-lactamase–producing and amoxicillin-clavulanate–resistant bacteria.[8]

Gram-negative organisms are responsible for over 70% of UTIs in KT recipients, with *Escherichia coli* being the most common isolate, and organisms are more likely to be resistant to trimethoprim-sulfamethoxazole and ciprofloxacin.[16] Thus, prompt initiation of broad-spectrum antibiotics is key in the acute

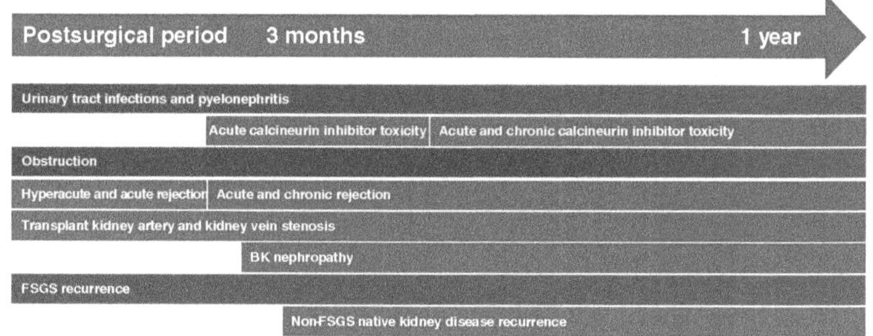

FIGURE 53.1: Etiologies of the most common causes of AKI in kidney transplant recipients by time after transplant. AKI, acute kidney injury; FSGS, focal segmental glomerulosclerosis.

setting and may be coupled with the decrease in immunosuppression if deemed appropriate by a transplant specialist.[17] A rare but life-threatening complication of acute pyelonephritis is emphysematous pyelonephritis, characterized by kidney parenchymal necrosis with gas accumulation.[18,19] Management is usually conservative, though interventions such as percutaneous nephrostomy and abscess drainage are used; however, transplant nephrectomy may be required.[18,20] In cases of recurrent UTIs, further evaluation for vesicoureteral reflux and consideration of long-term prophylactic antibiotics are warranted. The impact of pyelonephritis on short- and long-term patient and graft outcomes is variably reported in the literature and may differ based on when infection occurred relative to transplantation.[6,8,21]

Calcineurin Inhibitors

CNIs, cyclosporin A and tacrolimus, are the mainstay of immunosuppression therapy in kidney and other nonrenal transplants, but are known to cause long-term kidney injury as well as to contribute to the kidney's susceptibility to AKI.[22] CNIs cause afferent arteriolar vasoconstriction, decreasing renal blood flow and glomerular filtration, over time leading to arteriolar hyaline thickening, tubulointerstitial ischemia, and, eventually, interstitial fibrosis and tubular atrophy.[22-24] CNIs also reduce expression of the Na^+:K^+:2Cl^- cotransporter in tubuloepithelial cells, leading to polyuria, nephrocalcinosis, magnesium wasting, and hyperreninemic hyperaldosteronism.[25] Taken together, these effects predispose KT recipients to AKI, even from minor dehydration episodes. CNIs can themselves cause acute toxicity of the allograft, which manifests as AKI, electrolyte disturbances (e.g., hyperkalemia, hypomagnesemia, distal tubular acidosis), and, rarely, thrombotic microangiopathy. CNI toxicity is usually reversible with dose reduction.

CNIs are substrates of cytochrome P450 enzymes 3A4 and 3A5 and the P-glycoprotein transporter, leading to interactions with many drugs, herbs, food constituents, as well as susceptibilities to alterations in gut flora and function.[26] One single-center study of 138 KT recipients found that approximately 10% of hospital admissions were related to probable adverse drug reactions, of which 46% of cases were avoidable.[27] The most common drug interactions are identified in **Table 53.1**. It is important to consider drug interactions when beginning new medications in any patient on CNIs and to follow CNI drug levels closely during hospitalization.

Obstruction

Ureteral obstruction occurs in 2% to 10% of KT recipients, usually within the first 3 months of transplantation.[28] Ureteral ischemia accounts for up to 90% of cases and usually involves the distal ureter, which is furthest from the renal artery.[28] Other etiologies include long ureter (prone to ischemia and kinking), external compression (lymphocele, hematoma, seroma, urinoma, or abscess), calculi (donor-gifted or de novo), neurogenic bladder, ureteral stent blockage, and BK virus infection causing ureteral stricture. An asymptomatic rise in creatinine and decreased urine output should prompt evaluation by ultrasound, which has greater than 90% sensitivity for detecting urinary obstruction.[29] However, functionally nonsignificant mild-to-moderate hydronephrosis of the allograft is frequently seen owing to the lack of a ureteral valve, so further evaluation by renogram may be required to confirm the diagnosis.[30] Percutaneous nephrostomy and nephroureteral tube placement are often useful in the management of cases of obstruction, but prompt treatment of the underlying cause of obstruction is needed to preserve allograft function.

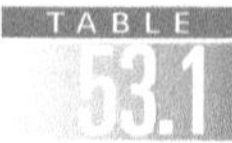

Most Commonly Noted Drugs, Foods, and Herbals Causing Calcineurin Inhibitor (CNI) Interaction

Agents That Increase CNI Levels	Agents That Decrease CNI Levels
Calcium channel blockers: diltiazem, verapamil	Antituberculosis medications: rifampin, rifabutin, isoniazid
Antifungals: ketoconazole, fluconazole, itraconazole[a]	Anticonvulsants: phenobarbital, carbamazepine, phenytoin
Protease inhibitors: ritonavir, indinavir	Antibiotics: nafcillin
Macrobid antibiotics[b]: erythromycin, clarithromycin	Non-nucleoside reverse transcriptase inhibitors: efavirenz, nevirapine
Amiodarone	Caspofungin
Suboxone	St. John's wort
Cimetidine	
Nefazodone	
Grapefruit	

[b]Dihydropyridine calcium channel blockers such as amlodipine and nifedipine do no cause CNI-level alterations.
[a]Azithromycin does not cause CNI-level alterations.

Transplant Renal Artery Stenosis

Transplant renal artery stenosis (TRAS) can cause AKI, hypertension, volume overload, pulmonary and peripheral edema, and graft failure, and its incidence ranges from 1% to 23%.[31,32] It is usually diagnosed within the first year of transplant, and known risk factors include older age, ischemic heart disease, and surgical technical errors.[31] Doppler ultrasonography is the main diagnostic screening test, whereas contrast-enhanced magnetic resonance imaging (MRI) is more specific and often used as a confirmatory test before intervention.[33] Treatment options include medical management, percutaneous intervention with angioplasty and/or stent placement, and surgical reconstruction (now very rare because of high success rates of other treatments). Medical management includes antihypertensive medications coupled with close monitoring of symptoms, renal function, and serial imaging when indicated. Although no randomized trials exist comparing treatment options, a single-center retrospective study found a high rate of stenosis recurrence when percutaneous angioplasty was used without stenting.[34] Transplant renal vein stenosis is much rarer than TRAS, but can present similar to TRAS and may also be found by Doppler ultrasonography or contrast-enhanced MRI.[35]

Rejection

The incidence of acute rejection has decreased significantly in recent years. In the 2015 to 2016 cohort of KT recipients, the incidence of rejection within the first year of KT was 9%, as opposed to 50% to 60% in the late 1980s.[36,37] However, acute rejection must still be considered a cause of AKI, especially in individuals who are at increased risk: those with high levels of preformed antibodies or donor-specific antibodies (DSAs), medication nonadherence, prior episodes of rejection, or delayed graft function. Rejection episodes vary from hyperacute rejection, leading to immediate graft loss within minutes of graft implantation (rarely seen), to acute and subsequent chronic rejection.[38] The current gold standard for rejection diagnosis is transplant biopsy with concurrent screening for DSAs, though recent developments in diagnostic testing include the use of assays for expression of rejection-specific genes and detection of cell-free donor-derived deoxyribonucleic acid (DNA).[39,40]

Although a thorough discussion of rejection diagnosis and treatment is beyond the scope of this book, what follows is a brief summary. Rejection can be classified according to Banff criteria into two types: cell-mediated and antibody-mediated rejection, although these can occur simultaneously.[41] Cell-mediated rejection is characterized by tubulitis, interstitial inflammation, and occasionally arteritis and can be treated with corticosteroids or antithymocyte globulin for more severe cases.[42] Acute antibody-mediated rejection is characterized by glomerulitis, peritubular capillaritis, and complement deposition in the endothelium (C4d staining positivity) in the setting of high levels of circulating DSAs. There may also be tubular necrosis and unexplained arteritis or thrombotic microangiopathy. Chronic antibody-mediated rejection is characterized by transplant glomerulopathy and is often accompanied by interstitial fibrosis and tubular atrophy.[41] Treatment for antibody-mediated rejection includes antibody clearance strategies such as therapeutic plasmapheresis, intravenous immunoglobulins (Igs), and B-cell therapies such as rituximab or bortezomib, though none of these therapies have strong evidence of efficacy.[42] Acute antibody-mediated rejection is noted to be associated with a 4-fold increase in graft loss as compared with T-cell–mediated rejection or no rejection, and recurrent rejection episodes are known to impair long-term graft survival.[43]

BK Virus Nephropathy

The BK virus is a polyomavirus in which an estimated 75% of the adult population has been exposed to and typically causes no symptoms in immunocompetent individuals.[44] However, in the setting of immunosuppression, BK virus (usually donor-derived) can replicate rapidly and cause nephropathy, ureteral stricture, or hemorrhagic cystitis.[44] BK virus nephropathy usually presents as an indolent decline in kidney function, occurs in 1% to 10% of KT recipients, typically within the first year of transplant, and seems to correlate with the degree of immunosuppression.[45] Most patients are asymptomatic early in the disease course, so transplant programs often test for BK virus levels empirically, but some patients may present with rapidly worsening creatinine levels, pyuria, or hematuria.[44] On biopsy, BK nephropathy is characterized by intranuclear viral inclusions, tubular injury and inflammation, and positive SV40 staining (100% specificity for polyomavirus).[45] The main treatment strategy is decreasing immunosuppression, typically starting with the antimetabolite (mycophenolate mofetil), followed by decreasing CNI dosage if there is no response to antimetabolite reduction. Immunosuppression reduction must always be balanced by the individual's risk for rejection, which has been reported to occur in concert with BK nephropathy, although it is unclear if this is related to immunosuppression reduction or challenges in rejection diagnosis when BK nephropathy is present.[45] Other treatment options include leflunomide, intravenous Ig, cidofovir, rapamycin, and ciprofloxacin, but good-quality data on these treatment strategies are limited.[46] BK nephropathy has been reported to cause a graft loss rate of 46% and has a recurrence rate of 15% in subsequent transplants.[47,48] Although BK viremia has been estimated to affect 5% of heart transplant recipients, progression to nephropathy in non-kidney solid-organ transplant recipients is rare.[49]

Recurrence of Native Kidney Disease

Recurrence of native kidney disease accounts for less than 2% to 4% of graft losses.[50,51] The causes of primary glomerulonephritis (in order of recurrence risk) are type II membranoproliferative glomerulonephritis (MPGN) (>80%), thrombotic thrombocytopenic purpura/hemolytic uremic syndrome (TTP/HUS) (60%), IgA nephropathy (20%-60%), focal segmental glomerulosclerosis (FSGS) (20%-50%), type I MPGN (20%-30%), membranous nephropathy (10%-30%), anti–glomerular basement membrane (GBM) nephritis (~12%), and lupus nephritis (2%-10%).[50,52-55] De novo glomerulonephritis is rare, but the most common entities include minimal change disease, MPGN, FSGS, membranous nephropathy, and IgA nephropathy.[55,56] An unexplained rise in creatinine, proteinuria, or hematuria should raise suspicion for recurrence of native disease. Kidney biopsy remains the gold standard for diagnosis. Workup and management are similar to those of native kidney disease but are tailored based on chronicity. Of note, unlike native kidney FSGS, plasmapheresis likely has a role in the treatment of recurrent FSGS in KT recipients.[57]

NON-KIDNEY TRANSPLANT RECIPIENTS

Although this chapter has focused on KT recipients, a few key points may also be applicable to recipients of a non-kidney solid-organ transplant. Recipients of non-kidney organ transplants are known to be at increased risk for chronic kidney failure (16.5% of non-kidney transplant recipients between 1990 and 2000), and AKI is known to contribute to that risk.[58] Because CNI therapy is a cornerstone of immunosuppression in non-kidney organ transplantation, issues related to CNI use are also common in the non-kidney organ transplant recipient. Non-kidney solid-organ transplant recipients are also at high risk of infection because of their immunosuppressed status, and urine remains a common infectious source, though pyelonephritis does not occur to the same frequency as with KT recipients.[59]

References

1. Voiculescu A, Schmitz M, Hollenbeck M, et al. Management of arterial stenosis affecting kidney graft perfusion: a single-centre study in 53 patients. *Am J Transplant.* 2005;5:1731-1738.
2. Mehrotra A, Rose C, Pannu N, et al. Incidence and consequences of acute kidney injury in kidney transplant recipients. *Am J Kidney Dis.* 2012;59:558-565.
3. Meier-Kriesche HU, Baliga R, Kaplan B. Decreased renal function is a strong risk factor for cardiovascular death after renal transplantation. *Transplantation.* 2003;75:1291-1295.
4. Mouloudi E, Massa E, Georgiadou E, et al. Course and outcome of renal transplant recipients admitted to the intensive care unit: a 20-year study. *Transplant Proc.* 2012;44:2718-2720.
5. Guinault D, Del Bello A, Lavayssiere L, et al. Outcomes of kidney transplant recipients admitted to the intensive care unit: a retrospective study of 200 patients. *BMC Anesthesiol.* 2019;19:130.
6. Sadaghdar H, Chelluri L, Bowles SA, et al. Outcome of renal transplant recipients in the ICU. *Chest.* 1995;107:1402-1405.
7. Fiorante S, Fernandez-Ruiz M, Lopez-Medrano F, et al. Acute graft pyelonephritis in renal transplant recipients: incidence, risk factors and long-term outcome. *Nephrol Dial Transplant.* 2011;26:1065-1073.
8. Sabe N, Oriol I, Melilli E, et al. Antibiotic treatment versus no treatment for asymptomatic bacteriuria in kidney transplant recipients: a multicenter randomized trial. *Open Forum Infect Dis.* 2019;6. doi:10.1093/ofid/ofz243
9. Graversen ME, Dalgaard LS, Jensen-Fangel S, et al. Risk and outcome of pyelonephritis among renal transplant recipients. *BMC Infect Dis.* 2016;16:264.
10. Kayler L, Kang D, Molmenti E, et al. Kidney transplant ureteroneocystostomy techniques and complications: review of the literature. *Transplant Proc.* 2010;42:1413-1420.
11. Bodro M, Sanclemente G, Lipperheide I, et al. Impact of urinary tract infections on short-term kidney graft outcome. *Clin Microbiol Infect.* 2015;21:1104.E1-1104.E8.

12. Choi YS, Kim KS, Choi SW, et al. Ureteral complications in kidney transplantation: analysis and management of 853 consecutive laparoscopic living-donor nephrectomies in a single center. *Transplant Proc.* 2016;48:2684-2688.
13. Carvalho JA, Nunes P, Antunes H, et al. Surgical complications in kidney transplantation: an overview of a Portuguese reference center. *Transplant Proc.* 2019;51:1590-1596.
14. Zavos G, Pappas P, Karatzas T, et al. Urological complications: analysis and management of 1525 consecutive renal transplantations. *Transplant Proc.* 2008;40:1386-1390.
15. Kotagiri P, Chembolli D, Ryan J, et al. Urinary tract infections in the first year post-kidney transplantation: potential benefits of treating asymptomatic bacteriuria. *Transplant Proc.* 2017;49:2070-2075.
16. Säemann M, Hörl WH. Urinary tract infection in renal transplant recipients. *Eur J Clin Invest.* 2008;38:58-65.
17. Goldman JD, Julian K. Urinary tract infections in solid organ transplant recipients: guidelines from the American Society of Transplantation Infectious Diseases Community of Practice. *Clin Transplant.* 2019:e13507.
18. Al-Geizawi SM, Farney AC, Rogers J, et al. Renal allograft failure due to emphysematous pyelonephritis: successful non-operative management and proposed new classification scheme based on literature review. *Transpl Infect Dis.* 2010;12:543-550.
19. Takahashi K, Malinzak LE, Safwan M, et al. Emphysematous pyelonephritis in renal allograft related to antibody-mediated rejection: a case report and literature review. *Transpl Infect Dis.* 2019;21:e13026.
20. Falagas ME, Alexiou VG, Giannopoulou KP, et al. Risk factors for mortality in patients with emphysematous pyelonephritis: a meta-analysis. *J Urol.* 2007;178:880-885; quiz 1129.
21. Fellstrom B, Jardine AG, Soveri I, et al. Renal dysfunction as a risk factor for mortality and cardiovascular disease in renal transplantation: experience from the Assessment of Lescol in Renal Transplantation trial. *Transplantation.* 2005;79:1160-1163.
22. Naesens M, Kuypers DRJ, Sarwal M. Calcineurin inhibitor nephrotoxicity. *Clin J Am Soc Nephrol.* 2009;4:481.
23. Liptak P, Ivanyi B. Primer: histopathology of calcineurin-inhibitor toxicity in renal allografts. *Nat Clin Pract Nephrol.* 2006;2:398-404.
24. Nankivell BJ, P'Ng CH, O'Connell PJ, et al. Calcineurin inhibitor nephrotoxicity through the lens of longitudinal histology: comparison of cyclosporine and tacrolimus eras. *Transplantation.* 2016;100:1723-1731.
25. Naesens M, Steels P, Verberckmoes R, et al. Bartter's and Gitelman's syndromes: from gene to clinic. *Nephron Physiol.* 2004;96:65-78.
26. Vanhove T, Annaert P, Kuypers DRJ. Clinical determinants of calcineurin inhibitor disposition: a mechanistic review. *Drug Metab Rev.* 2016;48:88-112.
27. Bril F, Castro V, Centurion IG, et al. A systematic approach to assess the burden of drug interactions in adult kidney transplant patients. *Curr Drug Saf.* 2016;11:156-163.
28. Kumar S, Ameli-Renani S, Hakim A, et al. Ureteral obstruction following renal transplantation: causes, diagnosis and management. *Br J Radiol.* 2014;87:20140169.
29. Duty BD, Conlin MJ, Fuchs EF, et al. The current role of endourologic management of renal transplantation complications. *Adv Urol.* 2013;2013:246520.
30. Nankivell BJ, Cohn DA, Spicer ST, et al. Diagnosis of kidney transplant obstruction using Mag3 diuretic renography. *Clin Transplant.* 2001;15:11-18.
31. Ngo AT, Markar SR, De Lijster MS, et al. A systematic review of outcomes following percutaneous transluminal angioplasty and stenting in the treatment of transplant renal artery stenosis. *Cardiovasc Intervent Radiol.* 2015;38:1573-1588.
32. Hurst FP, Abbott KC, Neff RT, et al. Incidence, predictors and outcomes of transplant renal artery stenosis after kidney transplantation: analysis of USRDS. *Am J Nephrol.* 2009;30:459-467.
33. Fananapazir G, Bashir MR, Corwin MT, et al. Comparison of ferumoxytol-enhanced MRA with conventional angiography for assessment of severity of transplant renal artery stenosis. *J Magn Reson Imaging.* 2017;45:779-785.
34. Chen LX, De Mattos A, Bang H, et al. Angioplasty vs stent in the treatment of transplant renal artery stenosis. *Clin Transplant.* 2018;32:e13217.
35. Granata A, Clementi S, Londrino F, et al. Renal transplant vascular complications: the role of Doppler ultrasound. *J Ultrasound.* 2014;18:101-107.
36. Hart A, Smith JM, Skeans MA, et al. OPTN/SRTR 2017 Annual Data Report: kidney. *Am J Transplant.* 2019;19:19-123.
37. Cecka JM, Terasaki PI. Early rejection episodes. *Clin Transpl.* 1989:425-434.
38. Bhatti AB, Usman M. Chronic renal transplant rejection and possible anti-proliferative drug targets. *Cureus.* 2015;7:e376.

39. Bloom RD, Bromberg JS, Poggio ED, et al. Cell-free DNA and active rejection in kidney allografts. *J Am Soc Nephrol.* 2017;28:2221-2232.
40. Roedder S, Sigdel T, Salomonis N, et al. The kSORT assay to detect renal transplant patients at high risk for acute rejection: results of the multicenter AART study. *PLoS Med.* 2014;11:e1001759.
41. Haas M, Loupy A, Lefaucheur C, et al. The Banff 2017 Kidney Meeting Report: revised diagnostic criteria for chronic active T cell-mediated rejection, antibody-mediated rejection, and prospects for integrative endpoints for next-generation clinical trials. *Am J Transplant.* 2018;18:293-307.
42. Linares L, Garcia-Goez JF, Cervera C, et al. Early bacteremia after solid organ transplantation. *Transplant Proc.* 2009;41:2262-2264.
43. Orandi BJ, Chow EH, Hsu A, et al. Quantifying renal allograft loss following early antibody-mediated rejection. *Am J Transplant.* 2015;15:489-498.
44. Lamarche C, Orio J, Collette S, et al. BK polyomavirus and the transplanted kidney: immunopathology and therapeutic approaches. *Transplantation.* 2016;100:2276-2287.
45. Bohl DL, Brennan DC. BK virus nephropathy and kidney transplantation. *Clin J Am Soc Nephrol.* 2007;2:S36-S46.
46. Johnston O, Jaswal D, Gill JS, et al. Treatment of polyomavirus infection in kidney transplant recipients: a systematic review. *Transplantation.* 2010;89:1057-1070.
47. Vasudev B, Hariharan S, Hussain SA, et al. BK virus nephritis: risk factors, timing, and outcome in renal transplant recipients. *Kidney Int.* 2005;68:1834-1839.
48. Hirsch HH, Brennan DC, Drachenberg CB, et al. Polyomavirus-associated nephropathy in renal transplantation: interdisciplinary analyses and recommendations. *Transplantation.* 2005;79:1277-1286.
49. Viswesh V, Yost SE, Kaplan B. The prevalence and implications of BK virus replication in non-renal solid organ transplant recipients: a systematic review. *Transplant Rev.* 2015;29:175-180.
50. Blosser CD, Bloom RD. Recurrent glomerular disease after kidney transplantation. *Curr Opin Nephrol Hypertens.* 2017;26:501-508.
51. Fairhead T, Knoll G. Recurrent glomerular disease after kidney transplantation. *Curr Opin Nephrol Hypertens.* 2010;19:578-585.
52. Golgert WA, Appel GB, Hariharan S. Recurrent glomerulonephritis after renal transplantation: an unsolved problem. *Clin J Am Soc Nephrol.* 2008;3:800-807.
53. de Fijter JW. Recurrence of glomerulonephritis: an underestimated and unmet medical need. *Kidney Int.* 2017;92:294-296.
54. Lingaraj U, Patil SR, Aralapuram K, et al. Recurrence of membranoproliferative glomerulonephritis post transplant—is this mere recurrence of pattern or recurrence of disease? *Saudi J Kidney Dis Transpl.* 2019;30:719-722.
55. Ponticelli C, Moroni G, Glassock RJ. De novo glomerular diseases after renal transplantation. *Clin J Am Soc Nephrol.* 2014;9:1479-1487.
56. Sener A, Bella AJ, Nguan C, et al. Focal segmental glomerular sclerosis in renal transplant recipients: predicting early disease recurrence may prolong allograft function. *Clin Transplant.* 2009;23:96-100.
57. Kashgary A, Sontrop JM, Li L, et al. The role of plasma exchange in treating post-transplant focal segmental glomerulosclerosis: a systematic review and meta-analysis of 77 case-reports and case-series. *BMC Nephrol.* 2016;17:104.
58. Ojo AO, Held PJ, Port FK, et al. Chronic renal failure after transplantation of a nonrenal organ. *N Engl J Med.* 2003;349:931-940.
59. Vidal E, Torre-Cisneros J, Blanes M, et al. Bacterial urinary tract infection after solid organ transplantation in the RESITRA cohort. *Transpl Infect Dis.* 2012;14:595-603.

What do we know about AKI episodes following kidney transplantation?

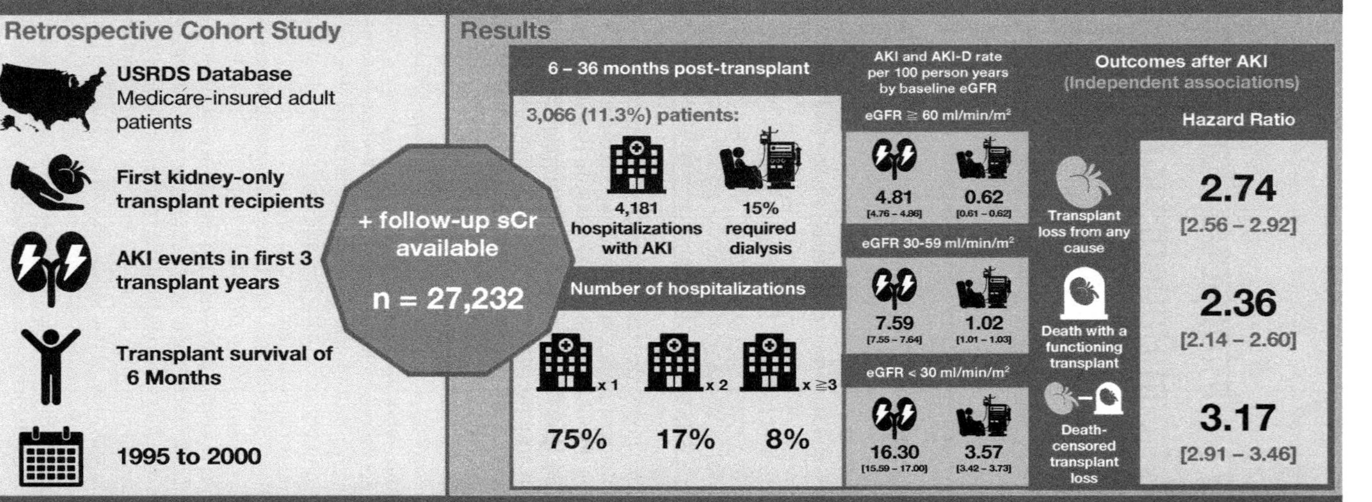

Conclusion: This cohort study revealed AKI and AKI-requiring dialysis (AKI-D) rates in a post-transplant population that were 20- and 45-fold higher than non-transplanted community-based patients.

Mehrotra A, Rose C, Pannu N, Gill J, Tonelli M, Gill JS. ***Incidence and consequences of acute kidney injury in kidney transplant recipients.*** Am J Kidney Dis. 2012;59(4):558-65.

VISUAL ABSTRACT 53.1

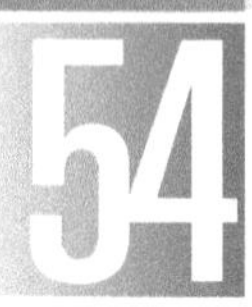

Infectious Complications in Patients with Kidney Transplant

Pratik B. Shah and Kathleen M. Mullane

INFECTIONS IN KIDNEY TRANSPLANT RECIPIENTS

Kidney transplant recipients (KTRs) are immunosuppressed and are at increased risk of conventional and opportunistic infections, which contribute to their morbidity and mortality.[1] Multiple pre- and post-transplant factors, operative procedural factors, and post-transplant factors place KTRs at increased risk of infection.[2,3] Post-transplant surgical site infections, respiratory infections, catheter infections (either intravenous [IV] or genitourinary [GU]), intra-abdominal infections including kidney and perinephric abscesses, graft-site candidiasis, as well as drug fever or acute rejection of the transplanted organs should also be considered when a transplant recipient returns with fevers or septic physiology.[4] Because immunosuppression is less aggressive in KTRs when compared to that required in hematopoietic cellular transplant recipients as well as in other solid-organ transplant recipients, fungal infections are less common.[5]

The etiology of the infection in KTR depends on the timeline from the transplant (see **Figure 54.1**). In the first month post-transplant, donor-derived and nosocomial infections are more common. In months 1 to 6 post-transplant, KTRs are at risk of opportunistic viral (community-acquired respiratory pathogens, gastrointestinal, and reactivation of latent viruses), fungal (reactivation of *endemic mycoses*, *Pneumocystis*, and *Candida* spp.), and parasitic (reactivation of *Strongyloides* or *Toxoplasma*) infections. After 6 months post-transplant, KTRs remain at higher risk of infection from community-acquired pathogens.[6,7] Because immunocompromised KTRs may not manifest classic clinical and radiologic features of infection, a high degree of vigilance and clinical suspicion is warranted. The use of prophylactic antimicrobials and exposure to the hospital environment may increase the risk of multiple antibiotic-resistant organisms as well as *Clostridium difficile* infection.

On presentation, source identification by serial physical examinations with special attention to the presence of central venous catheter–related infections, acquisition of a nosocomial or community-acquired respiratory infection, possible surgical site infections, and the presence of a Foley catheter or stents should be undertaken. Definite diagnosis with microbiology, multiplex panels, or next-generation sequencing technologies as well as tissue culture and histology with attention to obtaining special stains for fungal, viral, and acid-fast organisms should be pursued.[8] Serologies are not always positive nor are they helpful in the diagnosis of an acute infection. It must be remembered that consideration of noninfectious complications such as allograft rejection, drug toxicity or drug hypersensitivity reactions, and ischemic or thrombotic events may mimic the features of sepsis[3] (see **Figure 54.2**).

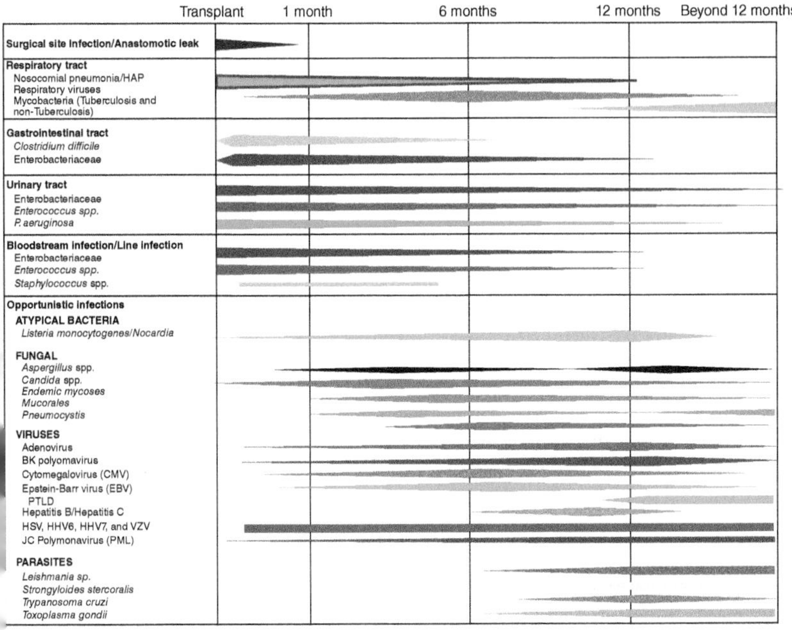

Transplant | 1 month | 6 months | 12 months | Beyond 12 months

Surgical site infection/Anastomotic leak

Respiratory tract
Nosocomial pneumonia/HAP
Respiratory viruses
Mycobacteria (Tuberculosis and non-Tuberculosis)

Gastrointestinal tract
Clostridium difficile
Enterobacteriaceae

Urinary tract
Enterobacteriaceae
Enterococcus spp.
P. aeruginosa

Bloodstream infection/Line infection
Enterobacteriaceae
Enterococcus spp.
Staphylococcus spp.

Opportunistic infections
ATYPICAL BACTERIA
Listeria monocytogenes/Nocardia

FUNGAL
Aspergillus spp.
Candida spp.
Endemic mycoses
Mucorales
Pneumocystis

VIRUSES
Adenovirus
BK polyomavirus
Cytomegalovirus (CMV)
Epstein-Barr virus (EBV)
PTLD
Hepatitis B/Hepatitis C
HSV, HHV6, HHV7, and VZV
JC Polymonavirus (PML)

PARASITES
Leishmania sp.
Strongyloides stercoralis
Trypanosoma cruzi
Toxoplasma gondii

FIGURE 54.1: Timeline of kidney transplant–related infections. HAP, hospital-acquired pneumonia; HHV6, human herpesvirus 6; HSV, herpes simplex virus; PTLD, post-transplant lymphoproliferative disorder; VZV, varicella-zoster virus. Adapted from Fishman JA. Infection in organ transplantation. *Am J Transplant.* 2017;17(4):856-879. doi:10.1111/ajt.14208; Van Delden C, Stampf S, Hirsch HH, et al. Burden and timeline of infectious diseases in the first year after solid organ transplantation in the Swiss Transplant Cohort Study. *Clin Infect Dis.* 2020;ciz1113. doi:10.1093/cid/ciz1113.

Sepsis in patients with kidney transplants

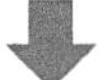

Physical assessment
Obtain blood and urine cultures; obtain cultures from suspicious sites
Initiate antimicrobial therapy, fluid and pressor support, stress dose steroids
Directed radiology assessment

Interventional radiologic or surgical drainage/debridement as indicated
Evaluate for noninfectious causes of sepsis
allograft rejection, drug toxicity/hypersensitivity reactions, ischemic and/or thrombotic events

Reduce immunosuppression as able
De-escalate or narrow antimicrobial therapy as able

FIGURE 54.2: Management of Sepsis in Patients with Kidney Transplants

Because delay in adequate antimicrobial therapy is associated with increased mortality, timely initiation of empiric broad-spectrum antimicrobial agents is the cornerstone of sepsis management. Given frequent exposure of KTRs to hospital- and health care–associated infections, a history of previous infections with multidrug-resistant organisms should be taken into consideration in the choice of empiric antimicrobial therapy with de-escalation once data from cultures and molecular diagnostic testing return. Fluid resuscitation with consideration of graft function and appropriate fluids as well as vasopressor support should be addressed based on current international guidelines.[9] Source control with directed image-guided or surgical drainage procedures, surgical debridement of infected/necrotic tissues, and removal of infected foreign objects should be undertaken in a timely manner. Appropriate stress-dose corticosteroid therapy should be considered in all KTRs at risk of adrenal insufficiency.[10] In the setting of sepsis, immunosuppression dose reduction or temporary withdrawal should be considered to improve the host immunologic response. This should be carefully balanced against the risk of allograft rejection. If the immunosuppressants are continued, drug level should be monitored, given pharmacodynamic and pharmacokinetic changes caused by sepsis.

CYTOMEGALOVIRUS INFECTION

Cytomegalovirus (CMV), a member of herpesvirus, is the most common opportunistic infection in KTR. Risk factors include CMV-seropositive donor (especially with CMV-seronegative recipient), use of antilymphocytic antibody for induction (e.g., thymoglobulin), rejection episodes, older donors, composite transplants, and impaired graft function.[11,12] CMV infection can develop as primary infection, infection with new CMV strain (donor-derived) different from latent strains present in the recipient, or reactivation of latent virus. CMV viremia is best detected by nucleic acid testing (NAT); CMV pp65 antigenemia assay is less sensitive and is rarely used. Viremia by NAT may be absent with colitis, pneumonitis, and retinitis; therefore, histopathologic confirmation may be necessary in some cases of suspected CMV end-organ disease. Universal prophylaxis with valganciclovir (VGCV) or preemptive therapy can be instituted for the prevention of CMV disease in intermediate- and high-risk KTR (see **Table 54.1**).

Based on 2019 Clinical Transplantation Consensus Statement and Recommendations, VGCV or IV ganciclovir (GCV) is recommended as the first-line treatment in adults for initial and recurrent episodes of CMV disease.[13] VGCV is recommended in patients with mild-to-moderate CMV disease who can tolerate and adhere to oral medication. IV GCV is recommended in life-threatening and severe disease. Oral GCV, acyclovir, or valacyclovir is not recommended for the treatment of CMV disease.

For CMV pneumonia and, possibly, more severe disease, addition of hyperimmune CMV immunoglobulin (Cytogam) may be beneficial. Reduction of maintenance immunosuppression should be considered to facilitate recovery from CMV disease. A 1 $\log_{10}$ decline in CMV viral load should be attained after 2 weeks of appropriately dosed antiviral therapy. If after 2 weeks CMV DNAemia or antigenemia increases more than 1 $\log_{10}$, it is considered refractory; if CMV DNAemia or antigenemia persists or increases less than 1 $\log_{10}$, it is considered probably refractory. These findings would warrant genotypic resistance testing

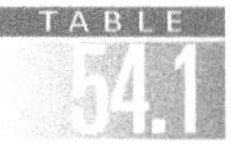

Clinical Effects of Cytomegalovirus

CMV Infection	**Evidence of CMV Replication Regardless of the Symptoms**
CMV disease	Evidence of CMV replication as well as the symptoms • CMV syndrome—fever, malaise, leukopenia, neutropenia, atypical lymphocytosis, and thrombocytopenia • Tissue invasive disease—pneumonitis, hepatitis, retinitis, gastrointestinal disease, nephritis
Indirect effects	Higher risk for other opportunistic infections (fungal, other herpesviruses), post-transplant lymphoproliferative disease (PTLD), post-transplant diabetes mellitus, transplant renal artery stenosis, and rejection of kidney allograft, resulting in decreased graft and patient survival

CMV, cytomegalovirus.

Adapted from Annane D, Renault A, Brun-Buisson C, et al. Hydrocortisone plus fludrocortisone for adults with septic shock. *N Engl J Med.* 2018;378(9):809-818. doi:10.1056/NEJMoa1705716; Brennan DC. Cytomegalovirus in renal transplantation. *J Am Soc Nephrol.* 2001;12(4):848-855.

for UL54 and/or UL97. If GCV resistance is documented or expected, therapy with foscarnet or cidofovir will need to be considered, both of which can cause nephrotoxicity.

BK VIREMIA/NEPHROPATHY

BK virus, a member of the polyomavirus family, is typically acquired in childhood but is clinically silent in immunocompetent patients. In immunocompromised KTRs, BK virus reactivation can occur, which can result in graft dysfunction (BK nephropathy or BKN) by tubulointerstitial inflammation and subsequent kidney fibrosis.[14] Occasionally, ureteral stenosis can be seen. When BKN is suspected, BK virus deoxyribonucleic acid (DNA) quantification in the blood and urine should be done by polymerase chain reaction (PCR). Transplant kidney biopsy may be needed to make a definitive diagnosis. Treatment of BK viruria, but no viremia, is not usually needed. The cornerstone for the treatment of BK viremia (BKV)/BKN is the reduction in immunosuppression, which needs to be carefully balanced against the risk of rejection of the graft. Leflunomide has been tried with varying success. There is no role of fluoroquinolones in the treatment of BKV/BKN.[15]

EPSTEIN-BARR VIRUS INFECTION

The risk is higher in Epstein-Barr virus (EBV)–seronegative KTRs who receive organ from EBV-seropositive donor. EBV disease has a wide spectrum. It can cause nonspecific febrile illness to specific organ involvement (hepatitis, pneumonitis, and gastroenteritis). It is also associated with post-transplant lymphoproliferative disorder (PTLD).[16] Diagnosis of PTLD requires histologic confirmation. Treatment of PTLD is based on the subtype and type of transplant and involves reduction of immunosuppression, immunotherapy with the CD20 monoclonal antibody rituximab, chemotherapy, and radiation therapy. Rituximab can be considered for prophylaxis of PTLD in patients who have significant EBV viremia.

There is no definite therapy to prevent EBV and PTLD. Limiting aggressive immunosuppression in low immunologic risk recipients and monitoring for plasma EBV viral load in EBV high-risk recipients are recommended. Preemptive treatment of PTLD at the time of viral reactivation with rituximab and reduced immunosuppression can be considered.

URINARY TRACT INFECTION

Epidemiology

Urinary tract infection (UTI) is the most common infectious complication in KTR. It accounts for 30% of all hospitalizations for sepsis in KTR. The incidence of UTI is highest in the first 6 months after kidney transplant (KT), although the risk persists throughout post-KT.[17] Risk factors for UTI are discussed in **Table 54.2.**[18-22]

Microbiology

Gram-negative bacteria account for more than 70% of UTI in KTR. *Escherichia coli* is the most common organism. Other common uropathogens include *Enterococcus, Pseudomonas, Klebsiella, Enterobacter*, and *Staphylococcus* species.[23] Urine cultures showing mixed flora are likely due to the contamination.

Clinical Manifestations and Treatment[24] (See Table 54.3)

CANDIDURIA

Candiduria is uncommon in KTR, with incidence rate accounting between 4% and 10%. *Candida glabrata* is the most common pathogen. Candiduria is asymptomatic in the majority of the KTRs, and antifungal treatment is not indicated.[25] Candiduria in the immediate post-transplant period, neutropenic patients, or those undergoing urologic interventions may be associated with an increased risk of complications, and antifungal treatment may be warranted in these settings.

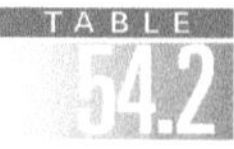

Risk Factors for Urinary Tract Infection

General Risk Factors	Transplant-Specific Risk Factors
Female gender	Induction with antithymocyte globulin
Older age	Presence of ureteral stent in early post-KT period
Diabetes	Episodes of acute rejection
Indwelling urinary catheter	Deceased donor transplant (compared to living donor)
Urologic abnormalities (neurogenic bladder, kidney stones or cysts, vesicoureteral reflux)	Duration of dialysis

KT, kidney transplant.

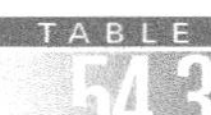

TABLE 54.3 Clinical Manifestations and Treatment of Urinary Tract Infection

Classification	Clinical Manifestation	Laboratory Investigations	Treatment
Asymptomatic bacteriuria	No urinary or systemic symptoms of infection	$>10^5$ CFU/mL uropathogen	No treatment is indicated.
Acute simple cystitis	Symptoms of lower UTI (dysuria, suprapubic pain, urinary frequency or urgency) in the absence of systemic symptoms and indwelling urologic device	>10 WBC/mm^3 $>10^3$ CFU/mL uropathogen	Third-generation oral cephalosporin or amoxicillin-clavulanate or ciprofloxacin or levofloxacin. Nitrofurantoin can be used if CrCl >40. Duration of treatment: 5-10 d
Acute pyelonephritis/ complicated UTI	Upper UTI symptoms (fever, chills, malaise, allograft or costovertebral angle pain), leukocytosis or bacteremia (without any other apparent cause), indwelling urologic device	>10 WBC/mm^3 $>10^4$ CFU/mL uropathogen	Piperacillin-tazobactam or cefepime or carbapenem. Once culture-susceptibility results are available, use the most narrow-spectrum antibiotic available. Duration of treatment: 14-21 d
Recurrent UTI	≥ 3 UTIs in prior 12-mo period	Urine studies as previously Consider further urologic workup (postvoid residual, kidney ultrasound/CT, voiding cystourethrography, urodynamic studies) to identify the etiology	Treat individual episode as previously. Prevention: Basic infection prevention measures (maintain hydration, frequent voiding, for females wipe from front to back), methenamine hippurate, antibiotic prophylaxis

CFU, colony-forming units; CrCl, creatinine clearance; CT, computed tomography; UTI, urinary tract infection; WBC, white blood cell.

References

1. Gotur DB, Masud FN, Ezeana CF, et al. Sepsis outcomes in solid organ transplant recipients. *Transpl Infect Dis.* 2019:e13214. doi:10.1111/tid.13214
2. Syu SH, Lin YW, Lin KH, Lee LM, Hsiao CH, Wen YC. Risk factors for complications and graft failure in kidney transplant patients with sepsis. *Bosn J Basic Med Sci.* 2019;19(3):304-311. doi:10.17305/bjbms.2018.3874
3. Schachtner T, Stein M, Reinke P. Sepsis after renal transplantation: clinical, immunological, and microbiological risk factors. *Transpl Infect Dis.* 2017;19(3). doi:10.1111/tid.12695
4. Haidar G, Green M, American Society of Transplantation Infectious Diseases Community of Practice. Intra-abdominal infections in solid organ transplant recipients: guidelines from the American Society of Transplantation Infectious Diseases Community of Practice. *Clin Transplant.* 2019;33(9):e13595. doi:10.1111/ctr.13595
5. Pappas PG, Alexander BD, Andes DR, et al. Invasive fungal infections among organ transplant recipients: results of the Transplant-Associated Infection Surveillance Network (TRANSNET). *Clin Infect Dis.* 2010;50(8):1101-1111. doi:10.1086/651262
6. Fishman JA. Infection in organ transplantation. *Am J Transplant.* 2017;17(4):856-879. doi:10.1111/ajt.14208
7. Van Delden C, Stampf S, Hirsch HH, et al. Burden and timeline of infectious diseases in the first year after solid organ transplantation in the Swiss Transplant Cohort Study. *Clin Infect Dis.* 2020;ciz1113. doi:10.1093/cid/ciz1113
8. Azoulay E, Pickkers P, Soares M, et al. Acute hypoxemic respiratory failure in immunocompromised patients: the Efraim multinational prospective cohort study. *Intensive Care Med.* 2017;43(12):1808-1819. doi:10.1007/s00134-017-4947-1
9. Rhodes A, Evans LE, Alhazzani W, et al. Surviving sepsis campaign: international guidelines for management of sepsis and septic shock: 2016. *Intensive Care Med.* 2017;43(3):304-377. doi:10.1007/s00134-017-4683-6
10. Annane D, Renault A, Brun-Buisson C, et al. Hydrocortisone plus fludrocortisone for adults with septic shock. *N Engl J Med.* 2018;378(9):809-818. doi:10.1056/NEJMoa1705716
11. Brennan DC. Cytomegalovirus in renal transplantation. *J Am Soc Nephrol.* 2001;12(4):848-855.
12. De Keyzer K, Van Laecke S, Peeters P, Vanholder R. Human cytomegalovirus and kidney transplantation: a clinician's update. *Am J Kidney Dis.* 2011;58(1):118-126.
13. Kotton CN, Kumar D, Caliendo AM, et al; The Transplantation Society International CMV Consensus Group. The Third International Consensus guidelines on the management of cytomegalovirus in solid-organ transplantation. *Transplantation.* 2018;102(6):900-931. doi:10.1097/TP.0000000000002191.
14. Bohl DL, Brennan DC. BK virus nephropathy and kidney transplantation. *Clin J Am Soc Nephrol.* 2007;2(suppl 1):S36-S46. doi:10.2215/CJN.00920207
15. Lee BT, Gabardi S, Grafals M, et al. Efficacy of levofloxacin in the treatment of BK viremia: a multicenter, double-blinded, randomized, placebo-controlled trial. *Clin J Am Soc Nephrol.* 2014;9(3):583-589. doi:10.2215/CJN.04230413
16. Karuthu S, Blumberg EA. Common infections in kidney transplant recipients. *Clin J Am Soc Nephrol.* 2012;7(12):2058-2070.
17. Razonable RR, Humar A. Cytomegalovirus in solid organ transplant recipients—guidelines of the American Society of Transplantation Infectious Diseases Community of Practice. *Clin Transplant.* 2019;33(9):e13512. doi:10.1111/ctr.13512
18. Le J, Durand CM, Agha I, Brennan DC. Epstein-Barr virus and renal transplantation. *Transplant Rev (Orlando).* 2017;31(1):55-60. doi:10.1016/j.trre.2016.12.001
19. Vidal E, Torre-Cisneros J, Blanes M, et al. Bacterial urinary tract infection after solid organ transplantation in the RESITRA cohort. *Transpl Infect Dis.* 2012;14(6):595-603.
20. Ariza-Heredia EJ, Beam EN, Lesnick TG, Kremers WK, Cosio FG, Razonable RR. Urinary tract infections in kidney transplant recipients: role of gender, urologic abnormalities, and antimicrobial prophylaxis. *Ann Transplant.* 2013;18:195-204.
21. Dantas SR, Kuboyama RH, Mazzali M, Moretti ML. Nosocomial infections in renal transplant patients: risk factors and treatment implications associated with urinary tract and surgical site infections. *J Hosp Infect.* 2006;63(2):117-123.
22. Lim JH, Cho JH, Lee JH, et al. Risk factors for recurrent urinary tract infection in kidney transplant recipients. *Transplant Proc.* 2013;45(4):1584-1589.
23. Saemann M, Horl WH. Urinary tract infection in renal transplant recipients. *Eur J Clin Invest.* 2008;38(suppl 2):58-65.
24. Goldman JD, Julian K. Urinary tract infections in solid organ transplant recipients: guidelines from the American Society of Transplantation Infectious Diseases Community of Practice. *Clin Transplant.* 2019:e13507.
25. Denis B, Chopin D, Piron P, et al. Candiduria in kidney transplant recipients: is antifungal therapy useful? *Mycoses.* 2018;61(5):298-304.

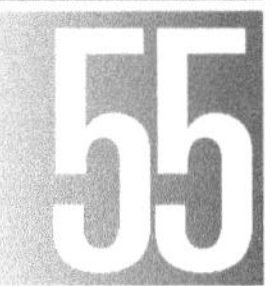

Care for the Brain-Dead Organ Donor

Aalok K. Kacha

INTRODUCTION

Organ transplantation is the treatment of choice for patients with end-stage disease. However, the supply of suitable organs constrains the ability to provide this therapy. The number of patients awaiting transplantation has expanded at a far greater rate than the supply of organs. There are multiple modifiable factors that can increase the supply of organs. These include expanded criteria to include older donors, donors with or at risk of specific infectious diseases, and ex vivo strategies to preserve or improve function.[1] Nationally determined societal models for donor consent also impact organ supply.[2]

In 1968, criteria defining irreversible coma were published, which facilitated the use of organs from brain-dead donors for transplantation.[3] Formal criteria for brain death have resulted in a robust process. Neurologic recovery after determination of brain death has not occurred, although complex motor movements or false-positive ventilator triggering may be observed. There is a legal and medical framework supporting the equivalence of brain death and circulatory death.[4] The determination of brain death in the comatose patient with identified, irreversible neurologic pathology and concordant imaging requires assessment of cerebral hemispheric and brainstem function in the absence of potentially confounding hypotension, hypothermia, sedative effect, acid-base, electrolyte, or endocrine derangements.

After brain death is determined, there is no obligation to provide continued supportive care in the United States, except in the state of New Jersey.[5] Despite the availability of published criteria from the American Academy of Neurology regarding brain death, there is substantial variation in hospital brain death policies in terms of clinical prerequisites for testing, types of health care professionals involved, clinical examination requirements, and methodology of apnea testing.[6] In addition to donation after neurologic determination of death (DNDD), donation after circulatory determination of death (DCDD) is another pathway to organ donation with specific ethical and policy issues. A joint white paper by the American Thoracic Society, Association of Organ Procurement Organizations and the United Network of Organ Sharing provides a deeper discussion of these issues.[7]

In the United States, consent for organ donation uses an opt-in process, with rates of donation comparable to systems with an opt-out process.[8] Patients may specify their wish to donate organs via family discussions, donor registry, driver's license notice, donor card, discussion with their physician, advance directive, or power of attorney document. Frequently, consent is obtained from the family. There is no consensus on the timing of discussions regarding organ donation and the determination of death, but informing the family of the patient's death has conventionally been independent from requests for organ donation. The organ procurement organization (OPO) should be notified prior to declaration of brain death, ideally as soon as a clinical circumstance with the potential for organ donation is identified. The Centers for Medicare and Medicaid Services (CMS) regulations require notification of the OPO within 1 hour of clinical triggers, such as diagnosis of irrecoverable devastating neurologic injury, intent to discuss a change in goals of care, or the consideration of brain death examination.

Conversion rates to organ donation are increased when requests for donation are made by specially trained personnel, as mandated by the CMS. Coordination of requests for donation between a nonphysician member of the care team and the OPO representative is associated with increased conversion rates.[9]

In 2001, family members, OPO staff, and health care practitioners (HCPs) involved in organ donation decisions were interviewed in a multicenter study at nine trauma hospitals. Factors associated with the decision to donate organs included families who had positive beliefs regarding organ donation and those with prior knowledge or the patient's wishes to donate. White ethnicity, younger age, male sex, and trauma as cause of death were associated with higher organ donation consent rates. HCP sociodemographic variables were not associated with consent rates, but HCPs' comfort with answering family questions was associated with donation, highlighting the importance of being informed on this topic.[10]

FAMILY AND CLINICAL FACTORS

Physicians and nurses often have concerns about burdening a family with a discussion about organ donation at a stressful time. Family members make organ donation decisions while experiencing grief, trauma, and shock. These decisions have life and death consequences for patients on transplant waiting lists. Understanding decision-making regarding organ donation is essential for clinicians.

The strongest predictor of authorization to donate is family knowledge of the potential donor patient's wishes. Family members report wanting more information about donation, brain death, the condition of the body after organ harvest, medical expenses, and funeral arrangements. Separating conversations about brain death and organ donation has been conventional practice, but broaching the topic of donation prior to death may be preferred by some. Families report a need for their relative to be treated with care and respect, including practitioners speaking with the patient as if he or she were conscious. The quality of communication between the treatment team, OPO staff, and family may have an impact on the psychological well-being of family members after the patient's death, highlighting the importance of these conversations in the intensive care unit (ICU).[11]

In a survey of family members who consented to organ donation, 50% of respondents reported that the sense that something good came out of a tragic event was a positive aspect of donation.[12] Many participants reported negative aspects of the donation process, which correlated with greater level of posttraumatic stress. A majority of respondents reported a comforting effect of the donation process, which correlated with fewer depressive symptoms. Owing to potential positive effects of organ donation, health care professionals may actually provide a benefit to the family by discussing donation.

The perception of organ donation by physicians and nurses affects how they communicate with family. France has an implied consent, opt-out system of organ donation. Standard practice includes discussing organ donation with family. Clinicians were surveyed, and their perception of the organ donation process was grouped into four categories: motivating (45.3%), stressful (20.7%), neutral (30%), and other (4%). Six domains were related to these perceptions: ICU culture surrounding organ donation, understanding of brain death, experience with interacting with family of brain-dead patients, professional experience with organ donation, personal feelings about donation, and sociodemographic characteristics of the respondents. In this French study, respondents who were younger rather than older or physicians rather than nurses were more likely to be identified as finding organ donation motivating.[13] Clinical staff may hold beliefs that lead to conflict between professional duties and personal feelings. These six domains may thus represent opportunities for education to relieve conflicts about organ donation in HCPs.

CRITICAL CARE MANAGEMENT OF ORGAN DONORS

Optimal management of the potential organ donor may improve organ supply. This is an area in which little research-derived information is available. There have been multiple barriers to conducting research on the management of deceased organ donors. Most US medical research consists of institutional review board (IRB)–regulated human subjects research falling under either Department of Health and Human Services (HHS) or Food and Drug Administration (FDA) regulations. A *human subject* is defined as a living individual; thus, deceased organ donors are not human subjects. The process for conducting organ donor research has been the subject of confusion. The potential harm that could occur from donor or organ research applies to the transplant recipient, and this is regulated by an IRB and appropriate consent should be obtained, unless waived.

The Uniform Anatomical Gift Act (UAGA) provides the legal basis for donation of all or part of the human body for therapy, research, and education. OPOs can facilitate donor research by including research as an intended use on the donation authorization form. A framework describing the oversight of deceased donor research has been proposed.[14] In 2017, the US National Academy of Medicine published a detailed report from the Committee on Issues in Organ Donor Intervention Research with goals to facilitate organ donor intervention research. Recommendations included development of a nationwide donor registry, clarification of gift intent for donors, and implementation of a coordinated system to consent wait list patients for the possibility of receiving a transplant from a donor or with an organ involved in a research study.[15]

One of the available studies is a retrospective, pre-post study demonstrating increased recovery of organs from potential donors after initiation of an intensivist-led organ donor support team. Local care for organ donors was transitioned from OPO coordinators to a team with dedicated intensivists working with the coordinators. The number of liver and heart grafts was similar before and after the implementation of the new donor management team. Most of the increase in organ supply was from a greater number of lungs and kidneys recovered.[16]

Active donor management likely improves the rate of organ retrieval. Potential organ donors are usually receiving supportive care prior to death. Ongoing support should continue the premortem care while compensating for the physiologic changes that accompany brain death. In 2015, a consensus statement on ICU care of the potential organ donor was published by the Society of Critical Care Medicine, the American College of Chest Physicians, and the Association of Organ Procurement Organizations.[9] A randomized controlled trial (RCT) to assess the effects of an evidence-based, goal-directed checklist for potential organ donor maintenance compared to standard care has been designed and may provide further information regarding donor management.[17] Prior studies have demonstrated that meeting donor management goals is accomplished in a minority of donors, but is associated with increased organ yield and decreased delayed graft function (DGF) of kidney allografts.[18-20]

PHYSIOLOGIC CARE OF THE ORGAN DONOR

Elevated intracranial pressure (ICP) and cerebral herniation resulting in brain death cause a biphasic hemodynamic response. The initial physiologic response to central nervous system (CNS) ischemia results in an autonomic storm with sympathetic stimulation resulting in hypertension and bradycardia, known as *Cushing reflex*. High levels of epinephrine, norepinephrine, and dopamine result in vasoconstriction, increased systemic vascular resistance, and additional myocardial oxygen consumption. Myocardial injury and stunning can result. In the kidney, this can cause ischemic injury and an upregulation in gene expression of inflammatory and heat shock proteins.[21] After brainstem function is lost, sympathetic tone, cardiac output, and vascular tone all decrease. This is often accompanied by hypovolemia resulting from physiologic changes associated with brain death such as diabetes insipidus (DI) and a systemic inflammatory response leading to capillary leak as well as predeath therapies to decrease ICP, such as hyperosmolar agents and loop diuretics.

To optimize end-organ perfusion, invasive monitoring with a central venous catheter or pulmonary artery catheter has traditionally been used in brain-dead donors. Modern ICU assessment of fluid responsiveness takes advantage of the dynamic relationship between changes in intrathoracic pressure during mechanical ventilation and resultant effects on cardiac filling. This can be measured by pulse pressure variation or systolic pressure variation, as further discussed in Chapter 1.[22] Global assessment of the adequacy of cardiac output can be assessed with central or mixed venous oxygen saturation, serum lactate, and base deficit. Echocardiography to assess valvular disease and ventricular function is routine for assessing the heart for transplantation. Assessment immediately after brain death may reveal global and regional abnormalities from catechol-mediated injury, so delayed echocardiography after weaning of vasoactive support may be preferred.

Fluid therapy should integrate inputs from measures of systemic perfusion, dynamic indices of volume responsiveness, and cardiac filling pressures. Prompt therapy after brain death to obtain adequate circulating volume can improve end-organ perfusion and decrease pressor requirements. Historically, fluid management goals for kidney function and lung function were thought to be at odds. More recent evidence suggests that management with lower central venous pressure (CVP) targets (such as <6 in one study) does not affect kidney graft function while improving heart and lung procurement, consistent with modern ICU management of other patients.[23-25]

Vasoactive therapy is closely linked to endocrine management consisting of hormone replacement therapy with vasopressin, steroids, and thyroid hormone. Destruction of the hypothalamic-pituitary axis occurs during brainstem herniation and often results in low levels of arginine vasopressin (AVP), hypothyroidism, and hypocortisolism. Thyroid hormone replacement may be beneficial when left ventricular ejection fraction is less than 45% or in hemodynamically unstable donors, although there are conflicting data in the literature.[26] Uncontrolled hyperglycemia is managed as in other ICU patients, but specific glucose targets are not defined for the deceased organ donor, so institutional or OPO protocols are usually followed.

Spontaneous hypothermia is common after brain death following cessation of brainstem function. The effect of temperature on organ function was evaluated in an RCT comparing targeted temperature management of brain-dead organ donors to either 34°C to 35°C or 36.5°C to 37.5°C. The primary outcome was DGF of kidney allografts, defined as a recipient requirement for dialysis in the first week after transplant. This study was terminated early based on an interim finding of efficacy of the intervention. DGF was reduced with mild hypothermia versus normothermia (28% vs 39%), with a significant effect in extended-criteria donors (**Visual Abstract 55.1**).[27] Lower donor temperature may be associated with worse outcomes after heart transplantation, but this finding results from retrospective analysis of a prior trial.[28]

High-dose methylprednisolone can improve liver graft function by attenuating the inflammatory cascade that follows brain death.[29] Steroids should only be administered after donor blood has been obtained for tissue typing because steroids can reduce cell-surface expression of human leukocyte antigens.[9] A meta-analysis of donor corticosteroid treatment including 11 RCTs and 14 observational studies examined the evidence for steroid administration. The authors noted that ten of the RCTs had neutral results, although the observational studies showed a benefit in terms of donor physiology, organ yield, and recipient outcomes, concluding that large-scale prospective trials are needed (**Visual Abstract 55.2**).[30] Steroid treatment of donors failed to decrease the incidence of dialysis in the first week after transplant in an RCT.[31]

Deficiencies in AVP may be present even in the absence of DI.[32] Treatment with AVP should be considered for refractory hypotension after volume resuscitation. Desmopressin is used for the management of DI, in the presence or absence of hypotension, to control urine output and correct hypernatremia.[9,33] Both drugs can be used in combination if needed. Dopamine has been the traditional vasoactive drug of choice for circulatory collapse following brain death. Norepinephrine is the first-line agent for vasodilatory shock in current ICU practice and may be an alternative to dopamine. Dopamine (4 μg/kg/min) has been studied as a hormonal therapy in hemodynamically stable (defined as norepinephrine $<$0.4 μg/kg/min) organ donors with a reduction in the need for dialysis in the first week after transplant, but not in 3-year graft survival (**Visual Abstract 55.3**).[34,35]

Contemporary ICU management of patients with acute respiratory distress syndrome includes low tidal volume, higher positive end-expiratory pressure (PEEP), measurement of driving pressure, and restrictive fluid management.[36] A multicenter RCT of potential organ donors compared standard management (tidal volume 10-12 mL/kg of predicted body weight, PEEP 3-5 cm H_2O) to lung protective ventilation (tidal volume 6-8 mL/kg of predicted body weight, PEEP 8-10 cm H_2O), apnea tests performed with continuous positive airway pressure, and closed circuit for airway suction. A greater percentage of potential donors in the lung protective group were eligible to donate lungs, whereas 6-month graft outcomes were similar between the two groups.[37]

OTHER FACTORS

Critical care management to achieve donor management goals is one avenue to expand the supply of organs. Another opportunity to increase supply is to utilize organs not previously used. Donor acute kidney injury (AKI) is associated with high rates of organ discard, but kidneys transplanted from donors with AKI are not associated with death-censored graft failure, although there is an increased incidence of DGF.[38] The use of kidneys from donors with AKI has resulted in favorable clinical outcomes with 3 years of follow-up.[39] The kidney donor risk index consists of donor and transplant or recipient factors and allows for the assessment of the risk of graft loss. It is used to help determine whether a particular organ offer is suitable for a specific patient.[40] Given the shortage of available organs relative to the number of patients awaiting transplantation, the use of organs from older donors or from donors with risk factors for infectious diseases may increase the supply by using organs previously discarded.[1,41] As the pool of potential donors expands, early recognition of potential organ donors and critical care management are important to enable the use of this latent supply of donor organs.

SUMMARY AND CONCLUSIONS

There is an increasing gap between organ supply and the demand from patients on transplant waiting lists. DNDD continues to be the primary source of organ gifts for transplantation. Brain death remains a difficult concept for many family members and health care workers to understand. Improved education about death by neurologic criteria and the process of organ donation may help meet ongoing needs. Optimal critical care management of deceased donors requires additional research to improve the supply of organs and the outcomes of transplant recipients. The management of the brain-dead donor relies on the application of supportive care guided by our understanding of the physiology of brain death.

References

1. Tullius SG, Rabb H. Improving the supply and quality of deceased-donor organs for transplantation. *N Engl J Med.* 2018;378(20):1920-1929.
2. Improving the supply and quality of deceased-donor organs for transplantation. *N Engl J Med.* 2018;379(7):691-694.
3. A definition of irreversible coma. Report of the Ad Hoc Committee of the Harvard Medical School to examine the definition of brain death. *JAMA.* 1968;205(6):337-340.
4. Wijdicks EF, Varelas PN, Gronseth GS, et al. Evidence-based guideline update: determining brain death in adults: report of the Quality Standards Subcommittee of the American Academy of Neurology. *Neurology.* 2010;74(23):1911-1918.
5. Russell JA, Epstein LG, Greer DM, et al. Brain death, the determination of brain death, and member guidance for brain death accommodation requests: AAN position statement. *Neurology.* 2019. doi:10.1212/WNL.0000000000006750
6. Greer DM, Wang HH, Robinson JD, et al. Variability of brain death policies in the United States. *JAMA Neurol.* 2016;73(2):213-218.
7. Gries CJ, White DB, Truog RD, et al. An official American Thoracic Society/International Society for Heart and Lung Transplantation/Society of Critical Care Medicine/Association of Organ and Procurement Organizations/United Network of Organ Sharing Statement: ethical and policy considerations in organ donation after circulatory determination of death. *Am J Respir Crit Care Med.* 2013;188(1):103-109.
8. Glazier A, Mone T. Success of opt-in organ donation policy in the United States. *JAMA.* 2019;322(8):719-720.
9. Kotloff RM, Blosser S, Fulda GJ, et al. Management of the potential organ donor in the ICU: Society of Critical Care Medicine/American College of Chest Physicians/Association of Organ Procurement Organizations Consensus Statement. *Crit Care Med.* 2015;43(6):1291-1325.
10. Siminoff LA, Gordon N, Hewlett J, et al. Factors influencing families' consent for donation of solid organs for transplantation. *JAMA.* 2001;286(1):71-77.
11. Kentish-Barnes N, Siminoff LA, Walker W, et al. A narrative review of family members' experience of organ donation request after brain death in the critical care setting. *Intensive Care Med.* 2019;45(3):331-342.
12. Merchant SJ, Yoshida EM, Lee TK, et al. Exploring the psychological effects of deceased organ donation on the families of the organ donors. *Clin Transplant.* 2008;22(3):341-347.

13. Kentish-Barnes N, Duranteau J, Montlahuc C, et al. Clinicians' perception and experience of organ donation from brain-dead patients. *Crit Care Med.* 2017;45(9):1489-1499.
14. Glazier AK, Heffernan KG, Rodrigue JR. A framework for conducting deceased donor research in the United States. *Transplantation.* 2015;99(11):2252-2257.
15. Liverman CT, Domnitz S, Childress JF. *Opportunities for Organ Donor Intervention Research: Saving Lives by Improving the Quality and Quantity of Organs for Transplantation.* National Academies Press; 2017.
16. Singbartl K, Murugan R, Kaynar AM, et al. Intensivist-led management of brain-dead donors is associated with an increase in organ recovery for transplantation. *Am J Transplant.* 2011;11(7):1517-1521.
17. Westphal GA, Robinson CC, Biasi A, et al. DONORS (Donation Network to Optimise Organ Recovery Study): study protocol to evaluate the implementation of an evidence-based checklist for brain-dead potential organ donor management in intensive care units, a cluster randomised trial. *BMJ Open.* 2019;9(6):e028570.
18. Malinoski DJ, Patel MS, Ahmed O, et al. The impact of meeting donor management goals on the development of delayed graft function in kidney transplant recipients. *Am J Transplant.* 2013;13(4):993-1000.
19. Malinoski DJ, Patel MS, Daly MC, et al. The impact of meeting donor management goals on the number of organs transplanted per donor: results from the United Network for Organ Sharing Region 5 prospective donor management goals study. *Crit Care Med.* 2012;40(10):2773-2780.
20. Patel MS, Zatarain J, De La Cruz S, et al. The impact of meeting donor management goals on the number of organs transplanted per expanded criteria donor: a prospective study from the UNOS Region 5 Donor Management Goals Workgroup. *JAMA Surg.* 2014;149(9):969-975.
21. Westendorp WH, Leuvenink HG, Ploeg RJ. Brain death induced renal injury. *Curr Opin Organ Transplant.* 2011;16(2):151-156.
22. Michard F. Changes in arterial pressure during mechanical ventilation. *Anesthesiology.* 2005;103(2):419-428.
23. Minambres E, Rodrigo E, Ballesteros MA, et al. Impact of restrictive fluid balance focused to increase lung procurement on renal function after kidney transplantation. *Nephrol Dial Transplant.* 2010;25(7):2352-2356.
24. Abdelnour T, Rieke S. Relationship of hormonal resuscitation therapy and central venous pressure on increasing organs for transplant. *J Heart Lung Transplant.* 2009;28(5):480-485.
25. Marik PE. Iatrogenic salt water drowning and the hazards of a high central venous pressure. *Ann Intensive Care.* 2014;4:21.
26. Venkateswaran RV, Steeds RP, Quinn DW, et al. The haemodynamic effects of adjunctive hormone therapy in potential heart donors: a prospective randomized double-blind factorially designed controlled trial. *Eur Heart J.* 2009;30(14):1771-1780.
27. Niemann CU, Feiner J, Swain S, et al. Therapeutic hypothermia in deceased organ donors and kidney-graft function. *N Engl J Med.* 2015;373(5):405-414.
28. Schnuelle P, Benck U, Kramer BK, et al. Impact of donor core body temperature on graft survival after heart transplantation. *Transplantation.* 2018;102(11):1891-1900.
29. Kotsch K, Ulrich F, Reutzel-Selke A, et al. Methylprednisolone therapy in deceased donors reduces inflammation in the donor liver and improves outcome after liver transplantation: a prospective randomized controlled trial. *Ann Surg.* 2008;248(6):1042-1050.
30. Dupuis S, Amiel JA, Desgroseilliers M, et al. Corticosteroids in the management of brain-dead potential organ donors: a systematic review. *Br J Anaesth.* 2014;113(3):346-359.
31. Kainz A, Wilflingseder J, Mitterbauer C, et al. Steroid pretreatment of organ donors to prevent postischemic renal allograft failure: a randomized, controlled trial. *Ann Intern Med.* 2010;153(4):222-230.
32. Chen JM, Cullinane S, Spanier TB, et al. Vasopressin deficiency and pressor hypersensitivity in hemodynamically unstable organ donors. *Circulation.* 1999;100(19 suppl):II244-II246.
33. Pennefather SH, Bullock RE, Mantle D, et al. Use of low dose arginine vasopressin to support brain-dead organ donors. *Transplantation.* 1995;59(1):58-62.
34. Schnuelle P, Gottmann U, Hoeger S, et al. Effects of donor pretreatment with dopamine on graft function after kidney transplantation: a randomized controlled trial. *JAMA.* 2009;302(10):1067-1075.
35. Schnuelle P, Schmitt WH, Weiss C, et al. Effects of dopamine donor pretreatment on graft survival after kidney transplantation: a randomized trial. *Clin J Am Soc Nephrol.* 2017;12(3):493-501.
36. Thompson BT, Chambers RC, Liu KD. Acute respiratory distress syndrome. *N Engl J Med.* 2017;377(6):562-572.

37. Mascia L, Pasero D, Slutsky AS, et al. Effect of a lung protective strategy for organ donors on eligibility and availability of lungs for transplantation: a randomized controlled trial. *JAMA.* 2010;304(23):2620-2627.
38. Liu C, Hall IE, Mansour S, et al. Association of deceased donor acute kidney injury with recipient graft survival. *JAMA Netw Open.* 2020;3(1):e1918634.
39. Hall IE, Akalin E, Bromberg JS, et al. Deceased-donor acute kidney injury is not associated with kidney allograft failure. *Kidney Int.* 2019;95(1):199-209.
40. Rao PS, Schaubel DE, Guidinger MK, et al. A comprehensive risk quantification score for deceased donor kidneys: the kidney donor risk index. *Transplantation.* 2009;88(2):231-236.
41. Aubert O, Reese PP, Audry B, et al. Disparities in acceptance of deceased donor kidneys between the United States and France and estimated effects of increased US acceptance. *JAMA Intern Med.* 2019;179(10):1365-1374.

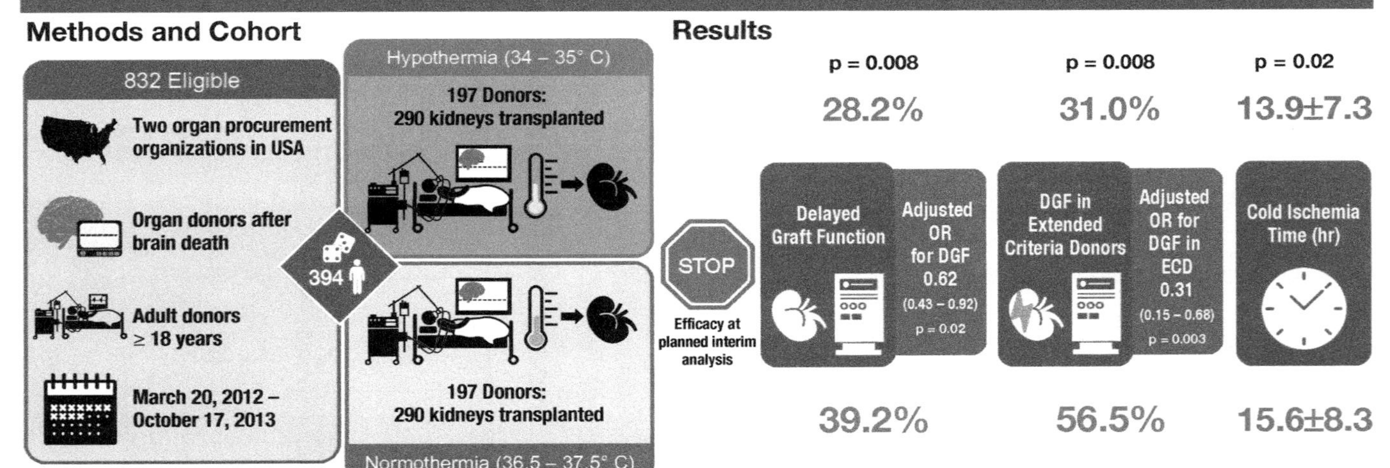

VISUAL ABSTRACT 55.1

Do corticosteroids used as pre-treatment in organ donors after brain death affect outcomes?

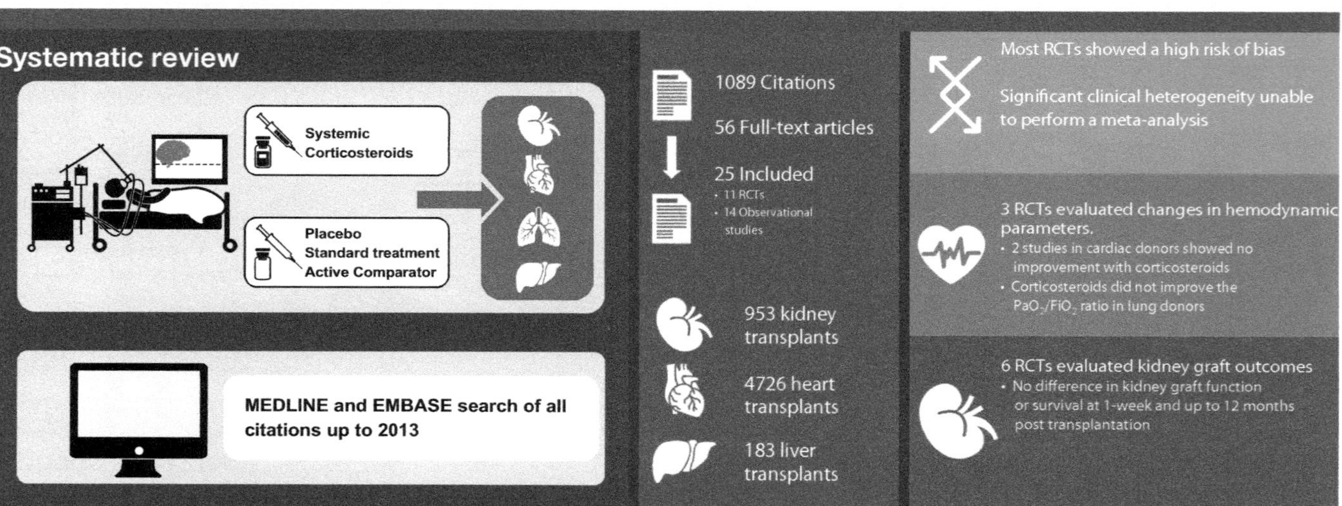

Conclusion: In a systematic review, which included 11 randomized controlled trials and 14 observational studies, evidence supporting the use of corticosteroids in the management of organ donors is conflicting

Reference: Dupuis S, Amiel JA, Desgroseilliers M et al. ***Corticosteroids in the management of brain-dead potential organ donors: a systematic review. Br J Anaesth.*** 2014;113(3):346-59.

VISUAL ABSTRACT 55.2

Does donor pre-treatment with dopamine affect graft outcomes after kidney transplantation?

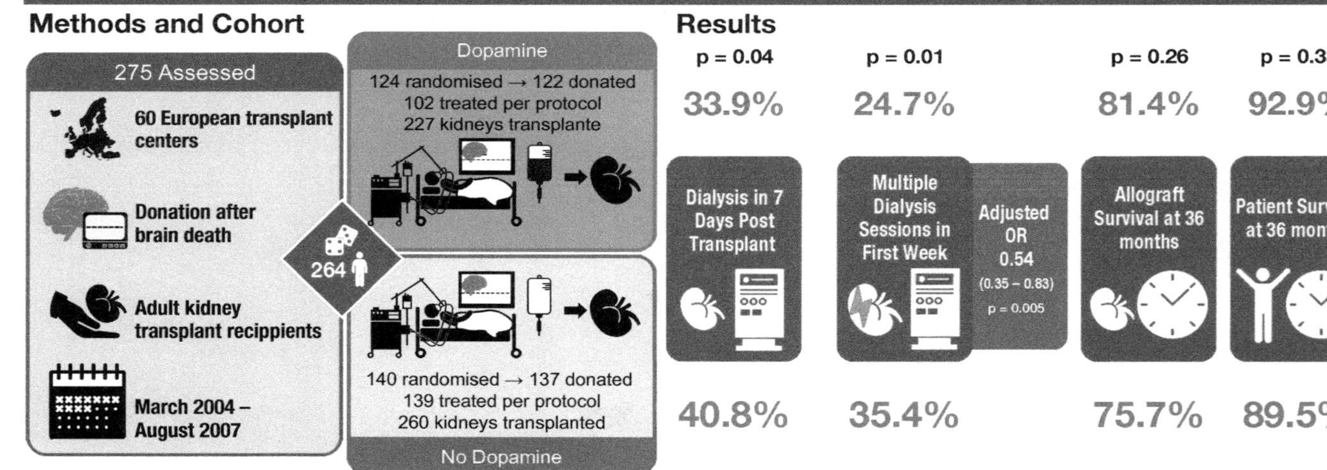

Conclusion: In a randomized controlled trial brain dead donors pre-treated with low-dose dopamine, the recipient has a reduced need for dialysis in the first week after kidney transplantation.

Reference: Schnuelle P, Gottmann U, Hoeger S, et al. ***Effects of donor pretreatment with dopamine on graft function after kidney transplantation: a randomized controlled trial***. JAMA 2009; 302(10):1067-75

VISUAL ABSTRACT 55.3

SECTION XI

Ethics/Palliative Care

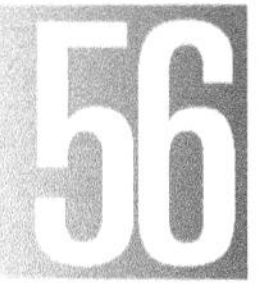

Shared Decision-Making/ Time-Limited Trials of Kidney Replacement Therapy

Alvin H. Moss

THREE CASES TO ILLUSTRATE THE RANGE OF ETHICAL ISSUES

Which older patients with acute kidney injury (AKI) in the intensive care unit (ICU) should be dialyzed? How should the decision be made? The following three cases illustrate the ethical issues at play.

Case #1: Large Sacral Ulcer, Septic Shock, and Anuric Acute Kidney Injury

A 68-year-old woman with diabetes, coronary artery disease, carotid artery disease status post (S/P) bilateral carotid endarterectomies, peripheral arterial disease s/p right above-the-knee amputation, morbid obesity weighing over 400 lb, and stage 3 chronic kidney disease (CKD) is admitted to the ICU with septic shock from a huge sacral pressure sore. She requires two vasopressors at maximum doses to maintain a mean arterial pressure above 65 mm Hg and develops anuric AKI. She is lethargic and lacks decision-making capacity. She had completed a living will and medical power of attorney. Her nutritional status is poor. The plastic surgeon says she would need a diverting colostomy if she were to have any possibility of healing the sacral wound, but he declines to operate, stating that she is not a surgical candidate. Her comorbidities make surgery risky, and her very poor nutrition makes healing of surgical wounds unlikely. Should the patient be started on dialysis? Is there anything else you would want to know first?

Case #2: Dialysis and Ventilator Dependence in a Patient With End-Stage Chronic Obstructive Pulmonary Disease

A 75-year-old woman with oxygen-dependent end-stage chronic obstructive pulmonary disease (COPD) and an ischemic cardiomyopathy with an ejection fraction of 35% is admitted to the ICU with pneumonia in respiratory failure. She is intubated and placed on mechanical ventilation, and she is started on vasopressors and antibiotics for septic shock. She becomes anuric and is started on hemodialysis several days after ICU admission. On day 11, the patient remains ventilator and dialysis dependent, and the ICU team approaches the husband for consent for a tracheostomy. The husband says, "my wife wouldn't want to be kept alive if dependent on machines, but we have made it this far after going through so much already ... we don't want to give up."[1] Should the patient undergo a tracheostomy? Should dialysis be continued?

Case #3: Multiple Comorbidities and Poor Functional Status in an Octogenarian

An 85-year-old man with stage 4 CKD, diabetes, coronary artery disease, heart failure, COPD, dementia, and hypercarbic respiratory failure is admitted to the ICU with pneumonia complicated by shock and new-onset atrial fibrillation with rapid ventricular response rate. He is intubated and started on medications to treat his infection and arrhythmia. His wife reports that he uses a walker at home and is unable to care for himself. His Karnofsky Performance Status score is 40%. He has been hospitalized about every 3 months for fluid overload. He develops oliguric AKI superimposed on his CKD, with estimated glomerular filtration rate (eGFR) of 22 mL/min. He has no advance directive. Should he be started on kidney replacement therapy (KRT)?

APPROACH TO ETHICAL DECISION-MAKING FOR TREATMENT OF PATIENTS WITH ACUTE KIDNEY INJURY IN THE INTENSIVE CARE UNIT

In their book *Clinical Ethics: A Practical Approach to Ethical Decisions in Clinical Medicine,* Jonsen et al[2] present a four-topic approach to organizing ethical reasoning for analyzing what should be done in particular cases. The four topics are presented in **Table 56.1**. The authors noted that medical indication is the first topic to be considered in an ethical analysis of a case and that an intervention is medically indicated when the patient's medical condition can be improved by its use. To preserve their professional integrity, physicians should not offer a treatment that is not medically indicated even if the patient wants it. For reasons that are discussed in Case #3, a treatment is not indicated if the likely harms outweigh the benefits.

When deliberating about whether dialysis should be offered, sometimes as in Case #1, the second topic, patient preferences, becomes determinative of what should be done in a particular case. Though the woman in Case #1 lacked decision-making capacity, she had expressed that if she lacked decision-making capacity and were dying, she would not want life-prolonging interventions. Prior to losing decision-making capacity, she had already refused intubation, mechanical ventilation, and cardiopulmonary resuscitation. All physicians involved in her care agreed that she was terminally ill from the complications of her sacral pressure sore and that her living will was in effect. With the agreement of her husband who was the patient's medical power of attorney representative, a comfort care plan was instituted, dialysis was not offered, and the patient died later that day. Ethical justifications for withholding or withdrawing dialysis are presented in **Table 56.2**. Case #1 satisfied the second justification in the table.

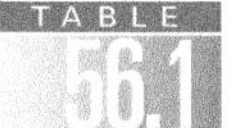

Approach to Ethical Case Analysis

Approach to Ethical Case Analysis
Medical indications—When benefits outweigh harms
Patient preferences
Quality of life
Contextual factors—Social, financial, legal, spiritual, public health

Adapted from Jonsen AR, Siegler M, Winslade WJ. *Clinical Ethics: A Practical Approach to Ethical Decisions in Clinical Medicine.* 8th ed. McGraw-Hill; 2015.

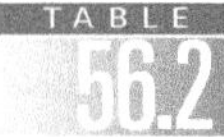

TABLE 56.2 Patients for Whom It Is Ethically Appropriate to Withhold or Withdraw Dialysis
Patients with decision-making capacity, who, being fully informed and making voluntary choices, refuse dialysis or request that it be discontinued
Patients who no longer possess capacity who have previously indicated refusal of dialysis in an oral or written advance directive
Patients without capacity whose health care proxy refuses dialysis or asks for it to be discontinued
Patients with irreversible, profound neurologic impairment

Reproduced with permission from Renal Physicians Association. *Shared Decision-Making in the Appropriate Initiation of and Withdrawal From Dialysis.* 2nd ed. Renal Physicians Association; 2010.

Case #2 is representative of the cascade of effects and clinical momentum that occurs for older patients with AKI in the ICU and for how the decision about dialysis is often tied to decisions about the use of other means of life support (**Figure 56.1**). In a study of critically ill older patients with AKI, Bagshaw et al found that those who were dialyzed were also more likely to have received mechanical ventilation and vasopressor support than those who were not.[3] The primary triggers for starting KRT were oligoanuria, fluid overload, and acidemia (**Visual Abstract 56.1**). Kruser et al noted that ICU care that is dictated by a cascade of effects can lead to a rapid accumulation of interventions without consideration and discussion with the patient and family of patient preferences

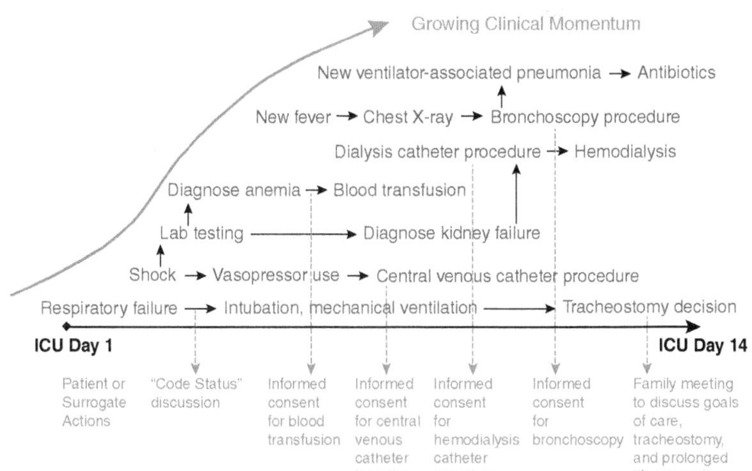

FIGURE 56.1: Clinical momentum and cascade of effects that occur for older patients with acute kidney injury in the intensive care unit (ICU). Reprinted with permission from Kruser JM, Cox CE, Schwarze ML. Clinical momentum in the intensive care unit. A latent contributor to unwanted care. *Ann Am Thorac Soc.* 2017;14(3):426-431.

based on likely outcomes.[1] Because of Case #2's life-limiting illness, COPD, apart from kidney disease and her uncertain outcome, her physicians would have been prudent to initiate treatment as a time-limited trial (TLT). Based on the husband's explanation of the patient's values, it does not seem that she would have wished long-term mechanical ventilation, which is what the tracheostomy would be preparing her for because she was unable to be weaned from respiratory support. Dialysis would be contributing to keeping the patient alive in a clinical scenario in which she did not want to be. Shared decision-making—the recognized preferred model for medical decision-making because it addresses the ethical need to fully inform patients about the risks and benefits of treatments, as well as the need to ensure that patients' values and preferences play a prominent role—at the outset of the ICU admission and every few days thereafter would have helped the husband to process that the course of treatment was headed in an unwanted direction.[4,5]

Case # 3 is one in which medical indications need to be carefully scrutinized. The "biomedicalization of aging" has led to the routinization of clinical interventions for older patients,[6] but this patient is one who can be predicted to do poorly based on the evidence even if dialysis is started. With his multiple comorbidities and poor functional status, he can be predicted to have a 90-day mortality of approximately 50% and to potentially spend much, if not most, of his remaining time in the hospital.[3,7] With his underlying stage 4 CKD, he is likely to be dialysis dependent for the rest of his life.[8] Nephrologists need to resist the technologic imperative—if you can do dialysis, you must do dialysis—because dialysis may not benefit all patients.

EVIDENCE OF OUTCOMES FOR OLDER PATIENTS WITH ACUTE KIDNEY INJURY STARTING DIALYSIS IN THE HOSPITAL

Older patients who start dialysis for AKI in the ICU are known to have a quite poor prognosis. In one study of patients who were predicted to have a 50% chance of dying within 6 months and who had a mean age of 61 years, a median of two comorbidities, dependence in at least one activity of daily living and a diagnosis of acute respiratory failure or multiorgan system failure with sepsis, the median survival after initiation of dialysis for AKI was 32 days with a 6-month survival of 27%.[9] In a study of Medicare beneficiaries aged 67 years or older who started dialysis in the hospital after a 2-week or longer hospital stay including an intensive procedure such as mechanical ventilation, feeding tube insertion, or cardiopulmonary resuscitation, the median survival was 0.7 year.[7] Older patients with AKI superimposed on CKD are 41 times more likely to develop end-stage kidney disease (ESKD).[8] In two studies, two-thirds or more of older patients with AKI superimposed on CKD developed dialysis dependence.[10,11] In a study of Health and Retirement Survey data for patients aged 65.5 years or older starting dialysis for AKI or ESKD between April 3, 1998, and December 21, 2014, after multivariate adjustment, factors significantly associated with higher 1-year mortality included activity of daily living dependence, age 85 years or older, inpatient dialysis initiation, and having four or more comorbidities. Survival at 6 months was 55.8% and at 1 year was 45.5% (**Visual Abstract 56.2**).[12] Case #3 has all the four major risk factors.

Based on the evidence and ethical considerations in evaluating the critically ill older patient with AKI in the ICU to determine whether dialysis should

Box 56.1 Questions to Evaluate the Critically Ill Older Patient With AKI in the ICU for Dialysis

- What is the patient's baseline kidney function?
- What is the age of the patient?
- What are comorbidities, and how severe are they?
- What is the patient's functional status? In nursing home?
- What is the patient's nutritional status?
- Is the patient decisionally capable?
- Are there advance directives? Who is the legal decision maker?
- Did patient specify treatments wanted/not wanted?
- What is most important to the patient: quality vs quantity of life?
- Is the patient at increased risk for dialysis-related complications?
- Will patient cooperate with dialysis process, and will it be safe?
- Is a time-limited trial of dialysis appropriate?
- What is the probability of ESKD?
- Is the patient a long-term dialysis candidate?

AKI, acute kidney injury; ESKD, end-stage kidney disease; ICU, intensive care unit.

be offered, clinicians might find helpful a series of questions that consider the patient's values, goals and preferences, and premorbid condition (**Box 56.1**).

TIME-LIMITED TRIALS TO ASSIST WITH DIALYSIS DECISION-MAKING

Dialysis decision-making for the critically ill older patient with AKI is complex. Clinicians need to consider not only the natural evolution of the patient's AKI within the context of the global prognosis (influenced by comorbidities and premorbid functional status) but also patients' values and goals and whether dialysis offers a realistic expectation of achieving patients' goals. Situations are often marked by prognostic uncertainty and clinical unknowns. It is in this setting that a TLT of dialysis may be particularly helpful. The clinical practice guideline on *Shared Decision-Making in the Appropriate Initiation of and Withdrawal from Dialysis* recommended a TLT for cases in which patients have an uncertain prognosis or in which there is conflict and a consensus cannot be reached about starting dialysis.[4]

A TLT requires knowledge of its structure and process to assist decision-making, strong communication skills, a patient-specific estimate of prognosis with the acknowledgment that it is just an estimate, elicitation of patient values, clear documentation, and, often, appropriate integration of palliative care consultation (**Figure 56.2**). A TLT of KRT is defined as a goal-directed trial with predetermined outcomes that are evaluated at planned intervals. TLTs allow the patient and family to assess what dialysis entails while providing the nephrologist with time to evaluate clinical response and the potential for benefit of continuing dialysis. Scherer et al have proposed four steps to a TLT: preparation, communication, initiation and conduct of the trial, and conclusion.[13]

In the preparation stage, the treating team and consultants reach agreement on the prognosis, what treatments would be likely to benefit, and milestones for

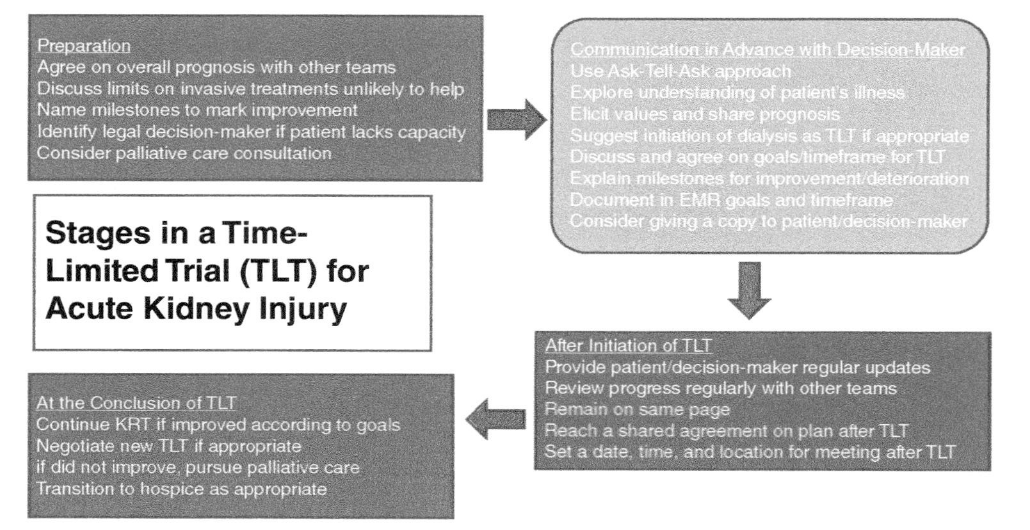

FIGURE 56.2: An approach to implementing a time-limited trial in the intensive care unit (ICU). AKI, acute kidney injury; IDFM, interdisciplinary family meeting; KRT, kidney replacement therapy; PC, palliative care; TLT, time-limited trial. Reprinted with permission from Scherer JS, Holley JL. The role of time-limited trials in dialysis decision making in critically ill patients. *Clin J Am Soc Nephrol.* 2016;11(2):344-353.

the trial. In the communication step, clinicians use the Ask-Tell-Ask approach to share estimated prognosis and to elicit patients' values and suggest initiation of dialysis as a TLT agreeing on goals to be achieved.

In the initiation and conduct of the TLT step, the treating and consulting teams would review the patients' progress regularly and reach agreement on the best course at the completion of the TLT, provide updates to the patient/legal agent, and set a date, time, and location for meeting after the TLT. In the conclusion step, the treating team and consultants meet with the patient/legal agent and reach agreement on whether milestones for the TLT were met. If the patient improved according to the goals, clinicians would continue KRT as needed for AKI. If the patient's condition improved but only slightly, then the clinicians might negotiate a new TLT. If the patient did not improve or deteriorated, then as agreed during the communication step, the clinicians would institute palliative care and hospice as appropriate. It is important to note that a TLT can be successful, whether the patient recovers or not, with clear communication and collaboration between the treating ICU team and consultants and with the patient/legal agent.

If conflict persists despite the use of a TLT, the dialysis decision-making guideline[4] recommends a systematic due process approach for conflict resolution if there is disagreement about what decision should be made with regard to dialysis (**Figure 56.3**). In talking with patients/legal agents, the nephrologist or other treating physician such as an intensivist should try to understand their views, provide data to support his/her recommendation, and correct misunderstandings. In the process of shared decision-making, the following potential sources of conflict have been recognized: (a) miscommunication or misunderstanding about prognosis, (b) intrapersonal or interpersonal issues, or (c) special values. If dialysis is indicated emergently, it should be provided while pursuing conflict resolution, provided the patient or legal agent requests it.

SUMMARY AND CONCLUSIONS

In light of the poor prognosis of many older critically ill patients with AKI, a shared decision-making conversation is particularly important before dialysis is started to enable them to determine their treatment goals. The clinical practice guideline on dialysis decision-making[4] and the Choosing Wisely Campaign of the American Society of Nephrology[14] both make this recommendation. As part of shared decision-making, depending on the patient's overall medical condition, older patients and their families/legal agents should be informed of the very real possibility with the initiation of dialysis of a prolonged hospitalization, the use of one or more intensive procedures in addition to dialysis, and limited life expectancy with a poor quality of life. The ethical principle of respect for patient autonomy, the basis for patient self-determination, requires that the treatments patients receive are aligned with their preferences as a result of informed decision-making.

In conclusion, to achieve good patient outcomes, nephrologists need to analyze the patient's overall condition, including comorbidities and functional status, prior to offering dialysis to older patients with AKI. For those in whom the benefit of dialysis for AKI is uncertain or who are not long-term dialysis candidates but the patient/legal agent is requesting dialysis, nephrologists ought to strongly consider starting dialysis as a TLT. Nephrologists can say "No" to offering dialysis when the burdens are predicted to substantially outweigh the benefits of dialysis. This is to preserve their professional integrity and honor their Hippocratic Oath. When dialysis can be predicted to be of little or no benefit, but the patient/family

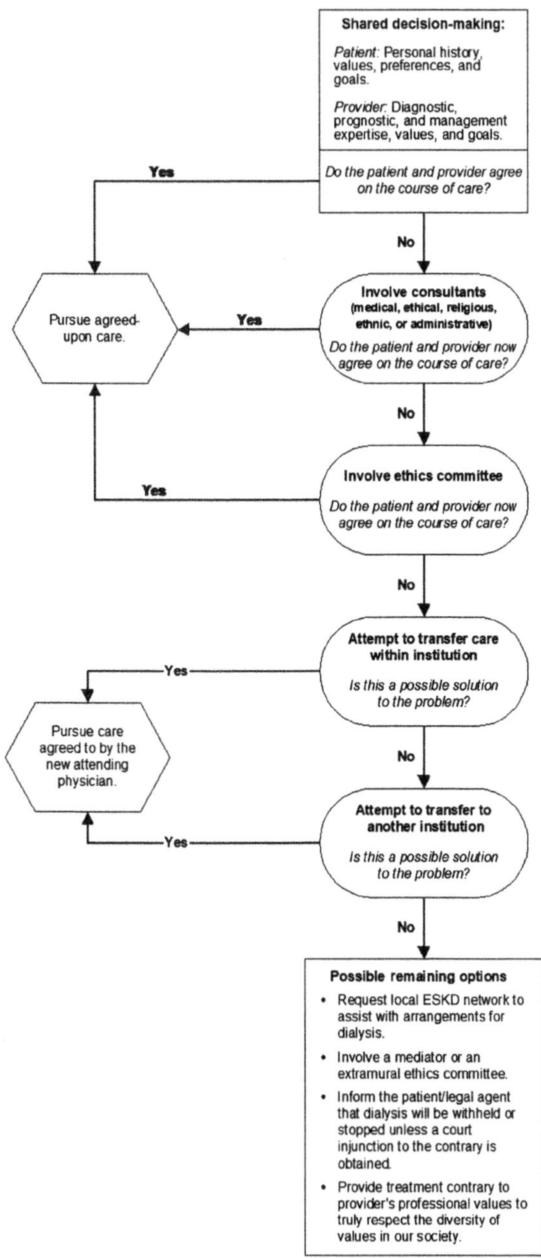

FIGURE 56.3: Systematic approach to resolving conflict between patient and kidney care team. ESKD, end-stage kidney disease. Reproduced with permission from Renal Physicians Association. *Shared Decision-Making in the Appropriate Initiation of and Withdrawal from Dialysis.* 2nd ed. Renal Physicians Association; 2010.

is/are requesting it, nephrologists ought to consider ethics/palliative/supportive care consultation for assistance with communication and conflict resolution.[15] Fortunately, there is a process for ethical decision-making with regard to offering dialysis in the ICU that has been outlined in this chapter and that can enable nephrologists and intensivists to handle situations when there is disagreement about the appropriate ethical course of action in patient care.

References

1. Kruser JM, Cox CE, Schwarze ML. Clinical momentum in the intensive care unit: a latent contributor to unwanted care. *Ann Am Thorac Soc.* 2017;14(3):426-431.
2. Jonsen AR, Siegler M, Winslade WJ. *Clinical Ethics: A Practical Approach to Ethical Decisions in Clinical Medicine.* 8th ed. McGraw-Hill; 2015.
3. Bagshaw SM, Adhikari NKJ, Burns KEA, et al. Selection and receipt of kidney replacement in critically ill older patients with AKI. *Clin J Am Soc Nephrol.* 2019;14(4):496-505.
4. Renal Physicians Association. *Shared Decision-Making in the Appropriate Initiation of and Withdrawal from Dialysis.* 2nd ed. Renal Physicians Association; 2010.
5. Barry MJ, Edgman-Levitan S. Shared decision making—pinnacle of patient-centered care. *N Engl J Med.* 2012;366(9):780-781.
6. Kaufman SR, Shim JK, Russ AJ. Revisiting the biomedicalization of aging: clinical trends and ethical challenges. *Gerontologist.* 2004;44(6):731-738.
7. Wong SP, Kreuter W, O'Hare AM. Healthcare intensity at initiation of chronic dialysis among older adults. *J Am Soc Nephrol.* 2014;25(1):143-149.
8. Ishani A, Xue JL, Himmelfarb J, et al. Acute kidney injury increases risk of ESRD among elderly. *J Am Soc Nephrol.* 2009;20(1):223-228.
9. Hamel MB, Phillips RS, Davis RB, et al. Outcomes and cost-effectiveness of initiating dialysis and continuing aggressive care in seriously ill hospitalized adults. SUPPORT Investigators. Study to Understand Prognoses and Preferences for Outcomes and Risks of Treatments. *Ann Intern Med.* 1997;127(3):195-202.
10. Palevsky PM, Zhang JH, O'Connor TZ, et al. Intensity of renal support in critically ill patients with acute kidney injury. VA/NIH Acute Renal Failure Trial Network. *N Engl J Med.* 2008;359(1):7-20.
11. Thakar CV, Quate-Operacz M, Leonard AC, et al. Outcomes of hemodialysis patients in a long-term care hospital setting: a single-center study. *Am J Kidney Dis.* 2010;55(2):300-306.
12. Wachterman MW, O'Hare AM, Rahman OK, et al. One-year mortality after dialysis initiation among older adults. *JAMA Intern Med.* 2019;179(7):987-990.
13. Scherer JS, Holley JL. The role of time-limited trials in dialysis decision making in critically ill patients. *Clin J Am Soc Nephrol.* 2016;11(2):344-353.
14. Williams AW, Dwyer AC, Eddy AA, et al. Critical and honest conversations: the evidence behind the "Choosing Wisely" campaign recommendations by the American Society of Nephrology. *Clin J Am Soc Nephrol.* 2012;7(10):1664-1672.
15. Chong K, Silver SA, Long J, et al. Infrequent provision of palliative care to patients with dialysis-requiring AKI. *Clin J Am Soc Nephrol.* 2017;12(11):1744-1752.

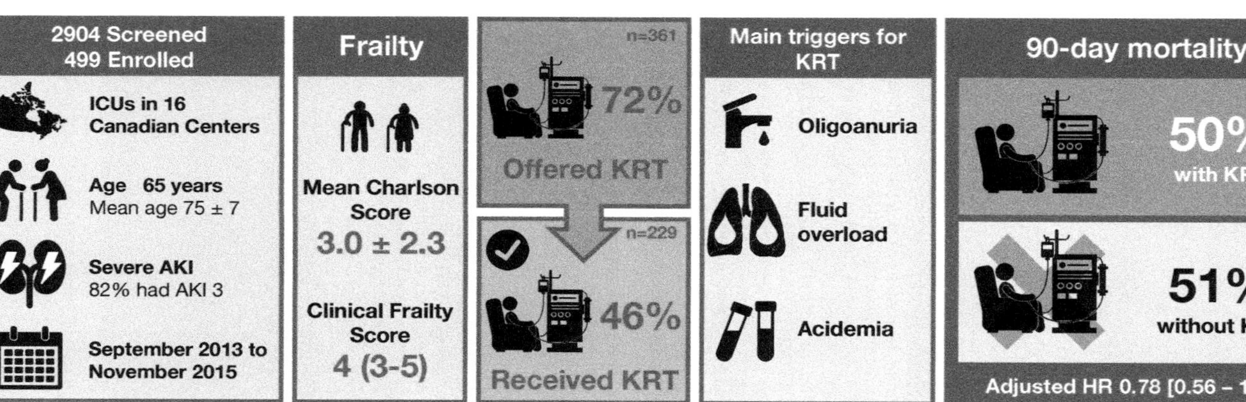

Conclusion: In this multicenter cohort study, clinicians were generally willing to offer kidney replacement therapy to the majority of older critically ill patients with severe AKI.

Bagshaw SM, Adhikari NKJ, Burns KEA, et al. ***Selection and Receipt of Kidney Replacement in Critically Ill Older Patients with AKI.*** Clin J Am Soc Nephrol. 2019;14(4): 496-505.

What is the one-year mortality in older adults after dialysis initiation?

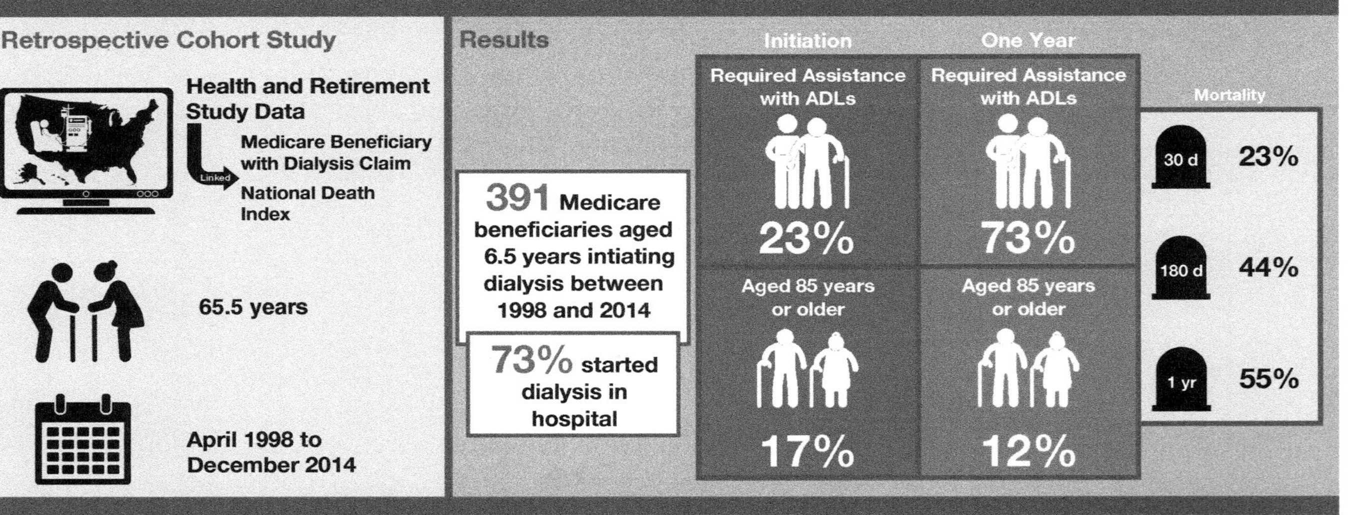

Conclusion: Using nationally representative data from the USA, 1 year mortality for patients over the age of 65.5 after dialysis initiation was 54.5%, almost double that reported for older adults in USRDS registry.

Wachterman MW, O'Hare AM, Rahman OK, et al. ***One-Year Mortality After Dialysis Initiation Among Older Adults.*** JAMA Intern Med. 2019;179(7):987-990.

VISUAL ABSTRACT 56.2

INDEX

Note: Page numbers followed by *b*, *f*, and *t* indicate material in boxes, figures, and tables respectively.

A

Abdominal compartment syndrome (ACS), 483–489
definition of, 483
diagnosis, 484
etiology, 483–484
natural history and sequelae, 486–487
cardiovascular, 487
gastrointestinal, 486–487
hepatobiliary, 486–487
kidney, 487
neurologic, 487
respiratory, 487
pathophysiology, 483–484
prevention, 485–486
abdominal wall compliance, 486
enteral and intraperitoneal volume, 486
fluid balance, 485
use of open abdomen, 486
ventilator management, 486
risk factors, 484, 485*t*
treatment, 487–488, 488–489*f*
Absolute hypovolemia, 12
ACE inhibitors. *See* Angiotensin-converting enzyme inhibitors, for hypertension
Acetaminophen, 295
Acetaminophen poisoning, hemodialysis in, 313–314, 314*t*
Acetazolamide, 135
Acid-base disorder, recognizing and determining the cause of, 275, 276*t*
Acid-base status, general considerations in the evaluation of, 275, 275*t*
ACS. *See* Abdominal compartment syndrome
activated partial thromboplastin time (aPTT), 376–377
Acute decompensated heart failure (ADHF), 213, 453
Acute dialysis, in LVAD patients, 467
Acute Disease Quality Initiative (ADQI), 475, 575
Acute fatty liver of pregnancy (AFLP), 439
Acute interstitial nephritis (AIN) from, 186
Acute kidney disease and disorders (AKD), 50*f*, 50–51, 50*t*
Acute kidney dysfunction, 172, 172*f*
Acute kidney injury (AKI)
acute kidney injury care bundles, 93, 94–96*t*
AKD, 50*f*, 50–51, 50*t*
anemia, 119
associations between acute kidney injury and adverse outcomes, 61–63
biomarkers of
acute tubular necrosis, 185
AIN from, 186
cirrhosis, 185, 185*t*
novel biomarkers for, 184
prognostic information, 186
SCr, 184–185
subclinical, 185
therapeutic interventions, 186
in burn patients, 520–523
extracorporeal therapies, 523
functional versus cellular damage, 521
management, 521–523
prevalence, staging, and impact, 520–521
causes of, 59–60
clinical test for urinary (TIMP-2)·(IGFBP7), 190
common etiologies of, 52–55
cardiac surgery–associated acute kidney injury, 53

Acute kidney injury (AKI) (*continued*)
contrast-associated acute kidney injury, 55
drug-induced acute kidney injury, 53, 53–54*t*
HRS, 55
hypoperfusion, 52
obstructive acute kidney injury, 55
primary kidney diseases, 55
rhabdomyolysis, 55
sepsis-associated acute kidney injury, 53
creatinine, 49
in decompensated cirrhosis, 474*f*
definition of, 58, 59*t*
definition of recovery from, 51
diagnostic criteria of, 47, 48*t*
in DKA, 432, 528–534
epidemiology, 528–529
etiology, 529–531, 530*t*
management, 533–534
pathophysiology, 531, 532*f*
risk factors, 531
dosing strategies, 286–290, 287–289*t*
drugs, 283–284
etiologies of, 51, 51–52*f*
furosemide stress test, 189
heterogeneous disease, 90
ICU, 81–87
blood pressure and vasopressors, 84
CA-AKI, 83–84
care bundles/systematic approach to, 84–86, 85*t*
ineffective interventions, 86–87, 86*t*
volume expansion and choice of intravenous fluid, 81–83
incidence of, 58–59, 60*t*
individualized treatment measures, 91–93
electrolyte management, 92
urea management, 93
volume management, 91–92
kidney biomarkers aid in, 191
kidney replacement therapy, 93, 97–98, 97*f*, 285
dosing of, 340–343
timing of, 348–354
limitations and challenges of, 49
limitations of urine output criteria, 50
in liver disease, 473–480
assessment, 473–475
definition of, 475
etiology, 475–477, 476*f*, 477*t*
pathophysiology, 473
prevention of, 477
treatment of, 478, 479–480*t*, 481–482
in LVAD patients, 467
metabolic management and nutrition of
metabolic management and nutrition support in patients, 173–176, 174–175*t*
monitoring of nutrition support, 176
stage 1, prevention and therapy of, 169–171, 170*t*
stage 2 and 3, infusion therapy and nutrition support in, 171–173, 172*t*
novel therapies, 98
older patients with, in ICU for dialysis, 630–631, 631*b*, 637
patient caring after, 575–581
chronic kidney disease/end-stage kidney disease, 577–578
follow-up, 575, 583–584
general aspects, 576–577, 577*t*
hypertension, 579
long-term complications, 576*t*
major adverse cardiovascular events, 579
mortality, 580
quality of life, 580
recurrent acute kidney injury, 578–579
requiring outpatient dialysis, 580–581
pharmacokinetic changes in, 284–285
in pregnancy
differential diagnosis of, 437–442, 438*f*
epidemiology of, 436
management of, 442
review of changes in, 437
risk factors for, 60–61, 60*t*
universal treatment measures, 90–91
appropriate dosing of medication, 91
avoidance of nephrotoxic insults, 90–91
maintenance of kidney perfusion, 90
Acute kidney injury care bundles, 93, 94–96*t*
Acute Kidney Injury Network (AKIN), 47, 416, 475, 520
Acute lithium toxicity, 90
Acute pancreatitis (AP), 114

Acute Physiology and Chronic Health Evaluation (APACHE), 68, 69*t*
Acute respiratory distress syndrome (ARDS), 112, 398, 408–411
  acute respiratory distress syndrome
    lung-kidney cross talk in, 37–38, 37*f*
    predictive biomarkers in, 38
  classification, 36–37
  definition, etiologies, and differential diagnosis, 36
  evidence-based acute respiratory distress syndrome therapy, 38–40
  KRT, 40
Acute tubular necrosis, 185
Acute/chronic, 259
ADHF. *See* Acute decompensated heart failure
Administration, 152
  vasoactive medications, extravasation injury of, 152
ADQI. *See* Acute Disease Quality Initiative
AFLP. *See* Acute fatty liver of pregnancy
AIN from. *See* Acute interstitial nephritis from
AKD. *See* Acute kidney disease and disorders
AKI. *See* Acute kidney injury
AKIKI trial. *See* Artificial Kidney Initiation in Kidney Injury trial
AKIN. *See* Acute Kidney Injury Network
ALBIOS. *See* Albumin Italian Outcome Sepsis
Albumin, 105–108, 109–110*t*
Albumin Italian Outcome Sepsis (ALBIOS), 107
Alcoholics, 267
American-European Consensus Conference in 1994, 36
Amount of volume expansion, 17
Angiotensin-converting enzyme (ACE) inhibitors, for hypertension, 516
Anion gap metabolic acidosis versus nonanion gap metabolic acidosis, 278
Antibody-mediated rejection, in KT recipients, 601
Anticoagulation, 465
  and KRT, 375–380
Antidotes, 295, 301
  acetaminophen toxicity, 295–297, 295–296*t*, 297–298*f*, 298*t*
  naloxone and flumazenil, 299
  toxic alcohols, 299–301, 300*f*
Aorta, 207–208
AP. *See* Acute pancreatitis
APACHE. *See* Acute Physiology and Chronic Health Evaluation
Apixaban, 165
aPTT. *See* activated partial thromboplastin time
ARDS. *See* Acute respiratory distress syndrome
Area Under the Curve (AUC), 6*t*
Argatroban, for CKRT, 380
Artificial Kidney Initiation in Kidney Injury (AKIKI) trial, 349, 350–351*t*, 352, 357
Assessment, Serial Evaluation, and Subsequent Sequelae in Acute Kidney Injury (ASSESS-AKI) study, 578
Asymptomatic, 246
Atrial fibrillation, 267
AUC. *See* Area Under the Curve
Azathioprine, 591

B

Bacillus polymyxa, 388
Balanced solutions, 108–111
Barbiturate poisoning, hemodialysis in, 316, 317*t*
Bedside evaluation, 14
Berlin definition, 36
β-lactam infusion time, 286
Bicarbonate, in DKA, 431
  N-acetylcysteine, 83
BigpAK trial, 85, 85*t*
Bilateral renal cortical necrosis, 438
Bisphosphonates, 250
BK viremia/nephropathy, 609
BK virus nephropathy, 601
Blood pressure (BP), 15
  and left ventricular assist devices, 465
  vasopressors, 84
Blood purification techniques, 387–393
  complications of, 392
  extracorporeal, 388*t*
  extracorporeal cytokine hemoadsorption, 390–391
  polymyxin B hemoperfusion, 388–389
  results from randomized clinical trials, 389–390
  therapeutic plasma exchange, 391

Body packers, 294
Body weight (PBW), 26
BP. *See* Blood pressure
Brain-dead organ donor, care for, 613–618
  corticosteroids use, 623
  critical care management, 615–616
  family and clinical factors, 614–615
  other factors, 617–618
  physiologic care, 616–617
  pre-treatment with dopamine, 621
  temperature management, 622
Braking phenomenon, 135
Bumetanide, for cardiorenal syndrome, 457
Bundles, 28

C

Calcimimetics, 251
Calcineurin inhibitors, in KT, 599, 600*t*
Calcitonin, 250
Calcium, 245–246
Calcium channel blocker and a-blocker overdose, 301–302, 302*t*
Calibration, 67
Candida glabrata, 610
Candiduria, 610
CAPD. *See* Continuous ambulatory peritoneal dialysis
Capillary refill time (CRT), 7
CAR T cell therapy. *See* Chimeric antigen receptor T cell therapy
Carbamazepine poisoning, hemodialysis in, 315, 315*t*
Cardiac, 206–208, 206–208*f*
Cardiac failure, ECMO for, 399–400, 399*t*
Cardiac output equation, 12, 13*t*
Cardiac surgery–associated acute kidney injury, 53
Cardiac toxicity, 303
Cardiogenic shock, 13
Cardiopulmonary resuscitation, 465
Cardiorenal syndrome (CRS), 453–459
  definition, 453
  epidemiology, 453
  management, 455–459
    diuretics, 457–458, 457*t*
    goals, 455–456, 455*f*
    improvement in volume status, monitoring for, 459
    inotropes, 456
    renin-angiotensin-aldosterone system, 459
    sympathetic nervous system, 459
    ultrafiltration, 458–459
    vasodilators, 456
  pathophysiology, 453–455, 454*f*
Care bundles
AKI, 93
systematic approach to, 84–86, 85*t*
CARRESS-HF trial, 457
Catheter insertion bundle, 333, 334*t*
Catheter site care, 333
Catheters, for KRT
  insertion bundle, 333, 334*t*
  location, 331–332, 337–339
    complications, 332
    function, 331–332
  minimizing complications, 333–334
    infections, 333–334
    mechanical, 333
  tip position, 332, 332*t*
  tunneled versus nontunneled, 333
"Ceiling"/plateau concentration, 135
Cell-mediated rejection, in KT recipients, 601
Centers for Medicare and Medicaid Services (CMS), 614
Central venous oxygen saturations (ScvO2), 6
Central Venous Pressure (CVP), 3, 4*f*, 17
Cerebral perfusion pressure (CPP), 546
Cerebral salt-wasting syndrome, 226
Chimeric antigen receptor (CAR) T cell therapy, 570–571
Chronic hyponatremia, 221
Circulatory shock, 12, 17
Cirrhosis, 185, 185*t*, 225
Citrate toxicity, 124, 125
CKRT. *See* Continuous kidney replacement therapy
CLASSIC study, 112
Clinical outcomes, 42
Clinical signs and symptoms, hypernatremia, 230
CMS. *See* Centers for Medicare and Medicaid Services
CMV infection. *See* Cytomegalovirus infection
Cockroft-Gault/Chronic Kidney Disease Epidemiology Collaboration (CKD-EPI), 91
Computed tomography (CT) scan, 91

Continuous ambulatory peritoneal dialysis (CAPD), 458–459
Continuous kidney replacement therapy (CKRT), 342–343, 346, 375
  advantages and disadvantages of, 365*t*
  anticoagulant
    dosing of, 376*t*
    selection of, 375*t*
  argatroban for, 380
  in burn patients, 522–523
    dosing, 522–523
    initiation of, 522
  convection versus diffusion in, 364
  and DKA, 433
  versus IHD, 365, 366*t*, 373
  modalities of, 360, 361*t*
    CVVH, 360–361, 362*f*
    CVVHD, 361, 363*f*
    CVVHDF, 361, 363–364*f*
  versus PD, 369
  versus PIKRT, 367, 374
  regional citrate anticoagulation for, 377–380, 378*f*, 379*t*, 384–386
  slow continuous ultrafiltration, 361
  unfractionated heparin for, 376–377
Continuous positive airway pressure (CPAP), 37
Continuous venovenous hemodiafiltration (CVVHDF), 361, 363–364*f*
Continuous venovenous hemodialysis (CVVHD), 361, 363*f*
Continuous venovenous hemofiltration (CVVH), 360–361, 362*f*, 375, 458, 522
  in burn patients, 527
Contracted extracellular volume, 225–226
Contrast-associated acute kidney injury (CA-AKI)
  gadolinium toxicology, 497
  incidence of, 491–492, 492*f*
  nephrogenic systemic fibrosis, 497–498
    epidemiology of, 497
    hemodialysis to prevent, 497–498
    phenotype of, 497
  outcomes associated with, 493–495, 494*t*
  pathophysiology, 491–492
  prevention of, 495–497, 503
    current recommendations for, 496–497
    pharmacologic agents, 495*t*
  risk factors for, 492–493, 493*t*
Convection versus diffusion, in CKRT, 364, 372
Correlation between central venous pressure (CVP), 9
Corticosteroids, 19
  for SA-AKI, 421
CPAP. *See* Continuous positive airway pressure
CPP. *See* Cerebral perfusion pressure
CrCl. *See* Creatinine clearance
Creatinine clearance (CrCl), 160, 161, 161*t*
Creatinine range, during gestation, 437*t*
Critical illness, biomarkers of
  heterogeneity conundrum, 192–194, 193*t*, 195*f*
  integration through enrichment, 197
  intensive care unit syndromes and novel biomarkers, 195–197, 196*f*
Critically ill patients
  anemia in, 118–122
    complications, 120, 121–122*t*
    definition of, 118
    indications for blood transfusions, 119–120
    intensive care unit patients, 118–119, 119*t*
    packed red blood cell preparation, 120
  thrombocytopenia in, 123–128
    assay-directed management of hemostasis, 126–128, 127*t*
    coagulation factor concentrates, 125–126
    indications for transfusions, 123
    massive transfusion protocol, 126
    plasma and cryoprecipitate content, 124
    plasma and cryoprecipitate, indications for use of, 124
    risks, 124–125
    risks of platelet transfusion, 123–124
CRS. *See* Cardiorenal syndrome
CRS. *See* Cytokine release syndrome
CRT. *See* Capillary refill time
Cryoprecipitate, 124
Crystalloids/colloids, 105
CT scan. *See* Computed tomography scan
Cushing reflex, 616
CVP. *See* Central Venous Pressure
CVP. *See* Correlation between central venous pressure

CVVH. *See* Continuous venovenous hemofiltration
CVVHD. *See* Continuous venovenous hemodialysis
CVVHDF. *See* Continuous venovenous hemodiafiltration
Cyclic antidepressants, 321–322
Cyclosporine, 591
Cytokine release syndrome (CRS), 570–571
Cytomegalovirus (CMV) infection, 608–609, 609*t*
CytoSorb, 390–391

D

DALYs. *See* Disability-adjusted life years
DCDD. *See* Donation after circulatory determination of death
DDS. *See* Dialysis disequilibrium syndrome
Denosumab, 250–251
Dexmedetomidine, for AKI, 447–448
Dextrose, 305
DI. *See* Diabetes insipidus
Diabetes insipidus (DI)
  central diabetes insipidus, 233–234
  drug-induced nephrogenic diabetes insipidus, 234
  electrolyte-induced nephrogenic diabetes insipidus, 234
  nephrogenic diabetes insipidus, 234
  recovery from AKI can cause NDI, 235
Diabetic ketoacidosis (DKA), 427–434
  diagnosis
    laboratory evaluation, 428–429
    signs and symptoms, 429
  epidemiology, 428
  management issues
    AKI, 432
    bicarbonate, 431
    hypercoagulable state, 432
    phosphorus, 431–432
    primary initiating event, 432
  pathology, 427, 428*f*
  special cases
    CKRT, 433
    end-stage kidney disease, 433–434
    euglycemic, 432–433, 433*t*
  treatment, 429–431
    insulin, 430–431
    potassium, 431
    volume, 429–430
Diagnosis, 232
Diagnostic specificity, 124–125
Dialysis decision-making, time-limited trials, 631–633, 632*f*, 634*f*
Dialysis disequilibrium syndrome (DDS), 541–544, 545*f*
  clinical spectrum of, 542*f*
  methods used to reduce risk of, 544*t*
  reverse urea hypothesis, 543*f*
  risk factors for, 542*t*
Dialyzability, of poisons, 311
Digoxin
  and other cardiac glycosides, 303, 303*f*, 304*t*
  for toxicity, 322–323
Direct oral anticoagulants
  dabigatran—direct thrombin inhibitor, 164
  direct xa inhibitors, 164–165
Disability-adjusted life years (DALYs), 528
Discrimination, 67
Diuretics and acute kidney injury
  assessment of tubular integrity in early acute kidney injury, use of furosemide for, 142
  classification, 131, 132–133*f*
  diuretic use for
    heart failure, 141
    management of generalized edema, 135–136
    patients with end-stage liver disease, 141–142
  loop diuretics and acute kidney injury outcome, 136–141, 137–140*t*
  pharmacology, 131–135
    k+ sparing diuretics, 134
    loop diuretics, 131–134
    mannitol, 134–135
    thiazide diuretics, 134
DKA. *See* Diabetic ketoacidosis
DNDD. *See* Donation after neurologic determination of death
Donation after circulatory determination of death (DCDD), 613
Donation after neurologic determination of death (DNDD), 613
Doppler mode, 202
DOSE trial, 457
Dosing strategies, 286–290, 287–289*t*
Drug concentration, 286
Drug-induced acute kidney injury, 53, 53–54*t*

Drug therapy, 284
Drugs, 283–284
antidotes, 295
acetaminophen toxicity, 295–297, 295–296*t*, 297–298*f*, 298*t*
naloxone and flumazenil, 299
toxic alcohols, 299–301, 300*f*
calcium channel blocker and a-blocker overdose, 301–302, 302*t*
digoxin and other cardiac glycosides, 303, 303*f*, 304*t*
gastrointestinal decontamination, 292–295
activated charcoal, 292–293, 293*t*
multidose activated charcoal, 293, 293*t*
orogastric lavage, 294, 294*t*
whole bowel irrigation, 294, 295*t*
sulfonylurea and insulin overdose, 303–306, 305*f*, 306*t*

E

Early goal-directed therapy (EGDT), 16
Early Use of Polymyxin B Hemoperfusion in Abdominal Septic Shock (EUPHAS) trial, 389, 395
Early versus Late Initiation of Renal Replacement Therapy in Critically Ill Patients with Acute Kidney Injury (ELAIN) trial, 349, 350–351*t*, 356
EBV infection. *See* Epstein-Barr virus infection
Echogenicity, 201
ECMO. *See* Extracorporeal membrane oxygenation
Edoxaban, 165
Effects of Hemoperfusion With a Polymyxin B Membrane in Peritonitis With Septic Shock (ABDO-MIX) trial, 389–390, 396
EGDT. *See* Early goal-directed therapy
EGDT. *See* Rivers trial on early goal-directed therapy
eGFR. *See* estimated glomerular filtration rate
ELAIN trail. *See* Early versus Late Initiation of Renal Replacement Therapy in Critically Ill Patients with Acute Kidney Injury trial
Electrolyte homeostasis/acid-base balance, 169–170
Electrolytes, 173
Elevated peak inspiratory pressure, differential diagnosis for, 28*t*
Emphysematous pyelonephritis, 598–599
Encephalopathy, 537, 540, 541*f*
End-stage kidney disease (ESKD), 433–434, 577–578
anemia, 119
Energy metabolism, 172
Epstein-Barr virus (EBV) infection, 609–610
ESKD. *See* End-stage kidney disease
estimated glomerular filtration rate (eGFR), 61
Ethical decision-making, for AKI patients in ICU, 628–630, 628*t*, 629*t*, 629*f*, 636
Euglycemic diabetic ketoacidosis, 432–433
EuLITE trial, 573
EUPHAS trial. *See* Early Use of Polymyxin B Hemoperfusion in Abdominal Septic Shock trial
EUPHRATES trial, 390, 397
Expanded extracellular fluid volume, 225
Extracorporeal blood purification techniques, 388*t*
Extracorporeal cytokine hemoadsorption, 390–391
Extracorporeal membrane oxygenation (ECMO), 39, 398–406
in burn patients, 523
complications, 402–403
components, 401–402
console, 402
heat exchanger, 402
membrane oxygenator, 401
pump, 401
tubing and cannulas, 401
configurations, 400–401
venoarterial, 400–401
venovenous, 400
contraindications, 400
history, 398–399
indication for, 399–400
in cardiac failure, 399–400, 399*t*
in respiratory failure, 399, 399*t*
and kidney, 403, 404–405*f*
managing kidney replacement therapy on, 406
weaning, 402
Extracorporeal therapy
for poisonings and intoxications, 309–323
dialyzability of, 311–312

Extracorporeal therapy (*continued*)
recommended against use of, for specific agents
cyclic antidepressants, 321–322
digoxin, 322–323
recommended use of, for specific agents
acetaminophen, 313–314, 314*t*
barbiturate, 316, 317*t*
carbamazepine, 315, 315*t*
lithium, 316–317, 317*t*
metformin, 320, 320*t*
methanol, 318–319, 319*t*
phenytoin, 316, 316*t*
salicylates, 312–313, 313*t*
thallium, 320, 321*t*
theophylline, 320–321, 322*t*
valproic acid, 314, 315*t*
types of
hemodialysis, 309–310
hemofiltration, 309–310
hemoperfusion, 310
plasma exchange, 310–311
Extracorporeal Treatments In Poisoning (EXTRIP), 309
Extrinsic PEEP, 26
EXTRIP. *See* Extracorporeal Treatments In Poisoning

F

Factitious Hypophosphatemia, 255
FACTT trail. *See* Fluid and Catheter Trial Therapy trial
Familial hypocalciuric hypercalcemia (FHH), 270
FDA. *See* Food and Drug Administration
FEAST trial, 112
FFP. *See* Fresh-frozen plasma
FFP transfusion, 124, 125
FHH. *See* Familial hypocalciuric hypercalcemia
Fibrinolysis, 128
Fluctuation, 5*f*
Fluid and Catheter Trial Therapy (FACTT) trial, 82, 141
Fluid challenge, 10
Fluid, choice of, 17
Fluid conservative strategy, 141
Fluid resuscitation, 15, 16–17
Fluid therapy, 616
Flumazenil, 299
Fomepizole, 301
Fondaparinux, 162
Food and Drug Administration (FDA), 185, 497
4-methylpyrazole (4-MP), 301
Fraction of inspired oxygen (Fio_2), 26
Fresh-frozen plasma (FFP), 124
Furosemide, 131
for cardiorenal syndrome, 457
for hypertension, 516
stress test, 92, 93

G

Gadolinium toxicology, 497
Gastrointestinal and diuretic-induced hyponatremia, 226
Gastrointestinal bleeding, in LVAD patients, 466
Gastrointestinal decontamination, 292–295
activated charcoal, 292–293, 293*t*
multidose activated charcoal, 293, 293*t*
orogastric lavage, 294, 294*t*
whole bowel irrigation, 294, 295*t*
General management, 223–225
Genome-wide association study (GWAS), 77
GFR. *See* Glomerular filtration rate
GI decontamination, 292
GI losses/renal losses, 266–267
Glomerular filtration rate (GFR), 47, 90
Glucocorticoids, 250
Goals of resuscitation, 15–16
GWAS. *See* Genome-wide association study

H

HCPs. *See* Health care practitioners
Health care practitioners (HCPs), 614
Health-related quality of life (HRQOL), 580
Healthy adult kidney, 228
Heart failure, 225
HeartMate 3 left ventricular assist device, 463–464, 464*f*
Hemodialysis, 214, 309–310
in acetaminophen poisoning, 313–314, 314*t*
in barbiturate poisoning, 316, 317*t*
in carbamazepine poisoning, 315, 315*t*
in lithium poisoning, 316–317, 317*t*
metformin poisoning, 320, 320*t*

methanol poisoning, 318–319, 319*t*
in phenytoin poisoning, 316, 316*t*
in salicylate poisoning, 312–313, 313*t*
thallium poisoning, 320, 321*t*
theophylline poisoning, 320–321, 322*t*
in valproic acid poisoning, 314, 315*t*
Hemodynamic kidney injury, 438
Hemodynamic parameters, 4
Hemodynamics, 446–447
prerenal, 183
Hemofiltration, 309–310
Hemoperfusion, 310
Hemophagocytic lymphohistiocytosis (HLH), 570–571
Henderson-hasselbalch simplified, 273–274, 274*t*
Heparin-induced thrombocytopenia (HIT), 160, 377
argatroban for, 380
Hepatic failure, 163
Hepatic veins, 207–208
Hepatorenal syndrome
definition of, 475
treatment of, 479*t*
Hepatorenal syndrome (HRS), 55
HES. *See* Hydroxyethyl Starch
Heterogeneity conundrum, 192–194, 193*t*, 195*f*
Heterogeneous disease, 90
HHS. *See* Hyperglycemic hyperosmolar state
High-volume hemofiltration (HVHF), 522–523
in adult burn patients, 526
Higher PEEP strategy, 39
HIT. *See* Heparin-induced thrombocytopenia
HLH. *See* Hemophagocytic lymphohistiocytosis
HRQOL. *See* Health-related quality of life
HRS. *See* Hepatorenal syndrome
Human subject, defined, 615
HVHF. *See* High-volume hemofiltration
Hydronephrosis, 202
Hydroxyethyl Starch (HES), 107–108
Hypercalcemia, 248–251, 249*t*
acute, 562–563
management algorithm, 565*f*
treatment, 564*t*
Hypercarbia, 37–38
Hyperglycemia, 170
Hyperglycemic hyperosmolar state (HHS), 427
Hyperkalemia, 92, 238–242, 240–241*t*, 241*f*, 303
Hypermagnesemia, 269–271, 269–270*t*
Hypernatremia, 232
cause of, 232
management
administer the fluid, 231–232
calculating ongoing losses, 231
calculating the fluid deficit, 231
increased water losses, look for and correct causes of, 232
Hyperphosphatemia, 258–261, 260–261*t*
HYPERS2S trial, 112
Hypertension, 579
Hypertensive emergency
defined, 504
diagnostic evaluation, 507–508, 507*b*
epidemiology, 506
etiology, 504–506, 505*b*, 506*f*
pathogenesis, 504–506
treatment of, 508–516, 517*t*
pharmacologic agents for, 509–511*t*
specific types of, 512–514*t*
Hypertonic saline, 111–112
Hypocalcemia, 246–248, 247*t*
Hypoechoic/anechoic, 201
Hypokalemia, 92, 236–238, 237*f*, 238*t*
Hypomagnesemia, 265–269, 265*t*, 268*t*
Hyponatremia, 218–228, 220–221*t*, 222*f*, 223*t*, 224*f*, 225, 227*t*, 232
cause-specific treatment, 223–226, 224*f*
clinical signs and symptoms, 220
management of asymptomatic hyponatremia, 221–223, 222*f*, 223*t*
management of symptomatic hyponatremia, 220, 220*f*
moderately severe symptoms, management of hyponatremia with, 221, 221*t*
severe symptomatic hyponatremia, 220–221
Hypoperfusion, 52
Hypophosphatemia, 254–258, 255–256*t*, 257, 258*t*
Hypotension, 3
Hypovolemic shock, 12–13
Hypoxemia, 37

I

IAH. *See* Intra-abdominal hypertension
IAP. *See* Intra-abdominal pressure
ICA. *See* International Club of Ascites
ICNARC. *See* Intensive Care National Audit and Research Centre
ICP. *See* Intracranial pressure
ICU. *See* Intensive care unit (ICU)
Ideal fluid, 231
Idiogenic osmole hypothesis, 542
IHD. *See* Intermittent hemodialysis
Immune-checkpoint inhibitors, 567, 570
Immunosuppression therapies, in kidney transplantation, 591
Impact analysis, 67
Inadequate circulation, 3–7
  assessment of resuscitation, 6–7
  clinical endpoints, 7
  dynamic markers, 4–6, 5*f*, 6*t*
  static markers, 3, 4*f*
Individualized treatment measures, 91–93
  electrolyte management, 92
  urea management, 93
  volume management, 91–92
Induction immunosuppression therapy, 591
Ineffective interventions, 86–87, 86*t*
Infections
  in kidney transplant recipients, 606–610
    BK viremia/nephropathy, 609
    candiduria, 610
    cytomegalovirus, 608–609, 609*t*
    Epstein-Barr virus, 609–610
    etiology of, 606, 607*f*
    sepsis management of, 606, 607*f*
    urinary tract infection, 610, 610*t*, 611*t*
  left ventricular assist device, 466
Inhaled nitric oxide (iNO), 153–154
Initial ventilator settings, 25–26
  Fio_2, 26
  positive end-expiratory pressure, 26
  respiratory rate, 26
  tidal volume, 25–26
Initiation of Dialysis Early versus Delayed in the Intensive Care Unit (IDEAL-ICU) trial, 350–351*t*, 352, 358
iNO. *See* Inhaled nitric oxide
Inotropes, 152–153
  dobutamine, 152
  levosimendan, 152–153
  phosphodiesterase inhibitors, 153
Inotropes, for cardiorenal syndrome, 456
INPRESS trial, 84
Institutional review board (IRB), 615
Insulin, for DKA, 430–431
Integration through enrichment, 197
Integrative ultrasound, 208–209
Intensive Blood Pressure Reduction in Acute Cerebral Hemorrhage Trial (INTERACT2), 515
Intensive Care National Audit and Research Centre (ICNARC), 68–70
Intensive care unit (ICU)
  acid-base management
    acid-base disorder, recognizing and determining the cause of, 275, 276*t*
    acid-base status, general considerations in the evaluation of, 275, 275*t*
    anion gap metabolic acidosis versus nonanion gap metabolic acidosis, 278
    henderson-hasselbalch simplified, 273–274, 274*t*
    lactic acidosis considerations, 279
    metabolic acidosis, 276–278, 279
    metabolic alkalosis, 279–280
    respiratory acid-base disorders, 280
  acute kidney injury and non–acute kidney injury risk scores in
    APACHE, 68, 69*t*
    external validation, 70
    external validations of, 72
    ICNARC, 68–70
    introduction to prediction models, 67
    limitations of intensive care unit mortality models, 70
    LODS, 70–71
    model performance, 67
    MODS, 71–72
    MPM, 68
    organ dysfunction scores, 70–72, 71*t*
    patients, mortality prediction in, 72, 73–74*t*
    recent acute kidney injury prediction studies and future directions, 72, 75–76*t*, 77, 77*f*
    SAPS, 68
    SOFA, 71
  anticoagulants in, 159*t*
    direct oral anticoagulants, 164–165

direct thrombin inhibitors, parenteral agents, 162–163
heparins, parenteral agents, 159–162, 161*t*
warfarin, 163–164
blood purification in, 387–393
complications of, 392
extracorporeal, 388*t*
extracorporeal cytokine hemoadsorption, 390–391
polymyxin B hemoperfusion, 388–389
results from randomized clinical trials, 389–390
therapeutic plasma exchange, 391
calcium management
critical care, epidemiology and significance of abnormalities in serum calcium in, 245–246
hypercalcemia, 248–251, 249*t*
hypocalcemia, 246–248, 247*t*
dyskalemias
hyperkalemia, 238–242, 240–241*t*, 241*f*
hypokalemia, 236–238, 237*f*, 238*t*
normal potassium homeostasis, 236
ECMO in, 398–406
hemodynamic monitoring, inadequate circulation, 3–7
hypernatremia
clinical signs and symptoms, 230
diabetes insipidus, 233–235, 233–234*t*
diagnosis, 232
management, 230–232
left ventricular assist devices in, 463–468, 470–472
magnesium management
hypermagnesemia, 269–271, 269–270*t*
hypomagnesemia, 265–269, 265*t*, 268*t*
normal magnesium levels, 264, 264*t*
MAP, 156
neurologic emergencies, 537–547
associated with kidney disease and dialysis, 538–539*t*
dialysis disequilibrium syndrome, 541–544, 542*f*, 542*t*, 543*f*, 544*t*, 545*f*
KRT in setting of reduced cerebral compliance/increased ICP, 544–547
uremic encephalopathy, 537, 540, 541*f*
phosphorus management
hyperphosphatemia, 258–261, 260–261*t*
hypophosphatemia, 254–258, 255–256*t*, 258*t*
role of intravenous fluids in, 103–105, 103–104*t*, 106*f*
sodium homeostasis and hyponatremia in
hyponatremia, 218–228, 220–221*t*, 222*f*, 223*t*, 224*f*, 227*t*
sodium physiology, 217–218, 219*f*
transfusion medicine in
anemia in critically ill patients, 118–122, 119*t*, 121–122*t*
thrombocytopenia in critically ill patients, 123–128, 127*t*
ultrasound imaging in
cardiac, 206–208, 206–208*f*
integrative ultrasound, 208–209
kidneys and bladder, 202, 203*f*
lung, 203–205, 204–205*f*
physics, 201–202
Intensive care unit syndromes and novel biomarkers, 195–197, 196*f*
Intermittent hemodialysis (IHD), 364–365, 365*t*
versus CKRT, 365, 366*t*, 373
versus PD, 369
Intermittent hemodialysis, 341, 342*t*
International Club of Ascites (ICA), 475
International Society of Peritoneal Dialysis (ISPD), 367, 369
Intra-abdominal hypertension (IAH)
causes of, 483–484
defined, 483
diagnosis of, 484
management algorithm, 488–489*f*
prevention, 485–486
Intra-abdominal pressure (IAP), 483
Intracranial pressure (ICP), KRT in setting of reduced cerebral compliance, 544–547
Ionized calcium fraction, 245
IRB. *See* Institutional review board
Isotonic saline solution, 108–112
ISPD. *See* International Society of Peritoneal Dialysis

K

K+ sparing diuretics, 134
KDIGO. *See* Kidney Disease Improving Global Outcomes
K_e, 217

Kidney
biopsy, 186
and bladder, 202, 203*f*
ECMO and CKRT for, 403, 404–405*f*
function, 271
infiltration, 561
mechanical ventilation, 38
Kidney Disease Improving Global Outcomes (KDIGO), 47, 72, 81, 92, 97, 108, 331, 333, 341, 416, 445, 475, 520
Kidney replacement therapy (KRT), 40, 82, 93, 97–98, 97*f*, 145, 255, 285
anemia, 119
anticoagulation and, 375–380
argatroban for, 380
regional citrate anticoagulation for, 377–380, 378*f*, 379*t*, 384–386
unfractionated heparin, 376–377
in burn patients, 522
catheters for
connection, 333, 335*t*
insertion bundle, 333, 334*t*
location, 331–332, 337–339
minimizing complications, 333–334
tip position, 332, 332*t*
tunneled versus nontunneled, 333
dosing of, 340–343
continuous, 342–343, 346
higher intensity dose, 347
intermittent hemodialysis, 341, 342*t*
optimal intensity of, 345
ECMO, 406
modality selection of, 360–369
continuous, 360–361, 362–364*f*
convection versus diffusion, 364, 372
intermittent hemodialysis, 364–365, 365*t*
peritoneal dialysis, 367, 369
nutrition support, 173
for postcardiac surgery acute kidney injury, 448
prolonged intermittent, 366–367
reduced cerebral compliance/increased ICP, 544–547
for rhabdomyolysis, 556
for SA-AKI, 421–422
time-limited trial of, 478, 480*t*
timing of, 348–354
recent randomized controlled trials, 349–353, 350–351*t*
remaining areas of uncertainty, 353
scope of problem, 348–349
for trauma-associated AKI, 534
Kidney transplant recipients (KTRs)
AKI in, 597–602
epidemiology, 597, 598*f*, 605
non recipients, 602
specific etiologies, 597–602
infections in, 606–610
etiology of, 606, 607*f*
sepsis management of, 606, 607*f*
perioperative management of, 589–594
immunosuppression, 591
operative details, 590–591
patient assessment, 589–590
post complications, 593–594
postoperative management, 591–593
KRT. *See* Kidney replacement therapy
KTRs. *See* Kidney transplant recipients

L

LA. *See* Lactic acidosis
Lactic acid, 6
Lactic acidosis (LA), 276
considerations, 279
Left ventricular assist device (LVAD), 463–468, 470–472
alarms, 464–465
complications
device infections, 466
gastrointestinal bleeding, 466
pump thrombosis, 466
right-sided heart failure, 465–466
stroke, 466
general mechanics, 464
indications and contraindications for, 463, 463*t*
and kidney
acute dialysis, 467
acute kidney injury, 467
maintenance dialysis, 467–468
patient care
anticoagulation, 465
blood pressure, 465
cardiopulmonary resuscitation, 465
types, 463–464
Levosimendan, for low cardiac output, 447
Liberation, mechanical ventilation, 29
Lithium poisoning, hemodialysis in, 316–317, 317*t*

LMWH. *See* Low-molecular-weight heparin
LODS. *See* Logistic Organ Dysfunction System
Logistic Organ Dysfunction System (LODS), 70–71
Loop diuretics, 131–134
  for myoglobin precipitation, 556
Low cardiac output states, 12–14, 19
Low-molecular-weight heparin (LMWH), 160–162, 161*f*
Low serum osmolality, 223
Low systemic vascular resistance states/ distributive shock, 14
Lung, 203–205, 204–205*f*
  and kidney interactions, 37*f*
Lung function/extrapulmonary-organ perfusion, 43
Lung point, 204
Lung sliding, 204
Lupus nephritis, 441
LVAD. *See* Left ventricular assist device
Lymphocele, 594

M

Mannitol, 134–135
Mannitol infusion, 134
MAP. *See* Mean arterial pressure
Massive transfusion, 126
MDAC. *See* Multiple dose activated charcoal
Mean arterial pressure (MAP), 12, 389
Mechanical ventilation, 24*t*
  initial ventilator settings, 25–26
    Fio_2, 26
    positive end-expiratory pressure, 26
    respiratory rate, 26
    tidal volume, 25–26
  liberation from, 29
  mechanically ventilated patient, 28–29, 29*t*
  modes of, 24–25, 25*t*
  noninvasive ventilation, 30–31, 35
    acute cardiogenic pulmonary edema, 30
    acute on chronic hypercapnic respiratory failure, 30
    hypoxemic respiratory failure, 30
    immunocompromised patients, 30–31
  for SA-AKI, 421
  ventilator, monitoring patients on, 26–28
    auto–positive end-expiratory pressure, 28
    ventilator waveforms, 26–28, 27*f*, 28*t*
Mechanically ventilated patient, 28–29, 29*t*
  ICU, 33
MELD score. *See* Model for End-Stage Liver Disease score
Metabolic acidosis, 276–278, 279
Metabolic alkalosis, 276, 279–280
Metformin poisoning, hemodialysis in, 320, 320*t*
Methanol poisoning, hemodialysis in, 318–319, 319*t*
Methylprednisolone, for liver graft function, 617
Mineralocorticoid deficiency, 226
MM. *See* Multiple myeloma
Model for End-Stage Liver Disease (MELD) score, 473–474
Model performance, 67
MODS. *See* Multiple Organ Dysfunction Score
MOST. *See* Multiorgan support therapy
Multiorgan support therapy (MOST), 523
Multiple dose activated charcoal (MDAC), 293
Multiple myeloma (MM), 562
Multiple Organ Dysfunction Score (MODS), 71–72
Mycophenolate mofetil, 591
Myeloma light-chain cast nephropathy, 562
MYRE trial, 574

N

N-acetyl-*p*-benzoquinoneimine (NAPQI), 297
N-acetylcysteine (NAC), 295
NAC. See N-acetylcysteine
Na_e, 217
NAPQI. See N-acetyl-p-benzoquinoneimine
Native kidney disease, recurrence of, 602
Nephrogenic systemic fibrosis, 497–498
  epidemiology of, 497
  hemodialysis to prevent, 497–498
  phenotype of, 497
Nephrolithiasis, ultrasonography versus computed tomography for, 212
Nephrotoxic agents, 90
Nephrotoxic Injury Negated by Just-in-Time Action (NINJA), 91
Nesiritide, for cardiorenal syndrome, 456

Neurologic emergencies, in intensive care unit, 537–547
  associated with kidney disease and dialysis, 538–539*t*
  dialysis disequilibrium syndrome, 541–544, 542*f*, 542*t*, 543*f*, 544*t*, 545*f*
  KRT in setting of reduced cerebral compliance/increased ICP, 544–547
  uremic encephalopathy, 537, 540, 541*f*
Neuromuscular hyperexcitability, 267
NINJA. *See* Nephrotoxic Injury Negated by Just-in-Time Action
NIV. *See* Noninvasive ventilation
Non-kidney transplant recipients, 602
Noninvasive ventilation (NIV), 30–31
  acute cardiogenic pulmonary edema, 30
  acute on chronic hypercapnic respiratory failure, 30
  hypoxemic respiratory failure, 30
  immunocompromised patients, 30–31
Nontunneled versus tunneled catheters, 333
Norepinephrine, for septic shock, 420–421
Normal magnesium levels, 264, 264*t*
Normal potassium homeostasis, 236
Normocaloric, 173
Novel agents, 19
Novel biomarkers for, 184
Novel therapies, 98
Nutrition, 169
Nutrition therapy, 170–171, 174–176, 175*t*

O

Obstetric acute kidney injury, 436–442
Obstructive nephropathy, 561–562
Obstructive shock, 13
ODS. *See* Osmotic demyelination syndrome
On-target, off-tumor toxicity, 571
Onconephrology emergencies, 561–571
  cancer and kidney injury, 561–562
    infiltration, 561
    myeloma light-chain cast nephropathy, 562
    obstructive nephropathy, 561–562
  metabolic complications of, 562–565
    hypercalcemia, 562–563, 564*t*, 565*f*
    tumor lysis syndrome, 563, 565, 566*t*, 567*f*
  treatment, 567–571, 568–569*t*
    chimeric antigen receptor T cells, 570–571
    immune-checkpoint inhibitors, 567, 570
OPO. *See* Organ procurement organization
Oral anticoagulants
  warfarin, 163–164
    dosing and use, 163
    pharmacology, 163
    safety and reversal, 163–164
Oral magnesium replacement, 269
Organ procurement organization (OPO), 613–614
Osmotic demyelination syndrome (ODS), 220–222
Osmotic dieresis, 430
Oxygenation, 16

P

Packed red blood cells (pRBCs), 118
Parenteral agents
  direct thrombin inhibitors, 162–163
    argatroban, 163
    bivalirudin, 162, 162*f*
    hirudin, lepirudin, and desirudin, 162
  heparins, 159–162
    LMWH, 160–162, 161*f*
    UFH, 159–160
Passive leg raise (PLR) test, 16, 115
PBW. *See* Body weight
PD. *See* Peritoneal dialysis
Peak inspiratory pressure (PIP), 26
PEEP. *See* Positive end-expiratory pressure
Peripheral venous pressure (PVP), 9
Peritoneal dialysis (PD), 367, 369, 458–459
  versus IHD and CKRT, 369
Perturbations, 245
pH, 273, 278
Pharmacokinetic changes in, 284–285
Pharmacologic therapy, for AKI, 478, 479*t*, 481–482
Phenytoin poisoning, hemodialysis in, 316, 316*t*
Phosphorus, in DKA, 431–432
Physics, 201–202
Piezoelectrics, 201
PIKRT. *See* Prolonged intermittent kidney replacement therapy
PIP. *See* Peak inspiratory pressure
Piperacillin/tazobactam, 283

PIVA signal, 3
Plasma biomarkers, 38
Plasma exchange (PLEX), 309–311
Pleural effusion, 205
PLEX. *See* Plasma exchange
PLR test. *See* Passive leg raise test
POCUS. *See* Point-of-care ultrasound
Point-of-care ultrasound (POCUS), 201
Polymyxin B hemoperfusion, 388–389
POSEIDON trial. *See* Prevention of Contrast Renal Injury with Different Hydration Strategies trial
Positive end-expiratory pressure (PEEP), 37
Post-transplant lymphoproliferative disorder (PTLD), 609–610
Postcardiac surgery acute kidney injury, 444–448
  drugs, 447–448
  hemodynamics, 446–447
  KRT, 448
  pathophysiology, 444–445
    kidney damage biomarker, 444–445
    subclinical acute kidney injury, 444–445
  preventive measures, 445
    KDIGO guidelines, 445
    remote ischemic preconditioning, 445
Postrenal acute kidney injury, 442
Potassium, for hyperglycemic crisis, 431
Potassium secretion, 241
Potassium-sparing diuretics, 131
PPV. *See* Pulse pressure variation
pRBCs. *See* Packed red blood cells
Preeclampsia/hemolysis, 438–439
Pregnancy, AKI in
  differential diagnosis of, 437–442, 438*f*
  epidemiology of, 436
  management of, 442
  review of changes in, 437
PRESERVE trial. *See* Prevention of Serious Adverse Events Following Angiography trial
PREV-AKI trial, 85, 85*t*
Prevention of Contrast Renal Injury with Different Hydration Strategies (POSEIDON) trial, 496
Prevention of Serious Adverse Events Following Angiography (PRESERVE) trial, 83, 495–496
Primary kidney diseases, 55
Prime time, 196
Prognostic information, 186
Prolonged intermittent kidney replacement therapy (PIKRT), 366–367, 368*t*
  versus CKRT, 367, 374
Propofol, for AKI, 447
Protein catabolism, 172
PTLD. *See* Post-transplant lymphoproliferative disorder
Pulse pressure variation (PPV), 3, 5
Pump thrombosis, 466
PVP. *See* Peripheral venous pressure
Pyelonephritis, 441, 598–599

Q

qSOFA screening criteria. *See* Quick Sequential Organ Failure Assessment screening criteria
quick Sequential Organ Failure Assessment (qSOFA) screening criteria, 14, 15*t*, 415–416

R

RAAS. *See* Renin-angiotensin-aldosterone system
Randomized parallel group feasibility trial, 82
Rating fluid response, 114–115, 115*t*
RCA. *See* Regional citrate anticoagulation
Recurrent acute kidney injury, 578–579, 585
Refeeding Syndrome, 254–255, 255*t*
Refractory shock, 19
Regional citrate anticoagulation (RCA), 377–380, 378*f*, 379*t*, 384–386
Rejection, in KT recipients, 600–601
Remote ischemic preconditioning (RIPC), 445
Renal artery thrombosis, 594
RENAL trial, 290
Renal vein thrombosis, 594
Renalism, 91
Renin-angiotensin-aldosterone system (RAAS), 459
Resorption of magnesium, 266
Respiratory acid-base disorders, 280
Respiratory component, 280
Respiratory failure, ECMO for, 399, 399*t*
"Restrictive" strategy of transfusion, 119
Resuscitation fluids, 113–114*t*
  intensive care unit, role of intravenous fluids in, 103–105, 103–104*t*, 106*f*
  questions, 105–112

Resuscitation fluids (*continued*)
albumin, 105–108, 109–110*t*
crystalloids or colloids, 105
isotonic saline solution, 108–112
rating fluid response, 114–115, 115*t*
Rhabdomyolysis, 55, 534, 550–558
clinical features, 553
etiologies of, 551–553, 551–552*t*
kidney replacement therapy, 556
management, 555–556, 557*t*
pathophysiology of, 550–551, 551*t*
prognosis, 554–555, 554*t*
RIFLE system. *See* Risk, Injury, Failure, Loss, and End-Stage Renal Disease system
Right-sided heart failure, 465–466
RIPC. *See* Remote ischemic preconditioning
Risk, Injury, Failure, Loss, and End-Stage Renal Disease (RIFLE) system, 416, 520
Rivaroxaban, 165
Rivers trial on early goal-directed therapy (EGDT), 112
Rumack-Matthew nomogram, 297

S

Salicylate poisoning, hemodialysis in, 312–313, 313*t*
SALT-ED trial, 83, 111
SAPS. *See* Simplified Acute Physiology Score
SCr. *See* Serum creatinine
"Scrub-the-hub" protocol, 333, 335*t*
SCUF. *See* Slow continuous ultrafiltration
Sepsis
BK viremia/nephropathy, 609
candiduria, 610
cytomegalovirus, 608–609, 609*t*
defined, 387, 415–416
Epstein-Barr virus, 609–610
management of, in KTRs, 607*f*
resuscitation, 420
urinary tract infection, 610, 610*t*, 611*t*
Sepsis-associated acute kidney injury (SA-AKI), 53, 415–422
detection of, 417
epidemiology, 417
pathophysiology, 417
prevention and medical treatment, 417–422, 418–419*t*
corticosteroids, 421
emerging therapies, 422
fluid selection, 420
kidney replacement therapy, 421–422
mechanical ventilation, 421
resuscitation, 420
vasoactive medications, 420–421
Septic shock, 11*b*, 15, 21–22, 158, 415–416
role of screening algorithms in, 14, 15*t*
Sequential Organ Failure Assessment (SOFA), 71, 389, 415–416, 416*t*
Serum creatinine (SCr), 49, 58, 184–185, 473–474
Serum lactate, 6, 15–16
Severe sepsis, defined, 415
Shock
evaluation, 14–15
bedside, 14
laboratory findings, 14–15
septic, role of screening algorithms in, 14, 15*t*
management, 15–19
fluid resuscitation, 16–17
goals of resuscitation, 15–16
refractory shock, 19
vasopressors/inotropes, 17, 18*t*
states, pathophysiology and differentiation of, 12–14
cardiac output equation, 12, 13*t*
low cardiac output states, 12–14
Shock, treatment of, 157
Shred sign, 205
SIADH. *See* Syndrome of Inappropriate Antidiuretic Hormone Secretion
Simplified Acute Physiology Score (SAPS), 68
Single-organ system, 194
SIRS. *See* Systemic inflammatory response syndrome
SLED. *See* Sustained low-efficiency dialysis
Slow continuous ultrafiltration (SCUF), 361, 458
SMART trial, 83
SNS. *See* Sympathetic nervous system
SOAP II trial, 147
Sodium-glucose cotransporter-2 (SGLT2) inhibitors, 458
Sodium physiology, 217–218
electrolyte free water clearance, 218, 219*t*

SOFA. *See* Sequential Organ Failure Assessment
Spine sign, 205
SPLIT-Plus, 111
SPLIT trial, 83
Spontaneous breathing trials, pressure support/T-piece ventilation, 34
SPRINT trial, 186
SPV. *See* Systolic pressure variation
Standard versus Accelerated initiation of Renal Replacement Therapy in Acute Kidney Injury (STARRT-AKI) trial, 352–353, 359
Stepwise approach, 163
Stroke, in LVAD patients, 466
Subclinical, 185
Sulfonylurea and insulin overdose, 303–306, 305*f*, 306*t*
Supportive therapy, 40
Surviving Sepsis Guidelines, 146, 147
Sustained low-efficiency dialysis (SLED), 366
Sympathetic nervous system (SNS), 459
Syndrome of Inappropriate Antidiuretic Hormone Secretion (SIADH), 226–228, 227*t*
Systemic inflammatory response syndrome (SIRS), 14, 15*t*
Systolic pressure variation (SPV), 3, 5

T

TACO. *See* Transfusion-associated circulatory overload
Tacrolimus, 591
TAPSE. *See* Tricuspid annular plane systolic excursion
Tezosentan, for cardiorenal syndrome, 456
Thallium poisoning, hemodialysis in, 320, 321*t*
Theophylline poisoning, hemodialysis in, 320–321, 322*t*
Therapeutic interventions, 186
Therapeutic plasma exchange (TPE), 391
Thiazide diuretics, 134
Third dimension, 193
Thrombotic microangiopathies, 439–441, 440*t*
Thymoglobulin, 591
Time-limited trials
  assist with dialysis decision-making, 631–633, 632*f*, 634*f*
  of kidney replacement therapy, 627–635
    dialysis decision-making, 631–633, 632*f*, 634*f*
    ethical decision-making, 628–630, 628*t*, 629*t*, 629*f*, 636
    ethical issues cases, 627–628
    older patients with AKI, in ICU for dialysis, 630–631, 631*b*, 637
TLS. *See* Tumor lysis syndrome
Torsemide, for cardiorenal syndrome, 457
Toxic alcohol ingestion, 299
TPE. *See* Therapeutic plasma exchange
Traditional fluid physiology, 105
TRALI. *See* Transfusion-related acute lung injury
Transfusion-associated circulatory overload (TACO), 125
Transfusion-related acute lung injury (TRALI), 124–125
Transfusion Requirements in Cardiac Surgery (TRICS) III trial, 119–120
Transfusion Requirements in Critical Care (TRICC) trial, 119
Transfusion Requirements in Septic Shock (TRISS) trial, 119
Transplant renal artery stenosis (TRAS), 600
TRAS. *See* Transplant renal artery stenosis
Trauma-associated acute kidney injury, 528–534
  epidemiology, 528–529
  etiology, 529–531, 530*t*
  management, 533–534
    kidney replacement therapy, 534
  pathophysiology, 531, 532*f*
  risk factors, 531
TRICC trial. *See* Transfusion Requirements in Critical Care trial
TRICS III trial. *See* Transfusion Requirements in Cardiac Surgery III trial
Tricuspid annular plane systolic excursion (TAPSE), 207
TRISS trial. *See* Transfusion Requirements in Septic Shock trial
Troponin-I, 197
Tumor lysis syndrome (TLS), 563, 565
  definition of, 566*t*
  management algorithm, 567*f*
Tunneled versus nontunneled catheters, 333

U

UAGA. *See* Uniform Anatomical Gift Act
UDT. *See* Urine dipstick test
UFH. *See* Unfractionated heparin
Ultrafiltration, 458–459
Ultrasonography/fluid responsiveness, 17
Unfractionated heparin (UFH), 159–160, 376–377
Uniform Anatomical Gift Act (UAGA), 615
Universal treatment measures, 90–91
  appropriate dosing of medication, 91
  avoidance of nephrotoxic insults, 90–91
  maintenance of kidney perfusion, 90
Uremia, 93
Uremic encephalopathy, 537, 540, 541*f*
Ureteral obstruction, in KT, 599
Urinary tract infection, 610, 610*t*, 611*t*
Urine dipstick test (UDT), 553
Urine output criteria, 50
Urologic complications, in post–kidney transplantation, 593
US Army Institute of Surgical Research (USAISR), 521
US Food and Drug Administration, 285
USAISR. *See* US Army Institute of Surgical Research

V

Valproic acid poisoning, hemodialysis in, 314, 315*t*
VANISH trial. *See* Vasopressin versus noradrenaline as initial therapy in septic shock trial
Vascular access, for kidney replacement therapy, 331–335
  catheter insertion bundle, 333, 334*t*
  minimizing catheter-associated complications, 333–334
    infections, 333–334
    mechanical, 333
  optimal catheter location, 331–332, 337–339
    complications, 332
    function, 331–332
  optimal catheter tip position, 332, 332*t*
  tunneled versus nontunneled catheters, 333
Vasoactive medications, 616
  administration, 152
    vasoactive medications, extravasation injury of, 152
  inotropes, 152–153
    dobutamine, 152
    levosimendan, 152–153
    phosphodiesterase inhibitors, 153
  for SA-AKI, 420–421
  vasodilators, 153–154
    carperitide, 153
    fenoldopam, 154
    iNO, 153–154
    recombinant natriuretic peptides, 153
  vasopressors, 145–151
    angiotensin ii, 148
    dopamine, 146
    epinephrine, 146
    norepinephrine, 146
    phenylephrine, 147
    vasodilatory shock, dopamine in, 147
    vasopressin, 147–148, 149–151*t*
Vasodilators, 153–154
  for cardiorenal syndrome, 456
  carperitide, 153
  fenoldopam, 154
  iNO, 153–154
  recombinant natriuretic peptides, 153
Vasopressin and septic shock trial (VASST), 147–148
Vasopressin versus noradrenaline as initial therapy in septic shock (VANISH) trial, 148
Vasopressors, 17, 18*t*, 145–151
  angiotensin ii, 148
  dopamine, 146
  epinephrine, 146
  norepinephrine, 146
  phenylephrine, 147
  vasodilatory shock, dopamine in, 147
  vasopressin, 147–148, 149–151*t*
VASST. *See* Vasopressin and septic shock trial
Velocity of ultrasound waves, 201
Venoarterial extracorporeal membrane oxygenation (V-A ECMO), 400–401
Venovenous extracorporeal membrane oxygenation (V-V ECMO), 400
Ventilator, monitoring patients on, 26–28
  auto–positive end-expiratory pressure, 28
  ventilator waveforms, 26–28, 27*f*, 28*t*
Volume expansion and choice of intravenous fluid, ICU, 81–83

Volume management, 169
Volume overload, 38, 91
von Willebrand factor–cleaving protease (ADAMTS-13) deficiency, 439

W

Warfarin, 160, 163, 164
Watchword, 91
Water intake, 228
Weaning, 402
World Society of the Abdominal Compartment Syndrome (WSACS), 483
WSACS. *See* World Society of the Abdominal Compartment Syndrome

Z

Zirconium cyclosilicate, 241